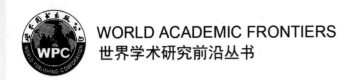

WORLD ACADEMIC FRONTIERS
世界学术研究前沿丛书

Tumor Research

肿瘤研究

"世界学术研究前沿丛书"编委会
THE EDITORIAL BOARD OF
WORLD ACADEMIC FRONTIERS

中国出版集团公司
世界图书出版公司
广州·上海·西安·北京

图书在版编目（CIP）数据

肿瘤研究：英文 / "世界学术研究前沿丛书"编委会编. 一广州：世界图书出版广东有限公司，2017.8
ISBN 978-7-5192-2461-5

Ⅰ. ①肿… Ⅱ. ①世… Ⅲ. ①肿瘤－研究－英文 Ⅳ. ①R73

中国版本图书馆 CIP 数据核字（2017）第 040982 号

Tumor Research © 2016 by Scientific Research Publishing

Published by arrangement with Scientific Research Publishing
Through Wuhan Irvine Culture Company

书　　名：肿瘤研究
　　　　　Zhongliu Yanjiu
编　　者："世界学术研究前沿丛书"编委会
责任编辑：张柏登　康琬娟
出版发行：世界图书出版广东有限公司
地　　址：广州市海珠区新港西路大江冲25号
邮　　编：510300
电　　话：（020）84460408
网　　址：http：//www.gdst.com.cn/
邮　　箱：wpc_gdst@163.com
经　　销：新华书店
印　　刷：广州市德佳彩色印刷有限公司
开　　本：787 mm×1092 mm　1/16
印　　张：49
插　　页：4
字　　数：930千
版　　次：2017年8月第1版　2017年8月第1次印刷
国际书号：ISBN 978-7-5192-2461-5
定　　价：598.00元

Preface

Oncology is a branch of medicine that deals with the prevention, diagnosis and treatment of cancer. Cancers are best managed by discussing in multi-disciplinary tumor board where medical oncologist, surgical oncology, radiation oncology, pathologist, radiologist and organ specific oncologists meet to find the best possible management for an individual patient considering the physical, social, psychological, emotional and financial status of the patients. It is very important for oncologists to keep updated of the latest advancements in oncology as changes in management of cancer are quite common.[1] Those who are interested in the field of oncology could read reviews and original articles in this book to gain a more systematic understanding of oncology.

In the present book, thirty typical literatures about oncology published on international authoritative journals were selected to introduce the worldwide newest progress, which contains reviews or original researches on medical science, oncology, genome biology, cytology, *ect*. We hope this book can demonstrate advances in oncology as well as give references to the researchers, students and other related people.

编委会：
- ✧ 伊娃·科里教授，华盛顿大学，美国
- ✧ 马库斯·J·赛贝尔教授，悉尼大学，澳大利亚
- ✧ 艾吉斯·西里瓦得纳教授，曼彻斯特大学，英国
- ✧ 詹姆斯教授，香港大学，中国
- ✧ 彼得·K·N，于教授，香港城市大学，中国
- ✧ 李亚明教授，博士导师，中国医科大学，中国

March 9, 2017

---

[1]From Wikipedia: https://en.wikipedia.org/wiki/Oncology

Selected Authors

Elaine Mardis, The Genome Institute at Washington University, Washington University, School of Medicine, 4444 Forest Park Blvd, St Louis, USA.

Debu Tripathy, University of Southern California, Keck School of Medicine, USC/Norris Comprehensive Cancer Center, 1441 Eastlake Avenue, NTT-3429, Los Angeles, USA.

Cihan Cetinkaya, Department of Immunology, Genetics and Pathology, Rudbeck Laboratory, Uppsala University, Uppsala, Sweden.

Bo Li, Program of Bioinformatics, University of Michigan, 5940A Buhl, Box 5618, Ann Arbor, USA.

Angabin Matin, Department of Genetics, The University of Texas M.D. Anderson Cancer Center, Houston, Texas, USA.

Kenneth Miles, Department of Diagnostic Imaging Princess Alexandra Hospital, Institute of Nuclear Medicine University College London, UK.

Michael Orth, Department of Radiotherapy and Radiation Oncology Ludwig-Maximilians-University of Munich, Germany.

Ralf Gallasch, Biocenter, Division of Bioinformatics, Innsbruck Medical University, Innsbruck, Austria.

Silvia Morbelli, PhD, Nuclear Medicine Unit, IRCCS AOU San Martino-IST, Department of Health Sciences, University of Genoa, Genoa, Italy.

Franco M. Buonaguro, Division of Molecular Biology & Viral Oncology, Department of Experimental Oncology Istituto Nazionale Tumori -IRCCS "Fond Pascale", France.

Contents

Tumor Heterogeneity: Next-Generation Sequencing Enhances the View from the Pathologist's Microscope

by Samuel Aparicio and Elaine Mardis

Next Generation Sequencing and Tumor Mutation Profiling: Are We Ready for Routine Use in the Oncology Clinic?

by Debu Tripathy, Kathleen Harnden, Kimberly Blackwell, et al.

Age Dependence of Tumor Genetics in Unfavorable Neuroblastoma: ArrayCGH Profiles of 34 Consecutive Cases, Using a Swedish 25-Year Neuroblastoma Cohort for Validation

by Cihan Cetinkaya, Tommy Martinsson, Johanna Sandgren, et al.

A General Framework for Analyzing Tumor Subclonality Using SNP Array and DNA Sequencing Data

by Bo Li and Jun Z. Li

Chapter 1

Tumor Heterogeneity: Next-Generation Sequencing Enhances the View from the Pathologist's Microscope

Samuel Aparicio[1,2], Elaine Mardis[3]

[1]Department of Molecular Oncology, BC Cancer Agency, 675 W10th Avenue, V5Z 1L3 Vancouver, British Columbia, Canada
[2]Nan and Lorraine Robertson Chair, Canada Research Chair, Department of Pathology and Laboratory Medicine, University of British Columbia, V6T 2B5 Vancouver, British Columbia, Canada
[3]The Genome Institute at Washington University, Washington University School of Medicine, 4444 Forest Park Blvd, St Louis, MO 63108, USA

Abstract: The term heterogeneity covers many aspects of the variability in tumor phenotypes, which are a characteristic of human malignancies. Morphologists of the late 19th century first described the multiple cell types composing tumors and began to recognize cancers of different types. Over the past half century the molecular underpinnings of the variability in human cancers has been gradually revealed but within the last 5 years there has been an explosion in our ability to determine and learn from cancer heterogeneity, through the use of next-generation sequencing and related methods. The complexity and variation in the structure of cancers can seem daunting, but important lessons in cancer biology and the approaches to therapy can be learned from studying how much of the complexity is subject to change and how much is a consequence of stochastic rather than deterministic processes. The evolution of clones, individual variation in response to therapy, distinct biological subtypes of cancer and tumor immune responses are all examples of the heterogeneous nature of human cancers. Self evidently, when heterogeneity is used to describe any aspect of a cancer, it is important to know which variational feature is being addressed.

1. Experimental Approaches to Heterogeneity

A review by Hiley et al.[1] sets the stage for the research studies of heterogeneity published in this special issue, by updating the reader regarding how the use of next-generation sequencing and clever experimental design have increased our understanding of genomic and regional heterogeneity in cancers. The special collection provides several research-based studies of tumor heterogeneity, encompassing the variation between individuals (the tumor subtype) in breast cancers (Ali et al.[2]) and, by contrast, the lessons that can be learned from longitudinal study of single patient ("N of 1") cases (Fisher et al.[3], Nadauld et al.[4]). These studies provide contrasts between the approaches needed to determine disease groupings in populations, where many hundreds or thousands of patients must be studied, with the approaches to pursuing the moving target of individual cancers. The latter can be effectively studied in smaller numbers with informative consequences when evolution is used to sift the features undergoing selection and fixation. An Opinion piece by Good et al.[5] provides a scientific and philosophical perspective on the N of 1 paradigm.

2. Methodological Approaches to Heterogeneity

Of equal importance to the experimental approaches used to study heterogeneity are the methods used to evaluate heterogeneity across the spectrum of variation that can be measured in cancer by different assay types. These encompass next-generation sequencing methods for analyzing tumor and normal cell composition, the analysis of clonal populations in cancers (Qiao et al.[6]), and methods addressing epigenetic plasticity (Zheng et al.[7]). Hence, several important tools and approaches are presented that facilitate answering critical questions about heterogeneity, and an opinion piece contributed by Russnes *et al.*[8] advocates for data integration to better interpret heterogeneity data.

3. Single Cell Approaches to Heterogeneity

Resolving structure and function with single cell approaches is also becoming important, both in studies of clonality as well as for functional assessment of tumor cell populations. Learning how to reconcile whole tumor cell-based population approaches with the single cell data will be important. Nicholas Navin's review[9] of single cell sequencing in cancer studies provides a survey of this rapidly developing area.

4. RNA-Based Studies of Heterogeneity

Next-generation sequencing-based studies of RNA populations from cancer cells are revealing important aspects of transcriptional activity and its role in cancer. A review by Patrick Nana-Sinkam and Carlo Croce[10] sets the stage by discussing the role of microRNAs in gene regulation in cancers. White *et al.*[11] present important new descriptions of long non-coding RNAs (lncRNAs) in lung cancers, and Wyatt *et al.*[12] describe transcriptomes in the context of therapy response in high-risk prostate cancers. The method for detecting allele-specific expression contributed by Mayba *et al.*[13] will also yield important insights into which variants detected by DNA sequencing are actually being expressed in the transcriptome of cancer cells. The role of the epigenome in contributing to the patterning of transcriptomes and the possibility of modulating RNA expression is emphasized in three primary research articles exploring this aspect of tumor heterogeneity (Lund *et al.*[14], Fleischer *et al.*[15], and Charlton *et al.*[16]).

5. Clinical Aspects of Heterogeneity

As our underlying knowledge about cancer genomics and heterogeneity improves, the need to translate this information into informed cancer care for patients is an obvious next step. Berger and Varghese have contributed an Opinion piece[17] to describe the translation of cancer genomics in the clinic, and contributions from de Bono[18] and Bardelli[19] outline the use of circulating tumour cells (CTCs) and circulating free DNA (cfDNA), respectively, as approaches to monitoring tumor progression. These blood-based or "liquid biopsy" approaches present an exciting new paradigm in contrast to conventional and less sensitive imaging-based approaches to monitor patients. Deininger also reviews[20] an important area to clinical therapeutics that is often identified by genomic information, providing an overview of therapy response and resistance to targeted therapies. The genomic variability between patients is highlighted in the research article of Ali et al.[2], delineating molecular subtypes in large cohorts of breast cancer patients.

6. Data and More Data

Finally, in the genomic era, sharing of data and complete descriptions of analytic methods, to the level of providing code in addition to data, will prove crucial to continued success. Boutros et al.[21] provide a novel look at crowd-sourcing algorithms for cancer analysis, and Bartha Knoppers and colleagues[22] present a critically important Opinion regarding the legal framework for genomic data sharing. Hence, the special collection provides a wide-ranging overview of cancer heterogeneity in its many manifestations, from fundamental methods-based approaches to study heterogeneity to the use of genomic information for response and progression monitoring. We think the breadth of cancer studies that have been impacted by next generation sequencing, including improved understanding and characterization of cancer heterogeneity, is setting the stage for major breakthroughs in our biological understanding of this vexing and complicated disease.

Competing Interests

The authors declare that they have no competing interests.

Acknowledgements

The guest editors would like to gratefully acknowledge the gracious and insightful contributions from all the authors who wrote reviews, opinions, or primary research manuscripts for the collection. We would also like to thank Rafal Marszalek for his tireless assistance, his encouragement, and his invaluable input toward the content of this special issue. Dr Mardis would like to acknowledge NIH/NHGRI 5U54HG003079 for support. Dr Aparicio is supported by the Canada Research Chairs program and the BC Cancer Foundation.

Source: Aparicio S, Mardis E. Tumor heterogeneity: next-generation sequencing enhances the view from the pathologist's microscope. [J]. Genome Biology, 2014, 15(9):463–463.

References

[1] Hiley C, de Bruin EC, Mc Granahan N, Swanton C: Deciphering intra-tumor heterogeneity and temporal acquisition of driver events to refine precision medicine. Genome Biol 2014, 15:453.

[2] Ali HR, Rueda OM, Chin SF, Curtis C, Dunning MJ, Aparicio SAJR, Caldas C: Genome-driven integrated classification of breast cancer validated in over 7,500 samples. Genome Biol 2014, 15:431.

[3] Fisher R, Horswell S, Rowan A, Salm M, De Bruin E, Gulati S, McGranahan N, Stares M, Gerlinger M, Varela I, Crockford A, Favero F, Quidville V, Andre F, Navas C, Gronroos E, Nicol D, Hazell S, Hrouda D, O'Brien T, Matthews N, Phillimore B, Begum S, Rabinowitz A, Biggs J, Bates PA, McDonald NQ, Stamp G, Spencer-Dene B, Hsieh JJ, et al: Development of synchronous VHL syndrome tumors reveals contingencies and constraints to tumor evolution. Genome Biol 2014, 15:433.

[4] Nadauld LD, Garcia S, Natsoulis G, Bell JM, Miotke L, Hopmans ES, Xu H, Pai RK, Palm C, Regan JF, Chen H, Flaherty P, Ootani A, Zhang NR, Ford JM, Kuo CJ, Ji HP: Metastatic tumor evolution and organoid modeling implicate TGFBR2 as a cancer driver in diffuse gastric cancer. Genome Biol 2014, 15:428.

[5] Good BM, Ainscough BJ, McMichael JF, Su AI, Griffith OL: Organizing knowledge to enable personalization of medicine in cancer. Genome Biol 2014, 15:438.

[6] Qiao Y, Quinlan AR, Jazaeri AA, Verhaak RGW, Wheeler DA, Marth GT: SubcloneSeeker: a computational framework for reconstructing tumor clone structure for cancer variant interpretation and prioritization. Genome Biol 2014, 15:443.

[7] Zheng X, Zhao Q, Wu HJ, Li W, Wang H, Meyer CA, Qin QA, Xu H, Zang C, Jiang P, Li F, Hou Y, He J, Wang J, Wang J, Zhang P, Zhang Y, Liu XS: MethylPurify: tumor purity deconvolution and differential methylation detection from single tumor DNA methylomes. Genome Biol 2014, 15:419.

[8] Russnes HG, Lønning PE, Børresen-Dale AL, Lingjærde OC: The multitude of molecular analyses in cancer: the opening of Pandora's box. Genome Biol 2014, 15:447.

[9] Navin NE: Cancer genomics: one cell at a time. Genome Biol 2014, 15:452.

[10] Nana-Sinkam SP, Croce CM: MicroRNA regulation of tumorigenesis, cancer progression and interpatient heterogeneity: towards clinical use. Genome Biol 2014, 15:445.

[11] White NM, Cabanski CR, Fisher-Silva JM, Dang HX, Govindan R, Maher CA: Transcriptome sequencing reveals altered long intergenic non-coding RNAs in lung cancer. Genome Biol 2014, 15:429.

[12] Wyatt AW, Mo F, Wang K, McConeghy B, Brahmbhatt S, Jong L, Mitchell DM, Johnston RL, Haegert A, Li E, Liew J, Yeung J, Shrestha R, Lapuk A, McPherson A, Shukin R, Bell RH, Anderson S, Bishop J, Hurtado-Coll A, Xiao H, Chinnaiyan AM, Mehra R, Lin D, Wang Y, Fazli L, Gleave ME, Volik SV, Collins CC: Heterogeneity in the inter-tumor transcriptome of high risk prostate cancer. Genome Biol 2014, 15:426.

[13] Mayba O, Gilbert HN, Liu J, Haverty PM, Jhunjhunwala S, Jiang Z, Watanabe C, Zhang Z: MBASED: allele-specific expression detection in cancer tissues and cell lines. Genome Biol 2014, 15:405.

[14] Lund K, Cole J, VanderKraats ND, McBryan T, Pchelintsev NA, Clark W, Copland M, Edwards JR, Adams PD: DNMT inhibitors reverse a specific signature of aberrant promoter DNA methylation and associated gene silencing in AML. Genome Biol 2014, 15:406.

[15] Fleischer T, Frigessi A, Johnson KC, Edvardsen H, Touleimat N, Klajic J, Riis MLH, Haakensen V, Wärnberg F, Naume B, Helland Å, Børresen-Dale AL, Tost J, Christensen BC, Kristensen VN: Genome-wide DNA methylation profiles in progression to in situ and invasive carcinoma of the breast with impact on gene transcription and prognosis. Genome Biol 2014, 15:435.

[16] Charlton J, Williams RD, Weeks M, Sebire NJ, Popov S, Vujanic G, Mifsud W, Alcaide-German M, Butcher LM, Beck S, Pritchard-Jones K: Methylome analysis identifies a Wilms tumor epigenetic biomarker detectable in blood. Genome Biol 2014, 15:434.

[17] Varghese AM, Berger MF: Advancing clinical oncology through genome biology and technology. Genome Biol 2014, 15:427.

[18] Mateo J, Gerlinger M, Rodrigues D, de Bono JS: The promise of circulating tumor cell analysis in cancer management. Genome Biol 2014, 15:448.

[19] Siravegna G, Bardelli A: Genotyping cell-free tumor DNA in the blood to detect residual disease and drug resistance. Genome Biol 2014, 15:449.

[20] Eiring AM, Deininger MW: Individualizing kinase-targeted cancer therapy: the paradigm of chronic myeloid leukemia. Genome Biol 2014, 15:461.

[21] Boutros PC, Margolin AA, Stuart JM, Califano A, Stolovitzky G: Toward better benchmarking: challenge-based methods assessment in cancer genomics. Genome

Biol 2014, 15:462.

[22] Kosseim P, Dove ES, Baggaley C, Meslin EM, Cate FH, Kaye J, Harris JR, Knoppers BM: Building a data sharing model for global genomic research. Genome Biol 2014, 15:430.

Chapter 2

Next Generation Sequencing and Tumor Mutation Profiling: Are We Ready for Routine Use in the Oncology Clinic?

Debu Tripathy[1], Kathleen Harnden[2], Kimberly Blackwell[2], Mark Robson[3,4]

[1]University of Southern California, Keck School of Medicine, USC/Norris Comprehensive Cancer Center, 1441 Eastlake Avenue, NTT-3429, Los Angeles, CA 90033, USA
[2]Duke Cancer Institute, Duke University Medical Center, 2301 Erwin Road, Durham, NC 27710, USA
[3]Memorial Sloan Kettering Cancer Center, Memorial Hospital, 1275 York Avenue, New York, NY 10065, USA
[4]Weill Cornell Medical College, 1275 York Ave, New York, NY 10065, USA.

Abstract: Next generation sequencing (NGS) coupled with sophisticated bioinformatics tools yields an unprecedented amount of information regarding tumor genetics, with the potential to reveal insights into tumor behavior. NGS and other multiplex genomic assays are rapidly spilling from the laboratory into the clinic through numerous commercial and academic entities. This raises the important question as to whether we are ready to use these data in clinical decision-making. While genetic lesions are clearly targeted by a new generation of biological cancer therapies, and certain regulatory approvals are actually coupled to single gene assays, we still do not know if the vast information on other genomic alterations is worth the added cost, or even worse, the inappropriate and unproven assignment of patients to treatment with an unapproved drug carrying potentially serious side effects. On the other hand, the trend toward a precision medicine pathway is clearly accelerating, and clinical trials validating pathway-driven personalized cancer therapeutics will be necessary in both the community and academic settings. Lower cost and wider availability of NGS now raises a debate over the merit of routine tumor genome-wide analysis.

Keywords: Breast Cancer, Next-Generation Sequencing, Oncology

1. Introduction: Are We Ready in the Clinic?

Debu Tripathy (**Figure 1**)

As with most new technologies and treatments, molecular diagnostics are entering the oncology arena in phases. However, these phases are not fully evidence-based or scientifically driven they are somewhat organic as physician and patient interest always seems to be a step or two ahead of the data. The concept of 'precision medicine', defined as therapy that is personalized to unique disease and host characteristics, has taken huge leaps in the cancer field with the advent of next generation sequencing (NGS)[1][2]. NGS encompasses several technologies that generate gene sequence as well as copy number alterations and translocation of numerous genes. However, as pointed out by Dr. Robson, the most evidence-based use of genomic-based therapy still relies on single gene analysis, such as EGFR mutations and ALK rearrangements for lung cancer, BCR-ABL translocation (both presence and transcript quantification) for chronic myelogenous leukemia (CML) and HER2 amplification for breast cancer[3]–[6]. The advantages of NGS are primarily the brute force of sequencing just about all expressed genes depending on the details of the platform, as well as the great 'depth', that is the number of 'reads' that allows for the detection of mutations that may be seen in only a fraction of cells (but are potentially the most dangerous ones). A disadvantage is the level of noise - mutations that may not be 'drivers' or may not be 'actionable', in that they do not clearly lend themselves to specific effective therapies. Several approaches have been devised to distinguish random (or 'passenger') mutations from true drivers, including direct testing of the genetic lesions in preclinical

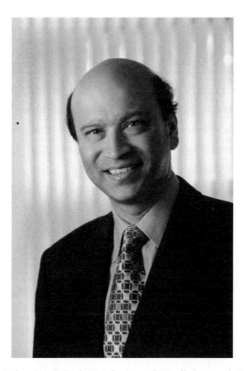

Figure 1. Debu Tripathy, MD is Professor of Medicine and Co-Leader of the Women's Cancer Program at University of Southern California/Norris Comprehensive Cancer Center and holds the Priscilla and Art Ulene Chair in Women's Cancer. His area of clinical research interest is novel therapeutics in breast cancer, specifically, growth factor receptor pathway targeting as well as biomarkers that predict sensitivity and resistance. He is also part of a transdisciplinary breast specialty team dedicated to patient-centered and personalized approaches to care, with an emphasis on translational clinical trials.

models or bioinformatics approaches that model the effects from the mutation sites and downstream biological pathways. We can also assume that more frequent mutations are those selected above the much rarer random ones due to their evolutionary selection as drivers of growth (or drug resistance in the case of those that may arise after treatment). Even mutations that can be biologically confirmed as mediators of malignancy and metastasis phenotypes and for which active drugs exist may not be clinically useful. This is evidenced by the successful targeting of BRAF mutation (V600E)-associated melanoma with BRAF and downstream MEK inhibitors, but the lack of efficacy in BRAF-mutated colorectal cancer, perhaps due to more genomic alterations and resultant bypass pathways[7][8].

NGS can generate results quickly since millions of pieces of small pieces of

DNA are read in parallel. But tiling, or aligning the reads to generate interpretable results, requires complex bioinformatics support and a significantly longer time. For many tumor types, NGS has no proven benefit, although the theoretical advantage is that it may identify a clinical trial or even drug approved for a different cancer type that MIGHT be helpful. Accordingly, for today's clinical practice, single gene assays suffice. However, as NGS become cheaper, it may be a simpler way to perform diagnostics on the small number of tumors in which several mutations, translocations or deletions are of proven benefit in decision-making, such as lung cancer or hematological malignancies. It also requires less tissue than multiple single gene tests. Also, customized panels for more commonly mutated genes in a specific cancer are becoming available that may offer focused multi-gene testing at a lower cost and yielding fewer 'uninterpretable or unactionable' findings.

NGS can also be applied to germline testing to detect heritable cancer susceptibility gene mutations and variants. It can also be helpful in the interpretation of tumor NGS results by excluding inherited variants that may be mono-allelic in the tumor. For familial genetic testing, NGS or multi-gene panel testing is being increasingly used as sequencing costs drop and can be informative in the setting of strong family histories without mutations seen in more common predisposition genes. In one series of patients, with a family history of breast cancer but no mutation seen in BRCA 1 or 2, a 42-gene panel assay found additional findings in 15 of 141 patients (11%), most of whom had breast cancer, with germline mutations/ variants seen in ATM, BLM, CDH1, CDKN2A, MUTYH, MLH1, NBN, PRSS1 and SLX4 genes[9]. This technology could therefore address the need to lower cost and expand the scope of gene susceptibility testing, but it also creates clinical dilemmas in the management of the carriers of these gene anomalies for whom we do not fully understand the natural history and cannot provide lifetime cancer risk estimates.

1.1. So When Should We Be Using NGS or Multi-Gene Testing?

From the standpoint of clinical utility, the bar is quite high, and has clearly not been reached that would require the demonstration that the actions based on the test actually result in clinical benefit compared to decisions made without its use. At this time, single gene assays meet that criteria, but not NGS. In fact, we have not even excluded harm an inappropriate or harmful decision from acting on a result of NGS given the vast amount of information contained in the result and the paucity of knowledge for most of the 'targets' listed. As an example, a recent trial for patients with advanced breast cancer that performed array comparative genomic hybridization for copy number variation and gene sequencing (AKT and PI3KCA only) and then assigned them to a panel of drugs that were known or presumed to address the genetic lesions. Of 423 patients enrolled, biopsies were obtained in 297, with genomic analysis feasible in 283, genomic alterations identified in 195, personalized' therapy available for 55, and in 43 patients treated with 16 different targeted regimens and evaluable for response, only 4 had objective responses and 9 had stability of disease[10]. These results illustrate the prematurity of using broad-based molecular testing routinely, but do point to the promise that these numbers can significantly improve with more comprehensive analysis and more experimental drugs available. Also, disease types with more "druggable" targets, such as lung cancer and hematological malignancies, could yield different results and several prospective consortia are testing this approach. Drs. Harnden and Blackwell appropriately emphasize that as more patients and their treating oncologists are able to access a growing number of mutation-guided clinical trials, NGS may be justifiable ideally as a formal part of such trials.

The future of genomically targeted cancer therapy will not only include NGS, but other high throughput technologies such as RNA sequencing that provides quantitative gene expression as well as mutational status and can also analyze micro and noncoding RNAs that modulate gene expression. Proteomic analysis can also provide functional information that lends itself to drug selection. Also, genomic analysis after treatment progression can be very productive as demonstrated with studies of imatinib-resistant CML harboring the difficult-to-treat T315 resistance-associated mutation in BCR-ABL and resistance-associated mutations in EGFR, such as T790M in lung cancer, where this knowledge has led to the development of new therapeutics (ponatinib approved for CML and several drugs in testing for EGFR-kinase inhibitor-refractory lung cancer)[11][12].

Importantly, a growing body of information regarding mutational analysis in large populations in the context of clinical outcome and response to therapies will assemble a more robust understanding of cancer genomics and systems biology that can elucidate critical vulnerabilities that can be tackled with specific targeted drugs, or more likely, combinations of drugs[13][14]. The availability of portals for patients and physicians to understand better the nature and consequences of genomic alterations, available therapies and open clinical trials (such as MyCancer-Genome)[15] will greatly aid in clinical decisions and trial referral. Finally, large trials with numerous available targeted drugs are planned, including the NCI Match demonstration trial across all solid tumors and the MASTER protocol as a regulatory approval pathway for second-line squamous cell lung cancer treatment[16]. Altogether, this spells for a bright future for this still nascent field that will lead to comprehensive and precision molecular cancer therapeutics.

1.2. Competing Interests

The author declares that he has no competing interests.

2. Tumor Mutation Profiling in Breast Cancer Is Ready for Routine Use in the Clinic

Kathleen Harnden and Kimberly Blackwell (**Figure 2** and **Figure 3**)

The foremost priority in cancer research is personalized treatment approaches offering the promise of more effective and better tolerated therapies. One major step towards offering personalized therapy is the use of genomic mutational analysis to help drive decision making in the clinic. Technologies such as NGS offer comprehensive analysis of specific mutations present in each patient's breast cancer. The argument to include NGS in clinical decision making is based on several concepts including: 1) Actionable mutations are well described in the literature and targeted therapies are now available in the approved or trial setting; 2) Mutations might provide predictive capabilities for certain types of standard and experimental therapies and, therefore, offer an enrichment strategy in designing clinical trials; and 3) Mutations might offer prognostic and/or predictive information in certain types of breast cancer, such as HER2+ and triple negative breast cancer. We will now discuss each of these points in some detail.

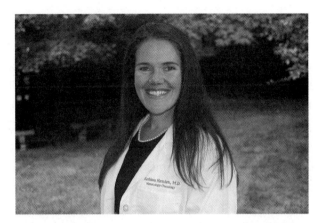

Figure 2. Kathleen Harnden, MD is a senior fellow at Duke University Medical Center. She graduated from Keck School of Medicine at University of Southern California and completed her internship and residency at Duke University Medical Center. Her research interests include breast cancer genetics and clinical trials in metastatic breast cancer.

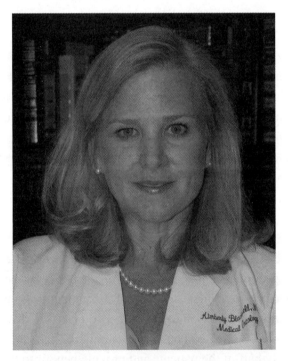

Figure 3. Kimberly Blackwell, MD is professor of medicine and assistant professor of radiation oncology at Duke University Medical Center and director of the breast cancer program at the Duke Cancer Institute, where she oversees all basic and translational research programs involving breast cancer patients. She has played a major role in two recently approved breast cancer drugs, lapatinib and T-DM1, both of which were studied in her laboratory and developed in trials in which she served as principal investigator.

There are many biologically meaningful and, therefore, actionable mutations described in cancer with currently available therapeutic options. These mutations are not confined to specific tissue origins. Instead, these mutations define subgroups of cancer in ways that we do not currently use clinically. The number of mutations with targeted therapies in breast cancer is ever increasing and currently includes genes such as poly (ADP-ribose) polymerase (PARP) (PARP inhibitors), p53 (vaccine therapy, gene therapy, Wee-1 inhibitors, Kevetrin), estrogen receptor alpha (ESR1) (alternative endocrine therapies), JAK1(JAK1 inhibitors), and mTOR (mTOR inhibitors)[17]. There are also new actionable mutations on the horizon that are not well described in breast cancer with developing targeted therapies, including mutated genes such as dynein (hsp90 inhibitors, HDAC inhibitors), MST1 (anti- MST1 receptor antibodies), ROS-1 (inhibitors), HGF (anti- bodies against c-met, c-met inhibitors), and ALDH8A1 (disulfiram). NGS empowers providers to identify and exploit driving mutations in breast cancer biology and to employ new real time therapeutic options in the clinic.

Additionally, NGS is ready for routine use in the oncology clinic as it could create a redesign in the way patients are enrolled in clinical trials. NGS identifies meaningful mutations, allowing improved and more rigorous enrollment in clinical trials. These actionable mutations allow providers to transform standard treatment plans to individualized approaches and match patients to clinical trials. As NGS becomes more readily available and affordable, it should allow for better enrichment strategies for enrollment into clinical trials. To use NGS to enrich trial populations should be a very attractive idea to both study sponsors and patients.

An example of using NGS for trial enrichment is found in the SAFIR01 study. In a prospective trial of more than 400 breast cancer patients, André et al. found a targetable genomic alteration in 46% of patients[10]. Of these patients, 25% had treatment driven by genomics and 28% of the patients who were treated with genomic-driven therapy had an objective response or stable disease for up to 10 months. In this heavily pretreated population of patients, the ability to find actionable targets in nearly half of the patients and provide benefit to the nearly 1/3 who received the treatment is clinically meaningful. Additionally, clinical trials of targeted agents in which patients would have been deemed ineligible using standard testing methods are now being designed to include NGS[18]. Patients with activating mutations of HER2 who were considered ineligible for standard HER2 based therapy now have new clinical trial options and therapeutic options based on se-quencing results[18].

Another example of how NGS can enrich trial populations is found in the NCI MATCH (Molecular Analysis for Therapy Choice) study[16]. In this study, 1,000 patients with common and rare tumors will be enrolled for NGS at the time of progression to elucidate resistance mechanisms and to choose single agent or combination targeted therapy for these patients. There are currently 20 'arms' of the study and more than 40 targeted agents pledged for use. The techniques, relia-bility and workflow are currently being optimized to streamline the NGS data for real time clinical impact.

A third reason that NGS is ready for the clinic is that it could better define prognosis (prognostic value) or potential compounds that have a higher likelihood of benefiting patients (predictive value). Each specific oncogenic event provides an opportunity for targeted therapy. If we can identify a molecular profile asso-ciated with greater therapeutic benefit we can prospectively select patients accor-dingly. Similar to the increased benefit of platinum therapy in metastatic triple-negative breast cancer in BRCA 1/2 positive patients[19] and a poorer prognosis in docetaxel and trastuzumab +/− pertuzumab therapy in HER2 amplified metastatic breast cancer in patients with a PIK3CA mutation[20], NGS can provide a founda-tion on which to maximize clinical benefit of highly targeted therapies based on tumor mutational signatures.

Finally, NGS could influence decision making in the clinic in determining prognosis in certain subtypes of metastatic breast cancer patients. O'Shaughnessy *et al*. found that extraordinary responders to lapatinib with trastuzumab prima-ry-refractory inflammatory breast cancer share a common cancer genotype[21]. These cancer genotypes and their response phenotype can be elucidated for innu-merable therapy regimens and used to make predictably beneficial treatment deci-sions in the clinic[22]–[25]. We presented data at the 2013 San Antonio Breast Cancer Symposium identifying gene mutations associated with progression free survival (PFS) in metastatic breast cancer[26]. Patients with WNK1 mutations had a median PFS of 1.4 months compared to 7.3 months (P = 0.03) in those with the wild type gene. Conversely, patients with mutated MST1 had improved PFS of 11.4 months compared to 6.2 months (P = 0.04) with the wild type gene. Likewise, several gene mutations conferred differences in overall survival. This prognostic information, obtained using NGS, could become incredibly valuable in counseling patients and in selecting appropriate therapies.

Although many of the therapeutic implications of NGS involve clinical trial participation, NGS is ready for the clinic. Some clinicians would argue it already is in the clinic. Our focus now should turn to bringing this revolutionary, therapy-altering and prognostic technology to all patients in an efficient, affordable way. In order to achieve this goal, scientists, bioinformatics specialists, clinicians and patients will need to work together to bring NGS to its full capacity.

Competing Interests

Dr. Harnden has no competing interests. Dr. Blackwell's Institution has received recent research funding from GSK, Bristol Meyer Squibb, Celgene and Genentech. Dr. Blackwell has served as a consultant to Novartis, Celgene and Genentech.

3. Tumor Mutation Profiling Is Not Ready for Routine Use Beyond the Research Setting

Mark Robson (**Figure 4**)

Cancer is a genetic disease, in the sense that the malignant phenotype arises, in large part, as a result of mutations in the DNA of the cancer cell. Massively parallel NGS offers the opportunity to define the pattern of genomic alterations in a patient's cancer quickly and affordably. This capability could, in theory, fulfill the promise of 'precision medicine' and allow treatment tailored to the specific drivers of the individual patient's disease. This promise has captured the imagination of oncology professionals, and a number of commercial and academic laboratories now offer tumor mutation profiling. Like any new technology, however, tumor mutation profiling with NGS is most appropriate for specific purposes. At this point, NGS is a tool for oncology research and does not yet have a place in routine clinical care.

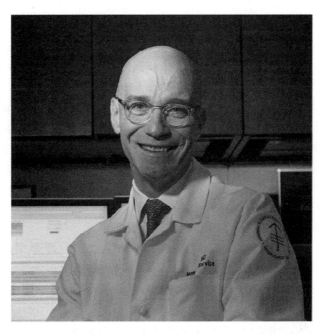

Figure 4. Mark Robson, MD is an Attending Physician of the Clinical Genetics and Breast Medicine Services in the Department of Medicine at Memorial Sloan-Kettering Cancer Center. His research is directed toward improving the integration of genetic information into the clinical management of women with breast cancer. He and his colleagues have conducted a number of studies examining outcomes in women with hereditary breast cancer to better define the risks and benefits of treatments such as breast conserving therapy and adjuvant chemotherapy in this group. He is currently conducting studies to evaluate the impact of intensive screening or surgical prevention upon women's quality of life and to develop new screening tools for breast cancer, such as serum peptide profiling.

There are three main ways that an oncologist could use information about the pattern of mutations in a patient's cancer. First, he or she could use the information to select a treatment that has been approved by regulatory authority for use in the setting of a particular genetic change. Second, the oncologist could use the information to identify patient eligibility for clinical trials of new targeted agents. Finally, the oncologist could use the information to select a targeted treatment for "off-study" and "off-label" use. At this time, it is not necessary to employ NGS for the first purpose, and inappropriate to utilize NGS for the last. There may be a limited role for NGS for the second purpose, at least in academic medical centers with early development programs, but in most clinical situations, more directed testing is more appropriate.

There are increasing numbers of agents that are approved for the treatment of cancers harboring specific genomic alterations. The canonical example, of course, is the use of imatinib in the treatment of chronic myelogenous leukemia harboring the BCR/ABL rearrangement[27]. A more recent example is the remarkable success of BRAF inhibitors in the treatment of malignant melanomas with BRAF V600E mutations[28]. Tumor mutation profiling can identify these mutations, of course, but the specific alterations appropriate for treatment with approved agents are well- defined, and there are usually specific companion diagnostic assays. There is no obvious benefit to using a NGS assay to identify an established mutation, and likely significant incremental cost. So, if there is a known target in a particular disease type, NGS profiling is not necessary.

At the other end of the spectrum is the hope that NGS may identify a therapeutic target that would not have been considered based on disease type, and that this knowledge will allow the oncologist to select an 'off the shelf ' treatment for a patient that will be superior to a more traditional physician-selected therapy. While this is the application that is the most logical in the popular imagination, it is also the one that is the least supported by data. Even if one identifies a mutation that confers sensitivity in a particular disease, it may not predict response in another context. An example is the relative insensitivity of BRAF-mutant colon cancer to BRAF inhibition, despite the presence of the same mutation that confers sensitivity in melanoma[8]. The situation becomes even more complicated when one attempts to predict response based upon non-canonical alterations in genes that could be plausible targets for existing drugs. If the platform evaluates tumor DNA alone, any identified sequence change may, in fact, be germ line (inherited) in origin. The mere fact that a variation is rare does not argue for pathogenic relevance, since most normal human variation is common, and even protein-truncating mutations are seen in the constitutional DNA of apparently healthy people[29][30]. To identify sequence variants that are present in tumor only, a number of laboratories now sequence tumor and normal samples simultaneously, and 'subtract' the germ line sequence from the somatic sequence in order to identify those variants that are unique to the tumor. However, even somatic variants may not be causative. Such variants may not be functionally significant, and the process of determining causality is both complex and partly subjective despite the best efforts of a number of groups to standardize the process of curation[31]. Even if causative, the variant may not be directly related to the cancer process ('passenger' rather than driver' mutation), in which case targeting the mutation will not have an effect on the growth of the tumor.

Even if a sequence variant is somatic, functional and related to the cancer process, targeting it may not be beneficial because it may not be present in the metastases that are threatening the patient. Genetic heterogeneity is an enormous challenge, both as a possible substrate for the development of resistance and as a source of variation between primary and metastatic sites (as well as between metastatic sites)[32]. Inadequate sampling may limit the ability to delineate the actual genomic changes that are most relevant to treatment.

Even if the variant is relevant in light of all of these considerations, it may not be targetable. There may not be an 'off the shelf' drug that can attack the vulnerability or tumor context may limit response (as discussed previously for BRAF inhibitors). Even if a drug is available, resistance to single agent targeted treatment often evolves quickly in solid tumors[33], and untested combinations of targeted agents are extremely unwise without careful delineation of toxicities in properly conducted clinical trials. Finally, even if a particular genomic alteration is relevant and targetable, the genomically-directed treatment may not be superior to conventional therapy, and foregoing a proven approach in favor of an unapproved targeted treatment may lead to inferior outcomes. The comparison of genomically-directed treatment to conventional therapy requires carefully designed, innovative clinical trials such as the recently announced Friends of Cancer Research-NCI Lung Cancer Master protocol[16][34].

While tumor mutation profiling does not yet have a role in determining treatment off-study, it may be a useful means of identifying patients who are candidates for studies of new genomically-directed therapies. At academic centers with extensive portfolios of new agents, it may be productive to conduct routine tumor profiling on patients with advanced disease in order to 'pre-form' cohorts of characterized patients who can be expeditiously directed towards appropriate studies when the time is right. Outside of the academic setting, however, patients may have limited geographic and financial access to trials, and it is not clear that it is helpful to them to learn about a study that they cannot travel to or afford. An alternative would be to conduct limited genomic characterization to determine eligibility for studies that are practical for the specific circumstance, rather than broad profiling.

In summary, then, somatic mutation profiling by NGS is not necessary for deployment of approved genomically-directed treatments and is not yet at the point where it can be used to direct off-protocol treatment. Profiling may be useful as a screening tool to determine trial eligibility but, for most patients, it may be more practical to employ a more limited approach to determine eligibility for specific studies of interest to the particular individual, given their clinical circumstances.

Competing Interests

The author declares that he has no competing interests.

Authors' Information

These debates were presented at the 31st annual Miami Breast Cancer Conference, March 2014.

Source: Tripathy D, Harnden K, Blackwell K, *et al*. Next generation sequencing and tumor mutation profiling: are we ready for routine use in the oncology clinic [J]. Bmc Medicine, 2014, 12(1):1–8.

References

[1] Chmielecki J, Meyerson M: DNA sequencing of cancer: what have we learned? Annu Rev Med 2014, 65:63–79.

[2] Garraway LA, Verweij J, Ballman KV: Precision oncology: an overview. J Clin Oncol 2013, 31:1803–1805.

[3] Eroglu Z, Tagawa T, Somlo G: Human epidermal growth factor receptor family-targeted therapies in the treatment of HER2-overexpressing breast cancer. Oncologist 2014, 19:135–150.

[4] Gridelli C, Peters S, Sgambato A, Casaluce F, Adjei AA, Ciardiello F: ALK inhibitors in the treatment of advanced NSCLC. Cancer Treat Rev 2014, 40:300–306.

[5] Jain N, O'Brien S: The frontline treatment of chronic myeloid leukemia in the chronic phase: current clinical decisions and future prospects for treatment. Expert

Rev Hematol 2013, 6:575–586.

[6]   Lee CK, Brown C, Gralla RJ, Hirsh V, Thongprasert S, Tsai CM, Tan EH, Ho JC, da
       Chu T, Zaatar A, Osorio Sanchez JA, Vu VV, Au JS, Inoue A, Lee SM, Gebski V,
       Yang JC: Impact of EGFR inhibitor in non-small cell lung cancer on progression-free
       and overall survival: a meta-analysis. J Natl Cancer Inst 2013, 105:595–605.

[7]   Flaherty KT, Infante JR, Daud A, Gonzalez R, Kefford RF, Sosman J, Hamid O,
       Schuchter L, Cebon J, Ibrahim N, Kudchadkar R, Burris HA 3rd, Falchook G, Algazi
       A, Lewis K, Long GV, Puzanov I, Lebowitz P, Singh A, Little S, Sun P, Allred A,
       Ouellet D, Kim KB, Patel K, Weber J: Combined BRAF and MEK inhibition in me-
       lanoma with BRAF V600 mutations. N Engl J Med 2012, 367:1694–1703.

[8]   Prahallad A, Sun C, Huang S, Di Nicolantonio F, Salazar R, Zecchin D, Beijersber-
       gen RL, Bardelli A, Bernards R: Unresponsiveness of colon cancer to BRAF(V600E)
       inhibition through feedback activation of EGFR. Nature 2012, 483:100–103.

[9]   Kurian AW, Hare EE, Mills MA, Kingham KE, McPherson L, Whittemore AS, Mc-
       Guire V, Ladabaum U, Kobayashi Y, Lincoln SE, Cargill M, Ford JM: Clinical eval-
       uation of a multiple-gene sequencing panel for hereditary cancer risk assessment. J
       Clin Oncol 2014, 32:2001–2009.

[10]   Andre F, Bachelot T, Commo F, Campone M, Arnedos M, Dieras V, Lacroix-Triki M,
       Lacroix L, Cohen P, Gentien D, Adélaide J, Dalenc F, Goncalves A, Levy C, Ferrero
       JM, Bonneterre J, Lefeuvre C, Jimenez M, Filleron T, Bonnefoi H: Comparative ge-
       nomic hybridisation array and DNA sequencing to direct treatment of metastatic
       breast cancer: a multicentre, prospective trial (SAFIR01/ UNICANCER). Lancet
       Oncol 2014, 15:267–274.

[11]   Cortes JE, Kim DW, Pinilla-Ibarz J, le Coutre P, Paquette R, Chuah C, Nicolini FE,
       Apperley JF, Khoury HJ, Talpaz M, DiPersio J, DeAngelo DJ, Abruzzese E, Rea D,
       Baccarani M, Müller MC, Gambacorti-Passerini C, Wong S, Lustgarten S, Rivera
       VM, Clackson T, Turner CD, Haluska FG, Guilhot F, Deininger MW, Hochhaus A,
       Hughes T, Goldman JM, Shah NP, Kantarjian H, et al: A phase 2 trial of ponatinib in
       Philadelphia chromosome-positive leukemias. N Engl J Med 2013, 369:1783–1796.

[12]   Lee HJ, Schaefer G, Heffron TP, Shao L, Ye X, Sideris S, Malek S, Chan E, Mer-
       chant M, La H, Ubhayakar S, Yauch RL, Pirazzoli V, Politi K, Settleman J: Nonco-
       valent wild-type-sparing inhibitors of EGFR T790M. Cancer Discov 2013,
       3:168–181.

[13]   Alexandrov LB, Nik-Zainal S, Wedge DC, Aparicio SA, Behjati S, Biankin AV, Big-
       nell GR, Bolli N, Borg A, Borresen-Dale AL, Boyault S, Burkhardt B, Butler AP,
       Caldas C, Davies HR, Desmedt C, Eils R, Eyfjörd JE, Foekens JA, Greaves M, Ho-
       soda F, Hutter B, Ilicic T, Imbeaud S, Imielinski M, Jäger N, Jones DT, Jones D,
       Knappskog S, Kool M, et al: Signatures of mutational processes in human cancer.
       Nature 2013, 500:415–421.

[14]   Ciriello G, Miller ML, Aksoy BA, Senbabaoglu Y, Schultz N, Sander C: Emerging land-
       scape of oncogenic signatures across human cancers. Nat Genet 2013, 45:1127–1133.

[15] My Cancer Genome. [www.mycancergenome.org]

[16] Abrams J, Conley B, Mooney M, Zwiebel J, Chen A, Welch JJ, Takebe N, Malik S, McShane L, Korn E, Williams M, Staudt L, Doroshow J: National Cancer Institute's Precision Medicine Initiatives for the new National Clinical Trials Network. Am Soc Clin Oncol Educ 2014, 71–76.

[17] Tinoco G, Warsch S, Gluck S, Avancha K, Montero AJ: Treating breast cancer in the 21st century: emerging biological therapies. J Cancer 2013, 4:117–132.

[18] Ellis MJ, Buzdar A, Unzeitig GW, Esserman L, Leitch AM, Dershryver K, Allred DC, Suman V, Hunt K, Olson JA: A randomized phase II trial comparing exemestane, letrozole, and anastrozole in postmenopausal women with clinical stage II/III estrogen receptor-positive breast cancer. J Clin Oncol 2010, 28(18, suppl): abstract LBA513.

[19] Isakoff SJ, Goss PE, Mayer EL, Traina TA, Carey LA, Krag K, Rugo HS, Liu MC, Stearns V, Come SE, Borger DR, Quadrino CA, Finkelstein D, Garber JE, Ryan PD, Winer EP, Ellisen LW: A multicenter phase II study of cisplatin or carboplatin for metastatic triple negative breast cancer and evaluation of p63/p73 as a biomarker of response. J Clin Oncol 2011, 29(15, suppl): abstract 1025.

[20] Baselga J, Majewski I, Nuciforo PG: PI3KCA mutations and correlation with pCR in the NeoALTTO trial (BIG 01-06). Eur Cancer Congress 2013, abstract 1859.

[21] O'Shaughnessy J: Extraordinary responders to lapatinib with trastuzumab in primary-refractory IBC share a common cancer genotype. San Antonio Breast Cancer Symposium 2013.

[22] Banerji S, Cibulskis K, Rangel-Escareno C, Brown KK, Carter SL, Frederick AM, Lawrence MS, Sivachenko AY, Sougnez C, Zou L, Cortes ML, Fernandez-Lopez JC, Peng S, Ardlie KG, Auclair D, Bautista-Piña V, Duke F, Francis J, Jung J, Maffuz-Aziz A, Onofrio RC, Parkin M, Pho NH, Quintanar-Jurado V, Ramos AH, Rebollar-Vega R, Rodriguez-Cuevas S, Romero-Cordoba SL, Schumacher SE, Stransky N, et al: Sequence analysis of mutations and translocations across breast cancer subtypes. Nature 2012, 486:405–409.

[23] Ellis MJ, Ding L, Shen D, Luo J, Suman VJ, Wallis JW, Van Tine BA, Hoog J, Goiffon RJ, Goldstein TC, Ng S, Lin L, Crowder R, Snider J, Ballman K, Weber J, Chen K, Koboldt DC, Kandoth C, Schierding WS, McMichael JF, Miller CA, Lu C, Harris CC, McLellan MD, Wendl MC, DeSchryver K, Allred DC, Esserman L, Unzeitig G, et al: Whole-genome analysis informs breast cancer response to aromatase inhibition. Nature 2012, 486:353–360.

[24] Shah SP, Roth A, Goya R, Oloumi A, Ha G, Zhao Y, Turashvili G, Ding J, Tse K, Haffari G, Bashashati A, Prentice LM, Khattra J, Burleigh A, Yap D, Bernard V, McPherson A, Shumansky K, Crisan A, Giuliany R, Heravi-Moussavi A, Rosner J, Lai D, Birol I, Varhol R, Tam A, Dhalla N, Zeng T, Ma K, Chan SK, et al: The clonal and mutational evolution spectrum of primary triple-negative breast cancers. Nature 2012, 486:395–399.

[25] Stephens PJ, Tarpey PS, Davies H, Van Loo P, Greenman C, Wedge DC, Nik-Zainal S, Martin S, Varela I, Bignell GR, Yates LR, Papaemmanuil E, Beare D, Butler A, Cheverton A, Gamble J, Hinton J, Jia M, Jayakumar A, Jones D, Latimer C, Lau KW, McLaren S, McBride DJ, Menzies A, Mudie L, Raine K, Rad R, Chapman MS, Teague J, et al: The landscape of cancer genes and mutational processes in breast cancer. Nature 2012, 486:400–404.

[26] Blackwell K, Hamilton EP, Marcom PK: Exome sequencing reveals clinically actionable mutations in the pathogenesis and metastasis of triple negative breast cancer. In Paper presented at: 36th Annual San Antonio Breast Cancer Symposium; December 10-14. San Antonio, TX; 2013: Abstract S4–03.

[27] Druker BJ, Sawyers CL, Kantarjian H, Resta DJ, Reese SF, Ford JM, Capdeville R, Talpaz M: Activity of a specific inhibitor of the BCR-ABL tyrosine kinase in the blast crisis of chronic myeloid leukemia and acute lymphoblastic leukemia with the Philadelphia chromosome. N Engl J Med 2001, 344:1038–1042.

[28] Chapman PB, Hauschild A, Robert C, Haanen JB, Ascierto P, Larkin J, Dummer R, Garbe C, Testori A, Maio M, Hogg D, Lorigan P, Lebbe C, Jouary T, Schadendorf D, Ribas A, O'Day SJ, Sosman JA, Kirkwood JM, Eggermont AM, Dreno B, Nolop K, Li J, Nelson B, Hou J, Lee RJ, Flaherty KT, McArthur GA, BRIM-3 Study Group: Improved survival with vemurafenib in melanoma with BRAF V600E mutation. N Engl J Med 2011, 364:2507–2516.

[29] Nelson MR, Wegmann D, Ehm MG, Kessner D, St Jean P, Verzilli C, Shen J, Tang Z, Bacanu SA, Fraser D, Warren L, Aponte J, Zawistowski M, Liu X, Zhang H, Zhang Y, Li J, Li Y, Li L, Woollard P, Topp S, Hall MD, Nangle K, Wang J, Abecasis G, Cardon LR, Zöllner S, Whittaker JC, Chissoe SL, Novembre J, Mooser V: An abundance of rare functional variants in 202 drug target genes sequenced in 14,002 people. Science 2012, 337:100–104.

[30] Tennessen JA, Bigham AW, O'Connor TD, Fu W, Kenny EE, Gravel S, McGee S, Do R, Liu X, Jun G, Kang HM, Jordan D, Leal SM, Gabriel S, Rieder MJ, Abecasis G, Altshuler D, Nickerson DA, Boerwinkle E, Sunyaev S, Bustamante CD, Bamshad MJ, Akey JM, Broad GO, Seattle GO, NHLBI Exome Sequencing Project: Evolution and functional impact of rare coding variation from deep sequencing of human exomes. Science 2012, 337:64–69.

[31] MacArthur DG, Manolio TA, Dimmock DP, Rehm HL, Shendure J, Abecasis GR, Adams DR, Altman RB, Antonarakis SE, Ashley EA, Barrett JC, Biesecker LG, Conrad DF, Cooper GM, Cox NJ, Daly MJ, Gerstein MB, Goldstein DB, Hirschhorn JN, Leal SM, Pennacchio LA, Stamatoyannopoulos JA, Sunyaev SR, Valle D, Voight BF, Winckler W, Gunter C: Guidelines for investigating causality of sequence variants in human disease. Nature 2014, 508:469–476.

[32] Gerlinger M, Rowan AJ, Horswell S, Larkin J, Endesfelder D, Gronroos E, Martinez P, Matthews N, Stewart A, Tarpey P, Varela I, Phillimore B, Begum S, McDonald NQ, Butler A, Jones D, Raine K, Latimer C, Santos CR, Nohadani M, Eklund AC, Spencer-Dene B, Clark G, Pickering L, Stamp G, Gore M, Szallasi Z, Downward J,

Futreal PA, Swanton C: Intratumor heterogeneity and branched evolution revealed by multiregion sequencing. N Engl J Med 2012, 366:883–892.

[33] Solit D, Sawyers CL: Drug discovery: How melanomas bypass new therapy. Nature 2010, 468:902–903.

[34] Lung Cancer Master Protocol Activation Announcement. Available at: http://www. focr.org/sites/default/files/Lung%20Cancer%20Master%20Protocol%20Activation% 20Announcement%20Slides.pdf. Accessed 27 May 2014.

Chapter 3

Age Dependence of Tumor Genetics in Unfavorable Neuroblastoma: ArrayCGH Profiles of 34 Consecutive Cases, Using a Swedish 25-Year Neuroblastoma Cohort for Validation

Cihan Cetinkaya[1,2], Tommy Martinsson[3], Johanna Sandgren[1,4], Catarina Träger[5], Per Kogner[5], Jan Dumanski[1], Teresita Díaz de Stáhl[1,4], Fredrik Hedborg[1,6]

[1]Department of Immunology, Genetics and Pathology, Rudbeck Laboratory, Uppsala University, Uppsala SE-751 85, Sweden
[2]Department of Surgical Sciences, Endocrine Unit, Uppsala University, University Hospital, Uppsala SE-751 85, Sweden
[3]Department of Clinical Genetics, Institute of Biomedicine, University of Gothenburg, Sahlgrenska Hospital, GöteborgSE-413 45, Sweden
[4]Department of Oncology-Pathology, Cancer Center Karolinska, CCK R8:04, Karolinska Institutet, Stockholm SE-171 76, Sweden
[5]Department of Women's and Children's Health, Childhood Cancer Research Unit, Karolinska Institutet, Karolinska Hospital, Stockholm SE 171 76, Sweden
[6]Department of Women's and Children's Health, Uppsala University, University

Hospital, Uppsala SE-751 85, Sweden

Abstract: Background: Aggressive neuroblastoma remains a significant cause of childhood cancer death despite current intensive multimodal treatment protocols. The purpose of the present work was to characterize the genetic and clinical diversity of such tumors by high resolution array CGH profiling. Methods: Based on a 32K BAC whole-genome tiling path array and using 50–250K Affymetrix SNP array platforms for verification, DNA copy number profiles were generated for 34 consecutive high-risk or lethal outcome neuroblastomas. In addition, age and MYCN amplification (MNA) status were retrieved for 112 unfavorable neuroblastomas of the Swedish Childhood Cancer Registry, representing a 25-year neuroblastoma cohort of Sweden, here used for validation of the findings. Statistical tests used were: Fisher's exact test, Bayes moderated t-test, independent samples t-test, and correlation analysis. Results: MNA or segmental 11q loss (11q-) was found in 28/34 tumors. With two exceptions, these aberrations were mutually exclusive. Children with MNA tumors were diagnosed at significantly younger ages than those with 11q- tumors (mean: 27.4 vs. 69.5 months; $p = 0.008$; $n = 14/12$), and MNA tumors had significantly fewer segmental chromosomal aberrations (mean: 5.5 vs. 12.0; $p < 0.001$). Furthermore, in the 11q- tumor group a positive correlation was seen between the number of segmental aberrations and the age at diagnosis (Pearson Correlation 0.606; $p = 0.037$). Among nonMNA/non11q- tumors ($n = 6$), one tumor displayed amplicons on 11q and 12q and three others bore evidence of progression from low-risk tumors due to retrospective evidence of disease six years before diagnosis, or due to tumor profiles with high proportions of numerical chromosomal aberrations. An early age at diagnosis of MNA neuroblastomas was verified by registry data, with an average of 29.2 months for 43 cases that were not included in the present study. Conclusion: MNA and segmental 11q loss define two major genetic variants of unfavorable neuroblastoma with apparent differences in their pace of tumor evolution and in genomic integrity. Other possible, but less common, routes in the development of aggressive tumors are progression of low-risk infant-type lesions, and gene amplifications other than MYCN. Knowledge on such nosological diversity of aggressive neuroblastoma might influence future strategies for therapy.

Keywords: High-Risk, Unfavorable, Neuroblastoma, Arraycgh, DNA Copy Number, Gain, Loss, Amplification, Age

1. Background

Neuroblastoma is a childhood malignancy that arises from embryonic cells of the sympathetic ganglia or the adrenal medulla[1]. It is mainly a disease of infants and toddlers; more than half of patients with neuroblastoma are diagnosed before two years of age and ~90 percent before age six[2][3]. This age dependence of the incidence of neuroblastoma may be a consequence of developmentally determined disappearance of the pool of immature cells from which neuroblastomas are thought to derive. The disease is clinically diverse, and ranges from cases with a very dismal prognosis, despite modern intensive multimodal therapy, to those with an excellent chance of survival[2]. This variation in clinical behavior is also highly age dependent: children who are diagnosed after two years of age suffer predominantly from aggressive forms. Neuroblastomas that are diagnosed during adolescence and young adulthood are rare, but they are of particular concern because they almost invariably progress, although with an indolent course[4][5]. In sharp contrast, tumors that are diagnosed before 18 months of age are generally associated with a favorable prognosis. Such tumors are usually less advanced, have a propensity for spontaneous involution or maturation, and respond well to mild chemotherapy[2].

These clinical differences correspond to clear differences in tumor genetics[2]. As a general rule, prognostically favorable tumors display numerical imbalances of entire chromosomes and have near-triploid DNA content, whereas higher-risk tumors present with segmental chromosomal aberrations (SCAs) and are often pseudodiploid. MYCN gene amplification (MNA) was one of the first genetic markers for highly aggressive neuroblastoma to be established[6], and remains a powerful prognostic indicator[7]. More recently, an independent prognostic value of a segmental deletion of 11q has also been recognized[7]–[9]. Both these aberrations are incorporated in the present International Neuroblastoma Risk Group (INRG) classification system for treatment stratification[10]. Several arrayCGH studies in the recent years support the MNA/segmental 11q loss dichotomy of high-risk neuroblastoma and indicate that any type of segmental numerical chromosomal aberration is a negative prognostic sign[11]–[13]. However, the representativeness of the studied tumor materials may be questioned because the tumors were from multiple sources and, hence, selection bias may have occurred. Therefore, the present study aims at characterizing the heterogeneity of genetic aberrations in aggressive neuroblastoma by exploiting a consecutive, population- based series of tumors, the representativeness of which was tested against data in the Swedish Childhood Cancer Registry. The most striking observations were related to age at tumor presentation: MNA tumors were associated with a particularly early age at diagnosis and low numbers of other chromosomal aberrations suggesting a rapid tumor evolution with few genetic hits involved, whereas 11q deleted tumors were diagnosed at older ages and showed significantly more SCAs, the numbers of which were positively correlated with the age at diagnosis, suggesting a chromosomal instability phenotype with a more stepwise tumor evolution. Other tumors seemed to be the result of late progression of low-risk neuroblastoma or of gene amplifications other than MYCN. This clinicogenetic diversity of unfavorable neuroblastoma is likely to reflect differences in tumor evolution and growth, which may have therapeutic implications.

2. Methods

2.1. Study Design

In order to obtain a representative view at high resolution of DNA copy number aberrations in aggressive forms of neuroblastoma a 32K BAC whole-genome tiling path array CGH platform was applied to a consecutive, population-based tumor material (described below). The representativeness of the tumor collection was analyzed by comparing the patients' ages at diagnosis and proportions of tumors in relation to the presence or absence of MNA with the corresponding data of neuroblastomas registered in the Swedish Childhood Cancer Registry during a 25-year period. For verification of the BAC array-based profiles high-resolution SNP array analyses were performed. Based on publically available gene expression data from neuroblastoma, expression profiles were compared between tumor groups for certain chromosomal regions of interest.

2.2. Patient Material

Fresh frozen specimens of neuroblastoma were collected consecutively during the period 1986-1994 at all Swedish centers at which pediatric tumor surgery is performed[14]. Samples collected between 1995 and 2010 at Uppsala University Hospital, which treats approximately 20 percent of Swedish patients with neuroblastoma, were also included. The inclusion criteria were: high-risk neuroblastoma, as defined by the INRG classification system[10], progression to disseminated fatal disease, and stage L2 tumors in children >12 years of age at diagnosis (one case). The INRG high-risk criteria applied here were: Stage M tumors in children >18 months of age at diagnosis and all tumors with MNA. Stage MS tumors were excluded. The individual clinical data of all 34 cases included in the study are shown in **Table 1**.

To ensure that the tumor specimens represented viable tumor tissue their quality was assessed from hematoxylin/eosin stained cryosections, requiring a tumor cell content of at least 60%–70%. Ethical approval was obtained from the Regional Ethical Review Board in Uppsala (approval 2007/069), and written informed consent was obtained from the parents.

There is an overlap between tumors included in this work and those of a similar Swedish report[15]. However, our study is based on another collection of biopsies from a partially different set of tumors. The previously reported Affymetrix SNP array data[15] was used for verification of our BA Carray results on tumors common to both studies (n = 15) and for verification of our data on presently unique tumors (n = 19) new original SNParray data was produced. Tumors in common with the aforementioned study are indicated in **Table 1** and information on their previous codes[15]; [Table S1] is given in the table legend.

2.3. Array-Based Comparative Genomic Hybridization

The 32K BAC array was established as reported previously[16]. High- quality DNA was obtained by standard methods[17]. DNA labeling, hybridization, washing, scanning of arrays, and data processing were performed as described earlier[16][18]–[20]. Experiments using 50K and 250K Affymetrix arrays were performed in accordance with the manufacturer's protocol (Affymetrix, Inc., Santa Clara, CA), and as described earlier[21].

2.4. Microarray Expression Data

Publically available gene expression data from high-risk metastatic neurob-

Table 1. Clinical data and main genetic findings of 34 unfavorable neuroblastomas.

ID	Age (mo)	Sex	Stage (INRGSS)	Outcome	Follow up (mo)	Survival median (mo)	Site	WCA (nr)	WCA (average)	SCA (nr)	SCA (average)	MNA	11q-	Array platform
52*	4	m	M	DOD	10		adr	0		6		+		32 K
55	8	f	M	DOD	16		adr	0		6		+		32 K, Affymetrix
106*	10	f	M	NED	265		adr	0		12		+		32K
123*	11	f	M	DOD	3		adr	0		6		+		32K, Affymetrix
241*	11	m	M	DOD	8		adr	1		3		+		32K, Affymetrix
244	14	f	M	*DOD*	22		adr	8		2		+		Affymetrix
212	15	m	M	DOD	5		adr	0		2		+		32K, Affymetrix
240*	21	f	M	NED	43		adr	0		3		+		32K, Affymetrix
135*	22	m	L2	DOD	3		adr	0		3		+		32K, Affymetrix
95*	26	f	M	DOD	15		adr	0		8		+		32K
238	30	f	M	DOD	24		adr	0		6		+		Affymetrix
207	37	f	M	DOD	7		adr	2		5		+		32K, Affymetrix
217	37	m	M	DOD	36		adr	0		8		+		32K
126	138	m	M	DOD	9		adr	0		7		+		32K, Affymetrix
MNA not 11q-						9.5			0.8		5.5			
68	41	m	M	DOD	12		adr	9		7		+	+	32K, Affymetrix
136*	48	f	L2	DOD	12		adr	1		8		+	+	32K
MNA & 11q-						12.0			5.0		7.5			

ID	Age	Sex	WCA	Status		Site				MNA	Platform
243	32	f	M	DOD	28	adr	2		10	+	Affymetrix
149	34	m	M	DOD	16	adr	0		12	+	32K, Affymetrix
112	40	m	M	DOD	18	adr	1		3	+	32K, Affymetrix
111*	42	f	M	NED	262	adr	0		7	+	32K
155	52	f	M	DOD	19	adr	3		13	+	32K, Affymetrix
32*	57	m	M	DOD	12	adr	2		15	+	32K, Affymetrix
110	60	m	M	DOD	12	adr	1		14	+	32K, Affymetrix
69*	60	m	L2	DOD	17	th	1		14	+	32K, Affymetrix
41*	77	f	M	DOD	8	th	2		15	+	32K, Affymetrix
49	82	m	M	DOD	14	adr	3		10	+	32K, Affymetrix
209	129	m	M	DOD	35	adr	2		10	+	32K, Affymetrix
229	169	m	L2	DOD	34	adr	1		21	+	32K, Affymetrix
					16.5		1.5		12.0		
11q- notMNA											
107*	23	m	M	DOD	10	adr	1		2	+	32K, Affymetriix
131	37	f	L2	DOD	21	adr	13		1	+	32K, Affymetriix
130	46	m	M	DOD	57	adr	0		3	+	32K, Affymetriix
208	59	m	L2	DOD	25	renal	4		3	+	32K
242*	90	f	M	SD	37	th	12		5	+	32K, Affymetriix
226*	91	m	M	SD	61	th	2		12	+	32K, Affymetriix
					23.0		5.3		4.3		
Not MNA not 11q-											

Cases are sorted on the basis of genetic category, as determined by the presence of MNA and segmental loss of 11q. Within each tumor category, cases are sorted according to age at diagnosis. Abbreviations: DOD: dead of disease; NED: no evidence of disease; SD: stable disease; WCA: whole-chromosome copy number aberration; SCA: segmental chromosomal copy number aberration; adr: adrenal; th: thoracic. Tumors marked with asterisk (*) with IDs: 52, 106, 123, 241, 240, 135, 95, 136, 111, 32, 69, 41, 107, 242, and 226 are reported also by Carén et al. [15] with the respective codes: 7, 14, 8, 2, 4, 13, 12, 37, 40, 42, 44, 39, 66, 73, and 63, as listed in [15; Table S1].

lastomas, series GSE13136[22], platform Affymetrix Human Genome U133 Plus 2.0, which were selected by the presence of MNA (GSM328993, GSM328996, GSM329000, GSM329006, GSM329007, GSM329008, GSM329011, GSM329012, GSM329013, GSM 329015) or segmental 11q loss (GSM328992, GSM328995, GSM328997, GSM328999, GSM329002, GSM329010, GS M329014, GSM329017) were downloaded from Gene Expression Omnibus (http://www.ncbi.nlm.nih.gov/geo/) and normalized in Expression Console v1.1 (3' Expression Arrays-RMA, Affymetrix).

2.5. The Swedish Childhood Cancer Database

Clinical data and the MYCN copy number status for neuroblastomas diagnosed in Sweden during the 25-year period of 1984-2008 were obtained from the Swedish Childhood Cancer Registry. The clinical criteria for inclusion were the same as for the array study. The limit for MNA was set at >4 copies of MYCN per haploid genome, as determined by FISH and/or SNP array.

2.6. Statistical Analysis

To analyze differences in DNA copy number among the tumor groups, Fisher's exact test was used within the Nexus Copy Number 5.0 analysis program (BioDiscovery, Inc., El Segundo, CA, USA). To search for genes that were differentially expressed among the tumor groups, an empirical Bayes moderated t-test was applied using the 'limma' package[23] and p-values were adjusted in accordance with the method of Benjamini and Hochberg[24]. Clinical data were processed using PASW Statistics 18.0 software (SPSS; Chicago, IL, USA). Mean differences in age were examined with the t-test for independent samples. Covariations were analyzed by correlation analysis, and the results were expressed as Pearson correlation coefficients.

3. Results

Identification of two major unfavorable neuroblastoma groups with different genomic signatures To visualize the results from the complete set of tumors, the percentages of tumors with copy number change were calculated and plotted relative to the position along the chromosomes [**Figure 1(A)**]. All individual profiles are also illustrated (Additional file 1: Figure S1). Partial or complete gain of one or two copies of the 17q arm was the most common aberration (88% of the tumors), followed by loss of 1p segments (56%), MNA (47%), and loss of 11q (47%; 14 tumors with segmental loss and 2 with loss of one entire chromosome 11) [**Figure 1(A)**] and Additional file 1: Figure S1). Subsequently, we examined the frequencies of copy number changes in tumor subgroups that were defined on the basis of the absence or presence of MNA and segmental 11q loss (11q-); hence, the tumors were separated into four subgroups: MNAnot11q-($n =1$ 4), 11q-notMNA ($n = 12$), MNA and 11q($n = 2$), and neither MNA nor 11q($n = 6$). The results are shown in **Figures 1(B)-1(D)** and Additional file 1: Figure S1. Selected profiles from each group are shown in **Figure 2**. Analysis using Fisher's exact test of differences between the MNAnot11q-and 11q-notMNA groups (which contained most of the samples, 26/34; 76%) revealed that loci on 1p, 2p, 3p, 5q, 7, 11, 12, 18p, and 20q were differentially altered between the two sets of tumors [**Figure 1(E)**]. These groups also differed in terms of the number of SCAs (mean 5.5 and 12.0, respectively; **Table 1**, $p < 0.001$, Wilcoxon's test), and with regard to an absence of numerical whole chromosomal aberrations, which was the case in 11/14 MNA-not11q- tumors, but in only 2/12 11q-notMNA tumors (**Table 1** and Additional file 1: Figure S1). Finally, tumors that showed neither MNA nor 11q- were more heterogeneous in terms of both segmental and whole chromosomal aberrations; two tumors showed aberrations in chromosome number for the majority of chromosomes (ID 131 and ID 242; **Table 1** and Additional file 1: Figure S1).

3.1. Age Dependence of Genetic Subgroups

As shown in **Table 1** and in **Figure 3**, MNA tumors were diagnosed early in life. In fact, 11 out of the 12 children who were youngest at diagnosis suffered from MNA tumors. If an outlier amongst the MNA group in terms of genetic profile and age (ID126; **Table 1** and Additional file 1: Figure S1) is disregarded, only two 11q-notMNA tumors were diagnosed in the same young age range as that of the remaining MNAnot11q- tumors (**Table 1** and **Figure 3**). Statistically, the ages at diagnosis of children with MNAnot11q-tumors differed highly significantly from those of children with 11q-notMNA tumors (mean age: 27.4vs. 69.5 months, respectively; $p = 0.008$; median age: 18 vs.58.5 months, respectively; $n = 14$ vs. 12).

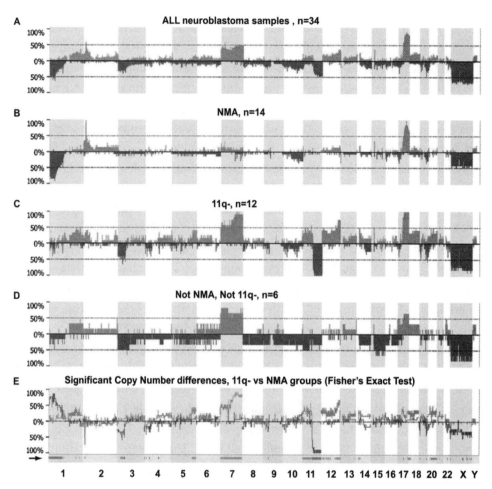

Figure 1. Genetic findings in unfavorable neuroblastoma. The frequency of copy number changes was calculated for all measurement points in the arrays and plotted relative to the position along the chromosome for: (A): all tumors, (B): MNA$^{not11q-}$ tumors, (C): 11q-^{notMNA} tumors, (D): neither MNA nor 11q loss tumors. The number of analyzed tumors is indicated (n). Green bars above the horizontal line indicate the percentage of tumors with copy gains and red bars below the horizontal line indicate the percentage of tumors with copy losses. Data for the X chromosome were normalized to female reference DNA and the respective proportion of boys in panels A-D were: 56%, 43%, 67%, and 67%, respectively (E): To search for copy number alterations that differ between the 11q-^{notMNA} and MNA$^{not11q-}$ groups, the frequency percentage difference between the two groups are plotted: Copy number gain difference (green graph): Values above baseline represent regions in which gains are more numerous among 11q-$^{not MNA}$ tumors, and vice versa for values below baseline. Deletion difference (red graph): Values above baseline represent regions in which losses are more common among MNA$^{not11q-}$ tumors, and vice versa for values below baseline. The regions significantly differentially altered between the groups, identified by using Fisher's exact test within Nexus copy-number software, (p < 0.05 and threshold difference in frequency >25%), are shown below the graph, as indicated by a black arrow.

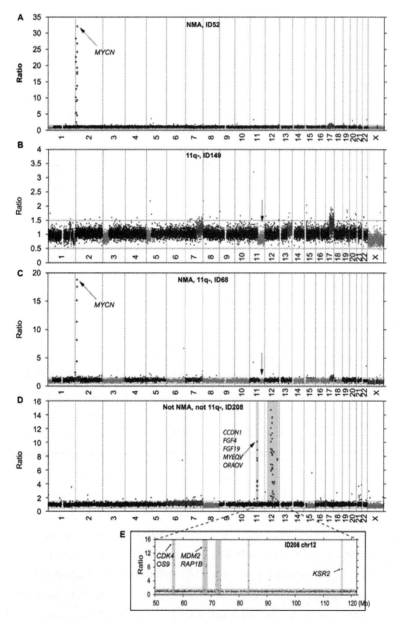

Figure 2. Examples of individual neuroblastoma profiles within genetic subgroups. (A) MNA^notllq-; (B) 11q-^notMNA; (C) combined MNA and segmental 11q loss; (D) neither MNA nor segmental 11q loss; (E) shows an expanded segment of chromosome 12 in panel (D). Amplified genes of particular oncogenic interest are indicated. Each individual clone was assigned a copy number class as follows: i) balanced: two alleles (blue dots); ii) gained: presence of three (red) or more (pink dots) alleles; or iii) deleted: hemizygous deletions (green dots). No homozygous deletions were found in these tumors. Black arrows indicate MNA amplification, 11q loss or other amplifications.

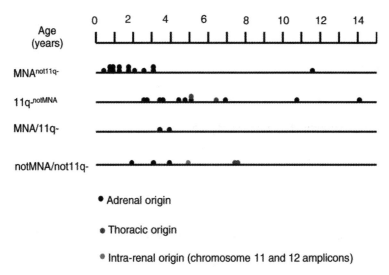

Figure 3. Age at diagnosis in unfavorable neuroblastoma (n = 34). Each tumor in the present study is plotted on a time axis according to age at diagnosis and genetic subgroup. Color symbols indicate the likely site of origin.

To test the validity of these findings in a larger sample, we utilized the Swedish Childhood Cancer Registry, which contained clinical information and data on the copy number of MYCN in tumors for 240 cases of neuroblastoma that were diagnosed during almost the same time period as the cases in the present study. Among these, 112 were unfavorable cases (100 high risk and 12 intermediate risk who suffered lethal tumor progression). Of the tumors included in the current study, 25 were represented among these 112 cases in the registry, and 11 of the 25 were cases with MNA. Given that 11q status is not registered consistently in the database, we compared the age at diagnosis of children with MNA tumors to those with non-MNA tumors. This analysis revealed highly significant differences both for the present study (MNA vs. non-MNA: mean: 29.5 vs. 65.6 months; p = 0.005; median age: 21 vs. 58 months; n = 16 vs. 18) and for cases of unfavorable neuroblastoma in the registry that were not included in the present study (MNA vs. non-MNA: mean age: 29.2 vs. 49.1 months; p = 0.001; median age: 24 vs. 43.5 months; n = 43 vs. 44). To determine whether the MNA cases included in our study might be biased towards a younger age range, we compared their ages at diagnosis to those of the other MNA cases in the registry and found no statistical difference (mean: 29.5 vs. 29.2 months; median: 21 vs. 24 months; p = 0.968; n = 16 vs. 43). There was also no statistically significant difference in the distribution of ages at diagnosis for non-MNA tumors (mean: 65.6 vs. 49.1 months; median:

58 vs. 43.5 months; p = 0.098; *n* = 18 vs. 44).

When the findings were merged, we were able to conclude that, among Swedish children who were diagnosed with unfavorable neuroblastoma during this time period, MNA tumors were almost four-fold more common than non-MNA tumors when diagnosis was made before two years of age (31 vs. 8), whereas this relationship was reversed in children who were diagnosed after 3.5 years of age (10 vs. 35; **Figure 4**).

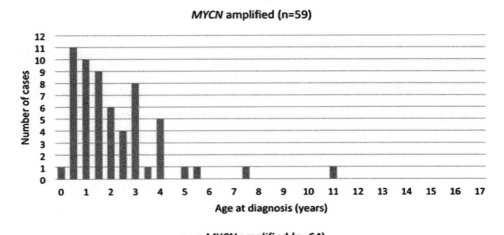

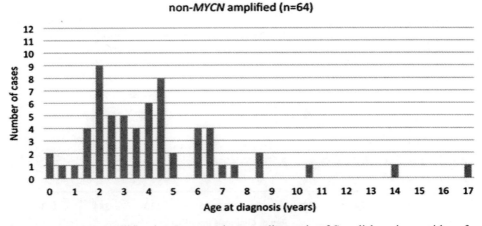

Figure 4. MYCN amplification status and age at diagnosis of Swedish patients with unfavorable neuroblastoma (n = 121). Present cases, representing the period 1986–2010, have been merged with all other cases of unfavorable neuroblastoma found in the Swedish Childhood Cancer Registry during the period 1984–2008. Data is presented in 6-month age intervals. Unfavorable criteria were: lethal tumor progression, MYCN amplification, INRGSS Stage M and >18 months of age at diagnosis, and INRGSS Stage L2 >12 years of age at diagnosis.

In view of the high number of SCAs that were found in tumors with segmental 11q deletion, we investigated the possibility of an age-dependence for the number of SCAs within this tumor subgroup and found a positive correlation with age at diagnosis (Pearson correlation 0.606; p = 0.037). When merging the four genetic groups the age dependence of SCA numbers was even more evident with a p-value of 0.001 (Pearson correlation 0.547; **Figure 5**).

3.3. High Copy Number Amplicons

In total, 17 tumors displayed amplified regions. The number of these amplified regions per tumor varied from one to seven, and their sizes ranged from 0.15 to 6.8 Mb. Of the 16 tumors with MNA, either the MYCN-containing amplicon was the only amplification event or it was accompanied by multiple amplified loci within 2p, and in one case by two amplified loci on chromosome 3q. The regions of amplification, their frequencies, and the genes encompassed are listed in **Table 2**. In one tumor with MNA and its associated cell line[15], a few novel amplicons

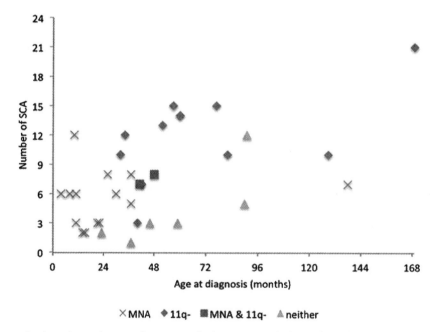

Figure 5. Age dependence of segmental chromosomal aberrations in unfavorable neuroblastoma (n = 34). Data are separated by genetic subtype, as indicated. X-axis: age at diagnosis (years). Y-axis: number of segmental chromosomal aberrations (SCA; amplicons not included).

Table 2. Regions of amplification in unfavorable neuroblastoma (n = 17).

Chr Region (Mb)	Cyto-band	Length(Mb)	Genes	Gene Symbols	Group	No of tumors
chr:2:0.366 - 0.793	p25.3	0.427	1	TMEM18	NMA	1
chr:2:2.304 - 6.219	p25.3 - p25.2	3.915	12	ADI1, ALLC, COLEC11, LOC150622, LOC400940, LOC730811, MYT1L, RNASEH1, RPS7, SOX11, TSSC1, TTC15	NMA	1
chr:2:3.605 - 4.280	p25.3	0.675	3	ALLC, COLEC11, RPS7	NMA	1
chr:2:5.708 - 7.439	p25.2 - p25.1	1.731	6	CMPK2, LOC150622, LOC400940, RNF144A, RSAD2, SOX11	NMA	1
chr:2:6.372 - 6.855	p25.2	0.483	0		NMA	1
chr:2:10.413 - 11.244	p25.1	0.831	10	ATP6V1C2, C2orf50, HPCAL1, KCNF1, NOL10, ODC1, PDIA6, PQLC3, ROCK2, SNORA80B	NMA	2
chr:2:11.622 - 11.878	p25.1	0.256	3	GREB1, LPIN1, NTSR2	NMA	1
chr:2:13.097 - 13.580	p24.3	0.483	0		NMA	1
chr:2:14.219 - 14.292	p24.3	0.073	0		NMA	2
chr:2:15.895 - 16.095	p24.3	0.200	2	MYCN, MYCNOS	NMA	16
chr:2:16.675 - 16.705	p24.3	0.030	1	FAM49A	NMA	6
chr:2:16.846 - 17.106	p24.3 - p24.2	0.260	0		NMA	6
chr:2:18.197 - 18.423	p24.2	0.227	0		NMA	3
chr:2:20.546 - 21.012	p24.1	0.466	3	C2orf43, GDF7, HS1BP3	NMA	1
chr:2:22.493 - 25.674	p24.1 - p23.3	3.181	21	ADCY3, ATAD2B, C2orf44, C2orf79, C2orf84, CENPO, DNAJC27, DNMT3A, DTNB, EFR3B, FKBP1B, ITSN2, KLHL29, LOC375190, MFSD2B, NCOA1, PFN4, POMC, SF3B14, TP53I3, UBXN2A	NMA	1
chr:2:26.853 - 27.169	p23.3	0.316	9	AGBL5, C2orf18, CENPA, DPYSL5, EMILIN1, KHK, LOC100128731, MAPRE3, TMEM214	NMA	2
chr:2:28.022 - 28.430	p23.2	0.408	1	BRE	NMA	2

Region	Cytoband	Ratio	Count	Genes	Status	N
chr:2:29.071 - 30.833	p23.2 - p23.1	1.762	8	ALK, C2orf71, CAPN13, CLIP4, FAM179A, LBH, LCLAT1, YPEL5	NMA	2
chr:2:38.841 - 39.010	p22.1	0.168	4	DHX57, GEMIN6, LOC100271715, MORN2	NMA	1
chr:2:45.742 - 46.467	p21	0.725	2	EPAS1, PRKCE	NMA	1
chr:2:47.379 - 47.698	p21 - p16.3	0.319	3	EPCAM, KCNK12, MSH2	NMA	1
chr:2:48.848 - 49.512	p16.3	0.664	1	FSHR	NMA	1
chr:3:170.768 - 1.72.093	q26.2	1.325	18	ARPM1, CLDN11, EIF5A2, GPR160, LOC100128164, LRRC31, LRRC34, LRRIQ4, MECOM, MYNN, PHC3, PRKCI, RPL22L1, SAMD7, SEC62, SKIL, SLC7A14, TERC	NMA	1
chr:3:173.047 - 173.459	q26.31	0.411	2	FNDC3B, TMEM212	NMA	1
chr:11:68.463 - 69.308	q13.2 - q13.3	0.845	9	CCND1, FGF19, FGF4, IGHMBP2, MRGPRD, MRGPRF, MYEOV, ORAOV1, TPCN2	Not NMA, not 11q-	1
chr:12:56.182 - 57.066	q13.3 - q14.1	0.884	23	AGAP2, AVIL, B4GALNT1, CDK4, CTDSP2, CYP27B1, DCTN2, DDIT3, DTX3, FAM119B, GEFT, KIF5A, LOC100130776, MARCH9, MARS, MBD6, METTL1, OS9, PIP4K2C, SLC26A10, TSFM, TSPAN31, XRCC6BP1	Not NMA, not 11q-	1
chr:12:67.060 - 68.692	q15	1.632	13	BEST3, CCT2, CPM, CPSF6, FRS2, LRRC10, LYZ, MDM2, NUP107, RAB3IP, RAP1B, SLC35E3, YEATS4	Not NMA, not 11q-	1
chr:12:71.578 - 73.413	q21.1	1.835	1	LOC552889	Not NMA, not 11q-	1
chr:12:83.287 - 83.563	q21.31	0.276	0		Not NMA, not 11q-	1
chr:12:116.476 - 116.802	q24.22 - q24.23	0.326	1	KSR2	Not NMA, not 11q-	1

Regions that involved at least two neighboring clones, with copy number count >3 and normalized fluorescence ratio >2 are shown. For amplicons with regions shared between tumors, the minimal overlapping region is shown. Genes of particular oncogenic interest in neuroblastoma are indicated in bold.

were found, which encompassed genes such as GDF7, FSHR, PRKCE, and TMEM18 (Additional file 2: Figure S2). Overall, 20% of the amplified loci did not encompass any gene (**Table 2**). One unusual case (ID 208) displayed multiple amplicons but not MNA. Genes of particular oncogenic interest within these loci were CCND1, FGF4, FGF19, IGHMBP2, MYEOV, and ORAOV1 on 11q13.2- q13.3 and CDK4, MDM2, andKSR2 on 12q13.3-q15 [**Figures 2(D)-2(E)** and **Table 2**].

3.4. Differentially Expressed Genes within Aberrant Regions of MNA and 11q-Deleted Tumors

Given that MNA and 11q-neuroblastomas present with divergent genomic signatures, we sought differences in gene expression profiles within the regions that differed most consistently between these two groups (1p, 2p, and chromosomes 7 and 11). For this purpose, we compared publicly available gene expression data for high-risk neuroblastomas with recorded MNA and 11q status (see Methods). Among the MNA tumors (n = 10), five tumor suppressor genes (among other genes) were underex-pressed within the distal 1p: CAMTA1, KIF1B, PRDM2, FABP3, and CDKN2C; whereas MYCNOS and MYCN were the two top differentially upregulated genes on 2p. Several constituents of the extracellular matrix or membrane proteins involved in cell adhesion, motility or proliferation that map to chromosome 7, namely PTN, CNTNAP2, ELN, HSPB1, SEMA3E, and COL1A2, were upregulated in the 11q-deleted group (n = 8). In the same group of tumors, CD44 was the top upregulated gene on 11p. Interestingly, on 11q, several tumor suppressor genes and genes encoding DNA-binding proteins involved in DNA repair and negative regulation of transcription were downregulated in the 11q-deleted tumors: C11orf30, RSF1, CREBZF, FAT3, MRE11A, ATM, CADM1, MLL, H2AFX, TBRG1, and CHK1.

4. Discussion

In this report, we describe the DNA copy number profiles of a consecutive series of neuroblastomas that were selected on the basis of unfavorable characteristics. The findings revealed considerable genetic heterogeneity within this clinically troublesome group, which was particularly evident when comparing tumors with MNA to those with segmental 11q deletions. With few exceptions, MNA and segmental 11q loss were mutually exclusive and defined two genetic subgroups of equal size that comprised more than three-quarters of the total samples. Such genetic dichotomy of advanced neuroblastoma has been well described previously[2][7][8][11][15] and both MNA and segmental 11q loss are included in the current INRG algorithm for pretreatment stratification of risk[10]. Less predictably, we also observed a clear clinical difference between these two genetic subgroups in relation to age: MNA tumors affected the youngest children of the series. It is surprising that this age dependence with respect to the tumor genetics of neuroblastoma has not received much scientific attention previously, although mentioned in several previous studies [9][11][15][25]. In view of the relatively moderate size of the present tumor series, it was important that we were able to confirm a generally low age at diagnosis for children with MNA tumors using independent data from the Swedish Childhood Cancer Registry; these data argued clearly against a bias in the present material. We conclude from the present findings that unfavorable neuroblastomas are predominantly of the MNA type when diagnosed under the age of 2 years, whereas tumors with loss of 11q and other genetic variants predominate after 3.5 years of age.

As the Swedish Childhood Cancer Registry, due to lack of records, could not be used to verify the older age at diagnosis for children with 11q-deleted tumors we searched the literature for this information: Spitz et al.[9] reported on segmental 11q deletions from a cohort of 611 neuroblastomas, found in 159 tumors. The median age at diagnosis of these 11q-deleted tumors was 3–5 years, constituting 59 percent of the tumors of this age range. Michels et al.[11] reported 48 and 28 months as median ages at diagnosis for ten 11q-deleted and 22 MNA tumors, respectively. In a meta study by Vandesompele et al.[25] poor risk neuroblastomas were separated into two genetic "clusters": The median age of 45 children belonging to the 11q deletion "cluster" was 41 months, although notably only 30 of the tumors were actually 11q deleted. The corresponding figures for 74 children belonging to the MNA "cluster" was 26.9 months median age with actual MNA seen in 51 tumors. Finally, Carén et al.[15] reported a median age of 42 months for 21 children with 11q-deleted tumors (four of which were common with our study) compared to 21 months for 37 children with MNA tumors (seven in common with our study). Together, these data consistently support an age difference between the two groups, although a certain bias towards older ages for 11q-

44

deleted tumors in the present study is observed (58.5 months median age).

Another difference that was observed between MNA and 11q-deleted tumors was the higher number of SCAs in the later group of tumors and a dependence of their prevalence on age, both of which imply a chromosomal instability phenotype, as suggested previously by Carén *et al.*[15]. Future analyses using larger sample sizes, including multiple tumor specimens (synchronous and metachronous), might be helpful in confirming such chromosomal instability. Also, deep sequencing might shed additional light on differences in genomic integrity at the DNA level among subsets of neuroblastoma. A recent report[26], based on whole-genome sequencing of 87 neuroblastomas of all stages, showed that the frequency of somatic amino-acid-changing mutations strongly correlated to tumor stage, survival, and age at diagnosis. However, no difference in frequency of such mutations was detected when comparing MNA tumors to high-stage non-MNA tumors. Hence, this aformentioned study reported a general age dependence of amino-acid-changing mutations in neuroblastoma, albeit the specific issue of DNA instability in tumors with deleted 11q, as compared to MNA tumors, was not addressed.

On the basis of the profile subtypes that were observed in the presently relatively limited series of tumors, and in view of previous data by others, we speculate on the existence of four genetic routes for the genesis of aggressive neuroblastoma:

4.1. The MNA Route

MNA neuroblastomas seem to fit into a model of rapid tumor evolution that involves only a few genetic events, which transform the progenitor cells into highly proliferative and primary metastatic tumor cells in a straightforward fashion. The likelihood of such few events to take place would, logically, be more proportional to the pool of cells of origin than for tumors requiring a larger sequence of genetic hits (e.g. 11q deleted tumors), hence explaining the early in life appearance of MNA tumors.

4.2. The 11q Route

It appears that the pathogenesis of tumors with segmental 11q loss accords with the traditional genetic model for adult cancer, which predicts a micro-evolutionary process of cancer development, with successive genetic hits affecting key cellular functions[27]. Acquisition of chromosomal instability might be fundamental in this process. Our analysis of differential gene expression in 11q-deleted tumors vs. MNA neuroblastomas pinpointed some candidate tumor suppressor/ DNA repair genes within the region of 11q that is deleted, such as ATM, MLL, H2AFX, and CHK1. Recently, the importance of aberrant gene expression within this region was underscored by the finding that decreased expression of genes within the region of interest at 11q was observed only in those 11q-deleted tumors with an aggressive clinical phenotype[28]. It is noteworthy, in this context, that a subgroup of 11q-deleted tumors with more favorable clinical characteristics has been described[28][29]. Apart from not showing a disproportionate downregulation of the expression of genes of the deleted region, such tumors were also reported to differ from unfavourable 11q-deleted tumors regarding microRNA expression profiles[29] and by having less SCAs[28]. It is therefore possible that the here suggested 11q route is not an important element in the pathogenesis of less aggressive tumors with 11q deletions.Evidently, our statistics on the present 11q-notMNA tumors represents the unfavorable type of 11q-deleted neuroblastoma since there was only one survivor in this group. It is noticeable in this context that our inclusion criteria would discriminate against tumors of the more favorable subtype.

4.3. The Tumor Progression Route

A third possibility in the evolution of aggressive neuroblastoma is progression from lower-risk tumors[13]. Although progression from a low-risk lesion to an aggressive tumor is considered in general to be a rare event, we think that three of the nonMNA/non11q deleted tumors in the present study might have evolved in this way. Two tumors showed genetic similarity to low-risk tumors in that they showed whole chromosome aberrations for more than half of the chromosomes and only few segmental gains or losses. It appears particularly likely that a third tumor (ID 226) was derived from a lower-risk tumor: on diagnosis at 7.5 years of age, it was revealed that a chest X-ray taken 6 years earlier already then showed the primary tumor. Genetically, the tumor had much in common with 11q deleted tumors, but 11q was intact.

4.4. Alternative Amplicon Driven Routes

An unusual genetic variant of the present study was a tumor with multiple amplicons on 11q and 12q. There are other examples in the literature of neuroblastoma cell lines and tumors with very similar amplified regions at 11q13[11]–[25] or 12q13–q15[11][21][30], respectively, and in two tumors synchronous amplification on both chromosomes have been reported[11][31][32], as in the present case. CCND1, IGHMBP2, ORAOV1, FGF4 on chromosome 11q13, and CDK4 and MDM2 on 12q13-15 are interesting oncogenes in this context. Generally, neuroblastomas with 11q13 amplicons were reported to be clinically aggressive and associated with an older age at diagnosis compared to children with MNA tumors of the present study. However, those 11q13 amplified neu-roblastomas which also displayed MNA were diagnosed at earlier ages[11]. Clinical information on 12q amplified neuroblastoma is sparse in the literature but indicates advanced disease[30][33][34]. MNA may occur also in 12q amplified neuroblastoma[21][30][31]. Amplicons of other chromosomal regions are described in single cases of poor outcome neuroblastoma, involving 16q.21, 4q.33, 6p12–21[25], 5q33.3[11], and the MYC containing 8q24 region[26]. Hence, with the support of these previously published data, it seems that our case harboring chromosome 11 and 12 amplifications is not totally unique and implies that such and other non-MYCN amplifications may underlie a minor subset of aggressive neuroblastomas.

5. Conclusions

On the basis of these categories, we suggest the following metaphor for the genesis of unfavorable neuroblastoma: MNA, segmental deletion of 11q, and low-risk precursor lesions provide an elevator, a staircase, and a first step of a staircase, respectively, towards unfavorable neuroblastoma. This metaphor builds on the notion that the first steps in tumor development take place during a common early developmental phase when the immature cells that are the source of neuroblastoma are still present in the sympathetic nervous system, whereas subsequent tumorigenic events differ in malignant effect between the genetic routes. Our speculations on main routes for the pathogenesis of unfavourable neuroblastoma are summarized in **Figure 6**, showing the four mentioned routes and adding also adolescent neuroblastoma as a separate, but still obscure, route. The present delineation

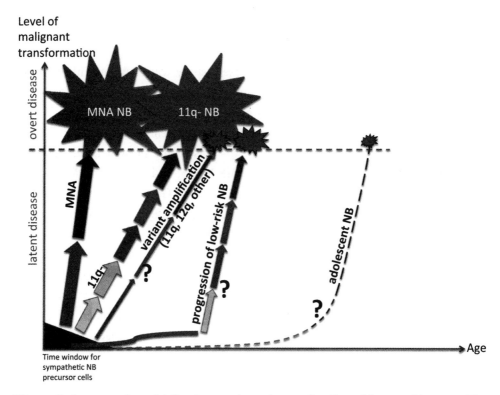

Figure 6. A proposed model for the age dependence of unfavorable neuroblastoma. The model builds on the assumption of an early common cellular origin of all neuroblastomas. Depending on genetic subtype the respective tumorigenic hits differ in type, number and degree of malignant effect most evident when comparing MNA and 11q- tumors. As tumors with alternative amplifications, putative low-to-high-risk progression, and adolescent presentation are poorly represented in the present study and in the literature these routes for tumor development are largely speculative, indicated by question marks. Abbreviation: NB: neuroblastoma; Symbols: Arrows: tumorigenic hits; Darkness of arrow: degree of malignant transformation; Arrow width/size of symbol for clinical disease: relative frequency of tumor subtype; Solid curved blue line: low-risk neuroblastoma development.

of genetic subsets of unfavorable neuroblastoma might have therapeutic implications. It would seem that MNA tumors are more proliferative, which calls for a dose-intensive treatment, and the relatively "clean" genetics of MNA neuroblastomas would appear to make them suitable for tailored treatments that target the functions of MYCN, e.g. apoptosis[35]. Novel therapeutic strategies specifically for 11q-deleted neuroblastoma are urgently needed, and the identification of novel subsets of neuroblastomas with non-MYCN amplifications may also have therapeutic consequences, but these will have to await more conclusive information on the genetic and clinical homogeneity of such tumors. Finally, the possibility of a transition from low to high-risk disease in some cases may have implications for the monitoring of low- risk rest tumors.

6. Additional Files

Additional file 1: Figure S1. Schematic representation of genetic profiles for neuroblastoma samples included in the study *(n = 34)*. Deleted and gained regions are represented by red and green bars, respectively. Cases are arranged according to genetic subgroup.

Additional file 2: Figure S2. Novel amplicons in association with MNA on 2p: 32K whole-genome array data are shown from: (A) the primary tumor of case ID55; (B) cell line U2715, which was established from this tumor.

7. Abbreviations

Adr: Adrenal; BAC: Bacterial artificial chromosome; CGH: Comparative genomic hybridization; DOD: Dead of disease; INRGSS: International Neuroblastoma Risk Group Staging System; MNA: MYCN amplification; NED: No evidence of disease; NB: Neuroblastoma; SCA: Segmental chromosomal aberration; SD: Stable disease; Th: Thoracic; WCA: Whole chromosomal aberration; 11q-: Segmental deletion on 11q.

Competing Interests

None of the authors have declared any financial or non-financial competing interests.

Authors' Contributions

CC performed DNA preparations and BAC array analyses, compiled the data, and participated in drafting the manuscript. TM was responsible for Affymetrix SNP array verification analyses and contributed with critical revision of the manuscript. JS contributed with important methodological assistance with the BAC array analyses and critical reading of the manuscript. CT contributed with the data from the Swedish Childhood Cancer Registry. PK contributed with tumor materials and clinical data and conceptually in the drafting of the manuscript, JD had chief responsibility for the development and use of the BAC array platform and contributed with critical revision of the manuscript. TDS had main responsibility for the design and realization of the study, including drafting of the manuscript. FH conceived of the study, participated in its design, was responsible for collecting tumor samples and clinical data throughout the years, and had main responsibility for the drafting of the manuscript. All authors read and approved the final manuscript.

Authors' Information

CC held a postdoc research position at the Department of Immunology, Genetics and Pathology, Uppsala University during the work. TM is a Professor of tumor genetics at the Department of Clinical Genetics, University of Gothenburg and a senior researcher on neuroblastoma. JS was a PhD student at the Department of Immunology, Genetics and Pathology, Uppsala University involved in the development of the BAC array platform and later holds a postdoc position at the Department of Oncology Pathology, Karolinska Institutet. CT is an MD, PhD, specialist in pediatric oncology and a senior researcher on neuroblastoma at Karolinska Institutet. PK is an MD, PhD, and specialist in pediatric oncology with national responsibilities for neuroblastoma treatment, and senior researcher on neuroblastoma at Karolinska Institutet. JD is a professor of experimental pathology at the Department of Immunology, Genetics and Pathology, Uppsala University. TDS is an associate Professor at the Department of Oncology-Pathology, Karolinska Institutet and formerly at the Department of Immunology, Genetics and Pathology, Uppsala University. FH is an MD, PhD, and specialist in pediatric oncology and senior researcher on neuroblastoma at the Department of Immunology, Genetics and Pathology and Women's and Children's Health, Uppsala University.

Acknowledgements

The authors thank: Johan Wadenbäck, Simin Tahmasebpoor, Inga Hansson and Ulrika Larsson for skilled technical support; Robin Andersson for developing SMAP within the LCB Data; Carl Bruder for decisive contributions in producing the BAC arrays; Sven Påhlman for collaboration in organizing the national collection of tumor specimens in 1986-1994; and the Swedish Childhood Cancer Foundation and Karolinska Institutet for financial support.

Source: Cetinkaya C, Martinsson T, Sandgren J, *et al.* Age dependence of tumor genetics in unfavorable neuroblastoma: arrayCGH profiles of 34 consecutive cases, using a Swedish 25-year neuroblastoma cohort for validation[J]. Bmc Cancer, 2013, 13(1):231.

References

[1]   Brodeur GM: Neuroblastoma: biological insights into a clinical enigma. Nat Rev Cancer 2003, 3(3):203–216.

[2]   Maris JM: Recent advances in neuroblastoma. N Engl J Med 2010, 362(23):2202–2211.

[3]   Park JR, Eggert A, Caron H: Neuroblastoma: biology, prognosis, and treatment. Hematol Oncol Clin North Am 2010, 24(1):6586.

[4]   Franks LM, Bollen A, Seeger RC, Stram DO, Matthay KK: Neuroblastoma in adults and adolescents: an indolent course with poor survival. Cancer 1997, 79(10):2028–2035.

[5]   Polishchuk AL, Dubois SG, Haas-Kogan D, Hawkins R, Matthay KK: Response, survival, and toxicity after iodine-131-metaiodobenzylguanidine therapy for neuroblastoma in preadolescents, adolescents, and adults. Cancer 2011, 117(18):4286–4293.

[6]   Brodeur GM, Seeger RC, Schwab M, Varmus HE, Bishop JM: Amplification of N-myc in untreated human neuroblastomas correlates with advanced disease stage. Science 1984, 224(4653):1121–1124.

[7]   Janoueix-Lerosey I, Schleiermacher G, Michels E, Mosseri V, Ribeiro A, Lequin D, Vermeulen J, Couturier J, Peuchmaur M, Valent A, *et al*: Overall genomic pattern is a predictor of outcome in neuroblastoma. J Clin Oncol 2009, 27(7):1026–1033.

[8]   Attiyeh EF, London WB, Mosse YP, Wang Q, Winter C, Khazi D, McGrady PW, Seeger RC, Look AT, Shimada H, *et al*: Chromosome 1p and 11q deletions and outcome in neuroblastoma. N Engl J Med 2005, 353(21):2243–2253.

[9]   Spitz R, Hero B, Simon T, Berthold F: Loss in chromosome 11q identifies tumors with increased risk for metastatic relapses in localized and 4S neuroblastoma. Clinical cancer research : an official journal of the American Association for Cancer Re-

search 2006, 12(11 Pt 1):3368–3373.

[10] Cohn SL, Pearson AD, London WB, Monclair T, Ambros PF, Brodeur GM, Faldum A, Hero B, Iehara T, Machin D, *et al*: The international neuroblastoma risk group (INRG) classification system: an INRG task force report. J Clin Oncol 2009, 27(2):289–297.

[11] Michels E, Vandesompele J, De Preter K, Hoebeeck J, Vermeulen J, Schramm A, Molenaar JJ, Menten B, Marques B, Stallings RL, *et al*: ArrayCGH-based classification of neuroblastoma into genomic subgroups. Genes Chromosomes Cancer 2007, 46(12):1098–1108.

[12] Mosse YP, Diskin SJ, Wasserman N, Rinaldi K, Attiyeh EF, Cole K, Jagannathan J, Bhambhani K, Winter C, Maris JM: Neuroblastomas have distinct genomic DNA profiles that predict clinical phenotype and regional gene expression. Genes Chromosomes Cancer 2007, 46(10):936–949.

[13] Schleiermacher G, Janoueix-Lerosey I, Ribeiro A, Klijanienko J, Couturier J, Pierron G, Mosseri V, Valent A, Auger N, Plantaz D, *et al*: Accumulation of segmental alterations determines progression in neuroblastoma. J Clin Oncol 2010, 28(19): 3122–3130.

[14] Hedborg F, Lindgren PG, Johansson I, Kogner P, Samuelsson BO, Bekassy AN, Olsen L, Kreuger A, Pahlman S: N-myc gene amplification in neuroblastoma: a clinical approach using ultrasound guided cutting needle biopsies collected at diagnosis. Med Pediatr Oncol 1992, 20(4):292–300.

[15] Caren H, Kryh H, Nethander M, Sjoberg RM, Trager C, Nilsson S, Abrahamsson J, Kogner P, Martinsson T: High-risk neuroblastoma tumors with 11q-deletion display a poor prognostic, chromosome instability phenotype with later onset. Proc Natl Acad Sci U S A 2010, 107(9):4323–4328.

[16] Diaz De Stahl T, Sandgren J, Piotrowski A, Nord H, Andersson R, Menzel U, Bogdan A, Thuresson AC, Poplawski A, Von Tell D, *et al*: Profiling of copy number variations (CNVs) in healthy individuals from three ethnic groups using a human genome 32K BAC-clone-based array. Hum Mutat2008, 29(3):398–408.

[17] Sambrook JFE, Maniatis T: Molecular Cloning; a Laboratory Manual. Cold Spring Harbor, NY: Cold Spring Harbor Laboratory Press; 1989.

[18] Ameur A, Yankovski V, Enroth S, Spjuth O, Komorowski J: The LCB data warehouse. Bioinformatics 2006, 22(8):1024–1026.

[19] Andersson R, Bruder CE, Piotrowski A, Menzel U, Nord H, Sandgren J, Hvidsten TR, Diaz de Stahl T, Dumanski JP, Komorowski J: A segmental maximum a posteriori approach to genome-wide copy number profiling. Bioinformatics 2008, 24(6):751–758.

[20] Yang YH, Dudoit S, Luu P, Lin DM, Peng V, Ngai J, Speed TP: Normalization for cDNA microarray data: a robust composite method addressing single and multiple

slide systematic variation. Nucleic Acids Res 2002, 30(4):e15.

[21] Caren H, Erichsen J, Olsson L, Enerback C, Sjoberg RM, Abrahamsson J, Kogner P, Martinsson T: High-resolution array copy number analyses for detection of deletion, gain, amplification and copy-neutral LOH in primary neuroblastoma tumors: four cases of homozygous deletions of the CDKN2A gene. BMC Genomics 2008, 9:353.

[22] Lastowska M, Viprey V, Santibanez-Koref M, Wappler I, Peters H, Cullinane C, Roberts P, Hall AG, Tweddle DA, Pearson AD, et al: Identification of candidate genes involved in neuroblastoma progression by combining genomic and expression microarrays with survival data. Oncogene 2007, 26(53):7432–7444.

[23] Smyth GK: Linear models and empirical bayes methods for assessing differential expression in microarray experiments. Stat Appl Genet Mol Biol 2004, 3:Article3.

[24] Benjamini YHY: Controlling the false discovery rate: a practical and powerful approach to multiple testing. J R Stat Soc 1995(Ser B 57):289–300.

[25] Vandesompele J, Baudis M, De Preter K, Van Roy N, Ambros P, Bown N, Brinkschmidt C, Christiansen H, Combaret V, Lastowska M, et al: Unequivocal delineation of clinicogenetic subgroups and development of a new model for improved outcome prediction in neuroblastoma. Journal of clinical oncology : official journal of the American Society of Clinical Oncology 2005, 23(10):2280–2299.

[26] Molenaar JJ, Koster J, Zwijnenburg DA, van Sluis P, Valentijn LJ, van der Ploeg I, Hamdi M, van Nes J, Westerman BA, van Arkel J, et al: Sequencing of neuroblastoma identifies chromothripsis and defects in neuritogenesis genes. Nature 2012, 483(7391):589–593.

[27] Hanahan D, Weinberg RA: Hallmarks of cancer: the next generation. Cell 2011, 144(5):646–674.

[28] Fischer M, Bauer T, Oberthur A, Hero B, Theissen J, Ehrich M, Spitz R, Eils R, Westermann F, Brors B, et al: Integrated genomic profiling identifies two distinct molecular subtypes with divergent outcome in neuroblastoma with loss of chromosome 11q. Oncogene 2010, 29(6):865–875.

[29] Buckley PG, Alcock L, Bryan K, Bray I, Schulte JH, Schramm A, Eggert A, Mestdagh P, De Preter K, Vandesompele J, et al: Chromosomal and microRNA expression patterns reveal biologically distinct subgroups of 11q- neuroblastoma. Clin Cancer Res 2010, 16(11):2971–2978.

[30] Chen QR, Bilke S, Wei JS, Whiteford CC, Cenacchi N, Krasnoselsky AL, Greer BT, Son CG, Westermann F, Berthold F, et al: cDNA array-CGH profiling identifies genomic alterations specific to stage and MYCN-amplification in neuroblastoma. BMC Genomics 2004, 5:70.

[31] Carr J, Bown NP, Case MC, Hall AG, Lunec J, Tweddle DA: High-resolution analysis of allelic imbalance in neuroblastoma cell lines by single nucleotide polymorphism arrays. Cancer Genet Cytogenet 2007, 172(2):127–138.

[32] Corvi R, Savelyeva L, Amler L, Handgretinger R, Schwab M: Cytogenetic evolution of MYCN and MDM2 amplification in the neuroblastoma LS tumour and its cell line. Eur J Cancer 1995, 31A(4):520–523.

[33] Rudolph G, Schilbach-Stuckle K, Handgretinger R, Kaiser P, Hameister H: Cytogenetic and molecular characterization of a newly established neuroblastoma cell line LS. Hum Genet 1991, 86(6):562–566.

[34] Su WT, Alaminos M, Mora J, Cheung NK, La Quaglia MP, Gerald WL: Positional gene expression analysis identifies 12q overexpression and amplification in a subset of neuroblastomas. Cancer Genet Cytogenet 2004, 154(2):131–137.

[35] Amati B, Littlewood TD, Evan GI, Land H: The c-Myc protein induces cell cycle progression and apoptosis through dimerization with Max. EMBO J 1993, 12(13):5083–5087.

Chapter 4

A General Framework for Analyzing Tumor Subclonality Using SNP Array and DNA Sequencing Data

Bo Li[1], Jun Z Li[2]

[1]Program of Bioinformatics, University of Michigan, 5940A Buhl, Box 5618, Ann Arbor, MI 48109–5618, USA

[2]Department of Human Genetics, University of Michigan, 5940A Buhl, Box 5618, Ann Arbor, MI 48109–5618, USA

Abstract: Intra-tumor heterogeneity reflects cancer genome evolution and provides key information for diagnosis and treatment. When bulk tumor tissues are profiled for somatic copy number alterations (sCNA) and point mutations, it may be difficult to estimate their cellular fractions when a mutation falls within a sCNA. We present the Clonal Heterogeneity Analysis Tool, which estimates cellular fractions for both sCNAs and mutations, and uses their distributions to inform macroscopic clonal architecture. In a set of approximately 700 breast tumors, more than half appear to contain multiple recognizable aneuploid tumor clones, and many show subtype-specific differences in clonality for known cancer genes.

1. Background

It has been recognized for nearly 40 years that cancer is a dynamic disease and its evolution follows a classical Darwinian process[1][2]. After the proposal of the two-hit model of oncogenesis[3], and especially after the discovery of the linear progression from benign polyps to colorectal cancer via a series of mutational events[4][5], it was briefly envisioned that cancer could be understood in most cases by simply finding the small number of events that act sequentially to drive step-wise clonal selection. However, initial efforts to sequence most coding genes in tumor DNA revealed remarkable heterogeneity between tumors in each cancer type examined[6]–[9]: typically, very few (<10) genes are mutated in >10% of tumors, but many (40 to 80) are mutated in 1% to 5% of tumors. Further, heterogeneity in cancer could manifest on other levels: not just among different patients, but also among tumors of different grades or organ sites in the same patient, as well as among different cells within a tumor[10][11]. Heterogeneity at any of these levels could confound diagnosis and treatment, and underlie the inherent evasiveness of this disease. Most genomic analyses to date, notably those led by the Cancer Genome Atlas (TCGA) Research Network[12]–[15] and the International Cancer Genome Consortium (ICGC)[16] have focused on inter-tumor heterogeneity. These studies analyze hundreds of tumors per cancer type, relying on bulk tissue samples, usually for one sample per patient. The data were primarily interpreted by regarding each tumor as a single population of cells with uniform character. Despite the inherent limitation of this assumption, as shown by the widely reported tumor-normal mixing[17]–[19], large-scale inter-tumor comparisons have led to important new insights into significantly mutated genes[12][13], recurrently perturbed pathways[20], mutation signatures[16][21], tumor subtypes[22][23], molecular predictors of outcome, and commonalities or distinctions among different cancer types[24]. However, these studies are not designed to adequately investigate intra-tumor heterogeneity. Ultimately, cancer genome evolution takes place at the single-cell level, and it is the cellular complexity and its dynamics that give rise to both intra- and inter-tumor heterogeneity. Currently, cytogenetic methods are of low throughput and often cannot assure representative sampling. And the cost of single-cell sequencing[25]–[28] remains prohibitively expensive for all but the proof-of-concept studies. Under such constraints, many groups have surveyed intra-tumor heterogeneity man by comparing multiple specimens from the same patient by longitudinal sampling or spatial sampling (mainly for solid tumors). Almost invariably, analyses of longitudinal samples have uncovered dramatic temporal changes of the cancer cell population that often correlate with disease progression, severity, and treatment resistance[29]–[32]. Similarly, multi-region comparisons have revealed extensive genomic variability across different geographic sectors of the tumor[33][34], or between the primary and metastatic tumors[35].

These studies, while using samples collected with a higher spatial or temporal resolution than those in TCGA and ICGC, often still contain heterogeneous populations of cells[35]-[37].

Fortunately, while bulk tissue data describe the global average of multiple subpopulations of cells, it is sometimes possible to statistically infer the number and genomic profile of such subpopulations. For example, when a sample is sequenced deeply, the somatic mutation frequencies sometimes cluster around a small number of distinct frequency "modes"[38][39], suggesting that somatic mutations of similar frequencies may reside in the same population of cells and these cells may have descended from the same founder cell. For this reason, these mutations are said to belong to the same "clone" or "subclones", the latter referring to a clonal population of a relatively small cellular fraction. This inference task, essentially a deconvolution problem (or Blind Source Separation Problem), pre- sents many analytical challenges, file of each need to be estimated simultaneously, and somatic copy number alterations (sCNAs) and somatic single- nucleotide variants (SNVs) often reside in the same region yet have unknown phase or genealogical order. Currently available methods often need to invoke simplifying assumptions and often focus on a subset of the issues. For example, ABSOLUTE[40] uses sCNA data to estimate the global mixing ratio of aneuploid and euploid cells, but only under a tumor-normal, two-population assumption, which involves a single tumor population of full clonality. When a sCNA or SNV is subclonal, ABSOLUTE makes the qualitative designation of "subclonal" without quantitatively estimating the clonality. Other methods also invoke other types of compromises, and we will defer the description of these limitations to the Discussion.

In this work, we developed Clonal Heterogeneity Analysis Tool (CHAT) as a general framework for estimating the cellular frequencies of both sCNAs and SNVs. It is suitable for analyzing genomewide SNP genotyping and DNA sequencing data for tumor-normal pairs (**Figure 1**). CHAT begins by identifying regions of sCNA or by partitioning the genome into bins; and for each sCNA or bin, it estimates a local mixing ratio, called segmental aneuploid genome proportion (sAGP), between a euploid population and a single aneuploid population carrying the local CNA. The assumption of local two-way mixing does not imply there are only two cell populations globally. It is akin to the infinite-site model in population genetics, stating that each locus experienced only one copy number alteration,

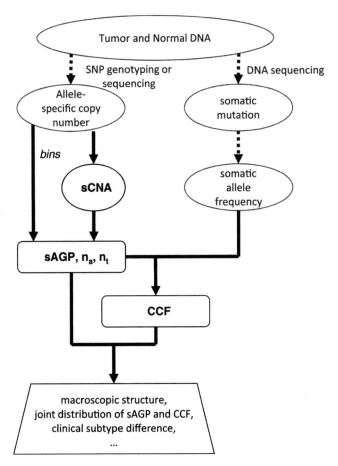

Figure 1. Schematics of CHAT pipeline. Tumor and Normal DNA samples are profiled for allele-specific copy number alterations by SNP arrays and somatic mutations by DNA sequencing. Gray texts and broken arrows (in the upper portion of the figure) indicate input data. CHAT offers two options to partitions the genome: by naturally identified sCNAs or by predefined bins. It then estimates sAGP for each partition (left side). Inference of CCF and timing-phase scenarios relies on sAGP of sCNA, copy number configuration (n_b, n_t), and SAF of the mutation (right side). CCF and sAGP can be used in a wide range of downstream analyses (bottom).

without a second over-riding alteration or the reversal to the original germline state (that is, back mutation). After calculating sAGP for every sCNA in the tumor, CHAT estimates the cellular prevalence of SNVs (also called cancer cell fraction, or CCF, as in[32]) by adjusting the observed somatic allele frequency (SAF) from sequencing data according to the background copy number status, while also considering the sCNA clonality (sAGP), the relative order of occurrence between the SNV and its associated sCNA, and their cisor trans-relationship. Through simulation we show that CHAT performs well in quantitatively recovering sAGP, CCF, and the underlying evolutionary scenario. We also show that it estimates CCF more accurately than EXPANDS and PyClone in most scenarios and CNA states. We have applied CHAT to calculate sAGP for sCNAs, and CCF for SNVs, across 732 human breast tumor samples previously analyzed for inter-tumor diversity by TCGA[14] (Materials and methods, Data access and sCNA identification), and we will present two vignettes of the results. Lastly, we discuss the model identifiability issue and compare the theoretical features of CHAT with that of several similar methods.

2. Results

2.1. Estimation of sAGP for sCNAs

The simplest form of intra-tumor heterogeneity is normal cell "contamination", that is, mixture of aneuploid cells in the tumor with euploid cells in the surrounding normal tissue, the latter carrying the full and balanced set of chromosomes found in germline DNA. In our previous work[18], we developed a method to calculate the overall fraction of the tumor cells, termed Aneuploid Genomic Proportion (AGP), assuming the global mixing of a tumor and a normal population. In brief, allelic intensity data from SNP genotyping arrays (or DNA sequencing) provide copy number information of the two parental chromosomes: n_a and n_b. Since n_a and n_b are both integers, the logarithm of total intensity ratio, LRR $\sim$ $\log(n_a + n_b)$, and the observed B allele frequency, BAF $= n_b/(n_a + n_b)$, adopt a finite number of discrete BAF-LRR combinations for different CNAs, and reside in "canonical positions" in the BAF-LRR plot. When aneuploid cells are mixed with euploid cells, logR-BAF positions of tumor sCNAs "contract" towards the euploid position; and different mixing ratios result in different degrees of contraction. Based on this feature we can quantitatively estimate a genome-wide tumor mixing ratio[18]. Our algorithm relies on the same type of information, and shares the same goal, as several other methods (for example, ASCAT and ABSOLUTE)[17][40]. All of these methods assume that there is a single tumor population and use the combined information from all CNAs.

However, intra-tumor heterogeneity may also manifest as the co-existence of multiple tumor cell populations, each with its own copy number profile[41]. One example is shown in **Figure 2(A)**, where the sCNA segments marked in red show stronger contractions to the diploid track, for both LRR and BAF, than those marked in black; whereas those marked in green show even stronger contractions [**Figure 2(A)** and **Figure 2(B)**]. As mentioned above, since all the sCNAs in black have similar cellular fraction values, we may infer the existence of a subclone, defined as a subpopulation of cells carrying the same set of events (the "black" sCNAs) due to their descent from a common ancestor tumor cell. This is the most parsimonious explanation why different somatic events in the genome could reach the same frequency. Meanwhile, another set of events, such as those in red, show a

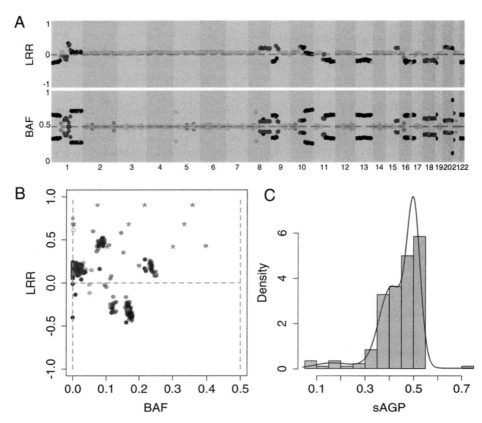

Figure 2. Example of intra-tumor heterogeneity (breast tumor sample TCGA-A1-A0SD). (A) BAF and LRR tracks for binned segments, showing different levels of contraction along the genome. Segments shown in the same color (black, red, green) have similar cellular fractions, and each may represent events in the same clonal population. (B) BAF-LRR plot for the same sample, showing different levels of contraction for segments of different colors. (C) MCMC fitting of sAGP distribution supports three modes, with peaks around sAGP = 0.5, 0.4, and 0.2. The distribution of sAGP is indicated by the light blue histogram, while the fitted three-Gaussian density is shown in dark green.

different cellular fraction values, suggesting the existence of a second sub- clone. Note that a subclone may be nested in a parental clone, and carry the events that are "older" and of higher frequency. These "parental events" may be shared between two sibling clones, each carrying its own unique set of newer events. Thus the sibling clones are disjoint (that is, non-overlapping) population of cells even when they share some events by common descent. Since the sCNA segments with different mixing ratios are interspersed along the genome, this regional variation of clonality motivates us to extend the earlier concept of genome-wide AGP to a new, segment-specific measure: sAGP.

A previous method[41] has attempted to simultaneously estimate the number of subpopulations, the copy number profile for each, and their mixing ratios. This deconvolution problem can be solved, in principle, via a general convex optimization algorithm, but in practice it is limited by computation burden, which increases quickly for more than several dozen events or more than three to four populations. Our method takes an alternative approach: CHAT estimates the mixing ratio for each sCNA (or bin) separately, postponing the question as to which events might belong to the same subclone by virtue of clustering around a similar sAGP, and how many subclones there might be. Thus, CHAT decouples the inference of local sAGPs from the subsequent clustering of sAGP, and is vastly more efficient: its computation time scales linearly with the number of sCNA events and there is nearly no time penalty when needing to consider an increasing number of subpopulations.

The estimation of sAGP follows a similar approach as estimating the global AGP[18], relying on the degree of contraction of each sCNA [**Figure 2(B)**, Materials and methods, sAGP inference]. The method has the implicit assumption that at each sCNA the mixing involves only two populations, one of which is euploid. This assumption is largely satisfied when the somatic genome has experienced relatively sparse copy number changes, without global doubling or multiple rounds of complex local aberration. In effect, it assumes that, even though different sCNAs in the genome may belong to multiple populations of aneuploid cells, at each sCNA region there is only one aneuploid state that is mixed with the euploid state. As such, sAGP is a local quantity inferred for each sCNA, and is naturally assigned zero in regions with no sCNA. The input can be either SNP array data or sequencing data as long as there is a sufficient density of sites with allele-specific copy number data. At this step there is no need to determine if a sCNA is clonal or sub-clonal. Also of note is that in ABSOLUTE[40], subclones CNA events were described by a global purity value and a real-valued copy fraction (not an integer copy number). In contrast, CHAT explicitly models the mixing of a euploid population and an aneuploid population, involving a real-valued local mixing ratio and integer copy numbers.

2.2. Macroscopic Clonal Structure

Before describing the next step in CHAT - using sAGP and the observed SAF values to estimate CCF - we introduce an important downstream inference based on the genome-wide distribution of sAGP values. When there are a sufficient number of sCNAs or bins covered by sCNA, CHAT produces a sufficient number of sAGP values; and their distribution could inform the clonal structure of the tumor. First, for some tumors the sAGP histogram may contain a single peak, potentially accompanied by a flat (nearly uniform) background distribution. This pattern can arise in a tumor containing a single clone that cover a large fraction of the sCNA-bearing portion of the genome, potentially with many other clones that cover much smaller portions of the genome and they are undiscernible in the sAGP spectrum. Second, for other tumors the histogram may follow a multi-modal distribution, representing a number of distinct clusters of somatic events, each with a different sAGP, with each cluster covering a comparable portion of the genome as to be recognizable in the histogram [an example is shown in **Figure 2(C)**].

In all, there are three attributes of each sAGP histogram. The number of the identifiable modes corresponds to the number of identifiable cell populations. (2) The position of each mode denotes the cellular frequency of the sCNAs in each cluster, and reflects the clonality of the cell populations carrying these sCNAs. The right-most peak represents the sCNAs with the highest sAGP values; and they suggest the existence of a population of cells with the highest cellular fraction in the tumor. This population is typically called the dominant clone. The peaks to the left represent sCNAs with lower sAGP values and they are carried by populations of cells with lower cellular fractions. These populations are often called subclone 1, sub-clone 2, and so on, but they may be nested within the dominant clone, and also carry the sCNAs in the right-most peak. (3) The areas under the peaks reflect the number of the sCNAs, or the regularly spaced bins, that belong to each peak. Note that the right-most peak may not have the largest area, thus the dominant clone may not carry sCNAs that cover the widest portion of the genome.

There are at least two ways to define the spatial unit in the sAGP analysis, and CHAT provides both options (Materials and methods, Data access and sCNA identification). The first is to calculate sAGP for regularly spaced bins, either for a fixed window width or for a fixed number of SNPs. The resulting sAGP values resemble the conventional genetic "markers"; and each tumor has a guaranteed number and density of such markers to construct the sAGP histogram, which is interpreted analogously to the allele frequency spectrum in population genetics studies. However, the bins do not match the naturally occurring sCNAs, which are highly variable in lengths, from tens of kb to entire chromosome arms. The sCNAs shorter than the bin width would have their true sAGP values "diluted" by flanking euploid segments in the same bin; whereas those longer than the bin width would generated a string of correlated sAGP values as the same sCNA is artificially divided into multiple adjacent bins, thus violating the assumption that sAGPs are independent. In the second option, CHAT will apply the identified sCNA as the naturally occurring spatial unit for sAGP calculation. While this has the advantage that all sAGPs are truly independent, there are two disadvantages. First, the longer (or shorter) sCNAs provide more (or less) precise estimates of sAGP, but this information of confidence was discarded, as it is also the case in[41]. Two, there will be large tumor-tumor variations in the number of sCNAs, and some tumors may not have enough sCNAs to construct an informative histogram for estimating clonal composition. In short, the per-bin sAGPs (option 1) are derived from segments of similar length and have similar confidence intervals they are identically distributed but not independent random variables. Conversely, the per-sCNA sAGPs (option 2) are independent, but are not identically distributed due to varying lengths. Rigorously speaking, neither is suited for analyzing macroscopic clonal architecture but can be applied in exploratory analysis, especially when there is no other data type such as the SNVs (see below).

When the primary goal of using CHAT is to accurately estimate CCF, which relies on accurate sAGP values, the user is advised to calculate sAGP using sCNAs as the spatial unit rather than the bins. Alternatively, when the primary goal is to explore clonal composition of a tumor, and if there are too few sCNAs and if most of them are very large, it is beneficial to increase the number of informative features, just as the detection of population stratification requires many ancestry informative markers. Here the user may choose regularly spaced bins to increase the number of available sAGPs. In fact, when sCNAs are few and large, it is more advisable to collect sequencing data; and if the mutation rate is high and/or the entire genome is sequenced (as opposed to small targeted regions), the number of SNVs may exceed that of sCNAs, and it is better to rely on the CCF histogram to estimate clonal structure. CCF distributions have the important advantage of meeting the condition of independent and identically distributed variable. Ultimately, the best approach is to integrate the sAGP and CCF distributions in estimating clonal structure.

CHAT fits the uni-modal pattern with a maximal likelihood framework, and the multi-modal pattern using a Bayesian Monte-Carlo Markov Chain (MCMC) approach, with Dirichlet Process prior to estimate a hierarchical Gaussian mixture model[42]. The approach is similar to those introduced in[32][38][39][43]. Details are provided in Materials and methods, Statistical modeling to infer macroscopic clonal structure. Model selection is based on the Bayesian Information Criterion (BIC)[44]. In Discussion we will further interpret the uni-modal and multi-modal patterns in terms of the likely evolutionary dynamics and the relationship to classic concepts such as punctuated equilibrium[45] and episodic evolution.

2.3. Estimating Cell Fractions of Somatic Mutations

2.3.1. Nature of the Problem

The next step of CHAT turns from estimating sAGP of sCNAs to estimating the frequency of cells carrying a specific mutation, that is, single nucleotide variant (SNV) or small insertion/deletion (indel). Here the method addresses the case where the tumor DNA has been sequenced, either for the whole genome or for a targeted subset, such as the exome. The input of the analysis is the observed number of reads in the sequence data containing the mutation as well as those containing the un-mutated allele. The relative fraction of mutation-bearing reads is termed somatic allele frequency (SAF). Following[32], we adopt CCF to denote the percentage of cells in the tumor sample carrying a specific somatic mutation. CCF is also termed cellular prevalence in[43]. The task is to use the observed SAF to estimate the unknown CCF.

If the mutation resides in a normal diploid region, it typically occurs on the background of one of the two parental chromosomes, contributing to about half the sequence reads in this region. In this simple case, as the fraction of cells carrying the mutation is CCF, the expected fraction of sequence reads carrying the mutation, SAF, is simply a binomial variable with an expected value of CCF/2. We therefore can estimate CCF by SAF $\times$ 2. However, if the mutation resides in a sCNA, the relationship between CCF and SAF depends on the copy number configuration (for example, copy neutral loss of heterozygosity (CN-LOH), deletion, amplification, and so on) and its sAGP. Further, it also depends on the chromosomal background in which the mutation occurs. For example, in a region of heterozygous amplification where one of the chromosomes has been duplicated, if the mutation occurs on the duplicated chromosome, it will contribute twice the number of sequence reads than the case where it occurs on the un-duplicated chromosome. Lastly, if the mutation occurs after the duplication has happened and the duplication-bearing clone is undergoing expansion, only a subset of the duplication-bearing cells will carry the mutation, and the relative size of this subpopulation can be any value in 0% to 100% and will also affect the relationship between CCF and SAF. In the following we systematically consider these possible scenarios. We will make the parsimonious assumption that each mutation only occurred once in the evolutionary history of the tumor cell population, therefore we will ignore the possibility of recurrent mutation at the same position, or simultaneous emergence of the same mutation is different subpopulations of cells. We will treat SNVs and indels equally, and use the term "mutation" to denote both.

2.3.2. Order-Phase Scenarios between sCNA and SNV

For a somatic mutation revealed by tumor DNA sequencing, with an observed SAF value, we consider the task of estimating CCF if this mutation resides in an sCNA, and the sCNA has been discovered by either SNP array genotyping data[17][40] or by sequencing data[32][38]. We assume that the sCNA has been well characterized, such that we already know n_a and n_b, the copy number of its major and minor alleles, respectively, that is, $n_a \geq n_b$ and $n_t = n_a + n_b$ is the total copy number. We also assume that its sAGP has been calculated using the method described above, and that SAF has been corrected for known sequencing errors and local biases[21][46]. Below we present the CCF estimation procedure for the case of heterozygous amplification ($n_a = 2$, $n_b = 1$). The two other common sCNA types, heterozygous deletion ($n_a = 1$, $n_b = 0$) and CN-LOH ($n_a = 2$, $n_b = 0$), are described in Materials and methods, CCF estimation and scenario identifiability for CN-LOH and deletion.

When a mutation resides in a sCNA region, there are three main scenarios that describe the possible mutation-sCNA combinations in terms of their relative temporal order and the chromosomal background of the mutation (**Figure 3**):

A. The mutation and sCNA emerged sequentially, with the mutation occurring first, and the sCNA occurring in a subset of mutation-bearing cells [**Figure 3(A)**].

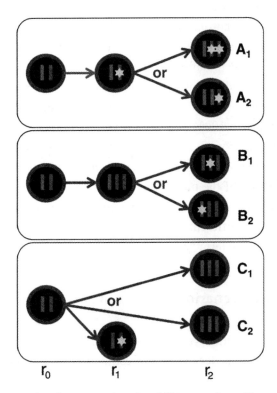

Figure 3. Lineage scenarios for a mutation that fall in a region of heterozygous amplification. In scenario A_1, the mutation (yellow star) occurred before the amplification, which doubled the mutation-bearing chromosome (shown in green). The three illustrated populations have fractions of r_0, r_1 and r_2, which sum up to 1. A_2 is similar to A_1, except that the un-mutated chromosome (in orange) was doubled. For scenario B, the amplification happened first, and the mutation occurred either on the amplified (B_1) or the unamplified (B_2) allele. For scenario C, the mutation and the sCNA occurred on independent lineages, and the amplification affects either the same (C_1) or the opposite chromosome (C_2) as the mutation. Blue arrow: mutation occurrence; red arrow: sCNA occurrence.

This led to the co-existence of three subpopulations: the original euploid mutation-free cells, with the population fraction of r_0; cells carrying the mutation only, with a fraction of r_1; and cellscarrying both the mutation and the sCNA (r_2). The last subpopulation has two alternative outcomes: A_1: the duplication occurred on the mutation-bearing chromosome, and A_2: the duplication occurred on the mutation-free chromosome. Intuitively, A_1 will have higher SAF than A_2 with the same (r_0, r_1, r_2) fractions.

B. Like A, the mutation and sCNA emerged sequentially; but unlike A, the sCNA occurred first, with the mutation occurring in a subset of sCNA-bearing cells [**Figure 3(B)**]. Again we have three subpopulations: the original cells (r_0), cells carrying only the sCNA (r_1) and those carrying both (r_2). The last subpopulation has two alternatives: mutation occurring on one of the duplicated chromosome (B_1) or the un-duplicated chromosome (B_2).

C. The mutation and sCNA emerged independently, that is, appearing in non-overlapping populations of cells [**Figure 3(C)**]. This also led to three subpopulations: the original cells (r_0), cells carrying only the mutation (r_1) and those carrying only the sCNA (r_2). Note that we do not consider the fourth population that carries both the mutation and the sCNA. This outcome would require that the mutation occurred twice, once in the original cells and again in the sCNA-bearing cells. Or it requires the sCNA to occur twice. Under the Maximal Parsimonious assumption, recurrent appearance of the same mutation or the same sCNA is highly unlikely in the same tumor.

The three scenarios outlined above covered all the possible mutation-sCNA combinations for one-copy amplification without recurrence. In Additional file 1: Figure S1 and Materials and methods, CCF estimation and scenario identifiability for CN-LOH and deletion, we show that heterozygous deletion and CN-LOH involve similar scenarios A, B and C, and each leads to a similar set of three subpopulations as described by r_0, r_1, and r_2, with $r_0 + r_1 + r_2 = 1$.

2.3.3. CCF as a Function of sAGP, SAF and the Underlying Scenario

When the (n_a, n_b) configuration and evolutionary scenario is known, CCF can be estimated from: (1) the preestimated sAGP of the sCNA (denoted p hereafter for simplicity) on which the mutation occurs; and (2) the observed allele frequency, SAF, of the somatic mutation (denoted f hereafter). In the following we derive the CCF estimation procedure for heterozygous duplication ($n_a = 2$, $n_b = 1$), and leave CN-LOH ($n_a = 2$, $n_b = 0$), and deletion ($n_a = 1$, $n_b = 0$) to Materials and methods, CCF estimation and scenario identifiability for CN-LOH and deletion.

For amplification, in scenario A_1, $n_t = 3$, the average total copy number $n_t = 2 \times (1 - p) + n_t \times p = 2 + p$. The sAGP $p = r_2$. The SAF $f = (r_1 + 2r_2)/(2 + p)$. This led to the expression $r_1 = f \times (2 + p) - 2r_2$. Since CCF $= r_1 + r_2$, we have

$$CCF^{A_1}\left(f, n_b, n_t, p\right) = f \times (2 + p) - r_2 = f \times (2 + p) - p \tag{1}$$

In A_2, the situation is similar to A_1 except that $f = (r_1 + r_2)/(2 + p)$. This led to $r_1 = f \times (2 + p) - r_2$, and

$$CCF^{A_1}\left(f, n_b, n_t, p\right) = f \times (2 + p) \tag{2}$$

In B_1 and B_2, the sAGP: $p = r_1 + r_2$. The SAF: $f = r_2/(2 + p)$. This led to $r_2 = f \times (2 + p)$. Since CCF $= r_2$, we have

$$CCF^{B}\left(f, n_b, n_t, p\right) = f \times (2 + p) \tag{3}$$

In C_1 and C_2, the sAGP: $p = r_2$. The SAF: $f = r_1/(2 + p)$. This led to $r_1 = f \times (2 + p)$. Since CCF $= r_1$, we have

$$CCF^{C}\left(f, n_b, n_t, p\right) = f \times (2 + p) \tag{4}$$

Note that Equations (2), (3), and (4) are identical. Thus even if we do not know how to distinguish among scenarios A_2, B, and C, CCF still has the same dependency on sAGP and SAF, and can be estimated as long as we can recognize A_1 and $A_2/B/C$. Thus CCF identifiability is easier to achieve than scenario identifiability.

Similar expressions for CN-LOH and deletion are presented in Materials and methods, CCF estimation and scenario identifiability for CN-LOH and deletion. In the general copy number configuration of n_a and n_b, for scenarios A_1, A_2, B, and C we have

$$CCF^{A_1}\left(f,n_b,n_t,p\right)=n_t \times f - p \times n_a + p \tag{5}$$

$$CCF^{A_2}\left(f,n_b,n_t,p\right)=n_t \times f - p \times n_b + p \tag{5}$$

$$CCF^{B/C}\left(f,n_b,n_t,p\right)=n_t \times f \tag{5}$$

with $n_t = 2 \times (1 - p) + n_t \times p$, is the averaged copy number at the locus.

Thus, for a given pair of mutation and sCNA, with known SAF and sAGP values, once we know which scenario applies we can use Equations (1), (2), (3), (4), (5), (6), and (7) to estimate CCF. The variance of CCF estimates can be calculated as in Materials and methods, Variance of CCF. In the following we turn to the question of how to determine which scenario applies.

2.3.4. Joint Distribution of (*p*, *f*) and Scenario Identifiability

By definition, f and p are both bounded by (0, 1). In any tumor, however, the possible range of f is constrained by p as well as by the sCNA type and the individual scenarios. For example, in scenario B of amplification, the mutation occurs in a subset of sCNA-bearing cells, thus f is always less than p (in this case it is always less than 0.5 p). As we show below, the attainable joint distributions of (*p*, *f*) differs among different scenarios and, importantly, this offers the possibility to infer the most likely scenario for a given sCNA-mutation pair based on their observed (*p*, *f*) values. Further, some "zones" of the (*p*, *f*) space overlap with multiple scenarios, thus if the observed (*p*, *f*) fall into these zones, it is impossible to unambiguously identify the exact evolutionary scenarios. Even then, however, because different scenarios sometimes have the same expression of CCF as a function of (*p*, *f*), CCF may still be uniquely estimated. In the following we derive the scenario-dependent (*p*, *f*) joint distributions using heterozygous amplification as example.

In A_1, for a given p, the observed f of the mutation depends on the relative abundance of the r_0 and r_1 populations (**Figure 3**). When $r_0 = 0$, the mutation occurred so early that all the diploid cells carry the mutation and belong to the r_1 subpopulation. $r_1 = 1 - p$, and f reaches its upper limit:

$$f_h^{A_1} = \frac{1 - p + 2 \times p}{n_t} = \frac{1 + p}{2 + p} \tag{8}$$

where $n_t = 2 \times (1 - p) + 3 \times p$, is the averaged total copy number for the sCNA. On the opposite end of the situation is $r_1 = 0$, when the sCNA occurred immediately after the mutation such that none of the diploid cells carries the mutation. The lower limit of SAF is reached:

$$f_h^{A_1} = \frac{2p}{2 + p} \tag{9}$$

If we plot the possible (p, f) combinations in an $p - f$ plot with f on the vertical axis, under scenario A_1, the observed f is bounded by $[2p/(2 + p), (1 + p)/(2 + p)]$, where $p \in (0,1)$, forming the zone marked A_1 in **Figure 4(A)**.

For A_2, we similarly obtain:

$$f_h^{A_2} = \frac{1 - p + p}{n_t} = \frac{1}{2 + p} \tag{10}$$

$$f_h^{A_2} = \frac{p}{2 + p} \tag{11}$$

The observed f for A_2 is bounded by $[p/(2 + p), 1/(2 + p)]$.

For B, f depends on the relative abundance of the r_1 and r_2 populations, and the expressions are

$$f_h^{B} = \frac{p}{n_t} = \frac{p}{2 + p} \tag{12}$$

70

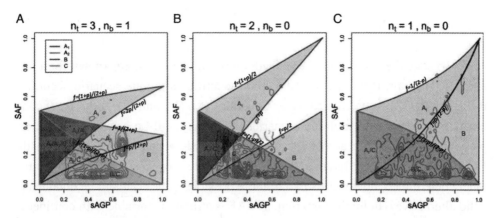

Figure 4. Identifiability zones in sAGP-CCF space, for amplification (A), CN-LOH (B) and deletion (C), with up to four scenarios described in the main text. Theoretically permissible areas of sAGP-CCF for different scenarios are marked by borders of different colors, and labeled with a single letter (such as "A_1") for uniquely occupied zones, and by two or more letters ("A_1/C") for overlapping zones. Regions of light gray support a unique CCF expression, whereas the regions of dark gray cannot unambiguously estimate CCF. The density contours (in orange) depict the distribution of 3,382 mutations in amplification regions (A), 2,008 in CN-LOH, and 4,662 in deletions representing 201 breast tumor samples with least data loss in sAGP estimation. Variants with coverage lower than 20 or SAF smaller than 0.05 were discarded. Only a very small portion of the mutations fall outside the theoretically predicted zones. Among the rest, approximately 48% belong to a unique scenario, but approximately 93% have a unique CCF estimation.

$$f_l^B = 0 \tag{13}$$

Thus f is bounded by $[0, p/(2 + p)]$.

For C, the upper limit of f is reached when $r_0 = 0$, $r_1 = 1 - p$, and

$$f_h^C = \frac{1-p}{n_t} = \frac{1-p}{2+p} \tag{14}$$

$$f_t^C = 0 \tag{15}$$

The f is bounded by $[0, (1 - p)/(2 + p)]$.

The results for CN-LOH and deletion are described in Materials and methods, CCF estimation and scenario identifiability for CN-LOH and deletion, and shown in **Figure 4(B)** and **Figure 4(C)**.

To state the full estimation procedure: when (f, n, n, p) are known for a mutation-sCNA pair, if the (p, f) combination identifies a unique scenario according to **Figure 4**, CCF is calculated using Equations (5), (6), and (7). If the (p, f) combination overlaps with multiple scenarios, CCF may still be calculated if the expressions are the same across the undistinguishable scenarios. Lastly, when the CCF expressions are different among the applicable scenarios, CCF cannot be uniquely determined, however its two or more possible values can still be obtained as valid alternatives. In implementation, as SAF is a random variable with confidence level depending on read depth, there is always uncertainty as to which scenario the observed (p, f) belongs. We formally calculate the probability of each scenario as described in Materials and methods, Probabilistic scenario identification.

2.3.5. Validation, Implementation, and Performance

To assess the performance of CHAT we simulated sCNA and SNV data for a range of copy number configurations, sAGP values, evolutionary scenarios, and CCF values. Details of the simulation procedures were described in Materials and methods, In silico validation and computation performance. For sCNAs, we evaluated the performance by reporting: (1) percent of cases of mistaken estimation of sCNA configuration (error in either n_b or n_t) [**Figure 5(A)**, top row] for dominant and minor clonal events; and (2) the median absolute deviation of the estimated sAGPs from the known sAGP values for the dominant and minor clones, for either the segments with correct (n_t, n_b) identification [**Figure 5(A)**, middle row], or all segments [**Figure 5(A)**, bottom row]. With all of these performance metrics, the errors are the largest when the clonal or subclonal sAGPs are small. The overall errors are small in most situations, suggesting that CHAT worked well in recovering the sAGP, n_b, and n_t values. For SNVs, we compared the estimated and the true CCF values in **Figure 5(A)**. Across all cases with different coverage and sCNA subclonal parameter settings, the Spearman's rank correlation coefficient between the known and the estimated CCF values was in the range of 0.946 to 0.97, indicating that CHAT makes accuracy CCF inference. To compare performance among SNVs in different sub-categories, we separated those falling in euploid regions from those in sCNAs, and for the latter, separated those in the major and minor subclone events, and those in different copy number status. As shown in **Figure 5(C)**, the

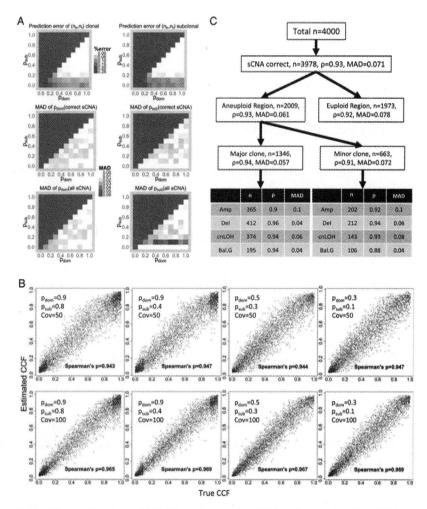

Figure 5. In silico validation of CHAT performance. (A) Performance of sAGP inferences. Upper row: percent of error in estimated n_b or n_t, for the dominant (left) and subclonal sCNAs (right), as described in Materials and methods, Performance of sAGP inference. Middle row: the median absolute difference (MAD) between estimated and simulated sAGP values for sCNAs with correctly identified (n_b, n_t), or for all sCNAs (Bottom row). The $p_{sub} = 0$ row of the lower-right and middle-right panels had zero error because when $p_{sub} = 0$ there is only one clone in the tumor population and all subclonal sCNA segments have correctly estimated sAGP = 0. (B) Performance of CCF inference. Shown are scatter plot of simulated and estimated CCF for four p_{dom} - p_{sub} cases and two coverage values: Cov = 50 (upper panels) and 100 (lower panels). (C) Comparison of CCF inference accuracy among different SNV categories: euploid vs. aneuploidy regions; and in the latter, between the dominant and the minor clones. Lastly, SNVs were divided by sCNA types. The tested case has the following parameter settings: $p_{dom} = 0.9$, $p_{sub} = 0.6$, coverage = 50, number of SNV sampled = 4,000, number of sCNA sampled = 200. ρ, Spearman's correlation coefficient between the true and the estimated CCF values. MAD: median absolution difference between the true and the estimated CCF values.

error rates are similar across these sub-categories, not affected by dominant/minor clonal events or different sCNA types.

CHAT is written in $R^{[47]}$ and available as a CRAN package. It can use SNP array-based copy number data and sequencing-derived mutation data, or can use sequencing data as a single input source. It is computationally efficient, taking approximately 1 CPU-hour to analyze every five tumor-normal samples profiled with 850 K SNPs genotying and exome sequencing at 30× (Materials and methods, Computational requirements).

2.3.6. Comparison with Previous Methods

We compared CHAT with two other methods, EXPANDS and PyClone, that also estimate cellular frequencies for somatic mutations. We simulated 488 mutations that reside in sCNA regions and correspond to different linear scenarios and copy number states (details described in Materials and methods, Comparison with EXPANDS and PyClone). **Figure 6(A)**, **Figure 6(B)**, and **Figure 6(C)** plots the CCF estimated by the three methods against the true CCF used to simulate the observed read counts. CHAT-based estimates have the highest correlation with the true CCF (Pearson's $r = 0.96$), followed by PyClone ($r = 0.94$) and EXPANDS ($r = 0.70$). As the four lineage scenarios were distinguished by different symbol colors, it can be seen that PyClone underestimates CCF in scenarios A_1 and A_2 [**Figure 6(B)**], likely due to the assumption that mutation and sCNA always co-occur. PyClone performs similarly to CHAT in scenarios B and C. Like PyClone, EXPANDS also fails to consider the sCNA-free cells carrying the mutation, thus underestimates CCF in scenarios A_1 and A_2. EXPANDS overestimates CCF in B and C [**Figure 6(C)**] because it ignores B and C by applying A_1 or A_2 instead. To assess the impact of CNA status we further stratified the simulated mutations by individual combinations of lineage scenarios and CNA states, including deletion (genotype A/B), copy-neutral LOH (AA/BB) and amplification (AAB/ABB) [**Figure 6(D)**]. PyClone actually has a slight underestimation in scenario B for CN-LOH and amplifications. The overestimation by EXPANDS in scenario C only occurs for deletions and amplifications. Overall, CHAT has the least bias and least variance in most combinations. Moreover, CHAT is the most efficient. It took CHAT approximately 1 s to analyze the 488 somatic mutations. EXPANDS needed 732s, and PyClone took 4,320s.

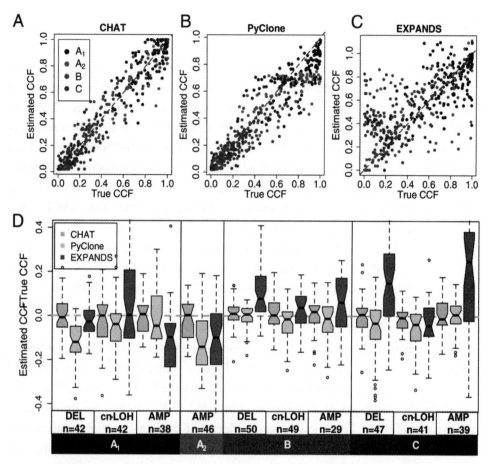

Figure 6. Performance comparisons of CHAT, EXPANDS, and PyClone. (A, B, C) Scatter plot of the CCF values estimated by the three methods against the known CCF values used in the simulation. The four lineage scenarios were distinguished by different symbol colors. (D) Boxplot showing the estimation errors for each of the three methods, stratified by both sCNA types and lineage scenarios, with the actual number of mutations simulated for each CNA type-scenario combination marked at the bottom of each panel. The sCNA types include heterozygous deletions (A/B), cn-LOH (AA/BB), and amplification (AAB/ABB). Mutations in balanced amplifications (n = 55) were not shown in order to reduce clutter.

2.4. Application to Human Breast Cancer

We applied CHAT to estimate sAGP for sCNAs identified using Affymetrix 6.0 single nucleotide polymorphism (SNP) array data for tumor and germline DNA samples from 732 breast cancer patients[14]. Of these, 445 also have whole-exome sequencing data available, and we estimated CCF for SNVs.

2.4.1. sAGP Distribution

We detected sCNAs using circular binary segmentation[48] of LRR and BAF data[18], resulting in the identification of an average of 261 sCNAs per tumor (range: 1 to 3,537). The median size of all sCNAs is 1.7Mb (range: 2.5Kb to 245Mb). On average, each tumor carries 125 sCNAs larger than 5Mb, a size corresponding to approximately 1,500 SNP markers in the 850K SNP array. Given this sCNA size range, we re-calculated sAGP for genomic bins containing 500 heterozygous SNPs in the germline DNA, a bin size that is approximately 5Mb, resulting in 502 bins per sample (range:404 to 794) and constructed the sAGP histogram for every tumor. Eighty-seven tumors (12%) had sCNAs for <50 bins, too few for analyzing the sAGP distribution patterns. For the remaining 645 tumors we fit the sCNAs distribution to either a unimodal + uniform distribution or a multi-modal distribution using methods described in Materials and methods, Statistical modeling to infer macroscopic clonal structure. In the example in **Figure 2(C)**, a three-mode distribution provides the best fit, with sAGP peaks around 0.5, 0.4, and 0.2. The highest peak corresponds to the black-colored sCNAs in **Figure 2(A)** and **Figure 2(B)**, while the second and third peaks correspond to the red- and green-colored sCNAs, respectively. In total we observed 392 samples (61%) with best fit by the multi-modal distribution, while 253 (39%) follow the uni-model + uniform distribution. This shows that a majority of the breast tumors analyzed by TCGA contain more than one recognizable aneuploid population, suggesting that the co-existence of more than one sub- clone is very common.

2.4.2. sAGP-CCF Joint Distribution for Known Cancer Genes

The 445 tumors with both SNP array and sequencing data have an average of 311 somatic mutations per tumor with CCF values (range: from 15 to 4,235, after counting the 8.8% loss due to sCNAs with un-estimable sAGP). While 48% of these mutations fall into a zone with overlapping scenarios, 93% of them have a unique mathematical expression and can produce a valid CCF estimate (Additional file 1: Figure S2). The remaining 7% are assigned missing CCF values due to scenarios with conflicting CCF estimates.

The calculation of sAGP for most sCNAs and CCF for most SNVs makes it possible to examine the joint distribution of clonality for these two types of genome aberrations. A "CCF vs. sAGP" plot can be created for all copy number and mutation events in a single tumor, or for events affecting a single gene of interest across many tumors. For a given gene, if a sample does not have any somatic mutation in the gene, we assign CCF = 0. Likewise if the copy number of the gene is normal, we assign sAGP = 0. **Figure 7(A)** shows a heatmap depicting the density of CCF and sAGP joint distribution for all events in a hypothetical sample (or for a hypothetical gene across all samples). In this two-dimension space, the "hot" peak near the origin (0, 0) is typical for most genes, affected by neither somatic mutation nor sCNA. The peak in the upper left (near the sAGP-axis) contains genes with highly clonal CNAs but carrying either no mutation or mutations of low clonality. A plausible interpretation is that for some of these genes, sCNA is a possible driver event. Similarly, the peak at the lower left (near the CCF-axis) contains genes with highly clonal somatic mutations and low-clonality sCNAs. Lastly, genes in the upper-right peak have both high sAGP and high CCF values, suggesting that both copy number changes and somatic mutations may have occurred at very early stages of tumor development, and their joint appearance may be necessary to act as a driver event.

Figure 7(B) allows close inspection of relative clonality between sCNA and mutations for four genes known to be related to breast cancer[14]: TP53, PIK3CA, and GATA3, which occurred in >10% of analyzed breast tumors, and MAP3K1, which had mutations enriched in the luminal A subtype. For TP53, there are two noticeable high-density "zones" in the heatmap: one along the sAGP-axis, the other at the upper right, indicating two groups of tumor samples: TP53 CNA-only and TP53 CNA/mutation, respectively. This pattern, when stratified by the four PAM50 subtypes[14][49] [**Figure 7(C)**], shows that the TP53 CNA/mutation group is enriched in the Basal and HER2 subtypes (accounting for 72 of 94 Basal and HER2 tumors), whereas the TP53 CNA-only group is enriched in the Luminal-A (94 of 105), and to a lesser degree, the Luminal-B subtypes (44 of 67). In comparison, the other three genes have not only the CNA-only and CNA/mutation groups, but also a third, mutation-only group near the CCF-axis. **Figure 7(D)** shows that for PIK3CA, the mutation-only group occurs almost exclusively in the Luminal-A and -B subtypes.

The CCF-sAGP plot can also be used to compare the clonality distribution between a pair of genes. In **Figure 8**, TP53 and PIK3CA are shown in red and blue symbols, respectively, with the lines linking the two genes for the same samples.

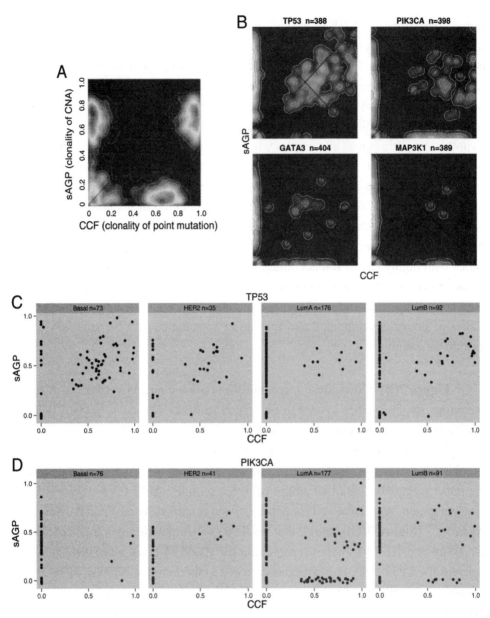

Figure 7. Comparison of clonality for SNVs and sCNAs of single genes in sAGP-CCF joint distribution heatmaps (A, B) or scatter plots (C, D). (A) sAGP-CCF 2D heatmap for a hypothetical sample, showing characteristic density peaks as explained in the main text. (B) Actual heatmaps for four breast cancer-related genes: TP53, PIK3CA, GATA3, and MAP3K1. Sample counts vary by gene, according to how many were removed due to missing values for either sAGP or CCF. (C, D) Scatter plot of sAGP-CCF for TP53 and PIK3CA, divided by PAM50 gene expression subtypes. We excluded seven Normal-like samples due to low count.

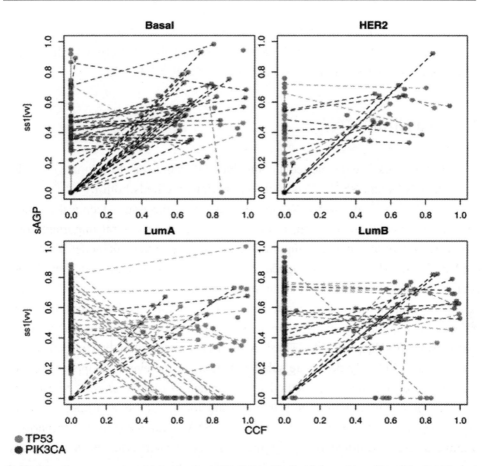

Figure 8. Two-gene comparison of sAGP-CCF distribution, with values for TP53 and PIK3CA in the same samples linked by lines, stratified by PAM50 gene expression subtypes. Groups with interacting co-occurrence patterns are shown by different line colors. Black: high CCF and sAGP in TP53, low in PIK3CA. Red and green: high sAGP for both genes, high CCR for TP53 (red) or high CCF for PIK3CA (green). Blue: high sAGP for TP53 and high CCF for PIK3CA.

There are three notable patterns of TP53-PIK3CA clonality. First, samples marked by the black lines have both sCNA and mutation in TP53 but no aberration in PIK3CA. Second, samples marked by the red and green lines tend to have sCNA for both TP53 and PIK3CA and at comparable sAGP, but only mutation in TP53 (red lines) or PIK3CA (green). Third, samples marked by the blue lines had high clonality for TP53 CNA, but not its mutation, and high clonality for PIK3CA mutation, but not its CNA, suggesting co-occurrence of aberrations of these two genes but involving different variant types. These patterns are subtype-specific: Pattern 1 is enriched in the Basal subtype (OR = 4.6 compared to the other three subtypes, P = 0.0001 by Fisher's exact test, for red; OR = 1.2, P = 0.67, for green), so is Pattern 2 (OR = 5.3, P = 6.4e−8,). Most remarkably, Pattern 3 is almost exclusively found in the Luminal A subtype (OR = 56, P = 4.4e−9).

3. Discussion

In this work, we developed a computational framework to estimate clonality for both sCNAs and SNVs. It is built on previous methods both by us[18] and by others[32][38][41][43][50]. While CHAT does not solve all the issues facing the cancer genome deconvolution problem, it attempts to overcome several important compromises or simplifying assumptions that underlie other methods. First, oncoSNP[51] and THetA[41] are designed to estimate sCNA clonality, but they do not address the clonality of somatic mutations. Second, Ding et al.[52] used a kernel density estimation method to characterize somatic mutations, but only focused on those in the euploid regions of genome, staying clear of the complicated relationship between SNV and sCNAs. Third, ABSOLUTE infers clonality for both sCNA and mutations but only designate subclonal status of the events, stopping short of quantitative estimation. This method was extended in Landau et al.[32] to estimate CCF for somatic mutations even if they are subclonal, but the algorithm only considers the case where sCNA occurred before SNV, equivalent to our scenario B (**Figure 3** and Additional file 1: Figure S1), and further assumes that the copy number was altered by only one in the sCNA. In this regard, CHAT considers a wider array of possible scenarios. Fourth, EXPANDS[50] works with next-generation sequencing data and jointly estimates the absolute DNA copy number, clonality of somatic mutations, and that of sCNAs. However, this method only considers scenario A, and without the r_1 population. In effect, it assumes that the mutation and sCNA occur at the same instance and are in phase. These assumptions explained its underestimation of CCF in scenario A and overestimation in B and C (**Figure 6**). Fifth, PyClone[43] infers clonality of somatic mutations and performs phylogenetic analysis. It receives as input the integer copy number profiles estimated from other methods, but only considers scenarios A and B, disregarding the possibility of a branching lineage (scenario C). Furthermore, for scenario A, it assumes co-occurrence of SNV and sCNA, thus ignoring the r_1 population. In sum, the first key contribution of CHAT is in providing a general mathematical framework that enumerates the complete set of scenarios covering the possible order and phase of the sCNA and the mutation.

Like many of the previous methods, CHAT has its own limitations, primarily in being unable to resolve extremely complex events such as three-way mixing or above. It models two-population mixing at each genomic region (a gene, a sCNA, or a bin) and works best when the tumor has not experienced extensive and repeated copy number alterations. In the TCGA breast tumor dataset we found that 9.3% of sCNAs do not follow the regional two-way mixing model and preclude sAGP estimation. For the other, permissible sCNAs, CHAT can proceed, and is able to infer the co-existence of two or more subpopulations by analyzing the distribution of sAGP or CCF values. We wish to re-emphasize that while CHAT invokes two-way mixing for each individual genomic region, it is not limited to infer the presence of only two populations of cells. Globally, the number of peaks in the sAGP or CCF distribution has no restriction, and can be very high when the signal-to-noise ratio is improved, such as with ultra-deep sequencing data, for example,[39].

A second contribution of CHAT is in systematically assessing the input data combinations that leads to "unidentifiable zones", in which the CCF, or "scenarios" (that is, the evolutionary order and phase of the sCNA and SNV), cannot be resolved even with perfect data. Importantly, we found that in many situations, even if the evolution scenario is undetermined, CCF can still be estimated. The ability to objectively evaluate the power of inference in any given dataset is an important part of method development. Our treatment of this topic therefore sets useful constraints for future development of similar analysis tools. We found that, with the TCGA breast tumor data, about 9.3% of the identified sCNAs cannot be explained by local two-way mixing and were assigned missing sAGP values. In the second step, about 7% of the SNVs have unidentifiable CCF because they fall in either an inadmissible sAGP-SAF zone or a region with conflicting CCF estimates. Thus 93% of SNVs are suitable for CCF estimation, despite the fact that 48% of them involve ambiguous scenarios.

When applying CHAT to the breast tumor dataset, we found that approximately 61% of the breast tumors in the TCGA cohort contain more than one recognizable sAGP peaks, suggesting that even in a tumor cohort collected for studying inter-tumor diversity there is opportunity to detect intra-tumor mixing of multiple populations of aneuploid cells. And the results show that extensive intra-tumor heterogeneity does exist. This observation expands the earlier view that tumor-normal mixing contributes to intra-tumor heterogeneity, and confirms the results from single-cell and multi-region analyses in other solid tumors, for example[25][33]. We wish to point out that the estimate of 61% was based on a specific analysis approach, and would vary with alternative parameter choices. For example, by using regularly spaced bins we found that 392 of 645 samples (61%) were multi-modal, yet by using the naturally occurring sCNAs, only 635 samples had sufficient number of events, and 373 of them, or 59%, were multimodal. More notably, of the 392 multi-modal samples called with bins, and the 373 multi-modal samples called with sCNAs, the overlap is 235, or about 60% for either method. This level of concordance is related to the inherent shortage of observations for many samples: when the number of sCNAs or bins is in the 50 to 100 range, and if the primary peak is far larger than the secondary peak, the inference is less stable. These data-derived limitations can be overcome in the future when more samples are analyzed with whole-genome sequencing, which will likely yield a far greater number of genealogically informative markers.

A useful downstream analysis of the inferred clonality measures is to assess the distribution patterns of cellular frequencies of somatic aberrations, and to detect frequency clusters when they do exist for a given tumor. CHAT provides the option of characterizing the macroscopic clonal structure by a cluster-based approach (**Figure 1**). It is important to emphasize that these frequency clusters, despite their many valid interpretations, cannot be equated to individual sub- clones. A subclone may carry somatic events in multiple clusters, and may share some events with another subclone if they are descendants of the same parental clone. The full deconvolution of the observed aggregate pattern into those contributed by individual subclones requires further mathematical modeling and involves additional challenges. Several methods have recently appeared to address this "Blind Source Separation Problem", or synonymously, "Feature Allocation Problem"[53]-[56]. CHAT can be applied in tandem with these methods, that is, the sAGP and CCF output from CHAT can serve as the input data for further feature allocation to component subclones.

The co-existence of multiple clonal populations in bulk tissues could be explained by several population genomics models that are not mutually exclusive. First, in a multi-region parallel-evolution model, the tumor tissue might contain geographically segregated "pure" populations, reflecting branched evolution of multiple clones of homogeneous tumor cells, each developing a different genomic profile that reflects its cell type of origin and adaptation to the local tissue habitat.

This model can only be tested by spatially restricted sampling. Second, even in the absence of spatial segregation, the non-spatial, sequential expansion model could still lead to multiple nested populations. In some episodes, a burst of mutations or copy number variants might occur in one cell, which subsequently expands to a detectable clonal size driven by its unusually high selective advantage[57]–[59]. Alternatively, even in the absence of such disruptive genomic crisis, the slow, successive replacement of mildly advantageous clones could also result in a series of partial sweeps, leading to co-existence of multiple clones at any given time[60][61]. In other words, episodic acceleration of cancer genome evolution can take place either via mutation rate "spikes" or simply through variabilities of selective advantage among driven events within a constant mutation regime. There are many routes that could lead from gradual evolution to punctuated equilibrium[62] in the history of each cell population; and this temporal heterogeneity is often further compounded in solid tumors by their spatial heterogeneity.

4. Conclusion

We developed an automated pipeline that estimates cellular fractions for both sCNAs and mutations, and uses their distributions to inform macroscopic clonal architecture. It considers a wider range of evolutionary scenarios than existing methods concerning the timing and phase relationship between a sCNA and a mutation it contains. Our method also explicitly evaluates model- and parameter-identifiability. When applied to a previously analyzed set of >700 breast tumors we found more than half of the tumors appear to contain multiple recognizable aneuploid tumor clones, and many show subtype-specific differences in clonality between sCNA and mutation in known cancer genes. This method adds to the available toolkit for examining intra-tumor heterogeneity using bulk tumor genomic data.

5. Materials and Methods

5.1. Data Access and sCNA Identification

From the Cancer Genome Atlas Data Portal[63] we downloaded: (1) the Level-2 copy number data derived from the Affymetrix Genome-Wide Human SNP Array 6.0 (the "XX-byallele.copynumber.data.txt" files) for 732 breast tumor DNA and their paired normal tissue DNA; and (2) the VCF files for whole-exome sequencing data for a subset of 522 tumor-normal samples analyzed by TCGA[14]. The IDs of the 732 samples are in Additional file 2. Of these, 445 samples have both SNP array and DNA sequencing available. The SNP array data were downloaded on 12 December 2012, while the sequencing data were downloaded on 22 March 2013. Each VCF file contains variant information for both the tumor and the paired normal sample. The procedures for variant calling and identification of somatic variants can be found in the Online Supplementary Methods of[14]. Counts for somatic and reference alleles of both tumor and normal samples were extracted for use in this study.

In addition, we also downloaded the clinical annotation file, including the PAM50 designations of all the involved patients, on 17 December 2012.

sAGP estimation (see below) can be performed on two types of user-selected spatial units: (1) genomic bins, predefined for each sample, typically consisting of 500 heterozygous markers in the germline DNA; (2) naturally observed sCNA segments, which we detect using the Circular Binary Segmentation (CBS) method[48], as follows. We independently perform segmentation on the LRR and the folded BAF (absolute value of BAF minus 0.5) values, using default parameters in the R package DNAcopy[46], except that minimal markers required was set to 5. With CBS results for both LRR and BAF, the two sets of change points are merged as follows: if a BAF change point falls within 5 markers of an LRR change point, either upstream or downstream, it is removed, that is, only the LRR breakpoint is kept, under the assumption that the two change points capture the same event, but the BAF change point is less accurately placed due to the greater sparsity of heterozygous markers.

After merging, the mean of LRR and folded BAF values are computed for each DNA segment (or the bin) in each sample, and used as input data for AGP and sAGP inference in the next step. For binned files, the bin length is on average 5.1 Mb, and each sample has an average of 502 bins.

5.2. sAGP Inference

As discussed in the main text, we jointly use BAF and LRR values to estimate sAGP for each sCNA, under the assumption of regional two-way mixing.

The algorithm has three steps:

1) Data pre-processing

We assume the allele-specific copy number data are already in bi-allelic format, with the following fields in the input file: SNP ID, chromosome, position, A allele count, B allele count. To note, the allele counts may not be integer numbers, but could be real-numbered values from the original CEL file. SNP markers are first grouped into either bins or merged sCNAs as described above. For each bin/sCNA, the median LRR and median folded BAF are calculated, and a segmentation file containing the above information for each segment is generated for each sample.

In the initial normalization of SNP array data the absolute LRR values depend on the genome-wide average ploidy, which is affected by the relative abundance of different copy number states in the genome. For example, in a tumor with a high fraction of cells undergone genome-wide doubling, the DNA segment located near the origin of the BAF-LRR plot are AABB, instead of the normal diploid configuration AB, and the global ploidy can be well above 2. The first step of sAGP estimation is therefore to ascertain the genotype of the sCNAs near the origin, following the procedures described in[18]. This allows unambiguous assignment (when possible) of copy number states for other sCNAs in the genome and the calculation of average ploidy. The deviation of BAF and LRR values of the baseline sCNAs from (x_0, y_0) is also used to quantify sd^2_{BAF} and sd^2_{LRR} for use in downstream analysis.

2) Estimate sAGP and absolute copy numbers

The method we used to estimate sAGP is extended from our AGP inference algorithm. For a sCNA with copy number configuration (n_b, n_t), where n_b is number of minor allele, and n_t number of total alleles, when mixed with a balanced diploid population its theoretical BAF and LRR values are:

$$BAF = \left| \frac{p \times n_b + 1 - p}{p \times n_t + 2 \times (1 - p)} - 0.5 \right| + x_0$$

$$LRR = \log_2 \left(p \times n_t + 2 \times (1 - p) \right) - 1 + y_0$$

where p is sAGP, and x_0, y_0 are the coordinates of the ($n_t = 2$, $n_b = 1$) state. When p changes, the points (BAF, LRR) follow a family of curved lines on the BAF-LRR plot, starting from the origin (x_0, y_0). Each line corresponds to a unique combination of (n_b, n_t) and is called a canonical line; and each point on this line uniquely corresponds to an sAGP value. The main task is to assign each observed segment to a canonical line. Due to noise, a sCNA does not locate precisely on a canonical line. Thus for each sCNA, we scan all possible canonical lines to find the one satisfying the following criteria:

a) Distance to the closest canonical line $\leq 2 \sqrt{sd_{BAF}^2 + sd_{LRR}^2}$; where sd2 BAF, and sd2 LRR are the estimated standard errors of BAF and LRR values.

Sometimes multiple lines satisfy (a) and result in multiple sAGP and n_t estimates. In such cases we apply

b) Choose sAGP = argmin($F = n_t -$ ploidy $+ |p_s - p|$); where p_s is sample-wide AGP and ploidy is the estimated global average ploidy from step 2). This criterion chooses the most probable canonical line as the one that results in a total copy number close to the genome-wide ploidy and an sAGP close to the global AGP.

If no canonical line can be found in (a), that is, the deviation is greater than the specified 2× scale of the standard deviations of BAF and LRR markers, we consider the sCNA not meeting the regional two-way mixing hypothesis, and its sAGP is assigned NA, its n_b and n_t are also treated as missing values in downstream analysis.

5.3. Statistical Modeling to Infer Macroscopic Clonal Structure

As explained in the main text, sAGP values can be calculated for either pre-defined genomic bins or identified sCNAs. In the per-bin analysis, the user can choose to filter out the non-sCNA bins or those with very small sAGP values, as true sCNAs with length shorter than the bin width tend to have reduced sAGP estimates due to the flanking euploid regions. In our analysis of the breast tumor data we applied two filtering steps. Firstly, we considered bins with median folded

BAF ≤ 0.04 and absolute median LRR ≤ 0.16 to be euploid, and assigned sAGP = 0. Secondly, before sAGP clustering, we removed bins with sAGP ≤ 0.05 to remove the contribution of the small sAGP values. At this step there is an average of $n = 224$ bins left per sample. The two models described in the main text are evaluated in a maximal likelihood framework. For Model-1, the log likelihood has a uniform and a normal component:

$$l = \sum_{i=1}^{n} \left(\frac{A}{range(Y)} + (1-A) \times Norm(y_i, \mu, \sigma) \right)$$

where Y is the observed sAGP vector for a given sample, with components y_i, $i = 1$, 2, $\cdots$, n, where n is the number of DNA segments after filtering. A is a scalar so that A/range provides the scaled uniform distribution. μ and σ are the mean and standard deviation of the single peak in the model following the normal distribution. We constrain A and μ in the range (0, 1). The parameters A, μ, and σ are estimated using the maximum likelihood approach, implemented in customized scripts (part of CHAT) written in the R statistical programming language[45].

Model-2 is fitted using a Dirichlet process Gaussian mixture model to infer the uncertain number of peaks and their relative abundances. The parameterization is as follows:

$$y_i \mid \mu_i, \sigma_i \sim Norm(\mu_i, \sigma_i), i = 1, 2 \cdots, n$$
$$\mu_i, \sigma_i \mid G \sim G$$
$$G \mid \alpha, G_0 \sim DP(\alpha G_0)$$
$$G_0 = Norm(\mu \mid \mu_1, \sigma \mid k_0) InvWishart(\sigma \mid v_1, \psi_1)$$
$$G_0 = Norm(\mu \mid \mu_1, \sigma \mid k_0) InvWishart(\sigma \mid v_1, \psi_1)$$
$$k_0 \mid \tau_1, \tau_2 \sim \Gamma(\tau_1/2, \tau_2/2)$$

Together these expressions describe a standard Dirichlet process mixture of normal model[40]. The implementation of the MCMC fitting is via R package DP package[56]. There are different ways to specify the prior parameters for the normal mixture model. The baseline Gaussian distribution G_0 relies on three prior parameters, μ_1, σ, and k_0, where σ is explicitly modeled by an Inversed Wishart distribution with priors v_1 and ψ_1, and k_0 follows a Gamma distribution. In practice, the hyperpriors, v_1, ψ_1, and k_0 can also be allowed to be random variables with a given prior distribution, and the model will have higher power to fit minor peaks in the data. In this work we used a conservative setting of prior parameters in terms of peak discovery sensitivity.

Model-1 cannot be included as a special case of Model-2, since when y is truly uniformly distributed, Dirichlet process tends to call multiple peaks instead of one peak, even with current conservative prior setting. Our solution is to fit both models, then numerically compute the likelihood of each model, and use Bayesian Information Criterion (BIC) to select the better model. Model-1 has three free parameters: A, μ, and σ, while Model-2 has seven: a_0, b_0, k_0, v_1, ψ_1, τ_1, and τ_2.

5.4. CCF Estimation and Scenario Identifiability for CN-LOH and Deletion

In the main text we presented how CHAT performs CCF estimation for the case of hemizygous amplifications ($n_b =1$, $n_t =3$). While this sCNA type has all four scenarios, Scenario B is not available for some other types of sCNAs, including LOH ($n_b = 0$, $n_t \geq 1$) and balanced allelic gains ($n_b > 1$, $n_t = 2n_b$). Below we will describe the cases of copy neutral LOH (CN-LOH) and hemizygous deletion.

5.4.1. CN-LOH

In Scenario A1 (Additional file 1: Figure S1A)

$$r_0 + r_1 + r_2 = 1$$
$$r_2 = p$$
$$f = \frac{r_1 + n_a \times r_2}{n_t} = \frac{r_1 + 2 \times r_2}{2}$$

where $n_t = 2 \times (1 - p) + n_t \times p = 2$ and CCF = $r_1 + r_2$. Using the above equations it is easy to show that

$$CCF^{A_1}\left(f, n_b, n_t, p\right) = n_t \times f - p \times n_a + p = 2 \times f - p$$

Scenarios A_2, B, and C have the same expression:

$$CCF^{A_2} = CCF^B = CCF^C = 2f$$

Note that A_2 and C not only have the same expression for CCF, they also have the same three-population composition, although the three populations emerge by different evolutionary routes. A previous study[32] failed to take A_1 into consideration and could have overestimated CCF under A_1, thus could have designated subclonal mutations as clonal when A_1 is the true evolutionary scenario.

The lower and upper limits of SAF in each scenario can be derived using the same process as in the main text. In scenario A_1, f reaches its upper limit when $r_0 = 0$, and $r_1 = 1 - r_2$.

$$f_h^{A_1} = \frac{1-p+2\times p}{n_t} = \frac{1+p}{2}$$

On the opposite side is r_1 is zero, when f reaches its minimum value:

$$f_l^{A_1} = \frac{2p}{2} = p$$

With p takes values from (0, 1), the areas defined by these limits are shown in **Figure 4(B)**.

For scenario B:

$$f_h^B = \frac{p}{N_t} = \frac{p}{2}$$
$$f_l^B = 0$$

And scenario C:

$$f_h^C = \frac{1-p}{N_t} = \frac{1-p}{2}$$
$$f_l^C = 0$$

5.4.2. Hemizygous Deletion

All four scenarios have the same expression:

$$CCF^{A_1} = CCF^{A_2} = CCF^B = CCF^C = f(2-p)$$

Similar to CN-LOH, A_2 and C not only have the same expression for CCF, they also have the same three-population composition.

The upper and lower limits for this sCNA type are:

$$f_h^{A_1} = \frac{1-p+p}{N_t} = \frac{1}{2-p}$$

$$f_l^{A_1} = \frac{p}{2-p}$$

$$f_h^B = \frac{p}{N_t} = \frac{p}{2-p}$$

$$f_l^B = 0$$

$$f_h^C = \frac{1-p}{N_t} = \frac{1-p}{2-p}$$

$$f_l^C = 0$$

The areas defined by these limits are shown in **Figure 4(C)**.

5.5. Variance of CCF

We use the same approach as described in[32] to estimate the standard deviation of CCF. The distribution of CCF is modeled as Binomial:

$$\Pr(CCF = x) \propto Binomi(S|N, G(x, p, \Theta))$$

where S is the read count for the somatic allele and N is the total read depth. $G(\cdot)$ is expected value of SAF given CCF value x, sAGP value p, and lineage scenario Θ. G is simply obtained by reversing the CCF expressions described in the main text [Equations (1), (2), (3), (4), (5), (6), and (7)]. We assume a uniform prior on x and the expectation and variance of CCF can be calculated as:

$$EXP(CCF) = \frac{\int_0^1 Binom(S|N,G)x\,dx}{\int_0^1 Binom(S|N,G)\,dx}$$

$$Var(CCF) = \frac{\int_0^1 Binom(S|N,G)x^2\,dx}{\int_0^1 Binom(S|N,G)\,dx - EXP(CCF)^2}$$

To note, the expectations of CCF are identical to the expressions in the main text [Equations (1), (2), (3), (4), (5), (6), and (7)].

5.6. Probabilistic Scenario Identification

The task is to use the observed somatic allele frequency (f) and sAGP value to determine the most likely scenario among the four scenarios described in the main text. We assume that f has a uniform prior, $U(0, 1)$, and we are interested in calculating the likelihood that the sSNV occurred before the sCNA, given the copy number configuration (n_b, n_t), known sAGP (p), and the observed allele counts. Let f_0 denote the true f. The probability of observing S count of the somatic allele is model by Binomial (f_0, N) and the likelihood of each scenario is the probability of observing S given the scenario is true, integrated over all the possible values of f_0:

$$
\begin{aligned}
p_X &= L\left(Scenario \quad X \,|\, p, n_b, n_t, N, S\right) \\
&= \Pr\{S|X, p, n_b, n_t, N\} \\
&= \int \Pr\{S|f_0, N\} \times \Pr\{f = f_0 | X, p, n_b, n_t\}\,df_0 \\
&= \int_{f_l^X}^{f_h^X} \Pr\{S|f_0, N\}\,df_0
\end{aligned}
$$

where X is A_1, A_2c scenarios, and f_h^X, f_l^X are computed according to Equations (8), (9), (10), (11), (12), (13), (14), and (15) in the main text and those in the section (CCF estimation and scenario identifiability for CN-LOH and deletion) above.

We then compute the summation of p_X:

$$P = p_{A1} + p_{A2} + p_B + p_C$$

and normalize each likelihood using P:

$$\widetilde{px} = \frac{px}{P}$$

We calculate the normalized probability for each scenario, as well as all the possible combinations of multiple scenarios. For example, the probability of either scenario A_1 or C is $\tilde{p}_{A1C} = \tilde{p}_{A1} + \tilde{p}_C$ There are in total $24 - 1 = 15$ possible combinations. If the normalized probability of any of the four scenarios is greater than 0.95, the SNV is assigned to the corresponding scenario. If none of the single-scenario probability exceeds 0.95, we ask if any of the six two-scenario combinations have probability >0.95. If this step fails, we next examine the four possible three-scenario combinations, and so forth. If all the above steps fail, we report the SNV scenario $A_1/A_2/B/C$, and no unique CCF can be estimated in this case.

5.7. In Silico Validation and Computation Performance

5.7.1. Performance of sAGP Inference

We first tested the performance of CHAT in sAGP estimation. We simulated LRR and BAF values for a series of sCNA datasets with two aneuploid tumor populations, which are mixed with the euploid population. The first population is the dominant clone, with an assigned sAGP value of $p_{\text{dom}} \sim [0.1, 0.2, \cdots, 1.0]$. The second population is a minor clone, with an assigned sAGP value of $p_{\text{sub}} \sim [0, 0.1, \cdots, p_{\text{dom}} - 0.1]$. The fraction of the euploid population is $1 - p_{\text{dom}} - p_{\text{sub}}$. In all, there are 55 $p_{\text{dom}} - p_{\text{sub}}$ combinations; and for each, we simulated 200 euploid segments ($n_b = 1$, $n_t = 2$, sAGP = 0) and 200 sCNA segments, of which 133 (about 2/3) were assigned to the dominant clone (sAGP = p_{dom}), and the remaining 67 were assigned to the minor clone (sAGP = p_{sub}). Within each clone, the sCNAs were assigned to one of four copy number configurations with the following ratios: 2/7 for deletion ($n_b = 0$, $n_t = 1$), 2/7 for CN-LOH ($n_b = 0$, $n_t = 2$), 2/7 for amplification ($n_b = 1$, $n_t =$

3), and 1/7 for balanced doubling ($n_b = 2$, $n_t = 4$). The BAF and LRR values were generated using the assigned sAGP and copy number configuration with the following formula:

$$BAF = \left| 0.5 - \frac{p \times n_b + 1 - p}{n_t} \right| + Normal\left(0, \sigma_{BAF}\right) \qquad (16)$$

$$LRR = \log_2 n_t - 1 + Normal\left(0, \sigma_{LRR}\right) \qquad (17)$$

where p stands for sAGP, and n_t is the averaged total copy number for the local segment: $2(1 - p) + n_t \times p$. σ_{BAF} and σ_{LRR} are the standard deviation values of the per- segment BAF and LRR, respectively. For the Affymetrix 6.0 platform, the per-SNP standard deviation for BAF is about 0.05, and for LRR is about 0.25 (our observation). Thus the choice of $\sigma_{BAF} = 0.01$ and $\sigma_{LRR} = 0.04$ is equivalent to the standard error of an sCNA of approximately 36 SNP markers. For a 1 million SNP platform, 36 SNPs cover approximately 110 kb, therefore ours are conservative choices for sCNAs 110 kb or longer, profiled by 1 million SNPs or more.

After generating the BAF and LRR values using Equations (16) and (17) for the 400 segments for each of the 55 $p_{dom} - p_{sub}$ combinations, we applied CHAT to estimate sAGP, n_b, and n_t for each simulated segment and reported the results in **Figure 5(A)**.

5.7.2. Performance of CCF Estimation

Of the 55 $p_{dom} - p_{sum}$ combinations described above we selectively tested CCF inference in four cases: $p_{dom} - p_{sum} \sim (0.9, 0.8)$, $(0.9, 0.4)$, $(0.5, 0.3)$, and $(0.3, 0.1)$. For each case, we simulated 4,000 SNVs, of which approximately 2,000 fall in the 200 euploid segments, and the other approximately 2,000 fall in the 200 sCNA regions, with the (sAGP, n_b, n_t) assignment implemented as described above. In effect we assume that the euploid intervals account for 50% of the genome. To make the test realistic, we used the sAGP, n_b, and n_t estimated by CHAT rather than the true values used in the initial simulation of the LRR and BAF data. If the SNV falls in a euploid region, the assigned SAF was randomly drawn from uniform (0, 0.5) and the corresponding "true" CCF = SAF $\times$ 2. If it falls in an aneuploid region, we randomly choose the lineage scenario from (A_1, A_2, B, C) according to the local copy number configuration. If the sCNA is a CN-LOH or balanced doubling region, we limit the scenarios to (A_1, B, C). The upper and lower limits of the chosen scenario were determined using Equations (8) to (15) in the main text and the equations in Materials and methods, CCF estimation and scenario identifiability for CN-LOH and deletion. SAF values were then randomly drawn from within this permissible range: uniform (f_l, f_h), where f_l and f_h were the lower and upper limits. "True" CCF values were computed using Equations (1) to (7) in the main text. Lastly, from the "true" CCF we simulated the allele counts in two steps. For a mean read depth k, the actual coverage at a given SNV, N, was sampled from $N \sim Poisson(k)$. With N and f (that is, CCF) thus assigned, the count of the somatic mutation allele was sampled from $Binomial(f, N)$. Based on the estimated sAGP, copy number configuration and the simulated somatic allele counts we used CHAT to estimate CCF. The estimated values were compared with the "true" CCF for both $k = 50$ and $k = 100$. For all eight cases (four $p_{dom} - p_{sub}$ combinations and two k values) we calculated the Spearman's rank correlation coefficient and/or the median absolute deviation (MAD) between the known and estimated CCF values [**Figure 5(B)** and **Figure 5(C)**].

5.7.3. Computational Requirements

We estimated the time and memory requirement of CHAT using the TCGA dataset for breast tumors. The time estimate below is based on allele-specific copy number data with 850K SNPs for tumor-normal pairs and whole-exome sequencing data with approximately 30× average coverage. For binned segmentation (approximately 500 heterozygous SNPs per bin), it takes 2min to complete the sAGP and CCF estimation for one tumor/normal pair, and it requires about 10 MB memory. For detected sCNAs, the computational time increases to an average of 12 min per sample pair. The above estimation is based on running R scripts with a single processor (AMD Opteron 6136, 2.4GHz with 4G RAM) and counting input file reading time. In CHAT, the user can apply the R package parallel to enable multi-thread processing. This allows the use of as many processors as available. On our server (32 AMD Opteron 6136 CPUs and 128G RAM), our test run used 14 processors on average, and it took 10h (140 CPU-hours) to complete the CBS segmentation, sAGP estimation for 732 breast tumor-normal samples and CCF estimation for 445 samples with downloaded VCF files.

5.7.4. Comparison with EXPANDS and PyClone

We simulated 200 CNA regions, with sAGP values randomly drawn from $U(0,1)$, and copy number configurations assigned by the ratio of 2/7 for deletion, 2/7 for CN-LOH, 2/7 for amplification, and 1/7 for balanced doubling, as described in Performance of sAGP inference. For each CNA, the LRR and BAF values were simulated as in Performance of sAGP inference. We then simulated 1,000 somatic mutations evenly across the "genome", with 488 that happened to fall in an sCNA region (with the rest falling in euploid regions). For these 488 somatic mutations, we assigned them to lineage scenarios with similar ratios across A_1, A_2-when possible, B, and C. The actual number assigned to each combination was shown in **Figure 6(D)**. For each mutation thus assigned, we sampled the somatic allele frequency (f) uniformly from its permissible range as described in Performance of CCF estimation, calculate the corresponding true CCF value, and simulated the sequencing read counts at the average coverage of $k = 50$, as described in Performance of CCF estimation. We applied CHAT to estimate (sAGP, n_t, n_b) from the simulated LRR and BAF data, then estimated CCF from the simulated read counts, sAGP and the estimated lineage scenarios and (n_t, n_b) status. In parallel, we applied PyClone to the same dataset, using the simulated read counts and the true (n_t, n_b) as input to estimate CCF. The choice of true (n_t, n_b) rather than the CHAT-estimated (n_t, n_b) should slightly favor PyClone as the errors in estimating (n_t, n_b) are not incorporated. Lastly, we applied EXPANDS to estimate CCF, using the simulated LRR and the observed somatic allele frequency as input. We compared the estimated CCF of the three tools with the known CCF in **Figure 6**. To make **Figure 6(D)** less cluttered we omitted balanced amplifications, thus only showing 423 mutations for the other CNA types.

5.8. Data Availability

CHAT source package is available at https://sourceforge.net/projects/clonalhetanalysistool/files/?. It is released underfully open source license, GPL ($\geq$2.0). It is also availableas a CRAN-R package. The breast tumor data were downloaded from the Cancer Genome Atlas Data Portal as described in Data access and sCNA identification. The TCGA IDs for the 732 tumors are in Additional file 2. The simulated data are available at http://sourceforge.net/projects/clonalhetanalysistool/files/simulations/ and as Additional file 3.

6. Additional Files

Additional file 1: Supplementary figures (Figure S1-S3) and legends describing additional information.

Additional file 2: TCGA Sample IDs for the 732 breast tumors we analyzed in this study.

Additional file 3: Simulated data used to compare CHAT, PyClone, and EXPANDS.

7. Abbreviations

CCF: Cancer cell fraction; CHAT: Clonal heterogeneity analysis tool.

ICGC: International Cancer Genome Consortium; SAF: Somatic allele frequency; sAGP: Segmental aneuploidy genome proportion; sCNA: Somatic copy number alteration; TCGA: The Cancer Genome Atlas.

Competing Interests

The authors declare that they have no competing interests.

Authors' Contributions

BL developed and implemented the algorithm; BL and JL wrote the manuscript; JL supervised the study. Both authors read and approved the manuscript.

Acknowledgements

The results presented here are in part based upon data generated by the TCGA Research Network: http://cancergenome.nih.gov/. We would like to thank a Rackham Predoctoral Fellowship (BL) and a Pilot Grant from the Center of Computation Biology and Medicine at University of Michigan (JL) for supporting this research. We thank Drs. Nancy Zhang, Kerby Shedden, and Sebastian Zoellner for helpful discussions.

Source: Li B, Li J Z. A general framework for analyzing tumor subclonality using SNP array and DNA sequencing data. [J]. Genome Biology, 2014, 15(9):473–473.

References

[1] Nowell PC: The clonal evolution of tumor cell populations. Science 1976, 194:23–28.

[2] Fidler IJ: Tumor heterogeneity and the biology of cancer invasion and metastasis. Cancer Res 1978, 38:2651–2660.

[3] Knudson AG Jr: Mutation and cancer: statistical study of retinoblastoma. Proc Natl Acad Sci U S A 1971, 68:820–823.

[4] Fearon ER, Vogelstein B: A genetic model for colorectal tumorigenesis. Cell 1990, 61:759–767.

[5] Vogelstein B, Kinzler KW: The multistep nature of cancer. Trends Genet 1993, 9:138–141.

[6] Sjoblom T, Jones S, Wood LD, Parsons DW, Lin J, Barber TD, Mandelker D, Leary RJ, Ptak J, Silliman N, Szabo S, Buckhaults P, Farrell C, Meeh P, Markowitz SD, Willis J, Dawson D, Willson JK, Gazdar AF, Hartigan J, Wu L, Liu C, Parmigiani G, Park BH, Bachman KE, Papadopoulos N, Vogelstein B, Kinzler KW, Velculescu VE: The consensus coding sequences of human breast and colorectal cancers. Science 2006, 314:268–274.

[7] Wood LD, Parsons DW, Jones S, Lin J, Sjoblom T, Leary RJ, Shen D, Boca SM, Barber T, Ptak J, Silliman N, Szabo S, Dezso Z, Ustyanksky V, Nikolskaya T, Nikolsky Y, Karchin R, Wilson PA, Kaminker JS, Zhang Z, Croshaw R, Willis J, Dawson D, Shipitsin M, Willson JK, Sukumar S, Polyak K, Park BH, Pethiyagoda CL, Pant PV, et al: The genomic landscapes of human breast and colorectal cancers. Science 2007, 318:1108–1113.

[8] Parsons DW, Jones S, Zhang X, Lin JC, Leary RJ, Angenendt P, Mankoo P, Carter H, Siu IM, Gallia GL, Olivi A, McLendon R, Rasheed BA, Keir S, Nikolskaya T, Nikolsky Y, Busam DA, Tekleab H, Diaz LA Jr, Hartigan J, Smith DR, Strausberg RL, Marie SK, Shinjo SM, Yan H, Riggins GJ, Bigner DD, Karchin R, Papadopoulos N, Parmigiani G, et al: An integrated genomic analysis of human glioblastoma multiforme. Science 2008, 321:1807–1812.

[9] Jones S, Zhang X, Parsons DW, Lin JC, Leary RJ, Angenendt P, Mankoo P, Carter H,

Kamiyama H, Jimeno A, Hong SM, Fu B, Lin MT, Calhoun ES, Kamiyama M, Walter K, Nikolskaya T, Nikolsky Y, Hartigan J, Smith DR, Hidalgo M, Leach SD, Klein AP, Jaffee EM, Goggins M, Maitra A, Iacobuzio-Donahue C, Eshleman JR, Kern SE, Hruban RH, *et al*: Core signaling pathways in human pancreatic cancers revealed by global genomic analyses. Science 2008, 321:1801–1806.

[10] Greaves M, Maley CC: Clonal evolution in cancer. Nature 2012, 481:306–313.

[11] Yates LR, Campbell PJ: Evolution of the cancer genome. Nat Rev Genet 2012, 13:795–806.

[12] The Cancer Genome Atlas Research Network: Comprehensive genomic characterization defines human glioblastoma genes and core pathways. Nature 2008, 455:1061–1068.

[13] The Cancer Genome Atlas Research Network: Integrated genomic analyses of ovarian carcinoma. Nature 2011, 474:609–615.

[14] The Cancer Genome Atlas Research Network: Comprehensive molecular portraits of human breast tumours. Nature 2012, 490:61–70.

[15] The Cancer Genome Atlas Research Network: Comprehensive genomic characterization of squamous cell lung cancers. Nature 2012, 489:519–525.

[16] Alexandrov LB, Nik-Zainal S, Wedge DC, Aparicio SA, Behjati S, Biankin AV, Bignell GR, Bolli N, Borg A, Borresen-Dale AL, Boyault S, Burkhardt B, Butler AP, Caldas C, Davies HR, Desmedt C, Eils R, Eyfjord JE, Foekens JA, Greaves M, Hosoda F, Hutter B, Ilicic T, Imbeaud S, Imielinski M, Jager N, Jones DT, Jones D, Knappskog S, Kool M, *et al*: Signatures of mutational processes in human cancer. Nature 2013, 500:415–421.

[17] Van Loo P, Nordgard SH, Lingjaerde OC, Russnes HG, Rye IH, Sun W, Weigman VJ, Marynen P, Zetterberg A, Naume B, Perou CM, Borresen-Dale AL, Kristensen VN: Allele-specific copy number analysis of tumors. Proc Natl Acad Sci U S A 2010, 107:16910–16915.

[18] Li B, Senbabaoglu Y, Peng W, Yang ML, Xu J, Li JZ: Genomic estimates of aneuploid content in glioblastoma multiforme and improved classification. Clin Cancer Res 2012, 18:5595–5605.

[19] Popova T, Manie E, Stoppa-Lyonnet D, Rigaill G, Barillot E, Stern MH: Genome Alteration Print (GAP): a tool to visualize and mine complex cancer genomic profiles obtained by SNP arrays. Genome Biol 2009, 10:R128.

[20] Sturm D, Witt H, Hovestadt V, Khuong-Quang DA, Jones DT, Konermann C, Pfaff E, Tonjes M, Sill M, Bender S, Kool M, Zapatka M, Becker N, Zucknick M, Hielscher T, Liu XY, Fontebasso AM, Ryzhova M, Albrecht S, Jacob K, Wolter M, Ebinger M, Schuhmann MU, van Meter T, Fruhwald MC, Hauch H, Pekrun A, Radlwimmer B, Niehues T, von Komorowski G, *et al*: Hotspot mutations in H3F3A and IDH1 define distinct epigenetic and biological subgroups of glioblastoma. Cancer Cell 2012, 22:425–437.

[21] Lawrence MS, Stojanov P, Polak P, Kryukov GV, Cibulskis K, Sivachenko A, Carter SL, Stewart C, Mermel CH, Roberts SA, Kiezun A, Hammerman PS, McKenna A, Drier Y, Zou L, Ramos AH, Pugh TJ, Stransky N, Helman E, Kim J, Sougnez C, Ambrogio L, Nickerson E, Shefler E, Cortes ML, Auclair D, Saksena G, Voet D, Noble M, DiCara D, *et al*: Mutational heterogeneity in cancer and the search for new cancer-associated genes. Nature 2013, 499:214–218.

[22] Verhaak RG, Hoadley KA, Purdom E, Wang V, Qi Y, Wilkerson MD, Miller CR, Ding L, Golub T, Mesirov JP, Alexe G, Lawrence M, O'Kelly M, Tamayo P, Weir BA, Gabriel S, Winckler W, Gupta S, Jakkula L, Feiler HS, Hodgson JG, James CD, Sarkaria JN, Brennan C, Kahn A, Spellman PT, Wilson RK, Speed TP, Gray JW, Meyerson M, *et al*: Integrated genomic analysis identifies clinically relevant subtypes of glioblastoma characterized by abnormalities in PDGFRA, IDH1, EGFR, and NF1. Cancer Cell 2010, 17:98–110.

[23] Curtis C, Shah SP, Chin SF, Turashvili G, Rueda OM, Dunning MJ, Speed D, Lynch AG, Samarajiwa S, Yuan Y, Graf S, Ha G, Haffari G, Bashashati A, Russell R, McKinney S, Group M, Langerod A, Green A, Provenzano E, Wishart G, Pinder S, Watson P, Markowetz F, Murphy L, Ellis I, Purushotham A, Borresen-Dale AL, Brenton JD, Tavare S, *et al*: The genomic and transcriptomic architecture of 2,000 breast tumours reveals novel subgroups. Nature 2012, 486:346–352.

[24] Garraway LA, Lander ES: Lessons from the cancer genome. Cell 2013, 153:17–37.

[25] Navin N, Kendall J, Troge J, Andrews P, Rodgers L, McIndoo J, Cook K, Stepansky A, Levy D, Esposito D, Muthuswamy L, Krasnitz A, McCombie WR, Hicks J, Wigler M: Tumour evolution inferred by single-cell sequencing. Nature 2011, 472:90–94.

[26] Shalek AK, Satija R, Adiconis X, Gertner RS, Gaublomme JT, Raychowdhury R, Schwartz S, Yosef N, Malboeuf C, Lu D, Trombetta JJ, Gennert D, Gnirke A, Goren A, Hacohen N, Levin JZ, Park H, Regev A: Single-cell transcriptomics reveals bimodality in expression and splicing in immune cells. Nature 2013, 498:236–240.

[27] Hou Y, Song L, Zhu P, Zhang B, Tao Y, Xu X, Li F, Wu K, Liang J, Shao D, Wu H, Ye X, Ye C, Wu R, Jian M, Chen Y, Xie W, Zhang R, Chen L, Liu X, Yao X, Zheng H, Yu C, Li Q, Gong Z, Mao M, Yang X, Yang L, Li J, Wang W, *et al*: Single-cell exome sequencing and monoclonal evolution of a JAK2-negative myeloproliferative neoplasm. Cell 2012, 148:873–885.

[28] Xu X, Hou Y, Yin X, Bao L, Tang A, Song L, Li F, Tsang S, Wu K, Wu H, He W, Zeng L, Xing M, Wu R, Jiang H, Liu X, Cao D, Guo G, Hu X, Gui Y, Li Z, Xie W, Sun X, Shi M, Cai Z, Wang B, Zhong M, Li J, Lu Z, Gu N, *et al*: Single-cell exome sequencing reveals single-nucleotide mutation characteristics of a kidney tumor. Cell 2012, 148:886–895.

[29] Keats JJ, Chesi M, Egan JB, Garbitt VM, Palmer SE, Braggio E, Van Wier S, Blackburn PR, Baker AS, Dispenzieri A, Kumar S, Rajkumar SV, Carpten JD, Barrett M, Fonseca R, Stewart AK, Bergsagel PL: Clonal competition with alternating domin-

ance in multiple myeloma. Blood 2012, 120:1067–1076.

[30] Ley TJ, Ding L, Walter MJ, McLellan MD, Lamprecht T, Larson DE, Kandoth C, Payton JE, Baty J, Welch J, Harris CC, Lichti CF, Townsend RR, Fulton RS, Dooling DJ, Koboldt DC, Schmidt H, Zhang Q, Osborne JR, Lin L, O'Laughlin M, McMichael JF, Delehaunty KD, McGrath SD, Fulton LA, Magrini VJ, Vickery TL, Hundal J, Cook LL, Conyers JJ, *et al*: DNMT3A mutations in acute myeloid leukemia. N Engl J Med 2010, 363:2424–2433.

[31] Durinck S, Ho C, Wang NJ, Liao W, Jakkula LR, Collisson EA, Pons J, Chan SW, Lam ET, Chu C, Park K, Hong SW, Hur JS, Huh N, Neuhaus IM, Yu SS, Grekin RC, Mauro TM, Cleaver JE, Kwok PY, LeBoit PE, Getz G, Cibulskis K, Aster JC, Huang H, Purdom E, Li J, Bolund L, Arron ST, Gray JW, *et al*: Temporal dissection of tumorigenesis in primary cancers. Cancer Discov 2011, 1:137–143.

[32] Landau DA, Carter SL, Stojanov P, McKenna A, Stevenson K, Lawrence MS, Sougnez C, Stewart C, Sivachenko A, Wang L, Wan Y, Zhang W, Shukla SA, Vartanov A, Fernandes SM, Saksena G, Cibulskis K, Tesar B, Gabriel S, Hacohen N, Meyerson M, Lander ES, Neuberg D, Brown JR, Getz G, Wu CJ: Evolution and impact of subclonal mutations in chronic lymphocytic leukemia. Cell 2013, 152:714–726.

[33] Gerlinger M, Rowan AJ, Horswell S, Larkin J, Endesfelder D, Gronroos E, Martinez P, Matthews N, Stewart A, Tarpey P, Varela I, Phillimore B, Begum S, McDonald NQ, Butler A, Jones D, Raine K, Latimer C, Santos CR, Nohadani M, Eklund AC, Spencer-Dene B, Clark G, Pickering L, Stamp G, Gore M, Szallasi Z, Downward J, Futreal PA, Swanton C: Intratumor heterogeneity and branched evolution revealed by multiregion sequencing. N Engl J Med 2012, 366:883–892.

[34] Sottoriva A, Spiteri I, Piccirillo SG, Touloumis A, Collins VP, Marioni JC, Curtis C, Watts C, Tavare S: Intratumor heterogeneity in human glioblastoma reflects cancer evolutionary dynamics. Proc Natl Acad Sci U S A 2013, 110:4009–4014.

[35] Yachida S, Jones S, Bozic I, Antal T, Leary R, Fu B, Kamiyama M, Hruban RH, Eshleman JR, Nowak MA, Velculescu VE, Kinzler KW, Vogelstein B, Iacobuzio-Donahue CA: Distant metastasis occurs late during the genetic evolution of pancreatic cancer. Nature 2010, 467:1114–1117.

[36] Campbell PJ, Yachida S, Mudie LJ, Stephens PJ, Pleasance ED, Stebbings LA, Morsberger LA, Latimer C, McLaren S, Lin ML, McBride DJ, Varela I, Nik-Zainal SA, Leroy C, Jia M, Menzies A, Butler AP, Teague JW, Griffin CA, Burton J, Swerdlow H, Quail MA, Stratton MR, Iacobuzio-Donahue C, Futreal PA: The patterns and dynamics of genomic instability in metastatic pancreatic cancer. Nature 2010, 467:1109–1113.

[37] McFadden DG, Papagiannakopoulos T, Taylor-Weiner A, Stewart C, Carter SL, Cibulskis K, Bhutkar A, McKenna A, Dooley A, Vernon A, Sougnez C, Malstrom S, Heimann M, Park J, Chen F, Farago AF, Dayton T, Shefler E, Gabriel S, Getz G, Jacks T: Genetic and clonal dissection of murine small cell lung carcinoma progression by genome sequencing. Cell 2014, 156:1298–1311.

[38] Nik-Zainal S, Van Loo P, Wedge DC, Alexandrov LB, Greenman CD, Lau KW, Raine K, Jones D, Marshall J, Ramakrishna M, Shlien A, Cooke SL, Hinton J, Menzies A, Stebbings LA, Leroy C, Jia M, Rance R, Mudie LJ, Gamble SJ, Stephens PJ, McLaren S, Tarpey PS, Papaemmanuil E, Davies HR, Varela I, McBride DJ, Bignell GR, Leung K, Butler AP, *et al*: The life history of 21 breast cancers. Cell 2012, 149:994–1007.

[39] Shah SP, Roth A, Goya R, Oloumi A, Ha G, Zhao Y, Turashvili G, Ding J, Tse K, Haffari G, Bashashati A, Prentice LM, Khattra J, Burleigh A, Yap D, Bernard V, McPherson A, Shumansky K, Crisan A, Giuliany R, Heravi-Moussavi A, Rosner J, Lai D, Birol I, Varhol R, Tam A, Dhalla N, Zeng T, Ma K, Chan SK, *et al*: The clonal and mutational evolution spectrum of primary triple-negative breast cancers. Nature 2012, 486:395–399.

[40] Carter SL, Cibulskis K, Helman E, McKenna A, Shen H, Zack T, Laird PW, Onofrio RC, Winckler W, Weir BA, Beroukhim R, Pellman D, Levine DA, Lander ES, Meyerson M, Getz G: Absolute quantification of somatic DNA alterations in human cancer. Nat Biotechnol 2012, 30:413–421.

[41] Oesper L, Mahmoody A, Raphael BJ: THetA: inferring intra-tumor heterogeneity from high-throughput DNA sequencing data. Genome Biol 2013, 14:R80.

[42] Escohar M, West M: Bayesian Density Estimation and Inference Using Mixtures. J AM Statist Assoc 1995, 90:12.

[43] Roth A, Khattra J, Yap D, Wan A, Laks E, Biele J, Ha G, Aparicio S, Bouchard-Cote A, Shah SP: PyClone: statistical inference of clonal population structure in cancer. Nat Methods 2014, 11:396–398.

[44] Schwarz G: Estimating the dimension of a model. Ann Stat 1978, 6:4.

[45] Gould SJ, Eldredge N: Punctuated equilibrium comes of age. Nature 1993, 366:223–227.

[46] Cibulskis K, Lawrence MS, Carter SL, Sivachenko A, Jaffe D, Sougnez C, Gabriel S, Meyerson M, Lander ES, Getz G: Sensitive detection of somatic point mutations in impure and heterogeneous cancer samples. Nat Biotechnol 2013, 31:213–219.

[47] Team RC: R: A language and environment for statistical computing; 2012.

[48] Olshen AB, Venkatraman ES, Lucito R, Wigler M: Circular binary segmentation for the analysis of array-based DNA copy number data. Biostatistics 2004, 5:557–572.

[49] Parker JS, Mullins M, Cheang MC, Leung S, Voduc D, Vickery T, Davies S, Fauron C, He X, Hu Z, Quackenbush JF, Stijleman IJ, Palazzo J, Marron JS, Nobel AB, Mardis E, Nielsen TO, Ellis MJ, Perou CM, Bernard PS: Supervised risk predictor of breast cancer based on intrinsic subtypes. J Clin Oncol 2009, 27:1160–1167.

[50] Andor N, Harness JV, Muller S, Mewes HW, Petritsch C: EXPANDS: expanding ploidy and allele frequency on nested subpopulations. Bioinformatics 2014, 30:50–60.

[51] Yau C, Mouradov D, Jorissen RN, Colella S, Mirza G, Steers G, Harris A, Ragoussis J, Sieber O, Holmes CC: A statistical approach for detecting genomic aberrations in heterogeneous tumor samples from single nucleotide polymorphism genotyping data. Genome Biol 2010, 11:R92.

[52] Ding L, Ley TJ, Larson DE, Miller CA, Koboldt DC, Welch JS, Ritchey JK, Young MA, Lamprecht T, McLellan MD, McMichael JF, Wallis JW, Lu C, Shen D, Harris CC, Dooling DJ, Fulton RS, Fulton LL, Chen K, Schmidt H, Kalicki-Veizer J, Magrini VJ, Cook L, McGrath SD, Vickery TL, Wendl MC, Heath S, Watson MA, Link DC, Tomasson MH, et al: Clonal evolution in relapsed acute myeloid leukaemia revealed by whole-genome sequencing. Nature 2012, 481:506–510.

[53] Hajirasouliha I, Mahmoody A, Raphael BJ: A combinatorial approach for analyzing intra-tumor heterogeneity from high-throughput sequencing data. Bioinformatics 2014, 30:i78-i86.

[54] Jiao W, Vembu S, Deshwar AG, Stein L, Morris Q: Inferring clonal evolution of tumors from single nucleotide somatic mutations. BMC Bioinformatics 2014, 15:35.

[55] Strino F, Parisi F, Micsinai M, Kluger Y: TrAp: a tree approach for fingerprinting subclonal tumor composition. Nucleic Acids Res 2013, 41:e165.

[56] Xu Y, Muller P, Yuan Y, Gulukota K, Ji Y: MAD Bayes for tumor heterogeneity - feature allocatioon with exponential family sampling. arXiv:14025090 [statME] 2014.

[57] Stephens PJ, Greenman CD, Fu B, Yang F, Bignell GR, Mudie LJ, Pleasance ED, Lau KW, Beare D, Stebbings LA, McLaren S, Lin ML, McBride DJ, Varela I, Nik-Zainal S, Leroy C, Jia M, Menzies A, Butler AP, Teague JW, Quail MA, Burton J, Swerdlow H, Carter NP, Morsberger LA, Iacobuzio-Donahue C, Follows GA, Green AR, Flanagan AM, Stratton MR, et al: Massive genomic rearrangement acquired in a single catastrophic event during cancer development. Cell 2011, 144:27–40.

[58] Rausch T, Jones DT, Zapatka M, Stutz AM, Zichner T, Weischenfeldt J, Jager N, Remke M, Shih D, Northcott PA, Pfaff E, Tica J, Wang Q, Massimi L, Witt H, Bender S, Pleier S, Cin H, Hawkins C, Beck C, von Deimling A, Hans V, Brors B, Eils R, Scheurlen W, Blake J, Benes V, Kulozik AE, Witt O, Martin D, et al: Genome sequencing of pediatric medulloblastoma links catastrophic DNA rearrangements with TP53 mutations. Cell 2012, 148:59–71.

[59] Molenaar JJ, Koster J, Zwijnenburg DA, van Sluis P, Valentijn LJ, van der Ploeg I, Hamdi M, van Nes J, Westerman BA, van Arkel J, Ebus ME, Haneveld F, Lakeman A, Schild L, Molenaar P, Stroeken P, van Noesel MM, Ora I, Santo EE, Caron HN, Westerhout EM, Versteeg R: Sequencing of neuroblastoma identifies chromothripsis and defects in neuritogenesis genes. Nature 2012, 483:589–593.

[60] Beerenwinkel N, Antal T, Dingli D, Traulsen A, Kinzler KW, Velculescu VE, Vogelstein B, Nowak MA: Genetic progression and the waiting time to cancer. PLoS Comput Biol 2007, 3:e225.

[61] Bozic I, Antal T, Ohtsuki H, Carter H, Kim D, Chen S, Karchin R, Kinzler KW, Vogelstein B, Nowak MA: Accumulation of driver and passenger mutations during tumor progression. Proc Natl Acad Sci U S A 2010, 107:18545–18550.

[62] Eldredge N, Gould SJ: Punctuated equilibria: an alternative to phyletic gradualism. In Models in Paleobiology. Edited by Schopf TJM. San Francisco, CA: Freeman Cooper; 1972.

[63] Cancer Genome Atlas Data Portal. [https://tcga-data.nci.nih.gov/tcga/ dataAccess-Matrix.htm].

Chapter 5

Oncogenes and Tumor Suppressor Genes: Comparative Genomics and Network Perspectives

Kevin Zhu[1], Qi Liu[2], Yubo Zhou[3], Cui Tao[4], Zhongming Zhao[2], Jingchun Sun[4], Hua Xu[4]

[1]Graduate School of Biomedical Sciences, The University of Texas Health Science Center at Houston, Houston, TX 77030, USA
[2]Department of Biomedical Informatics, Vanderbilt University, Nashville, TN 37203, USA
[3]National Center for Drug Screening, Shanghai Institute of Materia Medica, Chinese Academy of Sciences, Shanghai, China
[4]School of Biomedical Informatics, The University of Texas Health Science Center at Houston, Houston, TX 77030, USA

Abstract: Background: Defective tumor suppressor genes (TSGs) and hyperactive oncogenes (OCGs) heavily contribute to cell proliferation and apoptosis during cancer development through genetic variations such as somatic mutations and deletions. Moreover, they usually do not perform their cellular functions individually but rather execute jointly. Therefore, a comprehensive comparison of their mutation patterns and network properties may provide a deeper understanding of their roles in the cancer development and provide some clues for identification of novel targets. Results: In this study, we performed a comprehensive survey of TSGs and OCGs from the perspectives of somatic mutations and network properties. For comparative purposes, we choose five gene sets: TSGs, OCGs, cancer drug target genes, essential genes, and other genes. Based on the data from Pan-Cancer project, we found that TSGs had the highest mutation frequency in most tumor types and the OCGs second. The essential genes had the lowest mutation frequency in all tumor types. For the network properties in the human protein-protein interaction (PPI) network, we found that, relative to target proteins, essential proteins, and other proteins, the TSG proteins and OCG proteins both tended to have higher degrees, higher betweenness, lower clustering coefficients, and shorter shortest-path distances. Moreover, the TSG proteins and OCG proteins tended to have direct interactions with cancer drug target proteins. To further explore their relationship, we generated a TSG-OCG network and found that TSGs and OCGs connected strongly with each other. The integration of the mutation frequency with the TSG-OCG network offered a network view of TSGs, OCGs, and their interactions, which may provide new insights into how the TSGs and OCGs jointly contribute to the cancer development. Conclusions: Our study first discovered that the OCGs and TSGs had different mutation patterns, but had similar and stronger protein-protein characteristics relative to the essential proteins or control proteins in the whole human interactome. We also found that the TSGs and OCGs had the most direct interactions with cancer drug targets. The results will be helpful for cancer drug target identification, and ultimately, understanding the etiology of cancer and treatment at the network level.

1. Background

Cancer is the second disease leading to death worldwide[1]. It consists of more than 100 different diseases with diverse risk factors. Among these risk factors, genetic alternations play critical roles in the pathogenesis of the disease and provide fundamental clues for the identification of drug targets and the development of novel drugs[2]–[6].

Recently, several large-scale cancer genome projects produced multi-dimensional genome-wide big data such as The Cancer Genome Atlas (TCGA)[7], the Well come Trust Sanger Institute's Cancer Genome Project[8], and the International Cancer Genome Consortium (ICGC)[9]. These genome-wide data have dramatically advanced cancer research, especially in terms of its genetics and genomics[10], which enhances the accuracy and coverage of the identification of cancer-related genes that could drive or protect cancer development. However, though these large-scale sequencing data discovered thousands of mutations, they have not so far identified novel drug targets besides these previously identified[11]. Therefore, developing novel approaches to revealing the signal buried under the big data to discover the novel drug targets is necessary and critical for the development of effective treatment for cancer.

Among these cancer-related genes identified by high-throughput sequencing and small-scale traditional approaches, two classes of genes-tumor suppressor genes (TSGs) and oncogenes (OCGs) have been attracted much attention. Numerous studies demonstrated these genetic alternations involve the gain-of-function of OCGs together with the loss-of-function of TSGs determine the cell cycle processes that control the tumor formation and development[12][13]. Recently, protein-protein interaction (PPI) network based on computational methods have been used to identify disease-specific genes, modules, and cancer-subtype subnetworks [14]-[16]. Therefore, we hypothesized that comparative investigations of TSG and OCG mutation patterns and network properties would provide a number of novel insights into their functions in the tumorigenesis, which further offers valuable information for identification of novel drug targets for drug development.

As numerous genetic and genomic data in cancer become available, the list of OCGs and TSGs has been expanded through molecular, cellular, genomic, and computational studies including non-coding RNA genes[17][18]. Considering the gain-of-function of OCG mutations and loss-of-function of TSG mutations, TSGs and OCGs may be involved in the regulation of cellular functions in a yin-yang fashion[19]. For example, our previous study has shown that they have distinct and competitive regulatory patterns in ovarian cancer[20]. Furthermore, OCG mutations are usually dominant so that one mutant copy is enough to start switching on a cellular activity. TSG mutations tend to be recessive, so that they should follow the famous Knudson's "two-hit hypothesis": that both copies of tumor suppressor genes need mutate to cause loss of function. However, more and more evidence shows that even partial inactivation of TSGs could critically contribute to tumorigenesis[21]. Additionally, some genes' function could be switched between OCGs and TSGs, depending on the situation. Current therapeutic applications have shown that targeting OCGs and their related pathways is promising for developing novel drugs, including antibodies and small synthetic molecules[22]. Therefore, further understanding of OCGs and TSGs in the terms of networks will provide novel insights into their functions in the tumorigenesis. However, to our knowledge, there is no report that systematically investigates their relationships.

Thus, in this study, we compared five sets of proteins encoded by five sets of genes (TSGs, OCGs, drug target genes, essential genes, and other genes) with the perspectives of genomics and protein networks. We compared them using the somatic mutations from TCGA Pan-Cancer project[23] and network properties in human PPI networks[24]. Based on the genetic data from Pan-Cancer project, we found that TSGs had the highest mutation frequency in most tumor types and the OCGs second. For the network properties, relative to target proteins, essential proteins, and other proteins, both TSG and OCG proteins tended to have higher degrees, higher betweenness, lower clustering coefficients, and shorter shortest-path distances. In addition, both TSG and OCG proteins tended to have direct interactions with cancer drug target proteins. We further generated a TSG-OCG network and found that TSGs and OCGs connected strongly with each other. Our study first revealed that the OCGs and TSGs had different mutation patterns, but had similar and stronger protein-protein characteristics relative to the essential proteins or control proteins in the whole human interactome.

2. Materials and Methods

2.1. Somatic Mutations of the Cancer Genome

To explore the somatic mutation patterns, we obtained the somatic mutations from Supplementary Table 2 published by one Pan-Cancer analysis of TCGA project[23]. The study presents the data and analytical results for point mutations and small insertions/deletions from 3,281 tumours across 12 tumour types. The 12 tumours included bladder urothelial carcinoma (BLCA), breast adenocarcinoma (BRCA), colon and rectal adenocarcinoma (COAD/READ), glioblastoma (GBM), head and neck squamous cell carcinoma (HNSC), kidney renal clear cell carcinoma (KIRC), acute myeloid leukemia (LAML), lung adenocarcinoma (LUAD), lung squamous cell carcinoma (LUSC), ovarian cancer (OV), and uterine corpus endometrioid carcinoma (UCEC).

2.2. Human PPIs

To study the network properties of gene sets, we utilized the most recent version of the human PPI data from the Protein Interaction Network Analysis platform (PINA v2.0)[24]. After mapping the human protein IDs to their official gene symbols, we culled out the redundant connections and the self-interactions. The interaction network contains 12,978 nodes corresponding to human 12,978 genes and 101,219 edges.

2.3. Gene Sets

In this study, we choose TSGs and OCGs with high confidence from Davioli et al.[17]. Each set of TSGs and OCGs contains 50 genes that were selected from the Cancer Gene Census and have been implicated in tumorigenesis by experimental evidence in the literature[25].

To get cancer-related drugs, we utilized the Anatomical Therapeutic Chemical (ATC) Classification codes L01 (Antineoplastic Agents) to obtain the cancer drugs from Drug Bank[26]. We first downloaded the data from the Drug Bank database (version 4.0, June 2014) and extracted the drug-related information, such as the "Name," "Drug Targets," and "ATC Codes." Consequently, we obtained a total of 115 cancer drugs with their drug targets. These drug targets could map to 171 gene official symbols. We regarded them as cancer drug target genes.

For comparative purposes, besides TSGs, OCGs, and drug target genes, we included essential genes and other genes as controls. For the essential genes, we utilized the gene list that was predicted at the cellular level[17]. The other genes contained genes encoding proteins in the PINA PPI data set after excluding the OCGs, TSGs, targets, and essential genes. Overall, we investigated five gene sets in this study: TSGs, OCGs, target genes, essential genes, and others.

2.4. Network Properties

To explore network properties of these five sets of genes, we calculated four basic and important network properties: degree, betweenness, clustering coefficient, and shortest-path distance[27][28]. The degree (connectivity) of a node A is the number of other nodes that are directly connected to A by an edge. These nodes are neighbors of node A. A node with a higher degree will have a higher number of neighbors. The betweenness of a node A describes how many shortest paths between any two pairs in the network will pass through A. The clustering coefficient represents the ratio of the number of connections that occur between the immediate neighbors of A compared to the maximum number of connections that could occur among them. The shortest-path distance between two pair of nodes A and B is the smallest number nodes that must be passed through to get from A to B. This means that if A and B are neighbors, the shortest-path distance between them would be one. Given sets of nodes, we calculated the shortest-paths from a set of interest nodes to all other nodes in the network. Moreover, we calculated the shortest-path distances between target proteins to other interest gene set to measure their interrelationship. At the each distance, we calculated the proportion of interest proteins.

2.5. Subnetwork Generation

To better understand the interactions between OCGs and TSGs, we generated a subnetwork that contains OCGs and TSGs using the GenRev program[29] (version 1.0.1). Given a network and a set of interest nodes, GenRev enables calculate a subnetwork containing the interest nodes and non-interest nodes. The interestnodes are terminal nodes while the non-interest nodes are linker nodes that become part of the subnetwork based on the algorithm's criteria. GenRev offers three algorithms for generating subnetworks: the Klein-Ravi algorithm, the limited k-walk algorithm, and a heuristic local search algorithm. In this study, we utilized the Klein-Ravi algorithm to generate a node-weighted Steiner tree subnetwork. The algorithm enables to intertwine as many terminal nodes as possible through non-interest nodes (linkers) by calculating the shortest-path distance[30].

3. Results

3.1. TSGs Have the Highest Frequency of Mutations

In this study, we choose the 50 TSGs, 50 OCGs, and 145 essential genes,

171 target genes, and 12,315 other genes for investigation of mutation patterns. To compare the mutation frequencies of the tumor samples among the five gene sets, we performed the Kolmogorov-Smirnov (K-S) tests[31].

Figure 1(A) shows a comparison of a general mutation percentage of all samples in each gene set, and **Figure 1(B)** contains the average values and P-values of five gene sets. The TSGs had the highest average mutation frequency (4.34%), which was significantly higher than that of OCGs (2.36%, P = 0.002), target genes (1.32%, P = 1.04×10^{-10}), essential genes (0.59%, P = 2.08×10^{-20}), and other genes (0.98%, P = 7.29×10^{-17}). The OCGs had the second highest average mutation frequency (2.36%), which was significantly higher than that of target genes (P = 0.007), essential genes (P = 8.46×10^{-13}), and other genes (P = 4.53×10^{-17}), respectively. The target genes had the third highest average mutation frequency (1.32%), which was significantly higher than that of essential genes (P = 2.79×10^{-13}) and other genes (P = 4.15×10^{-6}). Interestingly, the essential gene had the lowest mutation frequency among the five gene sets.

We further examined the mutation frequency in the five gene sets across the 12 cancer types [**Figure 1(C)** and **Figure 1(D)**]. The mutation frequency in the TSGs was significantly higher than that of all other tumor types except for GBM, LAML, LUSC, and OV (p < 0.05). LAML had the lowest average mutation frequency (1.33%) and UCEC the highest (8.23%). The mutation frequency in the OCGs was significantly higher than that of essential genes and that of other genes (p < 0.05), respectively. Only in BRCA and LAML, the mutation frequency of the OCGs was significantly higher than that of the target genes. For the OCGs, OV had the lowest average mutation frequency (0.40%), and UCEC had the highest (6.20%).

In summary, these results indicated that TSGs had the highest mutation frequency in most tumour types, and the OCGs were the second. The essential genes had the lowest mutation frequency in all tumor types.

3.2. Network Properties

To explore the network properties, we mapped the five gene sets onto human PPI networks and obtained the 48 TSG proteins, 49 OCG proteins, 161 target

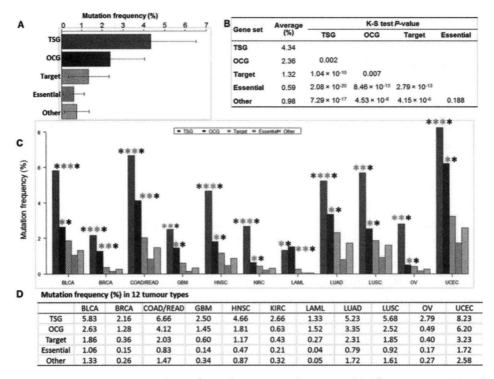

Figure 1. Percentage comparison of Pan-Cancer samples mutated in five gene sets (A and B) and across 12 tumor types (C and D). In Figure D, one star indicates a P-value less than 0.05 based on the Kolmogorov-Smirnov (K-S) test between the two gene sets. The star color indicates the corresponding gene sets. For example, in BLCA, the top of the TSG bar has four stars, which indicates that the percentage of samples with mutations in the TSG gene set was significantly higher than that of OCG genes (blue star), target genes (red star), essential genes (green star), and other genes (gray star). "TSG" represents the tumor suppressor genes, "OCG" represents the oncogenes, "Target" represents the genes encoding cancer drug targets, "Essential" represents the essential genes, and "Other" represents the other genes with mutation data that are part of the PPI data.

proteins, 141 essential proteins, and 12,315 other proteins. Then, we calculated four properties for each node in the network, including the degree, betweenness, clustering coefficient and shortest-path distance. To compare the network properties among the five sets of genes, we performed the K-S tests.

3.3. TSGs and OCGs Tended to Have Higher Degree and Betweenness

Figure 2(A) shows the degree distributions for the five pro-tein sets while

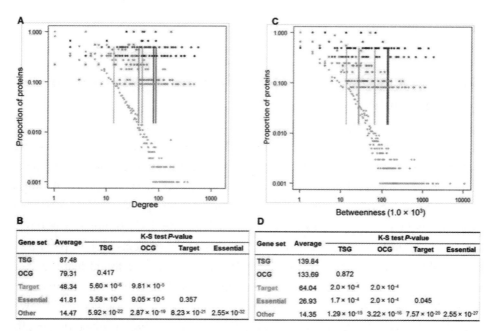

Figure 2. Comparison of degree and betweenness of five protein sets. (A) Degree distribution. (B) Summary of the average degree and the corresponding P-values of the Kolmogorov-Smirnov (K-S) tests for any two protein sets. (C) Betweenness distribution. (D) Summary of the average betweenness (1.0 × 103) and the corresponding P-values of the K-S tests for any two protein sets.

Figure 2(B) contains their average degrees and K-S test P-values. The average degree of the TSG proteins was 87.48, which was significantly higher than that of the target proteins (48.34, p = 5.60 × 10^{-5}), essential proteins (41.81, P = 3.58 × 10^{-6}), and other proteins (14.47, p = 5.92 × 10^{-22}). Similarly, the average degree of the OCGs was 79.31, which was also significantly higher than that of the target proteins (p = 9.81 × 10^{-5}), essential proteins (p = 9.05 × 10^{-5}), and other proteins (P = 2.87 × 10^{-19}). However, we did not observe any significant difference between TSG proteins and OCG protein (p = 0.417). The average degrees of the TSGs and OCGs were approximately 2.0 times that of the target proteins and essential proteins and about 6.0 times that of the other proteins. The latter ratio is higher than that (3.1 times) found in cancer proteins in a previous study[27].

Figure 2(C) shows the betweenness distributions and **Figure 2(D)** contains the average value and K-S test P-values for the five protein sets. The results for the betweenness were consistent with those for the degree. These observations indicated that TSG proteins and OCG proteins had the highest degree and betweenness in the human PPI network compared to other proteins.

3.4. TSGs and OCGs Tended to Have a Lower Clustering Coefficient

For each node, the clustering coefficient reflects the con-nectivity among its inte-ractors. The higher the clustering coefficient, the higher the connectivity of its neighbors has. **Figure 3** shows the distribution of the clustering coefficient values, the average value of each protein set, and the K-S test p-values among the five protein sets. The average clustering coefficient of the TSG proteins was 0.095, which was significantly lower than that of the essential proteins (0.131, p = 1.32 × 10^{-5}) and the other proteins (0.155, p = 0.020). Similarly, we found that the average clustering coefficient of the OCG proteins was 0.118, which was significantly lower than that of the essential proteins (p = 0.001), though only slightly lower than that of the other proteins (p = 0.087). We also found that the clustering coefficient of the essential proteins was significantly lower that of the other proteins(p = 0.004). To obtain the detailed distribution of clustering coefficients, we separated the clustering coefficients into different bins with an interval of 0.1 and calculated the proportion of the proteins in each bin. We found that, the proportion of the TSG proteins (68.8%) was higher than that of the OCG proteins (55.1%) at bin (0–0.1]. In contrast, at bin (0–0.2], the proportion of the TSG proteins (18.8%) was lower than that of the OCG proteins (32.7%).

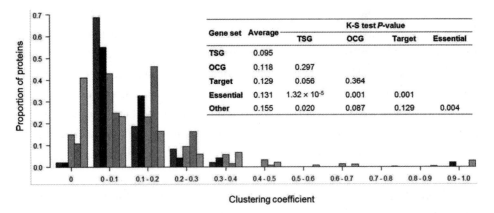

Gene set	Average	K-S test P-value			
		TSG	OCG	Target	Essential
TSG	0.095				
OCG	0.118	0.297			
Target	0.129	0.056	0.364		
Essential	0.131	1.32 × 10^{-5}	0.001	0.001	
Other	0.155	0.020	0.087	0.129	0.004

Figure 3. Distribution of clustering coefficient of five protein sets. The inserted table summarizes the average value of clustering coefficient for each protein set and the corresponding P-values based on the Kolmogorov-Smirnov (K-S) tests for any two protein sets.

3.5. TSGs and OCGs Tended to Have Shorter Shortest-Path Distance

For each node, the shortest-path distance (SPD) was calculated from the node to all other nodes in the human PPI network. To summarize the measure, we utilized the average value of all shortest path distances to represent its shortest-path distance to others. **Figure 4** shows the distribution of the SPD values, the average value of each protein set, and K-S test p-values among the five protein sets. The average shortest-path distance of the TSG proteins was 2.93, which was significantly shorter than that of the target proteins (3.18, p = 1.0 × 10^{-4}), or the other proteins (3.47, p = 5.03 × 10^{-18}). Interestingly, the average shortest-path distance of TSG proteins (2.93) was slightly lower than that of OCG proteins (2.98, p = 0.040). The average shortest-path distance of target proteins (3.18) was significantly longer than that of the essential proteins (3.00, p = 5.80 × 10^{-7}) but significantly shorter than that of the other proteins (3.47, p = 6.29 × 10^{-17}). While the proportion of shortest-path distances at each distance varied between the different sets, there were still a few similarities. In detail, from the shortest-path distance distribution at each distance, the proportion of proteins of different sets had much difference. For example, most proteins in each protein set have a shortest-path distance of 3.

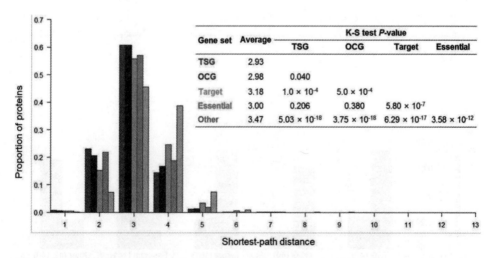

Figure 4. Distribution of shortest-path distance from five protein sets to the other nodes in human protein-protein interaction network. The inserted table summarizes the average value of shortest-path distance from each protein set to the rest nodes in human protein protein interaction network and the corresponding P-values based on the Kolmogorov-Smirnov (K-S) tests for any two protein sets.

3.6. From Targets to TSGs or OCGs in the Human PPI Network

Most drugs exert their therapeutic actions through interactions with specific protein targets. Moreover, the TSGs and OCGs play important roles in the cancer development. Then, we compared the shortest-path distances from targets to TSG proteins or OCG proteins with the shortest-path distances from targets to essential proteins and other proteins. **Figure 5(A)** shows the fraction of each protein set in the drug target neighborhood with a measure of shortest-path distance from zero to eight. Among the 161 drug target proteins, 13 also belong to the OCGs and 8 belong to essential proteins. The rest of the OCG proteins (73%) and all TSG proteins (100%) were enriched at the shortest-path distances 1 and 2 from target proteins, which is consistent with the previous results of drug targets to cancer genes[31]. Additionally, most of the TSG proteins (75%), OCG proteins (61%), and target proteins (75%) had direct interactions with protein targets while other proteins (22%) had less direct interactions with protein targets [**Figure 5(B)**].

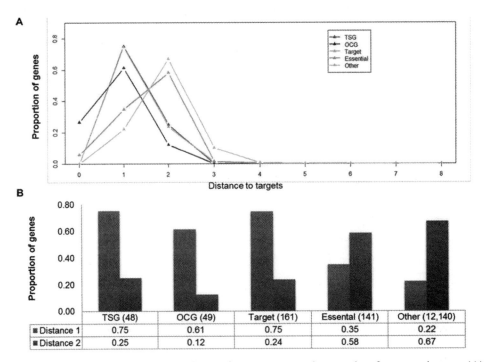

Figure 5. Network-based relationship between target proteins to other four protein sets. (A) Distribution of shortest-path distance of five gene sets. (B) Protein proportion at the shortest-path distance 1 and 2 from target proteins to TSG proteins or OCG proteins.

In summary, compared to the target proteins, essential proteins, and other proteins, both TSG and OCG proteins tended to have higher degrees, higher betweenness, lower clustering coefficients, and shorter shortest-path distances. Moreover, the TSG and OCG proteins did not have a significant difference with perspective of network topological properties. Both TSG proteins and OCG proteins tended to have more direct interactions with target proteins.

3.7. TSGs and OCGs Are Highly Connected

To further understand the relationship between TSG and OCG proteins in the local network organization and environment, we hypothesized that exploring TSG and OCG network would provide some novel insights. Then we generated one TSG-OCG network starting from the human PPI networks, 50 TSG proteins, and 50 OCG proteins.

The TSG-OCG network consisted of the 106 nodes and 303 edges (**Figure 6**). Among the 106 nodes, 48 belonged to the TSG proteins, which accounted for 96% of all the TSG proteins; 49 belonged to the OCG proteins, which accounted for 98% of all the OCG proteins; and 9 were linkers. The composition of the network indicated that the TSG-OCG network mainly consisted of the TSG and OCG proteins. Among the 303 edges, 89 links occurred among 42 TSG proteins, 51 among 36 OCGs, 117 among the 71 proteins (38 TSGs and 33 OCGs), and 46 between 9 linkers and 15 TSGs or 26 OCGs. Thus, 257 edges (84.8%) existed among TSGs and OCGs, suggesting that the TSG proteins and the OCG proteins were highly connected to each other in the context of protein-protein interaction networks. Moreover, the proportion of these links between the 38 TSGs and 33 OCGs (38.7%) were higher than that of interactions among the TSGs (29.5%) and that of interactions among OCGs (16.9%), respectively. Most of the TSGs (38, 79%) had at least one edge with OCGs. Similarly, most of the OCGs (67%) had at least one edge with TSGs.

To further explore the joint contribution of mutations in TSGs and OCGs, we integrated the mutation frequency of Pan-Cancer samples in each gene with the TSG-OCG network (**Figure 6**). The bigger node size represents the higher percentage of samples with mutations in Pan-Cancer project. The mutation frequency of the 106 genes encoding the 106 nodes in the TSG-OCG network ranged from

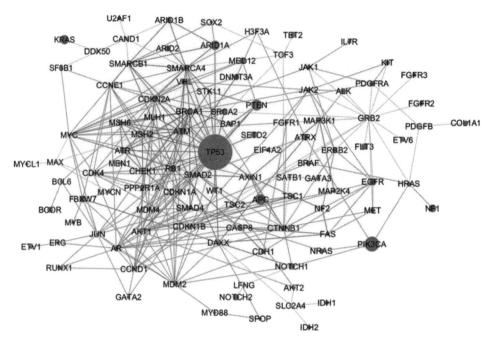

Figure 6. TSG-OCG network. Node color indicates the different protein sets: red for TSG proteins, blue for OCG proteins, and green for linkers that could link TSG proteins and OCG proteins. Edge color indicates protein-protein interaction among different protein sets: red for the interactions among TSG proteins, blue for the interactions among OCG proteins, dark green for the interactions between TSG proteins and OCG proteins, and gray for the interactions between linkers and OCG proteins or TSG proteins. Node size is corresponds to the mutation frequency in Pan-Cancer samples. The larger the node, the higher the frequency was.

0.33% to 46.15% with the average value of 3.14%. We further examined the correlation between the mutation frequency and degree of proteins using Pearson's correlation. We found that the mutation frequency and degree of proteins had a significant correlation (r = 0.30, P-value = 0.002). The observation indicated that the higher direct associations among these genes with higher mutation frequencies might contribute to the cancer development jointly. For example, TP53 had the highest mutation frequency in all samples and had 26 interactors. Among them, 21 were TSGs and four OCGs. Among the 21 TSGs, gene PTEN is another TSG gene with higher mutation frequency (11.27%), which might indicate that they might contribute to the cancer development together. In fact, several studies have demonstrated that that the PTEN and T53 genes jointly participate in the carcinogenesis o may malignancies[32]. Similarly, another example is the gene ARID1A that has an association with TP53 and had a higher mutation frequency (11.27%). One previous study has shown that one mutation in the gene associated with mismatch repair efficiency and normal p53 expression[33].

4. Discussion

Cancer is a genetically complex disease, which involves the combined functions of tumor suppressor genes (TSGs) and oncogenes (OCGs). TSGs and OCGs jointly play important roles in the cancer development through loss of function or gain of function. Most of them cannot trigger the cancer development by themselves. Numerous studies about genetic alterations of TSGs and OCGs, especially OCGs, have led to the identification of drug targets for cancer treatment. However, the identification of novel drug targets has become more challenging even though genome-wide sequencing data provide thousands of mutations. Therefore, development of novel approaches for identification of novel drug target is mandatory. To facilitate the development of novel approaches, in this study, we comprehensively compared TSGs and OCGs from the perspectives of somatic mutation and network properties. These broad comparative results allow us to address several questions that might be useful for the development of new methods: 1) Do TSGs and OCGs have similar or different mutation frequency patterns? 2) How do they relate to each other? 3) How do they relate to cancer drug target? 4) Do the TSGs and OCGs tend to link closely to each other? The results indicated that while the TSGs and OCGs had different mutation patterns, they had similar network characteristics. They were also not only related to each other closely, but also to cancer drug targets.

In this study, we mainly focused on the examination of the mutation patterns of TSGs and OCGs from the whole-genome wide data in the Pan-Cancer project[23]. It was different from the purpose of the Pan-Cancer analysis project. The study of Pan-Cancer analysis presents the data and analytical results for point mutations and small insertions/deletions from 3,281 tumours across 12 tumour types as part of the TCGA Pan-Cancer effort. They illustrated the distributions of mutation frequencies, types and contexts across tumour types, and establish their links to tissues of origin, environmental/ carcinogen influences, and DNA repair defects. However, they did not go further to examine the mutation patterns of TSGs and OCGs. In this study, we separated the mutation data of TSGs and OCGs from the rest genes and performed a comparison of five gene sets. We found that the TSGs had the highest mutation frequency in most tumour types and the OCGs second. The results might be interpreted by the theory that the gain-of-function mutations that convert proto-oncogenes to oncogenes acts dominantly while the loss-of- function mutation in tumor suppressor genes acts recessively. In addition, we observed that the essential genes had the lowest mutation frequency in all tumor types, which might reflect the fundamental roles in the survival of the essential genes.

However, we did not dive further to study the consequence of or causal relation to mutations for the function roles of TSGs and OCGs. As we know that TSGs and OCGs have different roles during the cancer development. However, it is not very clear how they work together. It will be very interesting and useful to further study the association between the mutation frequency and the roles of TSGs and OCGs. For example, we observed that the mutation frequency of TSGs was about two times of that of OCGs. It is not clear whether or not this mutation frequency difference influence or linked to their functional roles in the pathogenesis of cancer. Moreover, it is very challenging to assess the association between the mutation frequency difference and functional roles of TSGs and OCGs by both computational and experimental examination.

In this study, we compared the drug target genes with TSGs and OCGs in the view of mutation frequencies and network properties. We found drug target genes generally tend to have less mutations compared to TSGs and OCGs and also have lower degrees. These results suggested that the genetic contribution of drug target genes is not strong as TSGs and OCGs. Besides, we found both TSG and OCG proteins tended to have direct interactions with cancer drug target proteins. However, we did not further examine if the drug targets either suppress actions on oncogene activity or restore TSG functions through direct interaction or indirectly interactions. It might be very interesting to further examine if the mutations in OCGs or TSGs are necessary for both the establishment and maintenance of protein-protein interactions, which might lead to the identification of logical drug targets. However, to map the mutation to proteins for detecting the mutation-specific perturbations at the network level need much efforts including the development of protein structure-guided pipeline for extracting interacting protein sets specific to a particular mutation, which is beyond of the scape of this study. In the future, we will integrate the protein structure information with mutation information in the context of PPI network to further understand the connection of TSG and OCG proteins in the cancer development.

The study was mainly based on the data coming from both public data and predicted results. As most of the computational biology studies, it is very challenging to obtain the error-free or complete data. Therefore, in the analysis process, there still have several steps we could improve in the future, including the selection of gene sets, specification of protein function association data, and mutation data of cancer with less bias. For gene sets, we chose the genes with high confidence for analysis. The data set used here are far from complete and error-free. For the protein associations, we utilized the PPI data from PINA database, which includes the physical association, genetic association, and enzymatic reaction curated from six other databases. It is not clear about how these mutations alter the interaction relationship with their partners. For mutation data from cancer patients, we mainly utilized the data from TCGA, which might be biased by sequencing depth, platform, and sample size. However, our analysis still provided statistically significant characteristics of somatic mutations and networks of TSGs and OCGs. The list of TSGs and OCGs is updated frequently based on different methods. Therefore, the characteristics of TSGs and OCGs under investigation will not be exactly the same as those we concluded here. However, the tendencies we obtained in this study might provide some clues for further investigation of functional roles of TSGs and OCGs in carcinogenesis and identification of novel drug targets.

5. Conclusion

In this study, we explored the somatic mutation and network characteristics of TSGs and OCGs. Based on the mutation data from Pan-Cancer project, we found that the TSGs had the highest mutation frequency. Based on the human protein-protein interaction network, we found that TSG proteins and OCG proteins had similar global network topological characteristics and that the TSGs, OCGs, and drug targets had a tendency to interact with each other. Integration of mutation frequency with TSG-OCG network provided insights that TSGs and OCGs might jointly contribute to the cancer development. In summary, this study first comprehensively investigated TSGs and OCGs from the perspective of genetics and networks, which provides novel insight into the roles of TSGs and OCGs in cancer development and treatment.

Competing Interests

The authors declare that they have no competing interests.

Authors' Contributions

KZ, QL, JS conducted data collection and data analysis. YZ participated the data analysis. JS and HX conceived and designed the study. KZ, JS, YZ, CT, ZZ, and HX contributed to the writing of the manuscript. All authors read and approved the final manuscript.

Acknowledgements

This project is partially supported by a Cancer Prevention & Research Institute of Texas (CPRIT R1307) Rising Star Award to Dr. Hua Xu and R01LM011829 to Dr. Cui Tao.

Declaration

The publication funding came from Cancer Prevention & Research Institute of Texas (CPRIT R1307).

This article has been published as part of BMC Genomics Volume 16 Supplement 7, 2015: Selected articles from The International Conference on Intelligent Biology and Medicine (ICIBM) 2014: Genomics. The full contents of the supplement are available online at http://www.biomedcentral.com/bmcgenomics/supplements/16/S7.

Source: Zhu K, Qi L, Zhou Y, et al. Oncogenes and tumor suppressor genes: comparative genomics and network perspectives[J]. Bmc Genomics, 2015, 16(S7): 1–11.

References

[1] Society AC: Global cancer facts & figures 2nd edition. American Cancer Society 2011.

[2] Stratton MR, Campbell PJ, Futreal PA: The cancer genome. Nature 2009, 458(7239): 719–724.

[3] Cancer Genome Atlas Research Network: Comprehensive molecular characterization of urothelial bladder carcinoma. Nature 2014, 507(7492):315–322.

[4] Zhang L, Chen LH, Wan H, Yang R, Wang Z, Feng J, et al: Exome sequencing identifies somatic gain-of-function PPM1D mutations in brainstem gliomas. Nature Genetics 2014, 46(7):726–730.

[5] Hopkins AL, Groom CR: The druggable genome. Nat Rev Drug Discov 2002, 1(9):727–730.

[6] Eder J, Sedrani R, Wiesmann C: The discovery of first-in-class drugs: origins and evolution. Nat Rev Drug Discov. 2014, 13(8):577–587.

[7] Cancer Genome Atlas Research Network: Comprehensive genomic characterization defines human glioblastoma genes and core pathways. Nature 2008, 455(7216):1061–1068.

[8] Pleasance ED, Cheetham RK, Stephens PJ, McBride DJ, Humphray SJ, Greenman CD, et al: A comprehensive catalogue of somatic mutations from a human cancer genome. Nature 2010, 463(7278):191–196.

[9] International Cancer Genome Consortium, Hudson TJ, Anderson W, Artez A, Barker AD, Bell C, et al: International network of cancer genome projects. Nature 2010, 464(7291):993–998.

[10] Chin L, Hahn WC, Getz G, Meyerson M: Making sense of cancer genomic data. Genes Dev 2011, 25(6):534–555.

[11] Luo J, Solimini NL, Elledge SJ: Principles of cancer therapy: oncogene and non-oncogene addiction. Cell 2009, 136(5):823–837.

[12] Hahn WC, Weinberg RA: Modelling the molecular circuitry of cancer. Nature Rev Cancer 2002, 2(5):331–341.

[13] Chow AY: Cell cycle control by oncogenes and tumor suppressors: driving the transformation of normal cells into cancerous cells. Nature Education 2010, 3:7.

[14] Ideker T, Ozier O, Schwikowski B, Siegel AF: Discovering regulatory and signalling circuits in molecular interaction networks. Bioinformatics 2002, 18(Suppl 1):S233–S240.

[15] Hofree M, Shen JP, Carter H, Gross A, Ideker T: Network-based stratification of tumor mutations. Nat Methods 2013, 10(11):1108–1115.

[16] Akula N, Baranova A, Seto D, Solka J, Nalls MA, Singleton A, et al: A network-based approach to prioritize results from genome-wide association studies. PLoS One 2011, 6(9):e24220.

[17] Davoli T, Xu AW, Mengwasser KE, Sack LM, Yoon JC, Park PJ, Elledge SJ: Cumulative haploinsufficiency and triplosensitivity drive aneuploidy patterns and shape the cancer genome. Cell 2013, 155(4):948–962.

[18] Wrzeszczynski KO, Varadan V, Byrnes J, Lum E, Kamalakaran S, Levine DA: Identification of tumor suppressors and oncogenes from genomic and epigenetic features in ovarian cancer. PLoS One 2011, 6(12):e28503.

[19] Sun W, Qiao L, Liu Q, Chen L, Ling B, Sammynaiken R, Yang J: Anticancer activity of the PR domain of tumor suppressor RIZ1. Int J Med Sci 2011, 8(2):161–167.

[20] Zhao M, Sun J, Zhao Z: Distinct and competitive regulatory patterns of tumor suppressor genes and oncogenes in ovarian cancer. PLoS One 2012, 7(8):e44175.

[21] Berger AH, Knudson AG, Pandolfi PP: A continuum model for tumour suppression. Nature 2011, 476(7359):163–169.

[22] Osborne C, Wilson P, Tripathy D: Oncogenes and tumor suppressor genes in breast cancer: potential diagnostic and therapeutic applications. Oncologist 2004, 16(4):361–377.

[23] Kandoth C, McLellan MD, Vandin F, Ye K, Niu B, Lu C, et al: Mutational landscape and significance across 12 major cancer types. Nature 2013, 502(7471):333–339.

[24] Cowley MJ, Pinese M, Kassahn KS, Waddell N, Pearson JV, Grimmond SM, et al: PINA v2.0: mining interactome modules. Nucleic Acids Res 2012, 40(Database):D862–D865.

[25] Futreal PA, Coin L, Marshall M, Down T, Hubbard T, Wooster R, et al: A census of human cancer genes. Nature Rev Cancer 2004, 4(3):177–183.

[26] Knox C, Law V, Jewison T, Liu P, Ly S, Frolkis A, et al: DrugBank 3.0: a comprehensive resource for "omics" research on drugs. Nucleic Acids Res 2011, 39(Database):D1035–D1041.

[27] Sun J, Zhao Z: A comparative study of cancer proteins in the human protein-protein interaction network. BMC Genomics 2010, 11(Suppl 3):S5.

[28] Barabasi AL, Oltvai ZN: Network biology: understanding the cell's functional organization. Nature Rev Gen 2004, 5(2):101–113.

[29] Zheng S, Zhao Z: GenRev: exploring functional relevance of genes in molecular networks. Genomics 2012, 99(3):183–188.

[30] Sun J, Jia P, Fanous AH, van den Oord E, Chen X, Riley BP, et al: Schizophrenia gene networks and pathways and their applications for novel candidate gene selection. PLoS One 2010, 5(6):e11351.

[31] Yildirim MA, Goh KI, Cusick ME, Barabasi AL, Vidal M: Drug-target network. Nature Biotechnol 2007, 25(10):1119–1126.

[32] Janiec-Jankowska A, Konopka B, Goluda C, Najmola U: TP53 mutations in endometrial cancers: relation to PTEN gene defects. Int J Gynecol Cancer 2010, 20(2):196–202.

[33] Allo G, Bernardini MQ, Wu RC, Shih Ie M, Kalloger S, Pollett A, et al: ARID1A loss correlates with mismatch repair deficiency and intact p53 expression in high-grade endometrial carcinomas. Mod Pathol 2014, 27(2):255–261.

Chapter 6

Tumor Loci and Their Interactions on Mouse Chromosome 19 That Contribute to Testicular Germ Cell Tumors

Rui Zhu[1], Angabin Matin[2]

[1]Department of Systems Medicine and Bioengineering, Houston Methodist Research Institute, Houston, Texas 77030, USA
[2]Department of Genetics, The University of Texas M.D. Anderson Cancer Center, Houston, Texas 77030, USA

Abstract: Background: Complex genetic factors underlie testicular germ cell tumor (TGCT) development. One experimental approach to dissect the genetics of TGCT predisposition is to use chromosome substitution strains, such as the 129. MOLF-Chr 19 (M19). M19 carries chromosome (Chr) 19 from the MOLF whereas all other chromosomes are from the 129 strain. 71% of M19 males develop TGCTs in contrast to 5% in 129 strain. To identify and map tumor loci from M19 we generated congenic strains harboring MOLF chromosome 19 segments on 129 strain background and monitored their TGCT incidence. Results: We found 3 congenic strains that each harbored tumor promoting loci that had high (14%–32%) whereas 2 other congenics had low (4%) TGCT incidences. To determine how multiple loci influence TGCT development, we created double and triple congenic strains. We found additive interactions were predominant when 2 loci were combined in double congenic strains. Surprisingly, we found an example where 2 loci, both which do not contribute significantly to TGCT, when combined in a double congenic strain resulted in greater than expected TGCT incidence (positive interaction). In an opposite example, when 2 loci with high TGCT incidences were combined, males of the double congenic showed lower than expected TGCT incidence (negative interaction). For the triple congenic strain, depending on the analysis, the overall TGCT incidence could be additive or could also be due to a positive interaction of one region with others. Additionally, we identified loci that promote bilateral tumors or testicular abnormalities. Conclusions: The congenic strains each with their characteristic TGCT incidences, laterality of tumors and incidence of testicular abnormalities, are useful for identification of TGCT susceptibility modifier genes that map to Chr 19 and also for studies on the genetic and environmental causes of TGCT development. TGCTs are a consequence of aberrant germ cell and testis development. By defining predisposing loci and some of the locus interactions from M19, this study further advances our understanding of the complex genetics of TGCTs, which is the most common cancer in young human males.

Keywords: Congenic Strain, Chromosome Substitution Strain, M19, Testicular Germ Cell Tumor, Modifiers, Epistasis

1. Background

Testicular germ cell tumors (TGCTs) are the most common cancers that afflict young men. Higher incidence of TGCTs in certain ethnic groups and in men with a family history of TGCTs[1]–[3] indicates a strong genetic predisposition to this cancer. Some of the genes, genetic loci and signaling pathways that contribute to TGCTs have been identified[4]–[9]. These data indicate that multiple genetic defects contribute to TGCT development and that individual genes contribute with relatively modest effects. Thus additional genetic defects that contribute to TGCT predisposition are yet to be identified.

Most TGCTs initiate in utero even though the disease becomes evident decades after birth. The majority of testicular tumors originate from germ cells[10][11]. In mice, TGCTs occur on the 129 strain background and resemble the prepubertal, pediatric TGCTs that occur in humans[12]. 5% of 129/Sv (129S1/ SvImJ) males spontaneously develop TGCTs[13]–[16]. Defects in genes such as DMRT1 or KITLG are associated with TGCTs in both humans and mice[9][17]–[20] indicating that some of the underlying genetic causes of TGCT development is shared among mice and humans.

The present work is further extension of earlier studies in which a genome-wide linkage scan analysis revealed that multiple loci from MOLF chromosome (Chr) 19 contributed to TGCT development[21][22]. This result was initially surprising because the MOLF strain is TGCT resistant and not known to harbor TGCT predisposing loci. However, to verify the linkage result, a consomic mouse strain was made, the 129. MOLF-Chr 19 (or M19)[21][22]. In M19, Chr 19 of 129 is replaced with that of MOLF whereas all its other chromosomes are from the 129 strain. It is known that males of the 129 mouse strain are inherently susceptible to develop TGCTs at a low frequency whereas the MOLF strain is TGCT resistant. However, 71% of M19 males developed TGCTs[16][22], which confirmed the linkage analysis results. The MOLF strain, and thus Chr 19 from MOLF, belongs to the subspecies Mus musculus molossinus, whereas 129 strain is Mus musculus domesticus[23]. Thus the M19 strain, derived from interspecific crosses, shows a more extreme, transgressive phenotype compared to its parental strains[24]. This indicates that genes from MOLF Chr 19, when placed on a 129 strain background, contribute to TGCT development. More specifically, polymorphisms between MOLF compared to 129 genes on Chr 19 likely aberrantly affect germ cell and testicular development resulting in high rate of TGCTs in M19. In support of the role of Chr 19 in TGCT development, 3 genes that map to Chr 19 have been shown to positively or negatively impact TGCT development. Pten deficiency increases TGCT incidence in mice[25]. Dmrt1 deficiency increases TGCT incidence on the 129 strain background[19]. Thus, Dmrt1 is a modifier, that is, it magnifies TGCT incidence of the 129 strain but does not cause TGCTs in all strain backgrounds. Decreased Sf1 (Splicing factor 1) levels lowers TGCT incidence in mice[26]. Thus, the importance of mapping genetic loci as a first step towards the systematic identification of other genes on Chr 19 that contribute to TGCTs.

In an earlier study, we utilized a panel of congenic strains derived from the M19 strain to map TGCT loci on Chr 19[16]. Most of the congenics carried large segments (7 congenics carried 12cM to 34cM segments and 3 congenics had less than 10cM segments) of MOLF Chr 19 on the 129 background, and the MOLF segments in the different congenics overlapped to a great extent. Based on the tumor incidences of the congenics, we predicted that there are five MOLF-derived regions that harbor candidate TGCT modifier loci.

To further define the boundaries of TGCT modifier loci, in this study we generated congenic strains which carry smaller segments of MOLF Chr 19 and which lie within the predicted regions. Our results show that there are three TGCT susceptibility loci on Chr 19 that independently promote TGCT development. In addition, we find additive and epistatic interactions between loci that influence TGCT development in the M19. Interestingly, we found instances where 2 loci, both with either low or high TGCT incidences, when combined, contributed epistatically to higher or lower than expected TGCT incidences, respectively. Moreover, we found tumor loci that promote development of bilateral tumors (tumors that occur in both testes simultaneously) as opposed to loci that predispose tumor development in any one testis and loci that contribute to extremely high incidence of abnormal testes. Our results provide further novel insights into the complex genetics of TGCT development.

2. Results

2.1. Generation of Congenic Strains

For an earlier study, we made congenic mouse strains that carried large segments, mostly 12–34cM, of MOLF Chr 19 on a 129 background[16]. Based on the tumor incidences of these congenic strains, the data predicted the existence of 5 regions (regions I, II, III, IV and V) within Chr 19 that harbor TGCT susceptibility genes. The predicted regions I-V are indicated in **Figure 1(A)**. To test the predictions and to further map the extent of the TGCT susceptibility regions, we generated new congenic mouse strains that carry smaller (less than 10Mb or 8cM) MOLF Chr 19 segments on 129 background. The new congenic strains contain MOLF-derived segments that lie within Regions I, II and V and are named Congenic 5, 6 and 7. The MOLF segment in congenic 6 is slightly larger than predicted region II and in congenic 7 is smaller than predicted region V. Congenic 3 (also known as congenic-L1) which harbors 4.1Mb (3.7cM) region III[27] and B-81

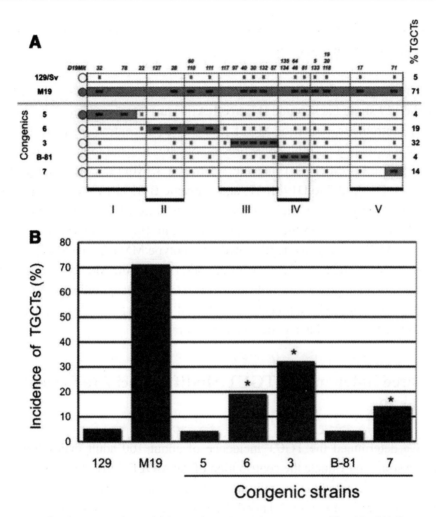

Figure 1. Single congenics within regions I to V on mouse Chr 19. (A) Representation of mouse chromosome 19 with centromere on left. Chr 19 of 129/Sv (represented in white), MOLF M19 (green) and MOLF segments (green) on 129/Sv background (white) in single congenic mouse strains. MOLF-derived segments are homozygous for MOLF alleles, represented by the MM genotype. 129-derived homozygous segments are represented by II genotype. Polymorphic SSLP markers between MOLF and 129 (starting at D19Mit32 near the centromere) used for genotyping, are shown on the top. Names of each congenic strain are listed on the left. TGCT incidence of 129/Sv, M19 and congenics are on the right. The five predicted regions (I-V) are aligned with markers and shown at the bottom of the figure. (B) Bar graph represents TGCT incidences of 129, M19 and single congenic strains. *Indicates that TGCT incidence is significantly different from that of 129.

with 1.4Mb (3cM) region IV[16] have been described previously and we include these strains in our analysis here.

The congenics 5, 6, 3, B-81 and 7 harbor consecutive regions of MOLF Chr 19 on the 129 strain background [**Figure 1(A)**]. Thus, congenic 5 harbors a 4.3Mb (2.3cM) centromeric region of MOLF Chr 19 (from centromere to D19Mit78), congenic 6 harbors a 9.4Mb (7.1cM) region of MOLF distal to that in congenic 5 (D19Mit127 to D19Mit111). Congenic 3 carries a 4.1Mb (3.7cM) region distal to congenic 6 (D19Mit97 to D19Mit57) and congenic B-81 has 1.4Mb (3cM) MOLF region (D19Mit135 to D19Mit81). Congenic 7 contains a 1.7Mb (0.6cM) region of MOLF from D19Mit71 to the telomere end of Chr 19. All congenics are homozygous for MOLF segments (represented as genotype MM) for the SSLP markers. Details regarding creation of congenics are described in the Methods Section. Because the previous study had indicated that TGCT susceptibility loci were not present between the SSLP markers D19Mit5 and D19Mit17 (10.2Mb, 8.0cM), this region is not represented in any new congenic strain[16].

2.2. Three Independent TGCT Modifier Loci Are Present on Chr 19

We determined the TGCT incidence of about 100 adult males from each congenic strain to evaluate the contribution of the MOLF-derived regions to tumor development. We noted the overall tumor incidence as well as the laterality of the tumors (unilateral tumor or bilateral testicular tumors) (**Table 1**). Our results showed that three of the five congenics had testicular tumor incidences higher than the expected background rate of tumor development found in the 129 strain [**Figure 1(B)**]. The tumor incidences of the males of Congenic 6, 3, and 7 were 19% (P < 0.01), 32% (P < 0.0001) and 14% (P = 0.062), respectively. In contrast, the tumor incidences of the males of Congenic 5 and B-81 were both 4%. (TGCT incidences of congenic 3 and B-81 have been reported previously[16][27]). A TGCT incidence of 4% is similar to that of the 129/Sv strain (5%) and is considered a "background" rate. The higher than background rate of TGCTs in congenics 6, 3 and 7 indicate that loci encompassing regions II, III and V harbor MOLF-derived TGCT predisposing genes which increase tumor incidence when present on the 129 strain background. Overall, these congenic strains clearly define three TGCT susceptibility, or modifier, loci that contribute to tumorigenesis.

Table 1. Incidence of testicular tumors and testicular abnormalities in the congenic strains.

Mouse strains	% TGCTs	No. with TGCT	% (no.) unilateral TGCTs	% (no.) bilateral TGCTs	% (no.) abnormal testes	No. of males examined
*129	5%	4	5% (4)	0	15% (12)	83
*M19	71%	85	39% (46)	33% (39)	5% (6)	119
Single congenics						
5	4%	4	3% (3)	1% (1)	24% (23)	96
6	19%	25	16% (21)	3% (4)	26% (35)	134
*3	32%	26	21% (18)	10% (8)	9% (7)	82
*B-81	4%	5	4% (5)	0	10% (13)	129
7	14%	18	12% (16)	2% (2)	5% (7)	133
Double congenics						
5 × 3	34%	47	26% (35)	9% (12)	12% (17)	137
5 × B-81	11%	14	9% (12)	2% (2)	16% (21)	133
5 × 7	8%	11	8% (10)	1% (1)	14% (18)	130
6 × B-81	10%	9	10% (9)	0	15% (13)	88
1	22%	38	20% (35)	2% (3)	6% (10)	171
3 × 7	26%	32	18% (22)	8% (10)	11% (13)	122
Triple congenic						
5 × 3× 7	37%	50	30% (40)	7% (10)	8% (11)	136

2.3. Negative and Positive Interactions between Congenic Regions

Next we examined whether the different regions of MOLF Chr 19 interact to additively increase TGCT incidence. The tumor incidences of congenic 6, 3 and 7 add up to 55% (see Methods for calculation), that is significantly less than the 71% TGCT incidence of M19 ($P < 0.05$). Thus, one possibility is that additional gene interactions likely account for the high TGCT incidence of M19. Alternately, although we followed the predictions of regions I-V to generate the new congenic strains, genes that map outside the MOLF segment boundaries and are not represented in the new congenics may affect TGCT susceptibility. In any case, to examine genetic interactions between the different regions, we combined the regions to create double and triple congenic regions and monitored TGCT incidences. First, we analyzed for interactions between two regions by calculating for expected additive effects and examining for any deviations from expected. A deviation from expected is considered an epistatic effect (interaction deviation)[28][29].

2.3.1. Primary Interactions of Region I (Congenic 5)

To test the interaction of region I with other loci, we generated the double congenics, 5 × 3 (meaning that the strain carries both congenic 5 and congenic 3 segments, homozygous for MOLF, in regions I and III), 5 × B-81 and 5 × 7 [**Figure 2(A)** and Additional file 1: Table 2]. We found that the TGCT incidence of congenic 5 × 3 (34%) was not significantly different from an expected additive effect of harboring regions I and III. The same was true for congenic 5 × 7 (Additional file 1: Table 2). Thus region I interacts additively with either regions III or V to increase TGCT incidences. In contrast, the double congenic strain 5 × B-81 had an elevated TGCT incidence (11%, P < 0.02) compared to the expected TGCT incidence (3%). This indicates a synergistic positive epistatic interaction between regions I and IV [**Figure 3(A)**]. Curiously, individually both regions I and IV (represented in congenics 5 and B-81, respectively) have low TGCT incidences (4% each).

2.3.2. Primary Interactions of Region II (Congenic 6)

In the double congenic 6 × B-81 (combining regions II and IV), the 10% tumor incidence can be accounted due to additive interactions between regions II and IV [**Figure 2(B)** and Additional file 1: Table 2].

2.3.3. Primary Interactions of Region III (Congenic 3)

Region III, in congenic 3, has the strongest independent effect on TGCT incidence compared to other regions (32% TGCT frequency). Region III interacts additively with either regions I or IV to increase TGCT incidences in congenic 5 × 3 and congenic 1, respectively [**Figure 2(A)**, **Figure 2(C)** and Additional file 1: Table 2]. However, there is negative epistatic interaction of region III with region

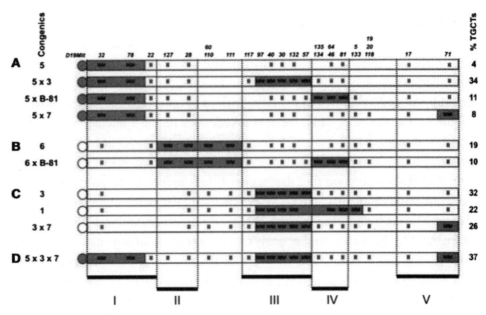

Figure 2. Single and double congenic strains. (A) Chr 19 of congenic 5 and derived double congenic strains 5 × 3, 5 × B-81 and 5 × 7. MOLF or 129-derived segments are in green and white, respectively. Homozygous MOLF and 129 alleles are indicated as MM and II, respectively. TGCT incidences of the congenics are on the right. (B) Chr 19 of congenic 6 and derived double congenic strains. (C) Chr 19 of congenic 3 and derived double congenic strains. (D) Chr 19 of triple congenic strain 5 × 3 × 7.

V resulting in lower than expected TGCT incidences (26% observed as opposed to 41% TGCT expected due to additive interaction, P < 0.02) in the double 3 × 7 congenic strain [**Figure 2(C)**]. Interestingly, individually both regions III and V (represented in congenics 3 and 7, respectively) have high TGCT incidences (32% and 14%, respectively).

2.3.4. Primary Interactions of Region IV (Congenic B-81) and Region V (Congenic 7)

The double congenics 5 × B-81, 6 × B-81, 1, 5 × 7 and 3 × 7 that test interactions of region IV and V, have been discussed above (**Figure 2** and Additional file 1: Table 2). The positive interaction of region IV with region I (in congenic 5 × B-81) and the negative interaction between regions V and III (congenic 3 × 7) have been described. Additive interactions account for increased TGCT incidences of the other double congenics.

2.3.5. Interactions between Multiple Loci

When multiple regions were present in a congenic strain as in 5 × 3 × 7 (which harbors regions I, III and V), the tumor incidence of 5 × 3 × 7 can be explained by an additive effect of the three regions [**Figure 2(D)** and Additional file 2: Table 3]. On the other hand, we also asked, does region I interact with regions III and V in congenic 5 × 3 × 7? The observed tumor incidence of congenic 5 (harboring region I) is 4% and congenic 3 × 7 (harboring regions III and V) is 26%. Using this observation, we find that region I does indeed show positive epistatic interaction with regions III and V [written as I (III, V)] as the observed TGCT incidence (37%) is higher than expected (25%, P < 0.04) (Additional file 2: Table 3 and Figure 3A). However, similar analysis for interaction of regions III with I and V [III (I, V)] and V with I and III [V (I, III)] show no unexpected interactions. Thus, positive epistatic interactions, between multiple regions in congenic strains, could contribute to higher than expected TGCT incidence and could be one reason for overall higher than expected incidence of TGCTs in M19.

2.4. Loci Promoting Bilateral Tumors

We evaluated the laterality of TGCTs in the panel of single, double and triple congenics (Additional file 3: Table 4). We compared the observed and expected unilateral and bilateral tumor incidences in each congenic and applied $\chi 2$ goodness-of-fit tests[16]. Two of the strains, congenics 5 and 3, showed significantly increased incidence of bilateral TGCTs (P < 0.04 and P < 0.03, respectively). This suggests that susceptibility loci for bilateral TGCTs are located within regions I and III. For example, in congenic 3, one out of every three affected males developed bilateral TGCTs. The double congenics which harbor region III, 5 × 3 and 3 × 7, also showed higher number of bilateral TGCT cases than would be expected. Although congenic 5 has a low TGCT incidence (4%), it was significant that 1 out of 4 males had bilateral TGCTs. In contrast, no bilateral tumors were observed when a similar sized cohort of 129/Sv and B-81 (both strains have 4% –5% TGCT incidence) were examined[16].

2.5. Incidence of Abnormal Testes in the Congenic Strains

While examining for testicular tumors, we observed that frequently males of

Table 2. Analysis for additive interactions between regions.

Region	Congenics	Observed incidence	Expected incidence	Test score ($\chi2$, P-value)
Region I				
I	5	0.04		
I.III	5 × 3	0.34	0.31	0.42, ns
I.IV	5 × B-81	0.11	0.03	5.96, P < 0.02
I.V	5 × 7	0.08	0.13	1.44, ns
Region II				
II	6	0.19		
II.IV	6 × B-81	0.10	0.18	2.28, ns
Region III				
III	3*	0.32		
III.I	5 × 3	0.34	0.31	0.42, ns
III.IV	1	0.22	0.31	3.37, ns
III.V	3 × 7	0.26	0.41	5.95, P < 0.02
Region IV				
IV	B-81*	0.04		
IV.I	5 × B-81	0.11	0.03	5.96, P < 0.02
IV.II	6 × B-81	0.10	0.18	2.28, ns
IV.III	1	0.22	0.31	3.37, ns
Region V				
V	7	0.14		
V.I	5 × 7	0.08	0.13	1.44, ns
V.III	3 × 7	0.26	0.41	5.95, P < 0.02

*Previously described congenic strains[16][27]; ns = no statistically significant difference between observed and expected values. Positive epistatic interactions are in green and negative epistatic interactions are in red.

some congenic strains had abnormal testes (**Table 1**). These testes were not tumorous but were grossly abnormal in shape or size. Often the abnormality affected one testis only. Histological examination of these abnormal testes frequently showed abnormal tubules and germ cells [**Figures 3(B)-3(D)**]. In congenics 5 and 6, close to a quarter (24% to 26%) of the males had abnormal testes. The abnormalities include cryptorchidism (undescended testes), atrophic calcified testes, dissociated dead testes, agonadism (missing testes), and hypoplastic testes with abnormal spermatogenesis [**Figure 3(D)**]. These abnormalities resemble human testicular defects[30][31] and our observations indicate that genes causing testicular abnormalities are localized in regions I and II of Chr 19. In other congenic strains, the incidence of abnormal testes ranged from 5% to 16%.

3. Discussion

Our previous study[16] had predicted the boundaries of multiple TGCT loci, additive effects and interactions between loci as well as a role for epigenetic modifications that result in high TGCT incidence in M19. However, the congenic mouse strains used in the previous study carried large MOLF segments making it difficult to ascertain the location and effects of TGCT-susceptibility loci with precision. In the present study, we generated and used congenic strains that carry smaller MOLF-derived segments so as to be able to test the predictions and define the effects and interactions of TGCT susceptibility loci with greater precision.

We first evaluated the regions I, II, III and V, which were previously predicted to harbor TGCT loci, by generating new congenic strains that harbor MOLF-derived segments encompassing these regions. Our results show that 3 regions, II, III, and V (in congenic strains 6, 3 and 7) contribute to higher than background frequencies of TGCTs. It is possible that genes located at the boundaries of regions I and V, which are not represented as MOLF segments in congenics 5 and 7, may harbor TGCT susceptibility genes. That could be one reason why congenic 5 (with region I) has low TGCT incidence of 4%. However, our analysis of double congenic strains show that although congenic 5 has low TGCT incidence, its MOLF segment interacts positively with other regions suggesting that this MOLF segment maps a "silent" region that under some circumstances can contribute to TGCT development. Congenic 7 has a 14% TGCT incidence, which is similar to the 16%–17% TGCT incidence predicted for region V[16]. This suggests that we have mapped this TGCT susceptibility loci to a 1.7Mb region between D19Mit71 to the telomere, in congenic 7.

When we analyzed for interactions between any two regions, we found that in most cases, tumor incidences were due to additive effects of two regions. This

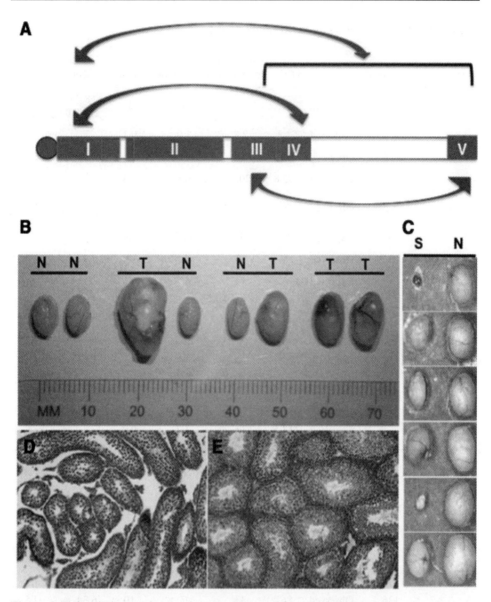

Figure 3. Epistatic interactions and testes abnormalities. (A) Epistatic interactions between regions. Bidirectional red arrows indicate positive epistatic interaction between regions I and IV and interaction of region I with (III.V). Bidirectional blue arrow indicates negative interaction between regions III and V. (B) TGCTs in congenic 3 mice. Specimens from left to right are: normal (N) pair of testes; tumor (T) in left testis and normal (N) right testis; normal left and tumor in right-testis; bilateral tumors in testes. (C) Abnormal testes from congenic 5 mice. Abnormal or small left testes (S) and normal (N) right testis. (D) Histological section of a small testis and (E) contralateral normal testis from congenic 5 mouse. In the small testes, spermatogenesis is arrested at specific stages. Few elongated spermatids are seen in the tubules.

Table 4. Laterality of TGCTs in the congenic strains.

Congenic strain	No. of males examined		No TGCT	Unilateral left tumor	Unilateral right tumor	Bilateral tumors	Test score	Left/ Right
5	96	Observed	92	2	1	1	8.76, P < 0.04	1.5
		Expected	91.3	2.8	1.9	0.1		
6	134	Observed	109	17	4	4	7.36, ns	2.7
		Expected	105.8	20.2	6.8	1.3		
3	82	Observed	56	10	8	8	8.97, P < 0.03	1.1
		Expected	51.2	14.4	12.8	3.6		
7	133	Observed	115	13	3	2	3.97, ns	2.8
		Expected	113.6	14	4.7	0.6		
5 × 3	137	Observed	90	20	15	12	8.37, P < 0.04	1.2
		Expected	84.4	25.2	21.1	6.3		
5 × B-81	133	Observed	119	8	4	2	5.73, ns	1.6
		Expected	116.2	10.1	6.1	0.5		
5 × 7	130	Observed	119	7	3	1	3.38, ns	2.0
		Expected	118.5	7.6	3.7	0.2		
6 × B-81	88	Observed	79	9	0	0	0, ns	All left
		Expected	79.2	8.8	0	0		
1	171	Observed	133	26	9	3	0.63, ns	2.4
		Expected	132	27	9.9	2		
3 × 7	122	Observed	90	12	10	10	16.98, P < 0.001	1.1
		Expected	84	18.4	16	3.5		
5 × 3 × 7	136	Observed	86	33	7	10	6.34, ns	2.5
		Expected	80.5	37.9	12	5.7		

ns = no statistically significant difference. Higher than Expected levels of Observed bilateral tumors are indicated in green.

was as predicted previously[16]. However, we also detected 2 unexpected epistatic effects. Regions I and IV interacted in a positive manner and the tumor incidence in double congenic strain 5 × B-81 was higher than expected. This was surprising, because individually regions I and IV (in congenic strains 5 and B-81) have low TGCT incidences Thus we name regions I and IV "silent regions" in terms of promoting TGCTs. These "silent regions" can interact with other regions to increase TGCT incidence. Interestingly, the presence of the "silent region" IV, but not I, was suggested in our previous study[16]. Overall, this indicates that TGCT mapping studies should be careful not to disregard loci with low tumor incidences because such regions could contribute with epistatic effects. Interestingly, males harboring the "silent" region I (in congenic 5) have higher incidence of testicular abnormalities and bilateral tumors, although the overall incidence of TGCT in this strain is low (4%). In an opposite example, regions III and V in double congenic strain 3 × 7 showed lower than expected TGCT incidence. Again this was surprising because individually both regions III and V have high TGCT incidences. Although we could only test double interactions of a limited number of regions, our results offer tantalizing insights regarding how widely separated regions on Chr 19 can interact additively or epistatically to affect tumor incidences.

When multiple regions were present within a congenic strain as in the triple congenic 5 × 3 × 7, the overall tumor incidence appears to be due to an additive effect. However, further analysis revealed that the tumor incidence could also be considered to be due to a positive interaction of region I (with inherently low TGCT incidence) with regions III and V. Again in this example, even though region I does not contribute significantly to TGCTs, this "silent region" appears to be important for epistatic interactions.

Thus, positive and negative interactions and the positive effect of "silent regions" likely contribute to the overall high incidence of TGCT in M19. At the molecular level, there are a number of reasons that could explain the unexpected positive or negative interactions between regions. For example, genes that have wide ranging effects such as transcription factors, splicing factors, miRNAs, etc., may account for the larger than expected increases or decreases in TGCT incidences when regions are combined. For example we identified Sf1[26], an alternate splicing factor from region I, that likely affects a broad range of targets in cells of the testes to modulate TGCT incidence. Thus, locus interactions likely reflect the overall cumulative effects of gene interactions between suppressors (such as Sf1) and enhancers of TGCT development (such as Dmrt1) that reside within the five regions mapped to Chr 19. However, most of the TGCT susceptibility genes from

M19 are yet to be identified.

Human genes involved in germ cell development, testicular dysgenesis, in-fertility and TGCT development likely reside in the orthologous regions mapped on mouse Chr 19. For example, region III is orthologous to human 9p24.1-9p24.3 (**Table 5**). Human disease loci which map to Chr 9p24 include DMRT1. Variants of DMRT1 have been shown to be associated with susceptibility to pediatric germ cell tumors as well as familial testicular germ cell tumors[20][32][33]. Dmrt1 is essen-tial for testes differentiation in vertebrates[34][35]. Deficiency of Dmrt1 in humans results in XY sex reversal and gonadal dysgenesis[36]-[39]. In mice, Dmrt1 null mu-tants on a C57BL/6 background develop severe testicular dysge- nesis but develop TGCTs on a 129 background[19]. Human genes related to gonadal dysfunction have so far not been reported to map to the other regions. In mice, a previous expression analysis study detected 3 transcripts, Sf1, D19Bwg1357 and Cox15, that were dif-ferentially expressed in the gonads of M19 compared to 129[27]. Sf1 maps to region I (congenic 5) and lowered Sf1 reduces TGCTs[26], which may be one reason why congenic 5 shows low TGCTs incidence. However, each locus may harbor more than one candidate TGCT gene. D19Bwg1357 and Cox15 map to region III (con-genic 3) and proximal to region V, respectively. The genetic effects of D19Bwg1357 or Cox15 on TGCT development are unknown.

In our earlier mapping study, loci encoding bilateral tumors were not de-tected[16]. We think that because the congenic strains harbored larger MOLF- de-rived segments harboring multiple regions, interactions among these regions likely masked the presence of loci encoding bilateral TGCTs. We found that loci for bi-lateral TGCT development are located in regions I and III. Our results

Table 5. Orthologous regions in the human genome corresponding to the five regions in mouse Chr 19.

Regions in mouse Chr 19	Mouse SSLP markers	Orthologous regions in humans
I	D19Mit32-D19Mit22	11q12.2-11q13.2
II	D19Mit22-D19Mit117	9q21.11-9q21.31
III	D19Mit117-D19Mit135	9p24.1-9p24.3
IV	D19Mit57-D19Mit5	10q23.1-10q23.32
V	D19Mit17-telomere	10q24.33-10q26.11

Source: www.ensembl.org.

indicate that unilateral and bilateral tumors are not caused by the same genetic factors. One possible scenario is that genes that cause development of unilateral or bilateral tumors affect primordial germ cells at different stages during germ cell migration. Germ cells are specified as a group of cells in the early embryo, which then proliferate and migrate through the embryo before splitting into two populations that each migrate towards the left or right genital ridges. Each genital ridge later develops into a testis. Genes causing bilateral tumors may be expressed and functional during early germ cell development and thus defects or polymorphisms in these genes would affect the entire germ cell population before they split to populate the left or right genital ridges. Thus, defects or disease-causing nucleotide polymorphisms in such genes is manifested as an excess of bilateral tumors. However, genes causing unilateral tumors may be expressed and function later during germ cell development, such as once germ cells have entered either the left or right genital ridges. Thus defects or polymorphisms in the late expressed genes likely manifests as unilateral tumors.

We observed that the TGCT frequency of the left testis is about 2-fold higher than that on the right (Additional file 3: Table 4). Most of the abnormal testes were also found on the left side, whereas the right-side was usually normal [**Figure 3(D)**]. The reason why left testes are more susceptible to abnormalities or TGCT development in mice is unclear. Our previous study[16] also detected a correlation between the length of MOLF-derived congenic segment in a strain and TGCT frequency, and that was suggested to be due to epigenetic modifications imposed by the 129 background on the MOLF-derived chromosome. However, when we examined whether MOLF-length is a significant predictor of TGCT frequency in our present study, we found only a moderate positive correlation (R = 0.42) between MOLF-length and TGCT frequency. The linear regression model of our current data suggests that MOLF-length is not a significant predictor of TGCT fre-quency (R^2 = 0.18; P = 0.17) (Additional file 4: Figure S1). One reason for the discrepancy between the two studies could be that the previous study used a total of 13 strains in which MOLF segments spanned 3cM to 52.6cM[16] and thus a correlation between length of MOLF segment and TGCT frequency was readily evident. In contrast, for the purpose of the present study, we utilized 12 strains (single, double and triple congenics) which harbored smaller MOLF regions (ranging from 0.6cM to 10.1cM). We think that because this study only examines a smaller, limited size range of MOLF-segments, the correlation between MOLF- length and TGCT frequency is not apparent.

The congenics reported here carry short segments of MOLF Chr 19 (10cM or less) and each has defined, quantitative incidences for TGCTs, bilateral tumors and testicular defects. Thus, these strains will be useful to study how exogenous agents can modulate TGCT incidences. As an example, congenic 3 has been used to study the role of radiation, endocrine disruptors and chemotherapeutic agents on TGCT incidences[40][41]. Moreover, detailed gene expression array analysis has identified a limited number of candidate TGCT genes that map to the different loci (data not shown) and future work will evaluate the contribution of these candidate genes to TGCT development and other testicular defects.

4. Conclusions

In summary, we have mapped three susceptibility loci on mouse Chr 19 that independently increases TGCT incidence. We found 2 regions on MOLF Chr 19 that contribute to bilateral TGCTs and 2 proximal regions that contribute to a very high incidence of testicular defects. Our results show that multiple loci on mouse Chr 19 together with their additive, negative and positive interactions affect germ cell and testes development to contribute to TGCTs. This study validates the use of chromosome substitution strain M19 to experimentally dissect the complex genetics of TGCT predisposition and further advances our understanding of the complex genetics of TGCTs, the most common cancer in young males.

5. Methods

5.1. Mouse Strains

The 129.MOLF-Chr 19 (M19)[22] and 129 (129S1/SvImJ; JR002448, Jackson Laboratory, Bar Harbor, ME, USA) strains have been described. Mice were maintained on a 12/12 hour light/dark cycle, and fed NIH-31 diet ad libitum.

5.2. Creation of Single, Double and Triple Congenic Strains

The single congenic strains were created as described[16][27]. Briefly the M19 strain was crossed to 129. Progeny were backcrossed to 129. Backcross progeny were genotyped for selected polymorphic SSLP markers that distinguish 129 and MOLF alleles, for example, marker D19Mit127 and D19Mit111 for generating congenic 6 [**Figure 1(a)**]. Mice whose genotypes were contiguously heterozygous for MOLF and 129 within the selected region and homozygous for 129 outside the region, were selected for further breeding. These selected mice were intercrossed to generate mice homozygous for MOLF containing segments. To verify the boundaries of the congenic regions, progeny were genotyped with additional SSLP markers spanning mouse Chr 19. SSLP markers used for genotyping are shown in **Figure 1(a)**. In **Figure 1(a)**, the homozygous MOLF regions on Chr 19 in each congenic strain are shown in green. For example, in congenic 6, markers D19Mit127 and D19Mit111 (and other SSLP markers in between) are homozygous for MOLF, indicated by genotype MM. Markers D19Mit22, D19Mit117 and others on Chr 19 are homozygous for 129 (indicated by genotype II) and are shown in white.

Double congenic and triple congenic strains harboring regions homozygous for MOLF (MM) alleles (**Figure 2**) were made by intercrossing appropriate single congenic strains followed by selection for homozygous pairs of F2 mice for further breeding and expansion of colony. For example, to create 5 × 7 strain, we first crossed congenic 5 female (homozygous for MOLF region 5) with congenic 7 male (homozygous for MOLF region 7). A pair of F1 male and female progeny (now heterozygous for MOLF-derived alleles in congenic region 5 and 7) were intercrossed. The F2 pups were genotyped and selected to identify pairs of males and females that were homozygous for both congenic 5 and congenic 7 MOLF-derived regions. Once selected, these homozygous 5 × 7 congenic male and female pairs were allowed to breed to produce homozygous 5 × 7 progeny and TGCT incidence in male progeny was assessed.

The experimental protocol was approved and conducted in compliance with Institutional Animal Care and Use Committee (IACUC) standards at MD Anderson Cancer Center.

5.3. Tumor Characterization

The 4–8 weeks old adult males were sacrificed and their testes examined for tumors. Tumors are usually detected visually at that age. In cases where it was unclear, testes were preserved in 10% phosphate-buffered formalin, sectioned and stained prior to microscopic examination for small tumors.

5.4. Statistical Testing for Interacting Loci on TGCT Susceptibility

$\chi 2$ goodness-of-fit tests were used to evaluate whether observed frequency of TGCT is statistically different from expected additive values. The expected additive TGCT frequencies were calculated based on the previously described equation[16]. A background, baseline TGCT incidence of the 129 strain of 5% was used. Briefly, the tumor incidence of a single congenic strain is the sum of the baseline effect and the effect of the MOLF congenic segment (QTL effect). Thus, a TGCT incidence of a single congenic of 10% = 5% (baseline) + 5% (QTL/due to MOLF congenic segment). The expected tumor incidence for double and triple congenic strains is the sum of the QTLs (due to congenic segments) plus the baseline effect. Thus the expected tumor incidence of combining 3 congenic regions (with QTL1, QTL2 and QTL3 of 10%, 15% and 20% respectively) in one mouse strain will be 35% (=5% QTL1 + 10% QTL2 + 15% QTL3 + 5% baseline).Thus expected additive incidence in mice with 2 QTLs (2 congenic regions) is calculated as: (observed QTL1-baseline) + (observed QTL2-baseline) + baseline. Similarly, the expected additive incidence of 3 QTLs (3 congenic regions) = (observed QTL1-baseline) + (observed QTL2-baseline) + (observed QTL3-baseline) + baseline. As one example, to estimate additive effects of region III with V in congenic 3 × 7, the TGCT incidences of congenic 3 (32%), congenic 7 (14%) and 129 background TGCT incidence of 5% was used. Therefore, the expected additive incidence is [(32%–5%) + (14%–5%) + 5%] = 41%. Because the observed TGCT incidence of congenic 3 × 7 (26%) is significantly lower than 41% (P < 0.02), this indicates that region III interacts epistatically with region V (Additional file 1: Table 2).

Interactions between multiple regions (Additional file 2: Table 3) were calculated in a similar manner but regarding multiple regions as one. For example, to test possible interaction of region I with regions III and V in congenic 5 × 3 × 7, the TGCT incidences of congenic 5 (4%) and congenic 3 × 7 (26%) were used.

Thus, the expected additive incidence of TGCTs by combining region I with III and V in [I(III.V)] is 25% = [(4%–5%) + (26%–5%) + 5%]. Because the observed TGCT incidence of congenic 5 × 3 × 7 (37%) differs significantly from 25% (P < 0.04), this indicates that region I interacts epistatically with regions III and V (Additional file 2: Table 3).

5.5. Statistical Testing for Effects on Tumor Laterality

The expected frequencies of unaffected, unilateral or bilateral TGCT cases in the congenic strains were calculated, as described in[16]. $\chi 2$ goodness-of-fit tests were performed to determine if bilateral TGCTs were occurring randomly or caused by distinct factors on Chr 19.

6. Additional Files

Additional file 1: Table S1. Analysis for additive interactions between regions.

Additional file 2: Table S2. Analysis for interactions between multiple regions.

Additional file 3: Table S3. Laterality of TGCTs in the congenic strains.

Additional file 4: Figure S1. Scatter plot of the length of MOLF-congenic segments (Mb) versus TGCT frequencies. The linear regression line: y = 1.485x + 8.704 is shown. (Residual standard error = 11.15 on 10 degrees of freedom; multiple R-squared = 0.178; adjusted R-squared = 0.09575; P-value = 0.172.).

7. Abbreviations

TGCTs: Testicular germ cell tumors; Chr: Chromosome; M19: 129. MOLFChr 19; SSLP: Simple sequence length polymorphism; cM: Centimorgan; Mb: Megabase.

Competing Interests

The authors declare they have no competing interests.

Authors' Contributions

RZ designed and performed the experiments, analyzed the data and wrote the manuscript. AM conceived the idea, designed the experiments, analyzed the data and wrote the manuscript. All authors read and approved the final manuscript.

Acknowledgements

We thank Glenda Seawood, Amatul Ali, Sara Ali and Ann Kong for assistance with mouse husbandry and genotyping. We thank J.H.Nadeau for reading the manuscript. This work was funded by David M. Carmines Cancer Research Fund, TC Hsu Faculty Research Award and funds from The Center for Stem Cell and Development Biology to AM.

Source: Zhu R, Matin A. Tumor loci and their interactions on mouse chromosome 19 that contribute to testicular germ cell tumors [J]. Bmc Genetics, 2014, 15(1): 1–12.

References

[1] Dieckmann K-P, Skakkebaek NE: Carcinoma in situ of the testis: review of biological and clinical features. Int J Cancer 1999, 83:815–822.

[2] Lutke Holzik MF, Sijmons RH, Sleijfer DT, Sonneveld DJ, Hoekstra-Weebers JE, van Echten-Arends J, Hoekstra HJ: Syndromic aspects of testicular carcinoma. Cancer 2003, 97(4):984–992.

[3] Hussain SA, Ma YT, Palmer DH, Hutton P, Cullen MH: Biology of testicular germ cell tumors. Expert Rev Anticancer Ther 2008, 8:1659–1673.

[4] Nathanson KL, Kanetsky PA, Hawes R, Vaughn DV, Letrero R, Tucker K, Friedlander M, Phillips K-A, Hogg D, Jewett MA, Lohynska R, Daugaard G, Richard S, Chompret A, Bonaïti-Pellié C, Heidenreich A, Olah E, Geczi L, Bodrogi I, Ormiston

WJ, Daly PA, Oosterhuis JW, Gillis AJ, Looijenga LH, Guilford P, Fosså SD, Heimdal K, Tjulandin SA, Liubchenko L, Stoll H: The Y deletion gr/gr and susceptibility to testicular germ cell tumor. Am J Hum Genet 2005, 77:1034–1043.

[5] Crockford GP, Linger R, Hockley S, Dudakia D, Johnson L, Huddart R, Tucker K, Friedlander M, Phillips KA, Hogg D, Jewett MA, Lohynska R, Daugaard G, Richard S, Chompret A, Bonaïti-Pellié C, Heidenreich A, Albers P, Olah E, Geczi L, Bodrogi I, Ormiston WJ, Daly PA, Guilford P, Fosså SD, Heimdal K, Tjulandin SA, Liubchenko L, Stoll H, Weber W: Genome-wide linkage screen for testicular germ cell tumour susceptibility loci. Hum Mol Genet 2006, 15:443–451.

[6] Linger R, Dudakia D, Huddart R, Easton D, Bishop DT, Stratton MR, Rapley EA: A physical analysis of the Y chromosome shows no additional deletions, other than Gr/Gr, associated with testicular germ cell tumour. Br J Cancer 2007, 96:357–361.

[7] Kanetsky PA, Mitra N, Vardhanabhuti S, Li M, Vaughn DJ, Letrero R, Ciosek SL, Doody DR, Smith LM, Weaver J, Albano A, Chen C, Starr JR, Rader DJ, Godwin AK, Reilly MP, Hakonarson H, Schwartz SM, Nathanson KL: Common variation in KITLG and at 5q31.3 predisposes to testicular germ cell cancer. Nat Genet 2009, 41:811–815.

[8] Rapley EA, Turnbull C, Al Olama AA, Dermitzakis ET, Linger R, Huddart RA, Renwick A, Hughes D, Hines S, Seal S, Morrison J, Nsengimana J, Deloukas P; UK Testicular Cancer Collaboration, Rahman N, Bishop DT, Easton DF, Stratton MR: A genome-wide association study of testicular germ cell tumor. Nat Genet 2009, 41:807–810.

[9] Turnbull C, Rapley EA, Seal S, Pernet D, Renwick A, Hughes D, Ricketts M, Linger R, Nsengimana J, Deloukas P, Huddart RA, Bishop DT, Easton DF, Stratton MR, Rahman N; UK Testicular Cancer Collaboration: Variants near DMRT1, TERT and ATF7IP are associated with testicular germ cell cancer. Nat Genet 2010, 42:604–607.

[10] Skakkebaek NE, Berthelsen JG, Giwercman A, Muller J: Carcinoma-in-situ of the testis: possible origin from gonocytes and precursor of all types of germ cell tumours except spermatocytoma. Int J Androl 1987, 10(1):19–28.

[11] Oosterhuis JW, Looijenga LHJ: Testicular germ-cell tumours in a broader perspective. Nat Rev Cancer 2005, 5:210–222.

[12] Rescorla FJ: Pediatric germ cell tumors. Semin Surg Oncol 1999, 16:144–158.

[13] Stevens LC, Hummel KP: A description of spontaneous congenital testicular teratomas in strain 129 mice. J Natl Cancer Inst 1957, 18:719–747.

[14] Stevens LC: Embryology of testicular teratomas in strain 129 mice. J Natl Cancer Inst 1959, 23:1249–1295.

[15] Stevens LC: Testicular teratomas in fetal mice. J Natl Cancer Inst 1962, 28:247–267.

[16] Youngren KK, Nadeau JH, Matin A: Testicular cancer susceptibility in the 129.MOLF-Chr 19 mouse strain: additive effects, gene interactions and epigenetic

modifications. Hum Mol Genet 2003, 12:389–398.

[17] Looijenga LH, Hersmus R, Gillis AJ, Pfundt R, Stoop HJ, van Gurp RJ, Veltman J, Beverloo HB, van Drunen E, van Kessel AG, Pera RR, Schneider DT, Summersgill B, Shipley J, McIntyre A, van der Spek P, Schoenmakers E, Oosterhuis JW: Genomic and expression profiling of human spermatocytic seminomas: primary spermatocyte as tumorigenic precursor and DMRT1 as candidate chromosome 9 gene. Cancer Res 2006, 66:290–302.

[18] Heaney JD, Lam M-YJ, Michelson MV, Nadeau JH: Loss of the transmembrane but not the soluble Kit ligand isoform increases testicular germ cell tumor susceptibility in mice. Cancer Res 2008, 68:5193–5197.

[19] Krentz AD, Murphy MW, Kim S, Cook MS, Capel B, Zhu R, Matin A, Sarver AL, Parker KL, Griswold MD, Looijenga LH, Bardwell VJ, Zarkower D: The DM domain protein DMRT1 is a dose-sensitive regulator of fetal germ cell proliferation and pluripotency. Proc Natl Acad Sci U S A 2009, 106:22323–22328.

[20] Kanetsky PA, Mitra N, Vardhanabhuti S, Vaughn DJ, Li M, Ciosek SL, Letrero R, D'Andrea K, Vaddi M, Doody DR, Weaver J, Chen C, Starr JR, Håkonarson H, Rader DJ, Godwin AK, Reilly MP, Schwartz SM, Nathanson KL: A second independent locus within DMRT1 is associated with testicular germ cell tumor susceptibility. Hum Mol Genet 2011, 20:3109–3117.

[21] Collin GB, Asada Y, Varnum DS, Nadeau JH: DNA pooling as a quick method for finding candidate linkages in multigenic trait analysis: an example involving susceptibility to germ cell tumors. Mamm Genome 1996, 7(1):68–70.

[22] Matin A, Collin GB, Asada Y, Varnum D, Nadeau JH: Susceptibility to testicular germ-cell tumours in a 129.MOLF-Chr 19 chromosome substitution strain. Nat Genet 1999, 23(2):237–240.

[23] Silver LM: Mouse genetics: concepts and applications. New York: Oxford University Press; 1995:32–61.

[24] Rieseberg LH, Archer MA, Wayne RK: Transgressive segregation, adaptation and speciation. Heredity 1999, 83:363–372.

[25] Kimura T, Suzuki A, Fujita Y, Yomogida K, Lomeli H, Asada N, Ikeuchi M, Nagy A, Mak TW, Nakano T: Conditional loss of PTEN leads to testicular teratoma and enhances embryonic germ cell production. Development 2003, 130:1691–1700.

[26] Zhu R, Heaney J, Nadeau J, Ali S, Matin A: Deficiency of Splicing Factor 1 (SF1) suppresses occurrence of testicular germ cell tumors. Cancer Res 2010, 70:7264–7272.

[27] Zhu R, Ji Y, Xiao L, Matin A: Testicular germ cell tumor susceptibility genes from the consomic 129.MOLF-Chr 19 mouse strain. Mamm Genome 2007, 18:584–595.

[28] Cordell HJ: Epistasis: what it means, what it doesn't mean. and statistical methods to detect it in humans. Hum Mol Genet 2002, 11:2463–2468.

[29] Frankel WN, Schork NJ: Who's afraid of epistasis? Nat Genet 1996, 14:371–373.

[30] Tollerud DJ, Blattner WA, Fraser MC, Brown LM, Pottern L, Shapiro E, Kirkemo A, Shawker TH, Javadpour N, O'Connell K, Stutzman RE, Fraumeni Jr JF: Familial testicular cancer and urogenital developmental anomalies. Cancer 1985, 55:1849–1854.

[31] United Kingdom Testicular Cancer Study Group U: Aetiology of testicular cancer: association with congenital abnormalities, age at puberty, infertility, and excercise. BMJ 1994, 308:1393–1399.

[32] Poynter JN, Hooten AJ, Frazier AL, Ross JA: Associations between variants in KITLG, SPRY4, BAK1, and DMRT1 and pediatric germ cell tumors. Genes Chromosomes Cancer 2012, 51:266–271.

[33] Kratz CP, Han SS, Rosenberg PS, Berndt SI, Burdett L, Yeager M, Korde LA, Mai PL, Pfeiffer R, Greene MH: Variants in or near KITLG, BAK1, DMRT1, and TERT-CLPTM1L predispose to familial testicular germ cell tumour. J Med Genet 2011, 48:473–476.

[34] Matsuda M, Nagahama Y, Shinomiya A, Sato T, Matsuda C, Kobayashi T, Morrey CE, Shibata N, Asakawa S, Shimizu N, Hori H, Hamaguchi S, Sakaizumi M: DMY is a Y-specific DM-domain gene required for male development in the medaka fish. Nature 2002, 417:559–563.

[35] Raymond CS, Murphy MW, O'Sullivan MG, Bardwell VJ, Zarkower D: Dmrt1, a gene related to worm and fly sexual regulators, is required for mammalian testis differentiation. Genes Dev 2000, 14:2587–2595.

[36] McDonald MT, Flejter W, Sheldon S, Putzi MJ, Gorski JL: XY sex reversal and gonadal dysgenesis due to 9p24 monosomy. Am J Med Genet 1997, 73:321–326.

[37] Veitia R, Nunes M, Brauner R, Doco-Fenzy M, Joanny-Flinois O, Jaubert F, Lortat-Jacob S, Fellous M, McElreavey K: Deletions of distal 9p associated with 46, XY male to female sex reversal: definition of the breakpoints at 9p23.3-p24.1. Genomics 1997, 41:271–274.

[38] Flejter WL, Fergestad J, Gorski JL, Varvill T, Chandrasekharappa S: A gene involved in XY sex reversal is located on chromosome 9, distal to marker D9S1779. Am J Hum Genet 1998, 63:794–802.

[39] Ogata T, Muroya K, Matsuo N, Hata J, Fukushima Y, Suzuki Y: Impaired male sex development in an infant with molecularly defined partial 9p monosomy: implication for a test is forming gene(s) on 9p. J Med Genet 1997, 34:331–334.

[40] Shetty G, Comish PB, Weng CC, Matin A, Meistrich ML: Fetal radiation exposure induces testicular cancer in genetically susceptible mice. PLoS One 2012, 7(2):e32064. doi:32010.31371/journal.pone.0032064.

[41] Comish PB, Drumond AL, Kinnell HL, Anderson RA, Matin A, Meistrich ML, Shetty G: Fetal cyclophosphamide exposure induces testicular cancer and reduced spermatogenesis and ovarian follicle numbers in mice. PLoS One 2014, 9(4):e93311.

Chapter 7

Familial Testicular Germ Cell Tumor: No Associated Syndromic Pattern Identified

Christine M Mueller[1], Larissa A Korde[2], Mary L McMaster[3], June A Peters[1], Gennady Bratslavsky[4], Rissah J Watkins[5], Alex Ling[6], Christian P Kratz[1], Eric A Wulfsberg[7], Philip S Rosenberg[8], Mark H Greene[1]

[1]Clinical Genetics Branch, Division of Cancer Epidemiology and Genetics, National Cancer Institute, National Institutes of Health, Bethesda, MD, USA

[2]Division of Medical Oncology, University of Washington/Seattle Cancer CareAlliance, Seattle, WA, USA

[3]Genetic Epidemiology Branch, Division of Cancer Epidemiology and Genetics, National Cancer Institute, National Institutes of Health, Bethesda, MD, USA

[4]Urologic Oncology Branch, National Cancer Institute, National Institutes of Health, Center for Cancer Research, Bethesda, MD, USA

[5]Westat, Inc, 6116 Executive Boulevard, Suite 400, Rockville, MD, USA

[6]Diagnostic Radiology Department, National Institutes of Health, Warren G. Magnuson Clinical Center, Bethesda, MD, USA

[7]Division of Human Genetic, Department of Pediatrics, University of Maryland School of Medicine, Baltimore, MD 21201, USA

[8]Biostatistics Branch, Division of Cancer Epidemiology and Genetics, National Cancer Institute, National Institutes of Health, Bethesda, MD, USA.

Abstract: Background: Testicular germ cell tumor (TGCT) is the most common

malignancy in young men. Familial clustering, epidemiologic evidence of increased risk with family or personal history, and the association of TGCT with genitourinary (GU) tract anomalies have suggested an underlying genetic predisposition. Linkage data have not identified a rare, highly-penetrant, single gene in familial TGCT (FTGCT) cases. Based on its association with congenital GU tract anomalies and suggestions that there is an intrauterine origin to TGCT, we hypothesized the existence of unrecognized dysmorphic features in FTGCT. Methods: We evaluated 38 FTGCT individuals and 41 first-degree relatives from 22 multiple-case families with detailed dysmorphology examinations, physician-based medical history and physical examination, laboratory testing, and genitourinary imaging studies. Results: The prevalence of major abnormalities and minor variants did not significantly differ between either FTGCT individuals or their first-degree relatives when compared with normal population controls, except for tall stature, macrocephaly, flat midface, and retro-/micrognathia. However, these four traits were not manifest as a constellation of features in any one individual or family. We did detect an excess prevalence of the genitourinary anomalies cryptorchidism and congenital inguinal hernia in our population, as previously described in sporadic TGCT, but no congenital renal, retroperitoneal or mediastinal anomalies were detected. Conclusions: Overall, our study did not identify a constellation of dysmorphic features in FTGCT individuals, which is consistent with results of genetic studies suggesting that multiple low-penetrance genes are likely responsible for FTGCT susceptibility.

Keywords: Familial Testicular Cancer, Dysmorphology, Developmental Anomalies

1. Background

Although testicular germ cell tumors (TGCT) account for only 1% of malignancies in males, it is the most common malignancy among men aged 20–35 years[1]. A familial predisposition has been well documented; sons of men with TGCT have a 4- to 6-fold increased risk compared with the general population and brothers of affected siblings have an 8- to 10-fold increased risk[2][3]. The higher relative risk of TGCT among siblings than among fathers/sons suggests both genetic heterogeneity and environmental influences, including possible intrauterine exposures. Cases of ovarian germ cell tumors have also been reported in Familial TGCT (FTGCT) kindreds[4]. FTGCT has not been definitively linked to any known hereditary cancer syndrome, and unraveling the genetic basis through traditional linkage studies has been difficult, in part because families with many affected individuals are exceedingly rare[5][6].

Autosomal dominant, autosomal recessive and X-linked patterns of inheritance are seen in FTGCT families, suggesting considerable genetic heterogeneity. An autosomal recessive model has provided the best data fit in the two segregation analyses performed to date, and several genomic regions of interest have been identified in linkage analyses, but no high-penetrance susceptibility genes have yet been identified[7]–[11]. We reported no disease-associated germline cytogenetic abnormalities in either the 28 FTGCT men we studied by high-resolution chromosome analysis and spectral karyotyping, or 17 previously-reported FTGCT men[12]. A Y-chromosome deletion (gr/gr) has been identified as conferring 2- and 3- fold increases in risk of sporadic and familial testicular cancers, respectively, in a small percentage of men, and reports have identified germline variants in PDE11A and DND1 as candidate modifiers of familial testicular cancer risk[13]–[15]. Three genomewide association studies (GWAS) of unselected testicular cancer patients have identified single nucleotide polymorphisms that are strongly associated with TGCT risk[16]–[19]. Kratz *et al.*, confirmed findings of BAK1, DMRT1, TERT-CLPTM1L, and KITLG variants in familial and bilateral cases of TGCT[20]. A recent meta-analysis of pooled GWAS data has identified 5 additional candidate susceptibility loci, one (UCK2) previously identified as of possible (but not statistically significant) interest in a prior GWAS, as well as 4 novel loci: HGPDS, MAD1L1, RFWD3 and 17q22.2[21][22].

Most recently, DAZL and PRDM14 have been implicated as well[23]. In addition, a strong correlation between LINE-1 methylation levels among affected father-son pairs suggested possible transgenerational inheritance of an epigenetic event that may be associated with disease risk[24]. Overall, these data suggest that a single major locus may not account for the majority of the familial aggregation of TGCT, but rather that multiple low-penetrance susceptibility loci acting in concert may be responsible for the genetic component of TGCT etiology.

Several additional risk factors have been described, including cryptorchidism, inguinal hernia, infertility and contralateral testicular cancer[25][26]. Previous case reports have linked TGCT with diverse congenital abnormalities including retroperitoneal anomalies (e.g. renal agenesis, duplicated collecting system, re-tro-aortic renal vein) and supernumerary nipples[27][28]. It has been postulated that TGCT stems from abnormal gonadal development during embryogenesis, and may be part of a "testicular dysgenesis syndrome," characterized by urogenital abnor-malities, subfertility, testicular microlithiasis, and testicular carcinoma in situ, and hypothesized as related to both environmental and genetic risk factors[29][30]. Fur-thermore, GCTs have been reported in a number of individuals with hereditary disorders or constitutional chromosome abnormalities, many of which also include other urogenital abnormalities[26][31].

Detailed physical examination for evaluation of minor morphologic abnor-malities in conjunction with detection of major congenital anomalies is a major tool for characterizing syndromes in clinical genetics and can be helpful in guiding molecular studies[32][33]. As part of our multidisciplinary, etiologically-focused at-tempt to refine the FTGCT phenotype, the putative intrauterine origin of TGCT led us to hypothesize the existence of unrecognized dysmorphic features or congenital anomalies in this syndrome[34]. Since no one had previously performed a syste-matic dysmorphology evaluation of FTGCT family members, we comprehensively evaluated men with FTGCT and their 1st-degree relatives in search of an excess of mild errors of morphogenesis and congenital anomalies to further define the FTGCT phenotype and to provide new insights into the genetic and/or environ-mental etiology of TGCT.

2. Methods

The objectives of the Clinical Genetics Branch Multidisciplinary Etiologic Study of Familial Testicular Cancer (NCI Protocol 02-C-0178; NCT-00039598; http://familial-testicular-cancer.cancer.gov) included identifying possible testicular cancer susceptibility genes and characterizing more precisely the clinical pheno-type of individuals with FTGCT[34]. In brief, families containing ≥2 family mem-bers with documented germ cell tumors were recruited. Families with a single male displaying bilateral TGCT were also included, because of its known associa-tion with FTGCT. To date, we have enrolled 665 members (including 203 FTGCT individuals) of 127 eligible families. Willing study participants were invited to the NIH Warren G. Magnuson Clinical Center for a research evaluation; 155 members (including 61 FTGCT individuals) of 37 families have elected to attend. For the current analysis, the first 38 TGCT cases and 41 first-degree relatives from 22 multiple-case families were studied with detailed dysmorphology examinations, physician-based medical history and physical examination, laboratory testing, ultrasound imaging of the testes and ovaries, computed tomography or ultrasound of the abdomen, and computed tomography of the chest. All participants completed detailed family history, medical history, and risk factor questionnaires. This study was reviewed and approved by the National Cancer Institute (NCI) Institutional Review Board (NCI Protocol 02-C-0178), and all participants provided written informed consent.

All dysmorphology examinations were performed by one of three trained clinical geneticists (EAW, MLM, CMM). A standardized data collection instrument was developed by two of these geneticists (EAW, MLM) to insure complete, systematic assessment of features. Diagnostic criteria were applied as described by Aase and Merks[32][35]. In the case of paired organs, no distinction was made between unilateral and bilateral occurrence. Height, weight, head circumference, inner and outer canthal distance, inter-pupillary distance, and hand lengths were measured with calipers and tape measure, and findings were compared with normal standards[36]. Clinical photographs of all subject's faces were obtained and reviewed by a single examiner (CMM) during data analysis, and no features were scored differently than previous examiners. We compared the prevalence of 11 major and 54 minor anomalies in individuals with FTGCT, their 1st-degree relatives, and those reported in 923 white school age children[37]. Fisher's Exact test was used for statistical comparisons, with a two-tailed p-value of <0.05 considered statistically significant. All statistical analyses were conducted using SPSS 15.0. Of note, retro-/micrognathia in the 923 school age children included individuals with retrognathia and micrognathia occurring separately or in combination.

3. Results

The study sample included 38 men with FTGCT and 41 of their unaffected first-degree relatives (21 males, 29 females) from 22 multiple-case white TGCT families (**Table 1**). Median age at TGCT diagnosis was 31 years (range: 15–56), and the usual mix of seminomatous and non-seminomatous tumors among the families was observed. Multiple patterns of inheritance were observed, including

157

Table 1. Composition of FTGCT families examined.

Family	Relationship among FTGCT family members	FTGCT family members examined	Unaffected 1st degree family members examined
1	Father/Son	1	0
2	Father/Son	1	1
3	Father/Son	2	0
4	Father/Son	2	0
5	Father/Son	2	4
6	Father/Son	2	7
7	Father/Son	2	2
8	Father/Son	1	2
9	Father/Son	2	0
10	Siblings	2	3
11	Siblings	2	2
12	Siblings	1	0
13	Siblings	2	3
14	Siblings	1	0
15	Siblings	3	0
16	Siblings	1	3
17	Siblings	2	4
18	Siblings	3	1
19	Cousins	2	1
20	Cousins	2	3
21	Uncle/Nephew	1	2
22	Bilateral	1	3

nine families with FTGCT brothers, 9 with FTGCT father-sons, 2 with FTGCT cousins, 1 with FTGCT uncle-nephew, and 1 bilateral FTGCT individual. We examined 41 unaffected first-degree relatives, 21 males and 20 females. Seven families did not have a first-degree relative available for examination. The median ages of FTGCT men, unaffected men, and women at the time of study were 40 (21–72), 31 (14–68), and 47 (15–67), respectively.

The prevalence of major abnormalities and minor variants did not significantly differ between either men with FTGCT or their first-degree relatives when compared with the normal population controls, except for tall stature, macrocephaly, flat midface, and retro-/micrognathia (**Table 2**). One mother had a previous diagnosis of Holt Oram syndrome (OMIM 142900), but otherwise no major abnormalities of the extremities or skeletal dysplasias were found in our cases or their relatives, so they are excluded from **Table 2**.

Table 2. Prevalence of congenital abnormalities in FTGCT individuals, first degree relatives, and normal school age children (%).

	FTGCT (N = 38)	1st degree relatives (N = 41)	Normal population (N = 923)
Major abnormality			
Short stature (proportionate)	0	0	2.0
Cleft lip	0	0	0
Cleft palate	0	0	0
Ear tags	0	0	0.3
Ear pits	2.6	0	1.1
Webbed neck	0	0	0
Supernumerary nipples	2.6	2.4	2.8
Talipes equinovarus	0	0	0
2,3 toe syndactyly	0	2.4	0.4
Joint hypermobility	0	0	10.3
Joint contractures	0	0	0
Minor variant			
Tall stature (proportionate) p = 0.05[††]	7.9	2.4	2.0
Macrocephaly* p = 0.01[††]	11.1	4.9	2.0
Microcephaly	2.6	0	2.0
Abnormal hair whorl	0	0	0.1
Widow's peak	5.3	2.4	6.7
Coarse face	2.6	2.4	0.5
Prominent forehead	0	0	2.4
Facial asymmetry p < 0.01[††††]	5.3	9.8	1.6
Flat mid-face p < 0.01[†††]	23.7	2.4	1.0
Hypertelorism	0	0	2.0
Hypotelorism	0	0	2.0
Telecanthus	0	0	0.4
Upslanting palpebral fissures	2.6	2.4	3.9
Downslanting palpebral fissures	5.3	2.4	0.8

Epicanthal folds	2.6	0	3.5
Ptosis	0	2.4	4.4
Broad nose	0	2.4	1.1
Short nose	2.6	0	9.3
Broad nasal tip	5.3	7.3	2.6
Anteverted nares	0	0	4.2
Hypoplastic alae nasae	0	0	0.7
Smooth philtrum	0	0	5.3
Prominent philtrum	5.3	0	1.8
Prominent upper jaw	0	0	2.1
Retro-/micrognathia p = 0.04[††]	7.9	4.9	1.7
Prominent lower jaw	0	0	0.3
Pointed chin	2.6	2.4	0.7
High-arched palate	2.6	4.9	6.2
Bifid uvula	0	0	0
Extra frenulae	0	0	0
Abnormally shaped teeth	2.6	0	1.6
Lowset ears	0	0	0.5
Posteriorly rotated ears	2.6	4.9	1.4
Overfolded helices	7.9	4.9	4.1
Darwinian tubercle	5.3	0	4.6
Ear lobe crease	2.6	2.4	0
Attached ear lobes	2.6	2.4	12.8
Pectus excavatum	5.3	7.3	2.3
Pectus carinatum	0	2.4	0.3
Gynecomastia	0	0	0.1
Absent/hypoplastic nipples	0	0	0
Wide-spaced nipples	2.6	0	0.4
Inverted nipples	2.6	0	4.1
Bridged palmar crease	0	2.4	2.7
Single transverse crease	0	2.4	2.3
Sydney crease	0	0	0.3
Clinodactyly	0	0	3.6
Partial 2,3 toe syndactyly	0	2.4	0.3
Hammer toes	2.6	0	0.2
2nd toe longer than 1st	7.9	7.3	3.1
Pes planus	0	2.4	2.6
Café-au-lait spots	13.2	12.2	13.5
Hemangiomas	2.6	2.4	0.7
Port wine stain	2.6	0	0.2

[††]Between FTGCT individuals and normal population. [†††]Between FTGCT individuals and normal population and FTGCT individuals and relatives. [††††]Between relatives and normal population. *36 FTGCT individuals measured.

The prevalence of tall stature, macrocephaly and retromicrognathia was significantly greater between men with FTGCT and the normal population, but not between men with FTGCT and their 1st-degree relatives. All individuals with macrocephaly were only mildly affected, and there was no evidence of familial aggregation for this trait. When head circumference was plotted against height, as suggested by Bushby *et al.*, only one affected male remained mildly macrocephalic, and this feature was no longer statistically significant[38]. Of note, retro-/ micrognathia included individuals with retrognathia and micrognathia occurring separately or in combination[37].

Flat mid-face was statistically significant between FTGCT individuals and the general population and their 1st-degree relatives. There was no familial aggregation among the 9 FTGCT individuals and 1 first-degree relative with flat mid-face. Facial asymmetry was seen more frequently in unaffected relatives than either their affected relatives or the normal population, and there was no evidence of familial aggregation. These 4 traits were not manifest as a constellation of features in any one individual or family.

Table 3 summarizes the prevalence of congenital genitourinary tract abnormalities in FTGCT males vs. unaffected males. By history, cryptorchidism was more frequent among cases than among unaffected men, 13% vs. 5% and, when compared with the highest estimates in the general population, 4%, was statistically significant[39][40]. The prevalence of congenital inguinal hernia was similar in FTGCT males vs. Unaffected family members (18.4% vs. 19%), statistically significantly higher than the occurrence in the general population, 5%[41]. One FTGCT male and one unaffected male from a different family had bilateral duplicated

Table 3. Prevalence of congenital genitourinary tract abnormalities (%).

Condition	FTGCT individuals (N = 38)	1st Degree unaffected male relatives (N = 41)	Normal population
Cryptorchidism* p < 0.05[††]	13.2	4.8	4.0
Congenital inguinal hernia* p < 0.01[†††]	18.4	19.0	5.0
Duplicated collecting system	2.6	2.4	1.0

*Includes only the 21 male 1st Degree relatives. [††]Between FTGCT individuals and normal population and FTGCT individuals and relatives. [†††]Between FTGCT individuals and normal population and relatives and normal population.

renal collecting systems (2.6% vs. 2.4%). This is one of the most common renal abnormalities, and occurs in approximately 1% of the population[42][43]. No other congenital renal retroperitoneal or mediastinal abnormalities were found in our thoraco-abdominal imaging studies.

4. Discussion

Our study provides the largest, most comprehensive descriptive analysis of formal dysmorphology evaluations in individuals from familial TGCT kindred. The current analysis is part of the only systematic, multidisciplinary etiologic study of extended multiple-case TGCT families being conducted in the world, and thus represents a unique opportunity to assess an important hypothesis: given the likely intra-uterine origins of testicular neoplasia, is there a dysmorphic and/or a congenital anomaly component to the FTGCT syndrome phenotype? We compared the prevalence of 11 major and 54 minor anomalies in 38 males from FTGCT families with those of 923 normal children. To assess familial aggregation and potential unidentified carriers of as yet unknown testicular cancer susceptibility genes, we also examined 41 available, unaffected 1st-degree relatives. No notable pattern of dysmorphic features was detected between FTGCT individuals and either their relatives or population controls, nor was there evidence of excess renal, retroperitoneal or mediastinal congenital anomalies.

Compared with the normal population, FTGCT men were more likely to have tall stature, macrocephaly, and retro-and/or micro-gnathia. They were also more likely to have these traits than their unaffected relatives, but these differences were not statistically significant. It is theoretically possible that clinically unaffected relatives displaying one or more of these traits are unidentified carriers of a familial TGCT phenotype. However, there was no familial aggregation of macrocephaly or retro-and/or micro-gnathia and no single individual manifested a constellation of these traits, making it difficult to identify a pattern of morphologic features that might be uniquely associated with familial TGCT. Furthermore, as familial aggregation of tall stature may occur in the general population, we also performed the analysis by excluding the one FTGCT individual and his daughter who were unusually tall, and tall stature was no longer statistically significant. The validity of the statistical significance of the prevalence of retro-micrognathia is difficult to discern, as the only available control data were comprised of retrognathia and micrognathia combined; typically, these are considered two distinct features[37].

Flat mid-face was significantly more common in affected males than either their relatives or the normal controls, suggesting that it might be a trait that is part of a familial TGCT phenotype. In addition, facial asymmetry was more common in unaffected relatives than the normal population or affected males. However, these traits are subjectively defined by the examiner and also may vary in any one individual depending on other physical features, such as weight and age at examination.

Previous reports have linked cases of TGCT with congenital abnormalities including retroperitoneal urinary anomalies and supernumerary nipples[27][28]. There were no differences in the prevalence of supernumerary nipples in any of the patient subsets. We also did not detect an increased frequency of renal, retroperitoneal or mediastinal abnormalities on thoraco-abdominal imaging in our families. We observed a higher prevalence of cryptorchidism among FTGCT cases than among unaffected relatives and the general population, as has been repeatedly described in sporadic TGCT. In addition, we observed a higher prevalence of congenital inguinal hernia in FTGCT cases and their unaffected relatives compared with the general population. FTGCT cases and their relatives with congenital genitourinary tract anomalies were not more likely to have the anomalies listed in **Table 2**.

The major strength of this study is that all participants underwent a comprehensive clinical evaluation by a small group of dysmorphologists who employed a standardized data collection form. In addition, study participants systematically provided detailed medical and family history information. This study is the first to examine men with FTGCT and their family members in sufficient detail to determine if there is a pattern of morphologic features common to this disorder.

The findings in our study are limited by the small sample sizes for both the affected males and their first-degree relatives, which results in minimal statistical power to detect differences between study sub-groups. In addition, our ability to detect differences in the subjective evaluation between examiners was limited by not having each participant evaluated by multiple examiners or having the photographs of participants evaluated by CMM scored by the other examiners. Furthermore, we might have been able to identify a larger number of abnormalities if we had access to all first-degree relatives of FTGCT individuals. Larger studies would be required to further characterize these traits in individuals with FTGCT but, pragmatically, it is unlikely that such data will be forthcoming in the foreseeable future. Comparing anomaly prevalence in our subjects to rates from a large, literature-based normal population may have been sub-optimal when evaluating traits that are subjectively defined by different examiners. In addition, the control population consisted of school age children from the Netherlands compared with our adult population from the United States; however, we believe that these white populations should be similar in morphological features and that minor differences that more commonly occur in adults compared with children (such as male pattern baldness or striae) were not included in our analysis. Finally, our study population may not be representative of all FTGCT families, since it was comprised of research volunteers who were willing to travel to the NIH Clinical Center for an in-person evaluation.

5. Conclusions

Our study did not identify a constellation of dysmorphic or congenital anomalies in affected males from multiple-case TGCT families or their unaffected close relatives. Based on the data that we were able to collect from this rare and unique population, it appears that this strategy would not be helpful in guiding ongoing molecular and etiologic studies. Furthermore, our findings are consistent with results of genetic studies that have been done to date, in that a single gene does not appear to account for the majority of the familial aggregation of TGCT; overall, the descriptive epidemiology of familial and sporadic testicular cancer are remarkably similar.

Our data provide further support for the hypothesis that multiple, common low-penetrance genetic variants are more likely responsible for FTGCT susceptibility rather than a rare, highly-penetrant gene of major effect.

Competing Interests

The authors declare that they have no competing interests.

Authors' Contributions

CMM, LAK, MLM, JAP, RJW, EAW, and MHG made substantial contributions to the conception and design of the study. CMM, MLM, and EAW designed the dysmorphology data collection and performed dysmorphology examinations. GB was responsible for genitourinary examination and AL and GB were responsible for radiologic examination review and contributed to the conception and design of the study. CMM performed data collection and statistical analysis. CMM, PSR, CPK, and MHG interpreted data and drafted the manuscript. All authors read and approved the final manuscript.

Acknowledgements

We acknowledge the contributions and support of Dr Marston Linehan, Dr Ahalya Premkumar, Susan Pfeiffer, and Jennifer Loud to the CGB Familial Testicular Cancer study. We also offer special thanks to our study participants, whose personal commitment has made this research possible. This work was supported by funding from the National Cancer Institute Intramural Research Program and by support services contracts NO2-CP-11019-50 and NO2-CP-65504-50 with Westat Inc., Rockville MD.

Source: Mueller C M, Korde L A, Mcmaster M L, *et al*. Familial testicular germ cell tumor: no associated syndromic pattern identified. [J]. Hereditary Cancer in Clinical Practice, 2014, 12(1):1–7.

References

[1] Edwards BK, Brown ML, Wingo PA, Howe HL, Ward E, Ries LA, Schrag D, Jamison PM, Jemal A, Wu XC, Friedman C, Harlan L, Warren J, Anderson RN, Pickle LW: Annual report to the nation on the status of cancer, 1975-2002, featuring population-based trends in cancer treatment. J Natl Cancer Inst 2005, 97:1407–1427.

[2] Dong C, Hemminki K: Modification of cancer risks in offspring by sibling and parental cancers from 2,112,616 nuclear families. Int J Cancer 2001, 92:144–150.

[3] Hemminki K, Li X: Familial risk in testicular cancer as a clue to a heritable and environmental aetiology. Br J Cancer 2004, 90:1765–1770.

[4]   Giambartolomei C, Mueller CM, Greene MH, Korde LA: A mini-review of familial ovarian germ cell tumors: an additional manifestation of the familial testicular germ cell tumor syndrome. Cancer Epidemiol 2009, 33:31–36.

[5]   Mai PL, Chen BE, Tucker K, Friedlander M, Phillips KA, Hogg D, Jewett MAS, Bodrogi I, Geczi L, Olah E, Heimdal K, Fossa SD, Nathanson KL, Korde L, Easton DF, Dudakia D, Huddart R, Stratton MR, Bishop DT, Rapley EA, Greene MH: Younger age-at-diagnosis for familial malignant germ cell tumor. Fam Cancer 2009, 8:451–456.

[6]   Mai PL, Friedlander M, Tucker K, Phillips KA, Hogg D, Jewett MA, Lohynska R, Daugaard G, Richard S, Bonaiti-Pellie C, Heidenreich A, Albers P, Bodrogi I, Geczi L, Olah E, Daly PA, Guilford P, Fossa SD, Heimdal K, Liubchenko L, Tjulandin SA, Stoll H, Weber W, Easton DF, Dudakia D, Huddart R, Stratton MR, Einhorn L, Korde L, Nathanson KL, et al: The International Testicular Cancer Linkage Consortium: a clinicopathologic descriptive analysis of 461 familial malignant testicular germ cell tumor kindred. Urol Oncol 2010, 28:492–499.

[7]   Crockford GP, Linger R, Hockley S, Dudakia D, Johnson L, Huddart R, Tucker K, Friedlander M, Phillips K, Hogg D, Jewett MAS, Lohynska R, Daugaard G, Richard S, Chompret A, Bonaiti-Pellie C, Heidenreich A, Albers P, Olah E, Geczi L, Bodrogi I, Ormiston WJ, Daly PA, Guildford P, Fossa SD, Heimdal K, Tjulandin SA, Liubchenko L, Stoll H, Weber W, et al: Genome-wide linkage screen for testicular germ cell tumour susceptibility loci. Hum Mol Genet 2006, 15:443–451.

[8]   Heimdal K, Olsson H, Tretli S, Fossa SD, Borresen AL, Bishop DT: A segregation analysis of testicular cancer based on Norwegian and Swedish families. Br J Cancer 1997, 75:1084–1087.

[9]   Nicholson PW, Harland SJ: Inheritance and testicular cancer. Br J Cancer 1995, 71:421–426.

[10] Rapley EA, Crockford GP, Teare D, Biggs P, Seal S, Barfoot R, Edwards S, Hamoudi R, Heimdal K, Fossa SD, Tucker K, Donald J, Collins F, Friedlander M, Hogg D, Goss P, Heidenreich A, Ormiston W, Daly PA, Forman D, Oliver TD, Leahy M, Huddart R, Cooper CS, Bodmer JG, Easton DF, Stratton MR, Bishop DT: Localization to Xq27 of a susceptibility gene for testicular germ-cell tumours. Nat Genet 2000, 24:197–200.

[11] Rapley EA, Crockford GP, Easton DF, Stratton MR, Bishop DT, International Testicular Cancer Linkage Consortium: Localisation of susceptibility genes for familial testicular germ cell tumour. APMIS 2003, 111:128–133.

[12] Mueller CM, Korde L, Katki HA, Rosenberg PS, Peters JA, Greene MH: Constitutional cytogenetic analysis in men with hereditary testicular germ cell tumor: no evidence of disease-related abnormalities. Cancer Epidemiol Biomarkers Prev 2007, 16:2791–2794.

[13] Horvath A, Korde L, Greene MH, Libe R, Osorio P, Faucz FR, Raffin-Sanson ML, Tsang KM, Drori-Herishanu L, Patronus Y, Remmers EF, Nikita ME, Moran J,

Greene J, Nesterova M, Merino M, Bertherat J, Stratakis CA: Functional phospho-diesterase 11A mutations may modify the risk of familial and bilateral testicular germ cell tumors. Cancer Res 2009, 69:5301–5306.

[14] Linger R, Dudakia D, Huddart R, Tucker K, Friedlander M, Phillips KA, Hogg D, Jewett MAS, Lohynska R, Daugaard G, Richard S, Chompret A, Stoppa-Lyonnet D, Bonaiti-Pellie C, Heidenreich A, Albers P, Olah E, Geczi L, Bodrogi I, Daly PA, Guilford P, Fossa SD, Heimdal K, Tijulandin SA, Liubchenko L, Stoll H, Weber W, Einhorn L, McMaster M, Korde L, et al: Analysis of the DND1 gene in men with sporadic and familial germ cell tumors. Genes Chromosomes Cancer 2008, 47:247–252.

[15] Nathanson KL, Kanetsky PA, Hawes R, Vaughn DJ, Letrero R, Tucker K, Friedlan-der M, Phillips KA, Hogg D, Jewett MA, Lohynska R, Daugaard G, Richard S, Chompret A, Bonaiti-Pellie C, Heidenreich A, Olah E, Geczi L, Godrogi I, Ormiston WJ, Daly PA, Oosterhuis JW, Gillis AJ, Looijenga LH, Guilford P, Fossa SD, Heim-dal K, Tjulandin SA, Liubchenko L, Stoll H, et al: The Y deletion gr/gr and suscepti-bility to testicular germ cell tumor. Am J Hum Genet 2005, 77:1034–1043.

[16] Kanetsky PA, Mitra N, Vardhanabhuti S, Li M, Vaughn DJ, Letrero R, Ciosek SL, Doody DR, Smith LM, Weaver J, Albano A, Chen C, Starr JR, Rader DJ, Godwin AK, Reilly MP, Hakonarson H, Schwartz SM, Nathanson KL: Common variation in KITLG and at 5q31.3 predisposes to testicular germ cell cancer. Nat Genet 2009, 41:811–815.

[17] Kanetsky PA, Mitra N, Vardhanabhuti S, Vaughn DJ, Li M, Ciosek SL, Letrero R, D'Andrea K, Vaddi M, Doody DR, Weaver J, Chen C, Starr JR, Hakonarson H, Rad-er DJ, Godwin AK, Reilly MP, Schwartz SM, Nathanson KL: A second independent locus within DMRT1 is associated with testicular germ cell tumor susceptibility. Hum Molec Genetics 2011, 20(15):3109–3117.

[18] Rapley EA, Turnbull C, Al Olama AA, Dermitzakis ET, Linger R, Huddart RA, Renwick A, Hughes D, Hines S, Seal S, Morrison J, Nsengimana J, Deloukas P, Rahman N, Bishop DT, Easton DF, Stratton MR, UK Testicular Cancer Collabora-tion: A genome-wide association study of testicular germ cell tumor. Nat Genet 2009, 41:807–810.

[19] Turnbull C, Rapley EA, Seal S, Pernet D, Renwick A, Ricketts M, Linger R, Nsen-gimana J, Deloukas P, Huddart RA, Bishop DT, Easton DF, Stratton MR, Rahman N: Variants near DMRT1, TERT, and ATF7IP are associated with testicular germ cell cancer. Nat Genet 2010, 42:604–607.

[20] Kratz CP, Han SS, Rosenberg PS, Berndt SI, Burdett L, Yeager M, Korde LA, Mai PL, Pfeiffer R, Greene MH: Variants in or near KITLG, BAK1, DMRT1 and TERT-CLPTM1L predispose to familial testicular germ cell tumor. J Med Genet 2011, 48:473–476.

[21] Chung CC, Kanetsky PA, Wang Z, Hildebrandt MAT, Koster R, Skotheim RI, Kratz CP, Turnbull C, Cortessis VK, Bakken AC, Bishop DT, Cook MB, Erickson RL, Fossa SD, Jacobs KB, Korde LA, Kraggerud SM, Lothe RA, Loud JT, Rahman N,

Skinner EC, Thomas DC, Wu X, Yeager M, Schumacher FR, Greene MH, Schwartz SM, McGlynn KA, Chanock SJ, Nathanson KL: Meta-analysis identifies four new loci associated with testicular germ cell tumor. Nat Genet 2013, 45:680–685.

[22] Schumacher FR, Wang Z, Skotheim RI, Koster R, Chung CC, Hildebrandt MAT, Kratz CP, Bishop DT, Casey G, Cook MB, Erickson RL, Fossa SD, Gjessing HK, Greene MH, Jacobs KB, Kanetsky PA, Kolonel LN, Loud JT, Korde LA, Marchand LL, Lewinger JP, Lothe RA, Pike MC, Rahman N, Rubertone MV, Schwartz SM, Siegmund KD, Skinner EC, Thomas DC, Turnbull C, *et al*: Testicular germ cell tumor susceptibility associated with the UCK2 locus on chromosome 1q23. Hum Mol Genet 2013, 22(13):2748–2753.

[23] Ruark E, Seal S, McDonald H, Zhang F, Elliot A, Perdeaux E, Rapley E, Eeles R, Peto J, Kote-Jarai Z, Muir K, Nsengimana J, Shipley J, Bishop DT, Stratton MR, Easton DF, Huddart RA, Rahman N, Turnbull C: Identification of nine new susceptibility loci for testicular cancer, including variants near DAZL and PRDM14. Nature Genet 2013, 45(6):686–689.

[24] Mirabello L, Savage SA, Korde L, Gadalla SM, Greene MH: LINE-1 methylation is inherited in familial testicular cancer kindreds. BMC Med Genet 2010, 11:77.

[25] Garner MJ, Turner MC, Ghadirian P, Krewski D: Epidemiology of testicular cancer: an overview. Int J Cancer 2005, 116:331–339.

[26] Lutke Holzik MF, Rapley EA, Hoekstra HJ, Sleijfer DT, Nolte IM, Sijmons RH: Genetic predisposition to testicular germ-cell tumours. Lancet Oncol 2004, 5:363–371.

[27] Holt PJ, Adshead JM, Filiadis I, Christmas TJ: Retroperitoneal anomalies in men with testicular germ cell tumours. B J U Int 2007, 99:344–346.

[28] Mehes K, Szule E, Torzsok F, Meggyessy V: Supernumerary nipples and urologic malignancies. Cancer Genet Cytogenet 1987, 24:185–188.

[29] Skakkebaek NE, Rajpert-De Meyts E, Main KM: Testicular dysgenesis syndrome: an increasingly common developmental disorder with environmental aspects. Hum Reprod 2001, 16:972–978.

[30] Skakkebaek NE, Holm M, Hoei-Hansen C, Jorgensen N, Rajpert-DeMeyts E: Association between testicular dysgenesis syndrome (TDS) and testicular neoplasia: evidence from 20 adult patients with signs of maldevelopment of the testis. APMIS 2003, 111:1–9.

[31] Lutke Holzik MF, Sijmons RH, Sleijfer DT, Sonneveld DJ, Hoekstra-Weebers JE, van Echten-Arends J, Hoekstra HJ: Syndromic aspects of testicular carcinoma. Cancer 2003, 97:984–992.

[32] Merks JH, van Karnebeek CD, Caron HN, Hennekam RC: Phenotypic abnormalities: terminology and classification. Am J Med Genet Part A 2003, 123A:211–230.

[33] Merks JH, Ozgen HM, Koster J, Zwinderman AH, Caron HN, Hennekam RC: Pre-

valence and patterns of morphological abnormalities in patients with childhood cancer. JAMA 2008, 299:61–69.

[34] Korde LA, Premkumar A, Mueller C, Rosenberg P, Soho C, Bratslavsky G, Greene MH: Increased prevalence of testicular microlithiasis in men with familial testicular cancer and their relatives. Br J Cancer 2008, 99:1748–1753.

[35] Aase JM: Diagnostic Dysmorphology. New York: Springer; 1990:320.

[36] Hall JG, Allanson JE, Gripp KW, Slavotinek AM: Handbook of Physical Measurements. New York: Oxford University Press; 2007:520.

[37] Merks JH, Ozgen HM, Cluitmans TL, van der Burg-van Rijn JM, Cobben JM, van Leeuwen FE, Hennekam RC: Normal values for morphological abnormalities in school children. Am J Med Genet Part A 2006, 140A:2091–2109.

[38] Bushby KM, Cole T, Matthews JN, Goodship JA: Centiles for adult head circumference. Arch Dis Child 1992, 67:1286–1287.

[39] Barthold JS, Gonzalez R: The epidemiology of congenital cryptorchidism, testicular ascent, and orchiopexy. J Urol 2003, 170:2396–2401.

[40] Berkowitz GS, Lapinski RH, Gazella JG, Dolgin SE, Bodian CA, Holzman IR: Prevalence and natural history of cryptorchidism. Pediatrics 1993, 92:44–49.

[41] Brandt ML: Pediatric hernias. Surg Clin N Am 2008, 88:27–43.

[42] Decter RM: Renal duplication and fusion anomalies. Pediatr Clin North Am 1997, 44:1323–1341.

[43] Hunziker M, Mohanan N, Menezes M, Puri P: Prevalence of duplex collecting systems in familial vesicoureteral reflux. Pediatr Surg Int 2010, 26:115–117.

Chapter 8

Integrating Genetics and Epigenetics in Breast Cancer: Biological Insights, Experimental, Computational Methods and Therapeutic Potential

Claudia Cava, Gloria Bertoli, Isabella Castiglioni

Institute of Molecular Bioimaging and Physiology (IBFM), National Research Council (CNR), Milan, Italy

Abstract: Background: Development of human cancer can proceed through the accumulation of different genetic changes affecting the structure and function of the genome. Combined analyses of molecular data at multiple levels, such as DNA copy-number alteration, mRNA and miRNA expression, can clarify biological functions and pathways deregulated in cancer. The integrative methods that are used to investigate these data involve different fields, including biology, bioinformatics, and statistics. Results: These methodologies are presented in this review, and their implementation in breast cancer is discussed with a focus on integration strategies. We report current applications, recent studies and interesting results leading to the identification of candidate biomarkers for diagnosis, prognosis, and therapy in breast cancer by using both individual and combined analyses. Conclusion: This review presents a state of art of the role of different technologies in breast cancer based on the integration of genetics and epigenetics, and shares some issues related to the new opportunities and challenges offered by the application of such integrative approaches.

Keywords: Future cities, Sustainability, Urbanisation, Environment, Innovations

1. Introduction

Breast Cancer (BC) is the most common cancer in women and the second most common cause of cancer mortality among females[1]. Classification of BC is currently based on histological types and molecular subtypes in order to reflect the hormone-responsiveness of the tumour. The three most common histological types include invasive ductal carcinoma, ductal carcinoma in situ and invasive lobular carcinoma. The molecular subtypes of BC, which are based on the presence or absence of estrogen receptors (ER), progesterone receptors (PR), and human epidermal growth factor receptor-2 (HER2), include luminal A (ER+ and/or PR+; HER2−), luminal B (ER+ and/or PR+; HER2+), basal-like (ER−, PR−, and HER2−), and HER2-enriched (ER−, PR−, and HER2+) subtypes[2][3]. This classification reflects the BC heterogeneity and the complexity of diagnosis, pro- gnosis, and treatment of BC.

High-throughput approaches allow today a tumour to be investigated at multiple levels: (i) DNA with copy number alteration (CNA), ii) epigenetic alterations, specifically, DNA methylation, histone modifications and microRNA (miRNA) expression level alterations, and (iii) mRNA, with gene expression (GE) de-regulation. These high-throughput approaches redefined the different types of BC in terms of classification, showing the presence of only two BC profiles with different prognosis[4]–[6].

Development of human cancer can proceed through the accumulation of genetic and epigenetic changes affecting the structure and function of the genome. Several studies have reported that the epigenetic silencing of one allele may act in concert with an inactivating genetic alteration in the opposite allele, thus resulting in total allelic loss of the gene[7][8]. Birgisdottir et al.[9] have reported hypermethylation and deletion of the BRCA1 promoter and suggested Knudson's two 'hits' in

172

sporadic BC[9]. Li *et al.*[10] were focused on the expression of beclin 1 mRNA and they demonstrated that loss of heterozygosity and aberrant DNA methylation might be the possible reasons of the decreased expression of beclin 1 in the BC. In BC, a biallelic inactivation of the FHIT gene could be a consequence of epigenetic inactivation of both parental alleles, or epigenetic modification of one allele and deletion of the remaining allele[11].

In 2006, Feinberg *et al.* suggested that epigenetics and genetics should be combined or integrated in order to achieve better understanding of cancer[12]. A systems biology approach has been employed to explore the functional relationships among multidimensional "omics" technologies. This approach has been demonstrated to be important for addressing a patient to the optimal treatment in a personalized way, in order to improve the efficacy of the treatment for that patient[13].

This review refers to current studies of genetic and epigenetic changes associated with BC, focusing in particular on the processes controlled by CNA, epigenetic alterations (DNA methylation, histone modifications and miRNAs), and GE. Several approaches combining genetic and epigenetic data, in particular regarding CNA and miRNA deregulation, have been considered with the final purpose to identify new biomarkers for BC diagnosis and prognosis suitable to be translated into a clinical environment. Furthermore, experimental and computation methods used for the study and the analysis of these biomarkers are presented. We also discuss the biological insights and clinical impact from such analyses as well as the future challenges of these combination approaches.

1.1. Copy Number Alterations in BC

1.1.1. Biological Insights

CNAs are alterations of the DNA of a genome that result in a cell having an abnormal number of copies of one or more sections of the DNA. They have been identified as causes of cancer diseases and developmental abnormalities (e.g.[14]). Changes in DNA copy number (CN) can occur in specific genes or involve whole chromosomes, usually genomic regions between 1kbp and 1Mbp in length[14].

Figure 1 shows an example of a wild type (WT) cell with two copies of DNA segments that suffer of alterations in tumour cells bringing deletions (CN = 0; CN = 1) or amplifications (CN = 3; CN = 4) of the DNA section.

The ability of cancer cells to accumulate genetic alterations is crucial for the development of cancer in order to inactivate tumour suppressor genes (TSGs) and activate oncogenes (OGs).

In BC, several genetic alterations have been found.

Frequent CN deletions between axillary lymph node metastasis and BC primary tumours were revealed, including aberrations at 6q15-16, containing the gene PNRC1 (a putative tumour suppressor)[15]. Amplification and overexpression of the HER2 (HER2/neu, ERBB2) oncogene on chromosome 17q12 has been observed in 15%–25% of invasive BC[16]. HER2-amplified (HER2+) has been associated with poor prognosis in BC[17], amplification of the HER2 gene leading to HER2 protein levels 10–100 times greater than normal levels[18].

EGFR amplification has been frequently associated with indices of poor prognosis in BC patients, such as large tumour size, high histological grade, high

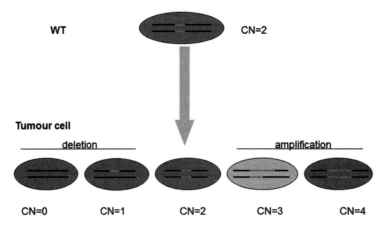

Figure 1. Copy Number alterations. WT cell, since diploid organisms, carry two copies of each gene (red segments). Deletions in tumour cells lead to no copy (CN = 0) or one copy (CN = 1) of this section of DNA, rather than two copies (CN = 2). Amplifications in tumour cells lead to three (CN = 3) or more copies (CN = 4) of DNA section.

proliferative index, HER2 negative, up-regulation of PR[19], and negative ER of the status[20].

In the same region of HER2 (17q12-21) other genes have been found co-amplified or deleted, e.g. topoisomerase (TOP2A)[21]. Different studies observed the possibility of guiding therapy based on TOP2A status[22][23].

A recent study has shown alterations of PIK3CA and MET in BC[24]. High CN of PIK3CA and MET was associated to a poor prognosis, and these alterations occur often in triple receptor negative BC[24]. Alterations were also found at 9q31.3-33.1, where the genes DBC1 and DEC1 (regulators of apoptosis) are located[15].

OGs activation by genomic amplification occurs in the members of different oncogene families, e.g. MYC and CCND. MYC is a key regulator of cell growth, proliferation, metabolism, differentiation, and apoptosis[25]. This oncogene is located on chromosome 8q24, and several mechanisms are implicated in its deregulation in BC, including gene amplification and traslocations. MYC amplification plays a role in BC progression because it has been detected in the more aggressive phenotype of ductal carcinoma in situ[26] or in invasive processes[27]–[29].

Gene amplification of CCND1 has been observed in a subgroup of BCs with poor prognosis and associated with resistance to tamoxifen[30]. Region of amplification is 11q13, and CCND1 acts as a cell cycle regulator, promoting progression through the G1-S phase[31].

Higher ESR1 gene amplification is found in BC with CCND1 gene amplification in comparison with tumours without CCND1 gene amplification[32]. Amplification of ESR1 has been associated with negative ER[32]. The gene TSPAN1 (on 1p34.1) has been found deleted in metastasizing BC and might represent an important TSG[33]. Another gene, EMSY was found involved in sporadic BC. EMSY amplification has been shown to be associated with a poor prognosis[34].

Compared to non-metastatic invasive ductal carcinoma, metastatic invasive ductal carcinoma showed a unique pattern of CNAs, including gains at 2p24-13, 2q22-33, 9q21-31, 12q21-23, 17 q23-25 and loses at 11q23-ter, 14q23-31, 20p11-

q12, 2q36-ter, 8q24-ter, 9q33-ter, 2p11- q11, and 12q13[35][36].

Table 1 reports a synthesis of the considered mutated genes in BC, with their genetic alterations due to CNs.

1.1.2. Experimental Methods

Current experimental methods for the identification of CNA include cytogenetic techniques, microarrays, and sequencing-based computational approaches.

Karyotyping is a cytogenetic technique performing a standardized and effective single cell screening in order to identify significant genomic aberrations in pathological and in normal samples.

In a standard karyotyping, a dye like Giesma or Quinacrine is used to stain bands on the chromosomes. Each chromosome presents banding pattern for detecting CNAs. Thus, any alteration in banding pattern represents a CNA[37].

Spectral karyotyping (SKY technique) is a novel technique for chromosome analysis[37], based on the approach of the fluorescence in situ hybridization

Table 1. Genes mutated and their alterations in BC.

Genes	Genetic alterations	References
MYC	Amplifications and translocations	[25]–[29]
CCND1	Amplifications and Translocations	[30]
HER2	Amplifications	[15]–[18]
TOP2A	Amplifications or Deletions	[22] [23]
PIK3CA, MET	Amplifications	[24]
PNRC1	Deletions	[15]
DBC1 and DEC1	Amplifications or Deletions	[15]
TSPAN1	Deletions	[33]
EGFR	Amplifications	[19][20]
ESR1	Amplifications	[32]
EMSY	Amplifications	[34]

technique (FISH). Sky refers to the multicolour-FISH technique where each chromosome is represented with different colours (a dye with different fluorophores). This technique is used to identify CNAs in cancer cells and in other disease conditions when other techniques are not enough accurate[37].

Resolution is the main limitation of both techniques, the chromosome profile obtained by karyotyping being not enough sensitive to notice short and relevant abnormalities[38].

Hybridization-based microarray approaches, including array comparative genomic hybridization (array CGH) and Single Nucleotide Polymorphism (SNP) microarrays, have been used as an alternative technology to conventional cytogenetic approaches[39]. They are able to infer CNAs (amplifications and deletions) compared to a reference sample. Array CGH platforms compare quickly and efficiently two labelled samples (different fluorophores test and reference). Denaturation of the DNA in single stranded allows the hybridization of the two samples to microarrays containing DNA sequence probes of known genome position (e.g. bacterial artificial chromosomes, cDNAs, or more recently, oligonucleotides). By using a fluorescence microscope and a dedicated computer software, the signal ratio of different coloured fluorescents is measured in order to identify chromosomal differences between the two sources. An important consideration is the consequence of the reference sample on the CN profile. A comprehensive-characterized reference is the key for the correct interpretation of array CGH data[40].

SNP-arrays have a higher resolution than CGH-arrays, and can be used to identify allele-specific information. SNP microarray has few key differences from CGH technologies. Probe designs are specific to single-nucleotide differences between DNA sequences.

Ultimately, next generation sequencing (NGS) have replaced microarrays as the platform for discovery and genotyping, and present considerable computational and bioinformatics challenges.

1.1.3. Computational Methods

We can summarize CNA analysis from microarray in three steps: 1) normalization, 2) probe-level modelling, and 3) CN estimation[41].

The target of normalization is to remove non relevant effects, such as the GC content of the fragment amplified by PCR, technical variations between arrays occurring from differences in sample preparation or labelling, and array production or scanning differences[42].

Probe-level modelling is usually performed at two levels: single locus and multilocus. Single locus modelling measures the CN of a specific target fragment or DNA probe locus in order to produce a raw fragment CN. Multilocus modelling combines the raw CNs of neighbouring fragments or DNA probe loci into a "meta-probe set" which determines the CN of the whole region[41][42].

Computerized methods to estimate CNs (e.g. segmentation) performs the detection of break points which separate neighbouring regions based on the Log ratio of probe intensity[41][42].

Several methods are suitable for analysing CNA on microarray data.

1) The first CNA analysis method has been developed by Affymetrix: Chromosome Copy Number Analysis Tool[43]. Normalization is performed by quantile normalization. Modelling uses robust multichip average. CN estimation can be done subsequently with an arbitrary algorithm.

2) DNA-Chip Analyzer (dChip)[44] normalizes using an invariant set method which corresponds to a normalization of the arrays based on the identification of a common baseline array and on adjustment of all the other arrays relative to the baseline array. Modelling is based on a model-based expression index (MBEI) for single-locus. This output is then used by a Hidden Markov Model (HMM) to infer CNs[44].

3) Copy Number Analyser for GeneChip arrays (CNAG)[45] normalizes the arrays in order to have the same mean signal intensity for all autosomal probes. This allows fragment probes comparable between arrays to be obtained. The signal intensity ratios is corrected for the differences in PCR product length and GC content. An HMM algorithm is applied to infer CNs along each chromosome.

4) Birdsuite's Birdseye[46] normalizes using quantile normalization. Modelling and segmentation are performed together at the multi-loci level. HMM estimates CNs.

5) Copy-number estimation using Robust Multichip Analysis (CRMA)[47] has been developed as an extension of the RMA model. Normalization is obtained by allelic cross-hybridization correction (ACC). Modelling uses robust multichip average (RMA). CNA analysis can be done using an arbitrary segmentation algorithm.

Given the different existing computational methods for CNA detection using SNP arrays, researchers have the problem to choose the optimal tool for their analyses.

With the aim of offering a support to bioinformatics researches and to answer to their emerging needs to choose among different CNA detection algorithms, the CNV Workshop was developed[48]. It represents the first cohesive and convenient platform for detection, annotation, and assessment of the biological and clinical significance of structural variants[48]. The purpose of the platform is to process data from a wide variety of SNP arrays, and to implement different normalization and CN estimation algorithms.

Since one of the main problems in the choice of the tool is the detection of discrepancies among different platforms[49], some studies have compared the different analysis using the same data set. Although limited to few methods, due to the high computational cost, several studies allowed the assessment of advantages and disadvantages of some techniques[49]–[51].

Baross et al.[49] found that CNAG, dChip, CNAT and GLAD are suitable for high-throughput processing of Affymetrix 100 K SNP array data for CN analysis. However, the tools revealed considerable variations in the numbers of putative CNA. dChip found more CNA than the other tested tools. The highest rate of false positive candidate deletion calls was produced by CNAG. In general, the performance of all tools in the detection of single copy deletions was better than that of single copy duplications. The authors recommend also the use of reference data set for accurate analysis, processed in the same laboratory and ideally from samples with an ethnic composition similar to the sample set.

Eckel-Passow *et al.*[50] provided a description of four freely-available software packages (PennCNV, Aroma. Affymetrix, Affymetrix Power Tools (APT), and Corrected Robust Linear Model with Maximum Likelihood Distance (CRLMM)) that are commonly used for CNA analysis of data generated from Affymetrix Genome-Wide Human SNP Array 6.0 platform. APT obtained the best performance with respect to bias. However, Penn CNV and Aroma. Affymetrix had the smallest variability associated with the median locus-level CN.

Zhang *et al.*[51] assessed four software programs currently used for CNA detection: Birdsuite (version 1.5.2), PennCNV-Affy (a trial version), HelixTree (Version 6.4.2), and Partek (Version, 6.09.0129). They evaluated the accuracy in detecting both rare and common CNVs in the Affymetrix 6.0 platform. They found considerable variations among the programs in the number of CNAs. Birdsuite obtained the highest percentages of known HapMap CNAs containing more than twenty markers in two reference CNA datasets. In the tested rare CNA data, Birdsuite and Partek had higher positive predictive values than the other tools.

Other methods exist for analysing CNA on NGS and they are not described in this review. However, most of the more recent algorithms for CNA discovery are modelled on computational methods which were first used to analyse capillary sequencing reads and fully sequenced large-insert clones[39].

1.1.4. Therapeutic Approach

A future challenging direction is the discovery of gene CN changes for the development of therapies. For example, duplication of one gene encoding a specific receptor can be associated with a particular pathology. Thus, compounds that down regulate receptor expression may lead benefit in patients.

Cancer is the prime case in which CNAs have been shown to drive disease[52] and therapies where overexpressed or amplified oncogenic drivers are targeted have been already considered. In particular, in BC, the gene encoding epidermal growth factor receptor (EGFR) results to be amplified, and small molecules such as gefitinib, erlotinib, lapatinib, and cetuximab have been applied to inhibit EGFR with benefits for patients[53][54].

ERBB2, encoding HER2, is amplified in 30% of BC[17][55]. In the therapy of HER2-amplified BC, trastuzumab, an anti-HER2 antibody, has been used[56]. Pertuzumab, a humanized monoclonal antibody, binds HER2, and like trastuzumab, it stimulates antibody-dependent, and cell mediated-cytotoxicity[57]. Pertuzumab and trastuzumab binds to different HER2 epitopes acting in the same way. When given together, they operate reinforcing antitumor activity[58].

These proven benefits, although limited to few genes involved in BC, raise the exciting possibility that targeting amplified disease drivers may offer opportunities for therapy development in BC where effective treatments are still limited.

2. Epigenetic Alterations in BC

2.1. DNA Methylation and Histone Modifications

DNA methylation and histone modifications play a crucial role in the maintenance of cellular functions and identity. In particular, the main cellular networks affected by epigenetics are cell cycle, apoptosis, DNA repair, detoxification, inflammation, cell adhesion and invasion.

In cancer, the DNA methylation and histone modifications are perturbed, leading to significant changes in GE, which confer to the tumoral cells advantages in proliferation and maintenance of tumoral phenotype. For instance, the genomic inactivation of a tumor suppressor gene (p53, BRCA1) or the activation of an oncogene (*i.e.*, Myc) contributes to the malignant transformation. Epigenetic changes differ from genetic changes mainly because they occur at a higher frequency than genetic changes; they are reversible upon treatment with pharmacological agents and occur at defined regions in a gene.

DNA methylation refers to the addition of a methyl group ($-CH_3$) covalently to the base cytosine (C) in the dinucleotide 5'-CpG-3'. CpGs islands are in the promoter region of many genes[59][60]. Most CpG dinucleotides in the human genome are methylated, and often leads to silencing of GE. The observation that

CpGs islands of housekeeping genes are mainly unmethylated, and the methylation is associated with loss of GE led to the hypothesis that DNA methylation plays an important role in regulating GE[59][60].

Figure 2 shows how DNA methylation affects GE. Methyl groups in the recognition elements of transcription factors inhibits the binding of transcription factors to DNA, thus resulting in reduced transcriptional activity.

Histones are considered DNA-packaging protein components of chromatin, able to regulate chromatin dynamics. In fact they are subjected to several post-translational modifications, occurring at the aminoterminal end of the histone tail protruding from the surface of the nucleosome[61]. The modifications of histone tails, including lysine acetylation, lysine and arginine methylation, lysine ubiquitylation, phosphorylation, sumoylation, and ribosylation, can significantly affect the expression of genes in a dynamic manner[61]. The most studied histone epigenetic alterations are acetylation/deacetylation, and methylation/demethylation. In BC, abnormal histone modification and DNA hypermethylation are frequently associated to epigenetic silencing of tumor suppressor genes and genomic instability[62][63].

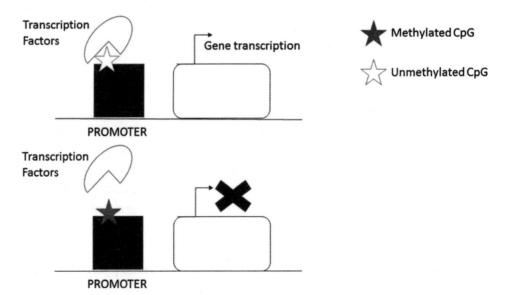

Figure 2. DNA methylation regulating GE. Methylated CpG restricts the binding between transcription factor and the gene promoter. Unmethylated CpG allows accessing of transcription factors to the gene promoter.

2.1.1. Biological Insights

The distribution of methylated and unmethylated CpGs in the genome shows different patterns of methylation confirming tissue-specific manner[64].

DNA methylation biomarkers for early detection and prognosis of cancer have been studied in the last years. **Table 2** shows genes differentially methylated in BC.

Fackler *et al.*[65] found that promoter methylation of 4 genes (RASSF1A, CCND2, TWIST, HIN1) was more frequently detected in tumor than in normal tissue. In another study[66], 4 genes CCND2, RASSF1A, APC and HIN1 were able to classify between invasive carcinomas, fibroadenomas, and normal tissue. 10 hypermethylated genes, APC, BIN1, BMP6, BRCA1, CST6, ESR-b, GSTP1, P16, P21 and TIMP3, were identified to distinguish between cancerous and normal tissues[67].

Table 2. Genes differentially methylated in BC.

Genes	Biologicaleffects	References
RASSF1A and CCND2	Significantly more methylated in the ER+ than ER−cancers	[69]
PGR, TFF1, CDH13, TIMP3, HSD17B4, ESR1 and BCL2	The inverse correlations were found between their hypermethylation and ER expression	[70]
ESR1, TGFBR2, PTGS2 and CDH13	They were associated with PR expression	[70]
FAM124B, ST6GALNAC1, NAV1 and PER1	The methylation status were quite different between ER+/PR+ and ER−/PR−BC	[71]
RASSF1A, CCND2, TWIST, HIN1	Low levels of methylation were detected in normal control samples	[74]
CCND2, RASSF1A, APC and HIN1	Able to distinguish between invasive carcinomas, fibroadenomas, and normal tissue	[66]
ITIH5, DKK3, and RASSF1A	Early detection of BC	[74]
APC, BIN1, BMP6, BRCA1, CST6, ESR-b, GSTP1, P16, P21 and TIMP3	Able to distinguish between cancerous and normal tissues	[67]
CST6	Differentially methylated between BC and control plasma samples	[75]

Several studies provide strong evidence of DNA methylation signatures with prognostic role. DNA methylation status of the PITX2 in BC cell lines is negatively associated with PITX2 mRNA expression and with poor prognosis[68].

Previous studies observed several candidate methylation sites that are associated with the hormone receptor status of BC. RASSF1A and CCND2 were significantly more methylated in the ER+ than ER− BC[69], whereas the inverse correlations were identified between hypermethylation of the PGR, TFF1, CDH13, TIMP3, HSD17B4, ESR1 and BCL2 genes and ER status[70]. Hypermethylation of the ESR1, TGFBR2, PTGS2 and CDH13 genes was associated with PR status[70].

Li et al.[71] used 27 K arrays in a small sample of ER/ PR+ and ER/PR BC samples, and identified and validated four genes: FAM124B and ST6GALNAC1 were significantly hypermethylated, and NAV1 and PER1 were significantly hypomethylated in ER+/PR+BC.

Fang et al.[72] used genome wide analysis to characterize BCs based on their metastatic potential. The study found a coordinated methylation of a large number of genes discovering a "methylator" phenotype. The methylator phenotype was associated with low metastatic risk and survival.

Identification of promoter methylation of biomarker genes in the DNA of bodily fluids, like serum or plasma, is a rapidly growing research field in cancer detection.

The principle is based on evidence that solid malignant tumors release significant amounts of cell-free DNA into the bloodstream through cellular necrosis or apoptosis[73].

The analysis of the methylation patterns of cell-free DNA by a blood-based test could become a screening tool. In particular, DNA methylation in circulating free DNA from blood of BC was investigated. ITIH5, DKK3, and RASSF1A promoter methylation from serum were identified as candidate biomarkers for the early detection of BC[74].

CST6 has been identified by two independent dataset as being differentially methylated between BC and control plasma samples[75].

SOX17 promoter is highly methylated in primary BCs, in circulating tumor cells isolated from patients with BC, and in corresponding cell-free DNA samples[76].

Similar studies on plasma identified hypermethylation status of KIF1A[77], and HYLA2 locus[78] in BC suggesting methylation level in blood having a power to distinguish very early BC cases from controls.

Non-invasive technique such as blood-test screening is a more suitable and cost-efficient methodology compared to mammography and magnetic resonance imaging.

Actually, in clinical use no specific methylation bio-marker has been yet validated, due to the reduced number of matched normal DNA samples in cohorts.

Characterizing more than 880 human BC, Elsheikh *et al.* have demonstrated that histone acetylation and methylation patterns represent an early sign of BC[79]. Low levels of acethylated lysine and methylated lysine and arginine were described to have prognostic value, *i.e.* of triple-negative carcinomas and HER2-positive BC subtype[79][80].

2.1.2. Experimental Methods

In recent years three major technologies have been employed in DNA methylation analysis: chemical treatment with bisulphite (BS), methylation-specific enzyme digestion, and affinity enrichment[81][82].

The first category includes an assay to characterize methyl cytosine by treatment of genomic DNA with BS. BS treatment converts unmethylated cytosine residues to uracil, without recognizing methyl cytosine residues, which are protected against this treatment.

Methylated and unmethylated DNA can be distinguished by the employment of sequence analysis (e.g. NGS, microarray). PCR amplicons created after BS conversion can be hybridized to microarrays containing methylation-specific oligonucleotides (MSO; 19–23 nucleotides) to query DNA methylation status[83]. BS-based methods cannot distinguish between methylcitosine and other variants (e.g. hydroxymethylcytosine)[84].

The second category includes methylation-sensitive restriction endonucleases, which distinguish sequences based on methylation status; furthermore methylcytosine could be identified by immunoprecipitation with antibodies or by affinity purification on methyl-binding protein beads.

Restriction endonucleases and microarray are also combined for high-throughput examination of the methylation status[85][86]. A limitation in utilizing restriction endonucleases is that enzymes identify only a limited fraction of genome CpG sites[81][82]. A methodology[87] with multiple enzyme-mediated restrictions was proposed, leads to a better coverage of all CpG dinucleotides in mammalian genomes.

A third category, enrichment techniques, include methylated DNA immune-precipitation (MeDIP). Genomic DNA is immunoprecipitated with a monoclonal antibody that specifically identifies 5-methylcytidine. The immunoprecipitated fraction can be detected by PCR in order to identify the methylation state of individual regions[88].

A combination approach of MeDIP and methylation-sensitive restriction endonucleases was developed, promising to quickly compare methylomes at lower cost[89]. Alternatively, MeDIP can be combined with large-scale analysis (e.g. microarrays)[88].

Many of the techniques proposed for DNA methylation profiling can be combined with NGS technologies[90].

2.1.3. Computational Methods

Bioinformatics research has been focused on the prediction of DNA methylation information with a dual purpose: i) accurate DNA methylation predictions could replace experimental data, and ii) DNA methylation prediction algorithms from training data can give additional information of an epigenetic mechanism.

A large number of computational predictive models have been developed to identify CpG dinucleotides methylated or unmethylated[91][92], CpG islands (or CpG-rich regions) methylated or unmethylated[93][94], and CpG islands (or CpG-rich regions) differentially methylated in different tissue/cell types or phenotypes[95]. Most of them use DNA sequence characteristics combined with a machine-learning algorithm.

Combination approaches of computational and experimental methods can speed up genome-wide DNA methylation profiling and detect crucial factors or pathways driving DNA methylation patterns. However DNA methylation prediction shows some difficulties: i) DNA methylation of the sampled cells need to be averages across cells, ii) there are differences across tissues, iii) DNA methylation can have unstable position, and iv) can be not well located in a genomic locus[96][97].

A key step for accurate computational predictive models is a correct features selection.

The features can be grouped into two categories: genetic and epigenetic features. Given a region of interest (a CpG island or a genomic region around a particular CpG dinucleotide), the genetic features include: i) general features of the region of interest (e.g., length, and distribution of the CpG dinucleotides in the region), ii) DNA sequence composition of the region of interest, iii) patterns of conserved transcription factor binding sites or conserved elements within or near the region of interest, iv) structural and physicochemical properties of the region of interest, v) functional annotations of nearby genes, vi) single nucleotide polymorphisms of the region of interest, and vii) the conservation of the region of interest among species[98].

Epigenetic features are also crucial in order to fully characterize DNA methylation status.

DNA methylation, as an epigenetic phenomenon, is affected by some other epigenetic factors, such as histone methylation and histone acetylation.

Statistical methods related to differential DNA methylation data analysis cover a number of different approaches. In particular, these methods are accessible to the user by Bioconductor/R. **Table 3** shows some methods and packages currently available for methylation differential analysis, such as Wilcoxon rank sum test (implemented in methyAnalysis package)[99], t-test (implemented in methyAnalysis, CpGAssoc, RnBeads, and IMA package[99]–[102]), Kolmogorov- Smirnov Tests ([100]), permutation test (implemented in CpGAssoc package[101]), empirical Bayes method (implemented in RnBeads, IMA and minfi package[101]–[103]), and bump hunting method (implemented in bumphunter and minfi package[104][105]).

Wilcoxon rank sum test detect statistically significant sites according to the absolute difference between the average methylation levels of the analysed groups[106][107]. This method can have a limitation in case of low or unbalance number of samples groups[107].

t-test is statistically inefficient in the presence of heterogeneity of methylation variability and shows many false positives, particularly for studies with smaller sample sizes[108][109].

Kolmogorov-Smirnov test is another commonly used test that quantifies distributional differences. However, the Kolmogorov-Smirnov test considers each CpG marker as a sampling unit and its naive application is not valid[110][111].

Permutation test is a resampling-based nonparametric test which permutes data following the null hypothesis of equal data distributions between groups[112].

Table 3. Packages and methods for methylation differential analysis.

Package	Method	References
methyAnalysis	Wilcoxon rank sum test	[100]
methyAnalysis, CpGAssoc, RnBeads, and IMA	t-test	[100]–[102]
-	Kolmogorov-Smirnov test	[104]
CpGAssoc	permutation test	[101]
RnBeads, IMA and minfi	empirical Bayes	[102][103][105]
bumphunter and minfi	bump hunting	[105][106]

Different number of empirical Bayes models were proposed for differential methylation analysis, with different statistical distribution assumptions[113]. Teng *et al.*[113] constructed five empirical Bayes models based on either a gamma distribution or a log-normal distribution, for the detection of differential methylated loci. They observed that log-normal, rather than gamma, could be a more accurate and precise method.

Bump hunting method used in bumphunter and minfi packages based the correlations of methylation levels between nearby CpG locus, and, for each locus, a linear model was used to estimate the coefficient of difference in methylation levels between the cancer group and the normal groups[105][107].

A comparison study among these six statistical approaches was proposed[114]. Finally, different approaches were recommended for different applications: the bump hunting method is better for small sample size; the empirical Bayes methods are suggested when DNA methylation levels are independent across CpG loci, while only the bump hunting method is suggested when DNA methylation levels are correlated across CpG loci. All methods are found suitable for medium or large sample sizes[114].

2.1.4. Therapeutic Approach

Cancer was the first group of diseases to be associated with DNA methylation. Numerous genes have been identified as being differentially methylated in BC, with crucial roles in DNA repair, apoptosis, hormone receptor, and cell cycle. These TSGs may be good therapeutic targets through regulation of methylation activity by DNA methyltransferase inhibitors. Human DNA methylation is catalysed by enzymes of the DNA cytosine methyltransferases family including DNMT1, DNMT3A, DNMT3B and DNMT3L[115]. A lower DNA methyltransferase activity increases expression of silenced genes such as TSGs reactivating expression of key genes.

Previous studies[116][117] were reported in BC focusing on action of DNA methyltransferase compound inhibitors.

Key targets for potential DNA demethylation agents are DNA methyltransferase inhibitor 5-aza-2′-deoxycytidine (decitabine), zebularine, and SGI-110[117]. The mechanism of action of these pro-drugs is similar since they need to be incorporated into DNA to act as inhibitors of DNMTs[115].

Decitabine shows activity against hematologic malignancy and low-dose correlates with changes in GE induced by a reduction in DNA methylation.

A phase I clinical and pharmacodynamic trial was proposed in order to assess the feasibility of delivering a dose of decitabine combined with carboplatin[116]. Decitabine showed some limitations for treatment of advanced solid tumors (e.g. BC): i) weak stability, ii) lack of specificity for cancer cells, and iii) rapid inactivation by the action of cytidine deaminase[117].

Zebularine and SGI-110 are more selective for cancer cells and have higher resistance to deamination. In particular, Zebularine[118] showed an antitumor effect in a mouse model. In zebularine-treated mices, the oral treatment with zebularine showed a significant delay in tumor growth[118]. In combination with decitabine, zebularine has proven a significant inhibitory effect on cell proliferation and colony formation in MDA-MB-231 BC cell line through induction of ER alpha and PR mRNA expression[119]. Unfortunately, toxicity remain its main limitation[118].

SGI-110[120], a 5′-AzapG-3′ dinucleotide, induces expression of the p16 tumor suppressor gene, and inhibit tumor cell growth. This short oligonucleotide is resistant to cytidine deaminase deamination which may potentially increase its resistance, enhance bioavailability, and make the drug more efficacious.

DNA methyltransferase inhibitors can have side effects as the concomitant activation of both TSGs and OGs. The combination of chemotherapeutic agents and of DNA methyltransferase inhibitors could be efficacious[115].

Although the benefits of DNA methyltransferase inhibitors were demonstrated, toxicity, lack of specificity and low stability are issues to be solved in order to improve BC treatment[121].

Histone acetylation process is controlled by the balanced activity of histone acetyltransferases and histone deacetylases (HDACs). The HDAC family is divided into zinc-dependent enzymes (classes I, IIa, IIb, and IV, of which there are 11 subtype enzymes) and zinc-independent enzymes (class III, also calledsirtuins), requiring NAD+ for their catalytic activity.Over the past decade, a number of HDAC inhibitors have been designed and synthesized, based on HDAC chemical structures. Some of these HDAC inhibitors are able to modify the chromatin structure, causing re-expression of aberrantly silenced genes, which in turn is associated with growth inhibition and apoptosis in cancer cells[122]. In ER-negative BC, the treatment with specific HDAC inhibitors reactivates ERα and progesterone receptor (PR) gene expression, which are known to be aberrantly silenced in BC. Preclinical studies of HDAC inhibitors combined with DNMT inhibitors or with anti-tumoral treatment (*i.e.*, tamoxifen) have demonstrated a higher safety, tolerability and clinical effectiveness than single treatment[123][124].

2.2. microRNA Deregulation in BC

2.2.1. Biological Insights

miRNAs are small noncoding RNAs (20–22 nucleotides long) that are excised from longer (60–110 nucleotides) RNA precursor[105][106] and act in different biological functions including development, proliferation, differentiation and cell death[125][126]. miRNAs are major regulators of GE. Many evidences indicate that their deregulation is associated to several steps of cancer initiation and progression. In comparison with other approaches targeting single genes, they are certainly more stable thanks to their small size[127], and are able to discriminate different BC subtypes.

Blenkiron *et al.* found deregulated miRNAs between basal and luminal BC[128]. Iorio *et al.*[129], Lowery *et al.*[130] and Mattie *et al.*[131] identified miRNAs that were able to classify ER, PR and HER2/neu receptor status, respectively. Gregory *et al.*[132] found miR-200 associated with the BC luminal subtype. Reduced expression of miR-145 and miR-205 was found to play a role in basal like triple negative tumours (ER-/PR-/HER2-) while are normally expressed in normal myoepithelial cells[133].

miRNAs can be also prognostic and predictive biomarkers. Zhou *et al.*[134] found mir-125b as useful indicator for poorly response to taxol-based treatments in vivo. The overexpression of miR-181a has been correlated with lymph node metastasis[135]. miR-106b-25 expression was proven significantly predictor of good relapse time[136], while miR-375 was found negatively regulate ER expression[137].

miRNAs with a role in metastasis in BC include miR-7[138][139], miR-17/20[140][141], miR-22[142]-[144], miR-30[145][146], miR-31[147]-[149], miR-126[150], miR-145[151], miR-146[152], miR-193b[153], miR-205[154], miR-206[155], miR-335[156], miR-448[157], miR-661[158] and let-7[159].

miRNAs can be easily extracted and detected from blood[160], circulating exomes[161], saliva[162][163], and even sputum[164][165]. Several studies demonstrated that circulating miRNAs reflect the pattern observed in the tumour tissues (e.g.[167]), thus opening the possibility to use circulating miRNAs as biomarkers for diagnosis and prognosis. Lodes *et al.*[166] provided an evidence on using serum miRNAs as biomarkers to discriminate between normal and patients in many cancer diseases including breast, prostate, colon, ovarian, and lung cancer. They showed that it is sufficient 1 mL of serum to detect miRNA expression patterns, without the need of amplification techniques. Recently, an analysis of circulating miRNAs have led to identify mir-21, miR-92a[167][168], miR-10b, miR-125b, miR-155, miR-191, miR-382[169] and miR-30a[170] as candidate biomarkers for early detection of BC. Circulating miR-NAs have also been associated with disease prognosis and response to treatment. Madhavan *et al.*[171] found circulating miRNAs as marker of disease free survival and overall survival. Plasma miR-10b and miR-373 were found associated with the development of metastases[172] while miR-125b[173] and miR-155[174] have been found correlated to chemotherapy response.

Table 4 reports a synthesis of the considered miRNAs deregulated in BC, with their principal biological effects.

2.2.2. Experimental Methods

Many technologies for detecting miRNAs have been developed, including RT-PCR, in situ hybridization, microarray, and NGS[7].

Table 4. miRNAs deregulated in BC.

MiRNAs	Biological effect	References
miR-200	It associated with the luminal subtype	Gregory et al.[132]
miR-145 and miR-205	It associated with basal like triple negative tumours	Sempere et al.[133]
miR-125b	It can predict poor response to taxol-based treatment in vivo	Zhou et al.[134]
miR-181a	It correlated with lymph node metastasis	Taylor et al.[135]
miR-106b-25	It can significantly predict a good relapse time	Smith et al.[136]
miR-31	It controls metastasis and increases the survival of patients	Valastyan et al.[147]
let-7	It suppressed metastasis	Yu et al.[159]
miR-375	It negatively regulate ER expression	de Souza et al.[137]
miR-10b, miR-155	They correlate with metastasis	Mar-Aguilar et al.[169]
miR-21	It associated with cell migration and invasion	Si et al.[168]

RT-PCR is a sensitive and precise technology but it is also an expensive and low-throughput method[7].

In situ hybridization is based on labelled complementary strands for the sequences of interest (e.g. miRNA) in a portion or section of tissue[175]. The small size of the mature miRNA presents problems for conventional in situ hybridization methods and it is semi-quantitative.

Microarrays have several limitations as those due to background or cross-hybridization problems. Moreover, microarrays and other techniques can provide analyses only on known miRNAs[7].

Contrarily, sequence-based methods allow the identification of unknown miRNAs and early overcome other methods. Stark et al.[176], by using deep sequencing, discovered and quantified new miRNAs. Similarly, Farazi et al.[177], generated a miRNA signature able to differentiate ductal breast carcinoma in situ, invasive ductal breast carcinoma and normal tissue.

Also deep sequencing may be a powerful method to study circulating miRNAs. Several studies investigated correlations among miRNAs in the serum of BC with clinicopathological indices[178] and found miRNAs associations with overall survival[179].

Despite the high potential and promising results of these methods in clinical applications, there are still some problems that need to be addressed, e.g. the lack of inconsistency for some results between different studies. Standardization of procedures for sample conservation, preparation and/or processing[180], and the use of different quality controls for data normalization[181] could be effective in reducing these limitations.

2.2.3. Computational Methods

There are two different approaches to examine both miRNA and mRNA expression profiles.

A first approach considers either a miRNA or an mRNA first, and then applies ad-hoc strategies, such as computational or experimental methods, in order to obtain miRNA-mRNA pair information[182][183].

A second approach examines miRNA and mRNA regulatory pairs together[184]-[187].

Computational methods play important roles in the identification of new miRNAs. These methods can be divided into three major categories: 1) sequence or structure conservation-based, 2) machine learning-based method, 3) and non-comparative methods.

Sequence or structure conservation-based methods are based on sequence/structure conservation as techniques to find miRNAs. The principle is the nature of conservation across different species for most of the known miRNAs. Comparative genomics filter out sequence/structure conservation that are not evolutionarily conserved in related species[188]. Examples of such computational methods, focusing on the secondary structure of RNA and looking for conserved hairpin structures between related species, are Srnaloop[189], MiRscan[190], and miRseeker[191]. One of the first study related to these methods was by Lee and Ambros[192]. The authors, using bioinformatics techniques, searched for sequences conserved between the C. elegans and C. briggsae genomes. They focused on premiRNA sequences and secondary structures with similar characteristics to lin-4 and let-7, the first two miRNAs found on that time.

Several web based software tools have been developed to find new miRNA genes, based on sequence and secondary structure similarities with known miR-NAs[189]–[191][193]. However, the limit of these approaches was demonstrated by Bentwich et al., showing the possibility that large quantity of nonconserved miRNAs could be missed by the use of this tool[194].

Free energy (or Gibbs free energy) can be used as feature for miRNA target prediction. It shows how strong the binding of a miRNA with its target is by predicting how the miRNA and its candidate target will hybridize. The free energy of miRNA-mRNA binding is normally assigned by the RNAfold program-Vienna RNA Package[195].

Machine learning-based methods do not necessarily depend on sequence conservation. A classifier is constructed on a training dataset, that contains a set of known miRNA sequences (positive training dataset), and on a set consisting of mRNAs, tRNAs and rRNAs (negative training dataset). The information given to the classifier can be, for instance, the position of the mature sequence or the folding energy. The classifier, by describing a candidate miRNA with this set of features, is able to predict true and false miRNA sequences[196]. The limit of this approach is the choice of negative set. As example, we do not know a priori if a particular sequence can generate functional miRNAs[197]. Several studies have tried to overcome this kind of problems with the use of only positive models[198, 199]. However, the results were poorer than those found by approaches that consider both positive and negative training sets[199].

Different classification methods are currently available based on machine learning, e.g. SVM, neural networks, HMM, and Naive Bayes (NB), and several tools based on machine learning have been developed and released to the research community, e.g. RNAmicro[200], MiRFinder[201], ProMir[202], MiRRim[203], SSCprofiler[204], HHMMiR[205] and BayesMiRNAFind[206].

Non-comparative methods use intrinsic structural features of miRNA, and include algorithms like PalGrade[207], Triplet-SVM[208], miPred[209], miR- abela[210], and HHMMiR[211]. These methods are able of detecting a large number of miRNAs that seem to be unique to primates.

Bentwich *et al.*[207] developed PalGrade by integrating bioinformatics pre-dictions with microarray analysis and sequence-directed cloning. This approach allowed the detection of 89 human miRNAs, 53 of them being not conserved beyond primates.

Xue *et al.*[208] proposed an ab initio classification of real pre-miRNA from other hairpin sequences with similar stem-loop features. SVM was applied on these features to classify real vs pseudo pre-miRNAs achieving 90% of accuracy.

Ng *et al.*[209] employed a Gaussian Radial Basis Function kernel (RBF) as a similarity measure for 29 global and intrinsic hairpin folding attributes. They tested the model on 123 human pre-miRs and 246 pseudo hairpins, reporting 84.55%, 97.97%, and 93.50% in sensitivity, specificity and accuracy, respectively.

Sewer *et al.*[210] developed miR-abela to detect human miRNAs. They fo-cused on particular properties of some genomic regions around already known miRNAs, and were able to predict between 50–100 novel pre-miRNAs, 30% of them already found as new in other studies.

2.2.4. Therapeutic Approach

miRNAs may have a crucial role in guiding treatment decisions. miRNAs can be therapeutic agents in cancer for two major characteristics: (1) their expres-sion is deregulated in cancer compared to normal tissues, and (2) cancer phenotype can be changed by targeting miRNA expression[196].

Compared to gene profiles, miRNA-based therapeutics have several advan-tages, as for example their ability to target multiple genes, frequently in the context of a network. miRNAs regulating the network of genes and cellular pathways play a crucial role in BC pathogenesis and therapy.

There are two strategies for developing miRNA-based therapies: i) by the introduction of miRNA-mimic oligonucleotides, which mimic miRNA expression, up-regulating miRNA, and ii) by the introduction of miRNA inhibitor oligonucleotides to inhibit the expression of the miRNA of interest. However, some major obstacles for the use of miRNA therapeutics exist, including the tissue-specific delivery[211][212], and the fact that erroneous targeting of miRNAs may cause toxic phenotypes[213].

For an effective drug-design of miRNA-targeted therapies in BC, it could be useful to understand the interplay between miRNAs and mRNAs leading to BC, thus studying the networks of gene controlled by each miRNA of interest. miRNA and their targets can form complex regulatory networks, and the comprehension of miRNA-target relation will help the development of personalized and tailored therapies[213].

2.3. Gene Expression Deregulation in BC

2.3.1. Biological Insights

GE profiling in BC has been widely demonstrated to generate different prognostic and diagnostic gene signatures. However, molecular tests have a potential not only for diagnosis but also for tailoring treatment plans, in particular with the aim of reducing resistance, non-response and toxicity[214]. Most of the tests either focus on gene expression microarrays or quantitative reverse transcription (qRT)-PCR analyses.

van't Veer *et al.*[215] obtained one of the prognostic signature for BC currently available on the market: MammaPrint. Microarray analysis of 78 BC patients with no systemic therapy led to the identification of a list of 70 genes able to predict the prognosis of the disease. The test was independently validated in a cohort of 295 early stage invasive BC, and results proved that the signature was an independent prognostic marker in BC[216]. A second independent validation study was performed by the TRANSBIG Consortium[217] in a cohort of 302 adjuvantly untreated patients, and was followed by additional validation studies[218]–[220]. MammaPrint was developed by Agendia, a laboratory in Amsterdam, approved in 2007 by the U.S. Food and Drug Administration (FDA) and then released commercially. This is a microarray-based test assessing the risk that a BC can metastasize to other parts of the body.

Paik et al.[221] developed Oncotype DX, a qRT PCR-based signature which measures the expression level of 21 genes (16 target + 5 reference genes). The test is able to predict chemotherapy benefits and the likelihood of distant BC recurrence. This is the first genomic biomarker assay which is commercially available for BC treatment as support of chemotherapy. Three separate studies containing 447 BC patients allowed to identify the 21-gene profile, which were divided into 16 target and 5 reference genes. The test was then validated using 668 node negative, ER positive, tamoxifen treated patients from NSABP B-14. An Oncotype DX Recurrence Score (ODRS) was defined and measured, as expression of a risk percentage for the development of distant metastases[222]. Oncotype DX was subsequently evaluated in the NSA BP-B20 trial, a study that explored the benefit of chemotherapy plus tamoxifen, and proved the accuracy of the biomarker. Currently, the Oncotype DX assay is performed in the licensed Genomic Health laboratory, which is the laboratory where the assay was developed.

Prediction Analysis of Microarray (PAM50), by using qRT-PCR assay, measures the expression of 55 (50 target and 5 reference genes) to identify the intrinsic subtypes of BC: luminal A, luminal B, HER2-enriched, and basal-like[223]. The gene signature was developed by analysing 189 BC samples, and was then validated on 761 BCs for prognosis and on 133 BCs for prediction of response to a taxane and anthracycline regimen[223]. Nano-String's Prosigna™ received a CE-mark designation for selling BC PAM50 in 2012, and received FDA clearance in 2013.

Genomic Grade Index (GGI)[4] is a 97 gene which measures the histological tumour grade. This test is based on the assumption that histological grade is a strong prognostic factor in ER positive BC. Sotiriou et al.[4] found that GGI gene signature is able to classify BC as histological grades I and III. They used 64 samples of ER-positive BC tumours to select genes that were differentially expressed

(DE) between histologic grade I and III tumours, and to generate the gene signature. Data from 597 independent tumours were then used to evaluate GGI and to also demonstrate that GGI can separate histological grade 2 BC into low or high categories with different clinical outcomes. The results of the BIG-1-98 study (55 endocrine-treated patients)[224] demonstrated that the GGI is also a potential predictor of relapse for endocrine-treated BC patients. Ipsogen launched the Map Quant Dx (TM) genomic grade test by incorporating GGI. The test is currently used, in particular when tumor grade information can be decisive for prescribing a chemotherapy.

Immunohistochemical (IHC) assay Mammostrat[225] uses 5 immunohis- tochemical markers (SLC7A5, HTF9C, P53, NDRG1, and CEACAM5) to stratify patients on tamoxifen therapy into different risk groups, in order to inform treatment decisions. In the validation study, an analysis was performed on two independent data sets of 299 and 344 BC samples[226]. Clarient launched on the market the Insight® Dx Mammostrat® Breast Cancer Recurrence test in 2010.

Table 5 reports the considered commercially available tests, with their principal characteristics (e.g. number of genes, validation data sets).

2.3.2. Experimental Methods

Understanding GE and how it changes under normal and pathological conditions is necessary to provide information about the expressed genes. Large scale GE data provide the activity of thousands of genes at once.

Several techniques exist for studying and quantifying GE.

Traditional methods focus on measuring the expression of one gene at a time, as, for example, the Northern Blotting and the Real-Time Quantitative Reverse Transcription PCR (RT-PCR).

Northern blotting (called also RNA blot) was the first tool used to measure RNA levels, and, until the end of the 1990s, it was used extensively. It allows to quantify levels of mRNA by electrophoresis, which is able to separate RNA samples by size. The RNA of interest is revealed by a hybridization probe complementary

Table 5. Current commercially available genetic test for BC and their principal characteristics.

	Author	N. genes	Samples used to generate BC signature	Independent validation study	Laboratory
MammaPrint	van't Veer et al.[215]	70	- 78 BC patients	- 295 early stage invasive BC. - 302 who had received loco-regional therapybut no systemic adjuvant therapy	Agendia
Oncotype DX	Paik et al. [221]	21	- 447 BC patients	- 668 node negative ER positive tamoxifen treated cases - 651 BC samples: 227 had been randomly assigned to tamoxifen adjuvant therapy and 424 to tamoxifen plus chemotherapy	Genomic Health
PAM50	Parker et al.[223]	50	- 189 BC patients	- 761 patients (no systemic therapy), 133 (neoadjuvant chemotherapy)	NanoString's Prosigna™
Genomic Grade Index (GGI)	Sotiriou et al.[4]	97	- 64 BC patients	- 597 BC - 55 endocrine-treated patients.	Ipsogen
Mammostrat	Bartlett et al.[225]	5	- 466 BC patients	- 299 BC, 344 BC	Clarient

to it. The first step of RNA blot is to denature the RNA into single strands. Hence, gel electrophoresis separates the RNA molecules according to their size. Subsequently, the RNA is transferred from the gel onto a blotting membrane, containing RNA bands originally on the gel. A probe complementary to the RNA of interest binds to a particular RNA sequence in the sample[227]. The RNA-probe complexes can thus be detected using a variety of different chemistries or radionuclide labelling.

RT-PCR is a major development of PCR technology, overcoming Northern blot as the method for RNA detection and quantification[228]. It enables to monitor and measure a targeted DNA molecule generated during each cycle of PCR process. In RT-PCR, the mRNA must be converted to a double-stranded molecule by using the enzyme reverse transcriptase. This phase is followed by quantitative

PCR (qPCR) on the cDNA with the detection and quantification of amplified products[229]. The quantity of each specific target is obtained by measuring the increase in fluorescence signal from DNA-binding dyes or probes, during successive rounds of enzyme-mediated amplification. The limitation of this technique is the quantification of few genes at a time[229].

Several technologies such as microarray, Serial Analysis of Gene (SAGE), Cap Analysis of Gene Expression (CAGE) and Massively Parallel Signature Sequencing (MPSS) allow the mRNA expression data for hundreds of genes to be obtained in one single experiment[230].

The most commonly used technology to profile the expression of thousands of transcripts simultaneously is microarray. DNA microarray is an array of oligonucleotide probes bound to a chip surface[231][232]. Labelled cDNA from a sample is hybridized to complementary probe sequences on the chip, and strongly associated complexes are identified by detection of fluorophore-, silver-, or chemiluminescence-labelled targets[231][232]. Many variables influence the outcome of the experiments in microarray analysis, thus contributing to experimental errors and biological variations (for more details see[233]).

In contrast to microarray methods, sequence-based approaches directly determine the cDNA sequence[234]. SAGE[235], CAGE[236], and MPSS[237], all tag-based sequencing approaches, are based on Sanger sequencing technology.

The development of novel high-throughput DNA sequencing methods, such as RNA-Seq (RNA sequencing), has provided new approaches for both mapping and quantifying transcriptomes. It has clear advantage over existing approaches: RNA-Seq is not limited to the detection of transcripts that correspond to existing genomic sequence, and it is suitable to discovery genomic sequences that are still unknown[234].

In RNA-Seq analysis, RNA is converted to a library of cDNA fragments with adaptors attached to one or both ends. Each molecule is then sequenced in a high-throughput way in order to obtain short sequences (reads 30–400 bp). Following sequencing, the resulting reads are mapped to the genome in order to produce a genome-scale transcription map consisting of both the transcriptional structure and the level of expression for each gene[234]. Although RNA-Seq has many advantages with respect to the other methods, other issues must be overcome to achieve best practices in the measurement of gene expression, for instance, the lack of accurate methods able to identify and track the expression changes of rare RNA isoforms from all genes[234].

Table 6 reports a synthesis of the considered experimental methods for studying and quantifying GE, with their principal advantages and limitations.

2.3.3. Computational Methods

Microarray or RNA-sequencing technologies, as above reported, produce an overall design of all the transcriptional activity in a biological sample. However,

Table 6. Principal experimental methods for GE quantification.

Method	Pros	Cons
Northern Blotting	- Inexpensive - detectingtranscript size	- low throughput - semiquantitative - RNAase contamination
RT-PCR	- high sensitivity - high sequence specific	- high variability - normalizaton methods
Microarray	- measurement of the activity of thousands of genes at once - rapid - don't require large-scale DNA sequencing - low Background noise	- high cost - analysis of Big data - high Background noise - only a portion of the transcript
Sanger sequencing technology		- isoforms are generally indistinguishable from each other - Low throughput
RNA-seq	- measurement of the activity of thousands of genes at once - require low amount of RNA - high reproducibility - Low Backgroundnoise	- High cost - Analysis of Big data

these methods necessarily produce a large amount of data to be visualized, evaluated for their quality, normalized, filtered and interpreted.

Hence, the data originated by platforms (such as microarrays or RNA-seq) must be pre-processed. Preprocessing step is crucial to normalize the data and to clean biological signal values from experimental noise[238][239].

Data must be also reduced prior to be used in advanced analysis, and this can be accomplished in two different ways: 1) by dimensionality reduction methods, that do not modify the original representation of data, and 2) by dimensionality reduction techniques which involve modification or loss of information from the original data. Among this second category, there are those methods based on projection (e.g. principal component analysis) or compression (e.g. using information theory)[240].

One of the most validated methods of the first category is feature selection technique. It is often used to identify key genes able to separate the samples into different classes (e.g. cancerous and normal cells), and to remove irrelevant genes. Golub et al.[241] showed indeed that most genes are not significant in a problem of samples classification. However, feature selection is also important in order to obtain faster and efficient classification models, and to avoid over fitting.

Three categories of feature selection methods can be used: filters, wrappers, and embedded methods[242][243]. Filter methods find subset of genes dependent on the class label, and do not consider the relevance of genes in combination with other genes[243]. Usually they are simple and fast.

Filter methods include correlation-based feature selection (CFS)[244], t-test[243][245], information gain[243][245], mutual information[246], entropy-based methods[247], Euclidian distance[245], signal to noise ratio[245], and significant analysis of microarrays[248].

Wrapper methods try to achieve the best combination of genes that may offer high classification accuracy. They include hybrid genetic algorithms[249], particle swarm optimization[250], successive feature selection (SFS)[251] and GA-KDE-Bayes[252]. However, this approach is less used, in particular in microarray analysis, due to its high computational costs[243].

Filter approach does not interact with the classifier, contrarily to wrapper and embedded techniques, usually resulting in lower performance.

An intermediate approach between the lowest results of the filter methods and the high computational cost of the wrapper methods is represented by the embedded method. With this method, the feature selection procedure is inbuilt to a classifier. Classification trees like ID3, random forest, and Support Vector Machine (SVM) based on Recursive Feature Elimination (RFE) are all examples of embedded methods[243][245].

The principle of the feature selection and validation techniques is shown in **Figure 3**. A pre-processing step is performed: i) the quality of data is evaluated, ii) outliers are removed, and iii) data are normalized. Feature selection is performed. Usually, original data are divided into two data sets: a training set, subjected to the feature selection, and a testing set, used to evaluate the feature selection of the model with different validation techniques. Feature selection finds a subset of genes of interest, (e.g. a gene signature), and the validation of genes is performed. The most used validation techniques are cross-validation or leave one out validation[243], even if several studies suggested the use of a 10-fold cross validation because they give a more biased but less variable estimate than the leave-one-out error (e.g.[253]). When the feature selection of the model satisfies the required validation performance, the genes are defined and can be interpreted.

2.3.4. Therapeutic Approach

Drug compounds that facilitate and control tightly therapeutic GE are a promising target. Transcriptional gene regulatory system has been encoded within several viral vectors (eg. Tetracycline-based systems can regulate GE of particular targets with the use of cell-type-specific promoters)[254].

The regulation of GE systems is an attractive target for gene therapy development, and potential applications have been assessed in a wide variety of preclinical laboratory models of disease. The first study was performed by Hallahan *et al.*[255], which described how TNF-a expression, under the control of the Egr-1

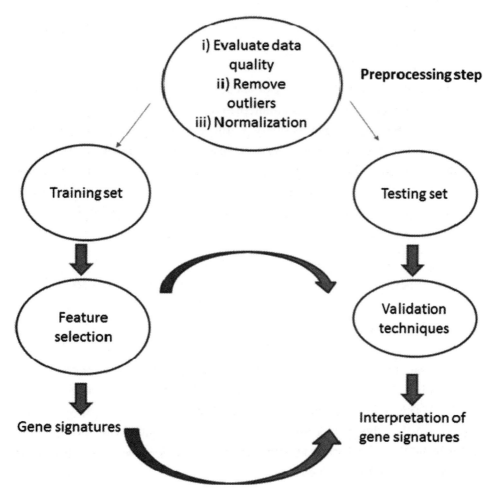

Figure 3. Feature selection model and validation. Feature selection acts on a training data set giving a gene signature. Gene signature is validated on a testing data set

promoter, could be increased in response to ionizing X-ray radiation. This increase of TNF-a expression was associated with an improved control of tumour growth in comparison with X-ray radiation alone[255]. Advantages from induction of GE by ionizing radiation include reduction of damage to adjacent healthy tissues[254].

Kan *et al.*[256] have constructed a novel retroviral vector (MetXia-P450) encoding CYP2B6. This vector was used to transfect the human tumour cell lines HT29 and T47D. CYP2B6 metabolizes the prodrug cyclophosphamide (CPA) to produce phosphoramide mustard that cross-links DNA, thus leading to cell death. In order to evaluate safety and clinical response, MetXia-P450 entered Phase I clinical trials for nine BC patients and three melanoma patients with cutaneous tumours, with encouraging results.

Although viral vectors are very efficient for gene transfer, their uses are still limited by safety concerns[257]. As an alternative, non-viral BC gene therapy (e.g. naked DNA) is growing due to its safety profile, easy preparation procedures, and moderate costs. β-galactosidase (LacZ) expressing plasmid DNA has been successfully delivered in three patients by a needle-free jet injection to skin metastases from primary BC, and also to melanoma lesions in 14 patients. No side effects were observed. The transgene was detectable at messenger RNA (mRNA) and at protein levels in all patients.

2.4. Copy Number Alterations and Gene Expression in BC

2.4.1. Biological Insights

Several studies demonstrated that changes in DNA CN are translated into corresponding changes in GE[258][259]. Although it is possible that changes in specific DNA sequences (*i.e.* centromeres or telomeres) can have directly negative consequences[260], the main responsible for the malignant phenotype has been proven to be the gene dosage hypothesis: alterations of gene copies change the expression levels of the involved gene[261].

Figure 4 shows the principle consequences of an altered gene dosage. Specifically, **Figure 4.1** shows: i) WT condition where a correct number and expression of A and B gives a correct production of C; ii) how the amplification/over expression of gene copies (e.g. B) can cause an increased dosage of a single gene (e.g. C), and iii) how a deletion/under expression of gene copies (e.g. B) can cause a decreased dosage of a single gene (e.g. C)[261]. **Figure 4.2** shows how altered gene dosage can influence stoichiometry of protein complex DE that produces F. An amplification/over expression of protein D can inhibit the formation of protein complex DE, thus altering the pathway activity and the correct production of F. A deletion/under expression of protein D do not produce protein complex DE[262].

While useful information has been revealed by analysing GE profiles alone

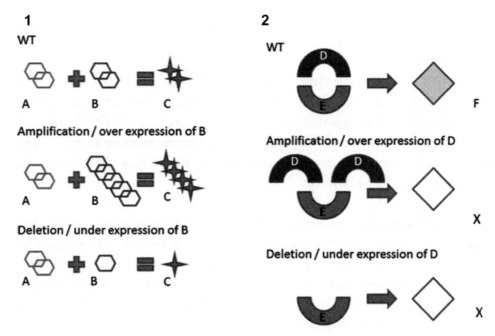

Figure 4. Consequences of gene dosage. 1) WT cell: a correct number of gene copies and expression gives a correct production of C. Amplification/Over expression of B can increase the output. Under expression of B can diminish the production of C. 2) WT cell: a correct number of gene copies and expression form a correct complex DE producing F. Amplification/Over-expression of D can interfere with stoichiometry of protein complex inhibiting F. Deletions/Under-expression of D not form complex DE and not produce F.

or CNA data alone, integrative analysis of CNA and GE data are necessary in order to have more information in gene characterization. Specifically, RNA data give information on genes that are up/down-regulated, but do not consider primary changes driving cancer from secondary modifications, such as proliferation and differentiation state. On the other hand, DNA data give information on amplifications and deletions that are drivers of cancer. Therefore, integrating DNA and RNA data can clarify genetic regulatory relationships in cancer cells[262]. It is interesting that transcriptional changes for 10%–63% of genes occur in amplified regions, and, for 14% –62% of genes, in regions of loss[263].

Several studies showed that gains (or losses) in DNA genomics have consequences in the expression levels of genes in the implicated regions, which are increases or decreased, respectively[264]–[266]. If we consider individual genes, the situation is more complicated. For instances, 14% of down-regulated genes can appear within regions of DNA gain, while 9% of up-regulated genes can occur in regions of DNA loss[266]. These findings suggest to take a particular attention in the integration of CNA and GE.

The Cancer Genome Atlas project[267] is generating multidimensional platforms including gene expression and CNA data for the same set of patients[263]. Although it is possible to perform analysis with unpaired data[263][268][269], the analysis is much more accurate when both types of data are available from the same patient. In this condition, the paired data analysis allows better statistical power and a reduction of false positives[270][271].

Some studies have shown that integrating CNA information with GE data can often provide a powerful tool for identifying functionally relevant genes in cancer[e.g.[275]–[282]]. Chen et al.[272] found a list of eighteen genes for which a strong correlation between CNA and GE exists, using signal-to-noise ratio (SNR). They found one particular gene, RUNX3, which is involved in the control of the in vitro invasive potential of MDA-MB-231.

Zhang et al.[273] identified an 81-gene prognostic CN signature that was found highly correlated with GE levels (Cox regression P < 0.05). This signature identified a subgroup of patients with increased probability of distant metastasis in an independent validation set of 113 patients.

Andre et al.[274] reported the level of mRNA expression, significantly correlated to the CAN, for VEGF, EGFR, and PTEN, using Algorithm Array CGH Expression integration tool (ACE-it). These genes could be targeted in triple-negative BC in clinical trials, and one of them, E2F3, can have a major role in a subset of triplenegative BC.

Hyman et al.[275] studied CNAs in 14 BC cell lines, and identified 270 differently expressed genes using signal-to-noise statistics (α value <0.05). 91 of the 270 genes represented hypothetical proteins or genes with no functional annotation, whereas 179 genes had available functional information.

Orsetti et al.[276] presented a study on CNA on chromosome 1, the prevalent target of genetic anomalies in BC, and the CNA consequences at the RNA expression level in BC. They identified 30 genes showing significant over-expression. A discriminating score was applied by comparing the expression levels of the subgroup of samples presenting amplification and the expression levels of the subgroup of samples without amplification.

Chin et al.[277] associated CNA and GE profiles of genes linked to poor treatment response. They identified 66 genes in these regions whose expression levels were correlated with CN, using Pearson's correlation (FDR < 0.01, Wilcoxon rank-sum test). Gene Ontology analyses of these genes showed that they are involved in nucleic acid metabolism, protein modification, signalling, and in the cell cycle and/or protein transport.

Chin SF et al.[278] evaluated genome-wide correlations between GE and CN by following an approach based on the Wilcoxon test. They showed strong statistical associations between either CN gain and over-expression (196 genes) or CN loss and under-expression (63 genes). Many well-known and potentially novel oncogenes and tumour suppressors were included in their analysis.

Table 7 reports a synthesis of the considered genes based on the integration of CNA and GE.

2.4.2. Computational Methods

No experimental methods actually exist giving, in one single analysis, results about the integration of CNA and GE.

Table 7. Gene signatures obtained by the Integration of CAN and GE.

Number of genes (gene signatures)	References
1	Chen et al.[272]
81	Zhang et al.[273]
4	Andre et al.[274]
270	Hyman et al.[275]
30	Orsetti et al.[276]
66	Chin et al.[277]
259	Chin SF et al.[278]

Computational integrative methodologies between CNA and GE include a two-step approach, and joint analysis. **Figure 5(A)** shows a two-step approach, combining the results from individual analysis of GE and CNA. **Figure 5(B)** shows a joint analysis obtaining directly the final result from the integration of GE and CNA.

There are different statistical measures to assess the CNA and GE relationship in order to quantify gene dosage effect. They include, in two-steps approaches, both regression and correlation-based analysis.

Regression approaches model the dependence of RNA levels from DNA CN, and consider RNA levels as responses and DNA CN as predictors[279]. These methods can be divided into: 1) univariate linear regression models, proposed to model the associations between individual CN and GE probes[280], 2) multivariate linear regression models, integrating statistical power across multiple probes targeting adjacent genes or chromosomal positions[281], and 3) nonlinear regression models.

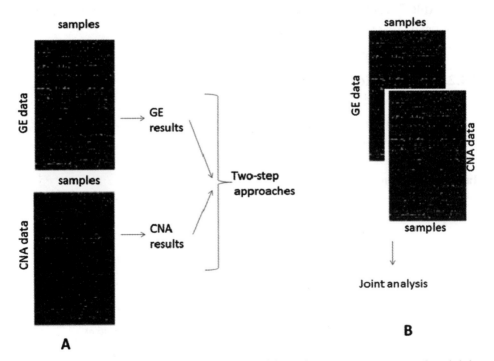

Figure 5. Integration approaches between GE and CNA data a two-step approaches, b joint analysis.

210

Most studies use linear regression models but regulatory mechanisms, contributing to gene expression changes (e.g. CNA, miRNA, DNA methylation), can give non linearity[282]. Non linear relationship between CNA and GE have been investigated by Solvang et al.[282], which focused on the identification of nonlinear relationships to explain the regulatory mechanisms of alteration of mRNA expressions in the cancer process.

Correlation-based approaches have been used to study the relationship between CNAs and GE. For each pair of co-measured data, a correlation matrix was estimated reflecting the strength of association[283]. Several studies have shown correlations between CNA and GE gene across samples e.g.[277]. Other studies, like Tsafrir et al.[284], identified a correlation along the genome by using filtered CNA and filtered GE. DR-Correlate[285], a modified version of the Ortiz-Estevez algorithm,[286] was used in a correlation-based analysis to examine the genome and to detect genes with high associations between CNA and GE. In order to improved correlation results, Schäfer et al.[287] replaced the sample means with the reference medians in the correlation test, while Lipson et al.[288] used a quantile-based analysis to obtain improved correlation coefficients.

Table 8 reports a synthesis of the considered two-step analyses and types.

Joint analysis uses CNA and GE data as paired data entries and not as separate structures. The discrepancy between the sample size and the number of genes

Table 8. Two step approaches to quantify gene dosage effect.

Analysis	Type	References
- regression	• univariate linear	[279]_[282]
	• multivariate linear	
	• nonlinear	
- correlation	• signal-to-noise ratio	[283]_[288]
	• Pearson's correlation	
	• Algorithm Array CGH Expression integration tool (ACE-it)	
	• discriminating score	

is a problem that can cause high noise. Techniques such as Singular value decomposition (SVD) or Principal Component Analysis (PCA) are the most popular ones for reducing the dimension of gene data[289][290]. However, GE and CNA data are separately analysed using these methods.

The generalized singular value decomposition (GSVD) is a popular regression framework used in joint analysis. With the purpose to identify variation patterns between two biological inputs, Berger et al.[291] applied an iterative procedure based on the GSVD, projecting CNA/ GSE data into different decomposition directions. GSVD was used in two BC cell lines and tumour datasets, thus obtaining gene subsets that were biologically validated.

Soneson et al.[292] applied PCA to reduce dimensions, and Canonical Correlation Analysis (CCA) to identify highly correlated CNA/GE pairs. Gonzalez et al.[293] implemented the regularized CCA to identify the correlation between paired datasets. iCluster is a method able to generate a single integrated cluster assignment based on a simultaneous inference analysis from multiple data types[294]. In BC, iCluster has been used to align concordant DNA CNA and gene GE changes, showing encouraging results[294].

Table 9 reports some software for the CNA and GE analysis and their method of integration type.

Table 9. Software for CNA and GE analysis.

Software	Integration type	References
Ace-it	two-step approaches	[295]
Magellan	two-step approaches	[296]
SODEGIR	two-step approaches	[297]
Edira	two-step approaches	[287]
CNAmet	two-step approaches	[298]
iCLUSTER	joint analysis	[294]
CONNEXIC	joint analysis	[299]
Remap	joint analysis	[281]
DR-Integrator	joint analysis	[285]

2.5. Integrating Genetics and Epigenetics in BC

The development of BC is mediated by the cooperation, directly or indirectly, between genetic and epigenetic alterations of the cell[300][301].

Sarkar *et al.* suggested that the epigenetic changes act as the initiating signal in the development of cancer progenitor cells and a combination of all genetic changes which are differentially expressed in the various cancer subtypes, could act on the cell vulnerable to epigenetic alterations[301].

Epigenetic mechanisms are tightly linked to one another and make the overall gene regulation system. The miR-29 family, for example, including miR-29a, miR-29b, and miR-29c, is a miRNA that collaborates with other epigenetic mechanisms. The expression of miR-29b is regulated by both histone modification[302] and DNA methylation[303]. miR-7/miR-218 can regulate DNA methylation and histone modification status by decreasing homeobox B3 (HOXB3) expression[304].

However, while classical epigenetic mechanisms, such as histone modification and DNA methylation, regulate expression at the transcriptional level, miRNAs act at the posttranscriptional level.

Elucidating the basic mechanisms of post-transcriptional regulation of GE is essential to gain a full understanding of how GE is regulated at different levels, of the interplay between these mechanisms, and of the extensive contribution of post-transcriptional dysfunction in cancer.

An impressive number of papers have been published on miRNAs increasing the number of scientific challenges, and we focused on the studies and methods applied to the combination miRNAs-mRNA, CNAs-miRNAs, and GE- genetic alterations-miRNAs.

2.6. Integrated Analysis of mRNA and miRNA in BC

2.6.1. Biological Insights

The miRNA profile is more accurately associated with cell differentiation and cancer progression when compared with GE expression profile.

The aberrant expression of miRNAs in cancer can lead to the altered expression of target mRNAs. miRNAs can also modulate multiple genes regulating entire networks. The interaction of a miRNA with its target mRNAs can lead to the repression or incentive of GE.

In general, integration study of miRNA and mRNA may allow the identification of both biomarkers and networks involved in the development of cancer[305][306].

Biomarkers Combination of miRNA and mRNA has still to be deeply explored in diagnostic and prognostic studies. Cascione et al.[307] proposed a large-scale analysis of miRNA and cancer-focused mRNA expression in normal, triple negative tumour, and associated metastatic tissues in BC. Two miRNA signatures were identified, predictive of overall survival (P = 0.05) and distant-disease free survival (P = 0.009), respectively. Volinia et al.[308] found 30 mRNAs and 7 miRNAs associated with overall survival, across different clinical and molecular subclasses of BCs. In addition, expression profiles from 8 BC datasets, different from those used for the miRNA extraction, were used for validation. Buffa et al.[309] matched mRNA and miRNA global expression profiling, and four miRNAs were found independently associated with DRFS in ER-positive BC (3 novel and 1 known miRNA-miR-128a) and six miRNAs in ER-negative BC (5 novel and 1 known miRNA; miR-210). Van der Auwera et al.[310] identified a set of 13 miRNAs whose expression differed between inflammatory BC (IBC) and non-IBC. Enerly et al.[311] demonstrated, from the joint analysis of miRNA and mRNA data, a central role for miRNAs in regulating particular pathways. Hannafon et al.[312] identified putative miRNAs by mRNA functional interactions in ductal carcinoma in situ: the three miRNAs miR-125b, miR-182 and miR-183, and six of their putative target genes, MEMO1, NRIP1, CBX7, DOK4, NMT2, and EGR1.

Luo et al.[313] performed an integrated analysis of miRNAs and mRNA expression profiles in 12 BC cell lines, identifying 35 functional target genes of three significantly down-regulated miRNAs in invasive cell lines (miR-200c, miR-205, and miR-375).

Several studies demonstrated the greater accuracy of miRNA expression levels compared with those of gene signatures. miRNA expression levels should directly represent the functional activity of the genes, while genes have to be translated to proteins to show their biological effects[314].

For a more detail review on the role of miRNAs and mRNA, see[315].

Table 10 reports a synthesis of the considered miRNAs biomarkers in BC as obtained by the integration of miRNA and mRNA.

Each miRNA can potentially regulate the expression of hundreds of genes, and a single gene can be targeted by multiple miRNAs[316].

Specific miRNAs has been identified as regulator of metastatic progression through miRNA regulatory networks. Yan *et al.*[317] found miR-21 as the most significantly up-regulated miRNA in BC when compared with normal adjacent tumour tissues (NAT). Its target prediction revealed the putative target genes by creating a small miRNA regulatory networks.

Table 10. miRNA deregulated by integration miRNA and mRNA.

Biomarker	Biological effect	References
miR-16, 155, 125b, 374a	predictive of overall survival (P = 0.05)	[307]
miR-16, 125b, 374a, 374b, 421, 655, 497	predictive of distant-disease free survival (P = 0.009)	[307]
miR-1307, 103, 328, 83, 874, 484, 148b	associated with overall survival across different clinical and molecular subclasses	[308]
miR-767-3p, 128a, 769-3, 135a, and miR-27b, 144, 210, 42, 150, 30c	associated with DRFS in estrogen receptor	[309]
miR-335, 337-5p, 451, 486-3p, 520a-5p, 548d-5p, 15a, 24, 29a, 30b, 320, 342-5p, 342-3p	associated with inflammatory breast cancer	[310]
miR-150, 155, 142	have strong positive correlation to the immune response module	[311]
miR-130b, 19a, 449a, 299, 154, 145	association with proliferation	[311]
miR-29c	associated with cell adhesion/extra cellular matrix	[311]
miR-125b, miR-182 and miR-183	highly overexpressed in ductal carcinoma in situ	[312]
miR-200c, miR-205, and miR-375	down-regulated miRNAs in invasive cell lines	[313]

Figure 6 shows mTOR and STAT3 signalling acting on miR-21 up-regulation in cancer[318] and miR-21 promoting cancer cell invasion and metastasis through suppression of BCL-2, PTEN, PDCD4,TPM1, maspin[319]. The introduction of anti-miR-21 to MCF-7 BC cells and in mouse model resulted in decreased cell growth (via increased apoptosis) and in reduced cell proliferation[319].

miR-10b was found highly expressed in BC metastatic cancer cells. In vivo studies demonstrated that miR-10b promotes cell migration and invasion[320][321] and initiates tumour metastasis[320][321]. miR-10b is induced by the transcription factor Twist. In turn, miR-10b inhibits HOXD10 and, through a cascade of cellular alterations, inhibits the expression of the prometastatic gene RHOC[320][321].

let-7 has been found poorly expressed or deleted in many cancers. Known oncogenic targets of let-7 are H-RAS, HMGA2, and BACH1. These genes result

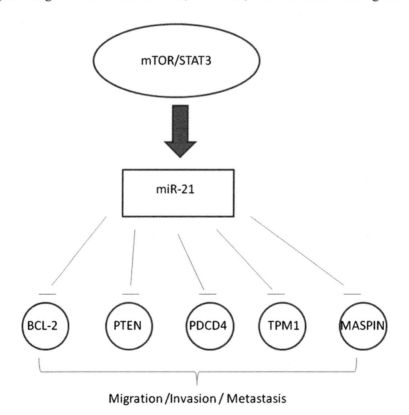

Figure 6. Example of miRNA regulatory networks.

down-regulated by let-7 over-expression[322]. HMGA2, and BACH1 promote the transcription of pro-invasive genes, suppress cell invasion and metastasis to the bone[323]. let-7 is regulated by LIN-28, MEK signalling, and RKIP[323].

miR-200 family is important in maintaining the tumour epithelial phenotype and in inhibiting the epithelial-to-mesenchymal transition (EMT). miR-200 family was found to inhibit cell migration by acting on the transcription factors ZEB1 and ZEB2, which suppress E-cadherin[324]. Furthermore, miR-200 was found silencing Sec-23a and promoting metastases by inhibiting TINAGL1 and IGFBP4[325].

Table 11 reports a synthesis of the considered mRNA-miRNA networks.

2.6.2. Experimental Methods

The most used experimental technique for determining miRNA targets is the transfection of mimic miRNAs or of miRNA inhibitors[329]. The consequences of the modulation of miRNAs on the expression levels are measured by using different tools, including RT-PCR or microarrays. The most important disadvantage of these techniques is that they are not able to discriminate between indirect and direct interactions[329]. Labelled miRNA pull-down (LAMP) assay system or luciferase report assays add reporters or labels to miRNAs on the 3'-UTR of transcripts of interest, allowing the identification and the analysis of direct interaction regions among miRNA and its target gene[7]. The disadvantage of reporter assays is that they are laborious, sensitive upon the region chosen for cloning, and that they require hard and complex work for trasfection[330].

Table 11. Example of network between miRNA and their targets in BC.

miRNA	Targets	Phenotype	Ref.
miR-21	BCL-2,PTEN, PDCD4,TPM1, maspin	Migration, invasion	[318][319]
miR-335	SOX4, Tenascin-C	Migration, invasion	[326]_[328]
miR-10b	HOXD10, RhoC	Migration, invasion	[320][321]
let-7	H-RAS, HMGA2, LIN28, PEBP1	Proliferation, differentiation	[322][323]
miR-200	BMI2, ZEB1, ZEB2, Sec-23a	Migration	[324]

2.6.3. Computational Methods

There are different approaches to examine both miRNA and mRNA expression profiles. In this paragraph we examine miRNA and mRNA regulatory pairs together[183][185][187][188]. Several studies showed that the miRNA-mRNA interactions varies with the development of disease[331][332].

Recently, in silico studies used expression profiles to decrease the number of false positives and to enhance the number of biologically relevant targets[333][334].

The integrative methods employ a three-step procedure: 1) Identification of DE miRNAs and mRNAs in the biological condition of interest. It can be done as reported in section 2 c); 2) Selection of putative miRNA-mRNA pairs (for instance, a prediction algorithm can be used to obtain the DE miRNA from DE mRNA. It can be done as reported in section 3 c); and 3) Identification of statistically significant miRNA-mRNA pairs. This last step needs the selection of an appropriate association measure, and the determination of its significance. The common assumption is based on the idea that regulatory relationship between any miRNA and its target mRNAs is an inverse correlation[335].

The mathematic tools consider simple correlation analyses (Pearson, Spearman)[336][337], mutual information[337], linear regression[338]-[340], regularized least squares[341][342] and bayesian inference[343][344]. These methods give a score for each interaction mRNA-miRNA.

van Iterson et al.[305] used the global test[345] to associateeach miRNA with the expression levels of a setof predicted mRNA targets. They suggest global tests tobe better suited for integrated analysis of miRNA andmRNA expression data, compared with either Pearsoncorrelation or lasso-based approaches.

Pearson Correlation is a measure of linear-dependency,widely used to show miRNA-mRNA showing a statisticallysignificant correlation[346]. There are several webtoolsthat employ Pearson correlation for miRNA-mRNAtarget research (e.g.[349]-[353]).

Non-parametric (Spearman) correlation coefficient canbe used as alternative measure of correlation. Usually itis chosen in case of outliers or with small number of measures. Contrary to Spearman correlations, Pearsoncoefficients require that both variables derive from a bivariatenormal distribution[348].

Mutual information is analogous to the Pearson Correlationbut it is sensitive not just to linear dependencies, and can define whether two given variables are independent[348].

Multiple linear regression can evaluate the interactionsbetween a set of miRNAs and a target mRNA, contraryto correlation measures which focuses on particularpairs interaction.

R-squared statistics is used for measuring the goodnessof the fit of the data . When the number of samples withGE profiles is smaller than the number of covariates(e.g. miRNA), partial least squares can be applied[351].This model gives those miRNAs explaining the maximumvariance in GE profiles by ensuring a good fit of the model.

Lasso-based approaches are used to deal with undetermined linear system[342].

Bayesian inference use a priori information to estimate parameters and predict values in a probability framework. Several studies use this method for scoring putative miRNA-mRNA targets based on miRNA and mRNA expression data[352]_[354].

Table 12 reports a synthesis of methods considered forthe integration analysis mRNA-miRNA.

2.6.4. Therapeutic Approach

In the context of a network, miRNAs are able to regulated istinct biological cell processes like apoptosis, proliferation or receptor driven pathways, thus suggesting their possible use also as therapeutic targets or tools[147]. The most important advantage, with respect to other approaches targeting single genes, is their ability to target multiple molecules.

Table 12. Methods for mRNA-miRNAs analysis.

Method	Ref.
global test	[243][282]
Pearson correlation	[346]–[350]
Spearman correlation	[348]
lasso-based approaches	[342]
Mutual information	[348]
Multiple linear regression	[338]–[340]
Partial least squares	[351]
Bayesian inference	[352]_[354]

There are two main approaches to target miRNA expression in cancer. Direct approaches involve the use of oligonucleotides or virus-based vectors to either block the expression of an oncogenic miRNA or to reintroducea TS miRNA lost in cancer. Indirect approaches involve the use of drugs to modulate miRNA expression by targeting their transcription and their processing.

We think that the miRNAs described in the following sections could be interesting for the development of possible therapies in BC.

Ma *et al.*[321] found miR-10b up-regulated in BC and explored a possible therapeutic application in an animal model of BC-bearing mice. The silencing of miR-10b with antagomiRs reduces miR-10b levels and increases miR-10b target, HOXD10. The therapy decreases metastases and was well tolerated by mice.

Multiple studies have also shown a significant association between miR-206 and ER in BC (e.g.[157]). In mouse models, the over expression of miR-206 was found significantly decreasing metastatic activity for 2BC cell lines: BOM1 (highly metastatic to bone) and LM2 (highly metastatic to lung)[355].

miR-125 was found to be significantly down regulated in BC patients[356]. Experimentally, over-expression of miR-125 reduces ERBB2 and ERBB3 cell motility, and also reduces invasiveness of other numerouscancers[357][358]

miR-34 is down regulated in BC cell lines and tissues, compared with normal cell lines and adjacent non-tumor tissues[359]. Expression of miR-34 was found correlated with p53 status. In fact, silencing of p53 in human tumour cell lines decreases in miR-34 level[360]. Moreover, as reported by Weidhaas *et al.*[361] miR-34 levels change levels significantly after irradiation. A potential use formiR-34 as radio sensitizing agent could be envisaged.

miR-155 is also linked to key cancer pathways as the gene is up-regulated by mutant p53 in BC, thus facilitating tumour cell invasion[362]. miR-155 hasalso attracted considerable interest as a putativetherapeutic target[363].

Table 13 reports a synthesis of the considered miRNAs, their potential target and function.

2.7. Integrated Analysis of CNA and miRNA in BC

2.7.1. Biological Insights

Many miRNAs are frequently located at fragile sites of the genome, which are usually either amplified or deleted inhuman cancer[364]. The aberrant miRNA expression in BC, in part, is due to these genomic alternations.

Zhang and colleagues studied 283 known human miRNAs in BC and showed that 72.8% of miRNAs are located in regions that reveal CNAs[365]. In a recent study, miRNAs were shown to be up-regulated in gain regions compared to copy-neutral regions in BC, although the effect on miRNA expression was not incisive[366]. Iorio *et al.*[129] compared BC CGH data with independent miRNA

Table 13. Potential therapeutic miRNAs.

miRNA	Potential Target	Function	References
miR-10b	RHOC	Invasion and metastasis	[321]
miR-206	ER	Metastasis	[155]
miR-125	ERBB2, ERBB3	Coordinate suppression	[356]–[358]
miR-34	p53, CCND1, CDK4 and CDK6,	cell cycle	[359]–[361]
miR-155	p53	cell cycle	[362][363]

expression by miRNA microarrays, and demonstrated that 81.8% of miRNAs increased expression level and showed high DNA CN, and that 60% of miRNAs exhibit decreased expression level with loss of DNA CN.

Several miRNAs have been associated with cancers due to CNA, suggesting that miRNAs can act either asoncomiRs or oncosuppressor miRNA[213]. **Figure 7** hows amplification of chromosomal regions of miRNA sencoding oncomiRs and leading to their up-regulation. OncomiRs can act silencing TSG thus making possible the development of cancer.

Biomarkers the first miRNA found to act as a mammalianoncogene is polycistron miR-17-92, also known asOncomiR-1 because it was the first identified oncomiR[367]. It is located in chromosome 13 and has been found amplified in human BC[368]. It acts as an antiapoptoticmiR cluster by targeting intrinsic apo- ptoticprotein Bim in B-cell lymphoma subtypes[369].

Other oncomiRs have been described since the first discovery. miR-21 is located in 3'UTR of VMP1 (vacuolemembrane protein 1) gene at chromosome

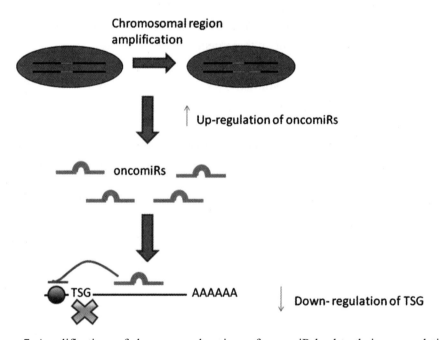

Figure 7. Amplifications of chromosomal regions of oncomiR lead to their up-regulation. These oncomiRs would then silence the TSG leading to the development of cancer.

17q23.2, a region amplified in BC and also in neuroblastomas, colon and lung cancers[370]. miR-151a-5p is located on8q24.3, a genomic site frequently associated with gain inBC[371]. High expression of miR-151a-5p has been associated with gain, and functional experiments showedthat over-expression induce cell proliferation and also increase the levels of p-AKT[372].

As for oncomiRs, also several miRNAs with oncosuppressor functions have been described. **Figure 8** shows deletion of chromosome region of oncosuppressor miRNAsleading to their down-regulation. Down-regulation of oncosuppressor miRNAs results in up-expression of target oncogenes.

Chromosome 11 is frequently altered in BC and mirR-125b, that is located at 11q23-24, results one of the most frequently deleted regions[373]. In a study of

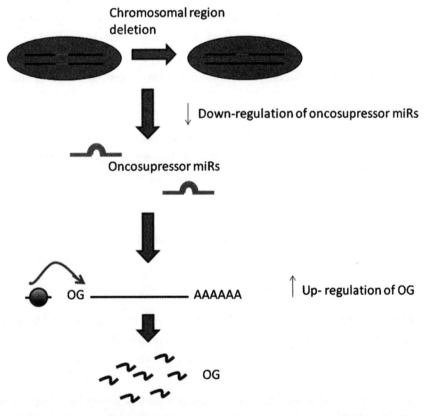

Figure 8. Deletions of chromosomal regions of oncosuppressor miRNAs lead to their down-regulation. Down-regulation of oncosuppressor miRNAs results in up-regulation of oncogenes and thus proliferation of cancer cells.

Muller *et al.*[374], mir-320 has been found to be located in regionswith DNA CN loss in BC. The predicted target of miR-320 is MECP2 which is up-regulated in BC and serves asan oncogene promoting cell proliferation. Genetic deletion could contribute to miR-100 down-regulation[375] inducing epithelial-mesenchymal transition.

In several cancer types, including BC, genomic deletionor loss of heterozygosis of the region of the miR-34a have been described[376]. miR-34a is highly expressed in normal tissues. Its expression level is under the control of the TS gene product p53 and it acts as aTS inducing cell cycle arrest in G1-phase, senescence and apoptosis[377].

Wang *et al.*[378] showed that CN deletion is an important mechanism leading to the down-regulation of expression of specific let-7 family members in BC. AlsomiR-33 expression was found to be strongly associated with the genomic alteration[128]. Furthermore, the expression of the cluster miR-145/miR-143 family, miRNA located on a region involved in several types of translocations and deletions, has been found reduced or absent in various types of cancers, including BC[152][368].

Table 14 shows the principal oncomiRs and oncogenes with their alterations considered in this section. Networks miRNAs that are silenced or amplified from CNA can have a cascade effect on the expression of different genes regulating entire pathways.

In the following paragraph, we give examples of important miRNAs that are altered in BC and of the consequences of their down regulation in the functional pathway.

Figure 9(A) shows miR-335 that suppresses BC metastasis by targeting SOX4 and Tenascin-C which promotecancer cell migration, invasion and ultimately metastasis[326]–[328]. miR-335 is silenced through CN deletions[328].

mir-320 is found to be located in regions with CN lossin BC. The predicted target of miR-320 is methyl CpGbinding protein 2 (MECP2), which is up-regulated in BC and is an oncogene promoting cell proliferation[374].

Table 14. miRNAs altered obtained by the integration miRNA and CAN.

miRNA	Genetic alterations	Ref.
miR-125b	Deletions	[373]
mir-320d	Deletions	[374]
let-7 g	Deletions	[378]
miR-34a	Deletions	[376]
miR-100	Deletions	[375]
miR-145	Deletions	[112]
miR-143	Deletions	[112]
OncomiR-1	Amplifications	[367]
miR-21	Amplifications	[369]
miR-155	Amplifications	[368]
miR-151a-5p	Amplifications	[370][371]

In a study of Volinia *et al.*[368] miR-21 was found as the only miRNA up-regulated in all six types of solidcancers (BC, colon, lung, prostate, stomach carcinomasand pancreas exocrine tumours). **Figure 9(B)** shows miR-21 network: it modulates gemcitabine-induced apoptosisby PTEN-dependent activation of PI 3-kinase and byactivation of AKT/mTOR signalling[379]. Inhibition ofthis miRNA should result in cell death[370].

2.7.2. Computational Methods

Several studies showed that miRNA levels are influenced by CNAs.

No-experimental methods are usually used for their integration. Individual studies from miRNA and CNA are combined with statistically and/or computational analysis.

de rinaldis *et al.*[380] analysed association between miRNA expression and CNAs in a large triple-negative BC data set. This association was evaluated using Spearman correlation. In addition, for each miRNA-encoding DNA locus identified as altered in any of the samples, aseparate non-parametric Wilcoxon rank sum test was applied to measure differences in expression between samples with deletions

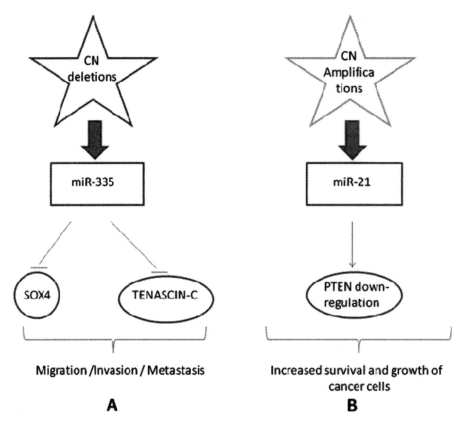

Figure 9. Examples of CNAs regulatory network. (a) Deletions of miR-335 produces effect that appear as promoting migration, invasion, and metastasis. In particular, it has been shown to be an important negative regulator of SOX4, and TENASCIN-C (b) Amplifications of miR-33 produce effects that appear as dyseregulation of PTEN pathway.

and amplifications, compared to samples with no CNAs. 64 miRNAs were found with statistically significant miRNA-CNA correlation, showing an overall influence of genetic alterations (amplifications and deletions) on the expression of the miRNAs.

Aure et al.[372] investigated individual and combined effects of CN and methylation on miRNA expression in BC. They identified 70 miRNAs whose expression was associated with CNAs or methylation, or with both conditions.24 miRNAs were associated mainly with CNAs, 22 miRNAs with methylation aberrations and 24 miRNAs with acombination of CN and methylation aberrations. In orderto identify miRNAs associated with hypomethylation oramplification, each miRNA in each patient was allocated toone of the two groups 'altered' or 'non- altered' based on CNA and DNA methylation. A Wilcoxon rank-sum testwas used for each miRNA to underlie whether the miRNA expression was significantly different in the two groups.

Srivastava *et al.*[381] showed that H2AX was negatively correlated with miR-24-2 and not in accordance with the CNA status, both in cell lines and in sporadic BC tissues. The authors tried to explain the possible mechanisms of such non concordant relationship between expression and number of gene copies based on specific miR regulation of expression. They discussed a role of miR-24-2 in guidingH2AFX GE in the background of the differential status of CNA.

2.8. Combination of Gene Expression, Genetic Alterations and miRNAs in BC

Fearon and Vogelstein[382] proposed that accumulation of genetic alterations could determine a malignantphenotype and accompany cancer progression. However, this theory does not explain the great heterogeneity of observed genetic alterations, even within homogeneoushistological groups[12].

Normal cells evolve progressively to a neoplastic state, based on a multistep process to acquire the traits that enable them to become tumorigenic and ultimately malignant. Tumors are not only masses of proliferating cancer cells, but complex tissues composed of multiple distinct molecular types that participate in an interaction with one another[383][384].

The transitions in the malignant cancer progression are dynamic and reversible steps between multiple phenotypicstates (e.g. epithelial and mesenchymal phenotype)[385]. These reversible transitions are based on complex epigenetic regulatory mechanisms (e.g. the induction of changes in the modifications of chromatin-associated histones) during epithelial-mesenchymal transitions[385][386].

Sarkar *et al.*[387] reported a review based on the role of epigenetic regulation in the steps from normal cell to cancer progenitor cells that, after growing, undergo anepithelial-mesenchymal transition. Epigenetic drugs could potentiate traditional therapeutics by inhibiting both the formation and growth of cancer progenitor cells[387].

We argue that tumour heterogeneity is due not only toa simple accumulation of genetic alterations but can be the cause of the combined effect of genetic and epigeneticalterations. Furthermore, Alfred Knudson[388] hypothesized that hereditary retinoblastoma involves two mutations, the first one in the germ line. Thus, non-hereditaryretinoblastoma should be due to two somatic mutations, an hypothesis known as Knudson "two-hit" hypothesis. The two-hit hypothesis proposes that loss of a single functionalallele, which may potentially results in expression ofa truncated or mutated product, is insufficient to involvecellular functions.

Several studies support the validity of the "two hittheory" in BC. Meric-Bernstam et al.[389] applied this hypothesis in BC, and suggested that the second hitdoes not need to be a point of mutation or somaticloss, but it may be the epigenetic silencing of a gene.

Konishi et al.[390] showed that cell lines carrying onemutant and one normal copy of BRCA1 have a normalcell phenotype, and they are normal until the second alleleis lost through somatic mutation or epigenetic silencing.

Genetic and epigenetic events are two complementary mechanisms that are involved in carcinogenesis. It is not clear at all how these mechanisms influence GE during tumorigenesis.

In BC, integration analysis of GE, genomic changes and miRNA expression was adopted in a limited number of studies (e.g.[397]–[399]). Eo et al.[391] proposed apathway-based classification of BC which integrates data on DE genes, CNA and miRNA. Pathway information was incorporated in a condition-specific manner. A 215-genesignature was found from 327 tumours. By using an independent data set, this gene signature was validated.

Cancer Genome Atlas Network[392] analysed BC bygenomic DNA CN arrays, DNA methylation, exome sequencing, messenger RNA arrays, microRNA sequencing and reverse-phase protein arrays. They found biomarkers for gene expression subtypes and the presence of fourmain BC classes.

Kristensen *et al.*[393] used an integrated approach to identify and classify BC according to the most deregulated path ways that provide the best predictive value with respect to prognosis, and identified key molecular and stromal signatures.

In a combined analysis of miRNA and mRNA expression data, Blenkiron *et al.*[128] found a number of miRNAsDE among molecular tumour subtypes. Furthermore, they found that changes in miRNA expression correlate with genomic loss or gain.

PARADIGM was tested using CN and mRNA expression data[394], as well as with the addition of methylation and miRNA expression data[393].

Cava *et al.*[5] assessed the potential of a new triple approach by integrating mRNA expression profile, CNAs, and miRNA expression levels to select a limited number of genomic BC biomarkers and to obtain a more accurate classification of BC grade.

CNAs have been demonstrated to be able also to identify genes DE between drug-sensitive and -resistant BC cells when integrated to GE and microRNA expression profiles.

Yamamoto *et al.*[395] focused on miRNAs and geneslocated on the genome-amplified and -deleted regions. These genes showed also an altered expression in GEprofiles. The authors analysed MCF7 and a parental BCcell line drug-resistance MCF7-ADR. miR-505 was identified as a tumour suppressor, whose genomic region was found to be deleted in doxorubicin-resistant cells. Furthermore, miR-505 seems to be regulated by its predictedtarget Akt3 (an anti-apoptotic gene), by mRNA profiling coupled with downstream validation studies.

3. Discussion

Despite promising initial results about the possible clinical implications of GE profiling, a more recent source of concern has been that gene signatures derived from the various studies show little overlap and poor reproducibility. This can be explained, from one side, by the complexity of the human genome which provides that different genes can be indices of the same message with identical outcomes. From the other side, one explanation can be the use of different types of arrays (of different sample quality) and the different parameters considered for the data analysis. However, GE analysis measures mRNA expression, which, by the central dogma of molecularbiology, results from the transcription of DNA. Specifically, GE analysis give information on DE genes among different conditions, but do not consider primary alterations of DNA from secondary effects of disease, such as, in the case of cancer, proliferation and differentiation state. On the other hand, studies of DNA CNA allow important indices to be derived as drivers of cancer. Therefore, integrating DNA and RNA data has been proposed to clarify genetic some regulatory relationships in cancer cells.

Since 2001, a new term "microRNA" was introduced into the scientific literature, challenging the centraldogma of molecular biology. miRNAs are segments of RNA that are transcribed from DNA in a way similar to mRNA but they are not translated into proteins. In short, instead of producing a protein, miRNA can blockm RNA directly. Evidences demonstrated that their deregulation is associated to several steps of cancer initiation and progression. However, we think that the association of miRNAs and their mRNA targets is amore favourable approach to study cell differentiation and cancer progression when compared with GE expression or miRNA profile alone. It is therefore of great concern for researchers to investigate how miRNA expression is linked to known BC markers. Several advantages can be envisaged by miRNA analysis: i) miRNAs are certainly more stable due to their small size when compared to long mRNAs[127], ii) miRNA expression levels can characterize the functional activity of the target gene while genes have to be translated to proteins to be biologically functional iii) miRNA-based therapeutics have the ability to target multiple genes.

Misregulation of genes with consequence disruption of the gene function is often induced by epigenetic and genetics events. The epigenetic silencing of one allele may act in concert with an inactivating genetic alteration in the opposite allele, thus resulting in a total allelic loss of the gene[7][8]. From this viewpoint a gene subjected to a different possible alterations (such as CNAs and target of miRNAs) and that presents DE levels between two conditions is a "weak" point of DNA and could be a key element for cancer development. In our opinion each cancer should have a signature with the description of a specific set of alterations. Based on these observations, targeting specifically and simultaneously multiple path ways sub-jected to different alterations may confer a greater therapeutic efficacy.

We argue that useful information has been revealed by analysing GE pro-files alone, CNA data alone but or miRNAs, however, in order to have compli-mentary information in gene characterization, an integrative analysis of CNA and GE data and miRNA is necessary.

However, integrative analyses have some limitations: the most fundamental challenge is dimensionally, considering that more levels in the analysis increase the computational time and the dimension of unknown parameters[396]. In addition, at every step, there are problems of compatibilityof the data, such as normalization to the same scale, batch effects, and use of different platforms.

Large-scale integration is possible only for few projects worldwide, given the high cost for all analyses to be carried out simultaneously and on the entire data set.

In referring to current studies of genetic changes associated with BC, we focused in particular on the processes controlled by CNA. However, DNA changes include other genomic rearrangements, such as somatic point mutations.

The analysis of the genomes of 100 tumours revealed more than 7400 so-matic point mutations in 21416 protein-coding genes[397]. These mutations affect many of the well-established cancer related genes, such asBRCA1, RB1, TP53, PTEN, AKT1, CDH1, GATA3, PI3KCA. These genes control apoptosis, prolifera-tion and cell cycle, and transcription. Other somatic mutations affect genes in-volved in signal transduction (APC, KRAS, MAPK2K4, SMAD4, CASP8, CDKN1B...). Somaticmutation in three main genes (TP53, PI3KCA, andGATA3) shows more than 10% incidence across all BC[397]. One of the most commonly mutated TSG in BCis P53[398]. It is localized to chromosome 17p13 and its inacti-vation is important also in other cancer diseases Several studies have investigated the predictive power ofP53 for response to treatments and outcome of BC pa-tients[399]–[401]. Bertheau *et al.*[401] reported that P53 base-pair substitutions are highly linked to specific BC molecularsub types, being found in 26% of luminal tumours (17% of luminal A, 41% of luminal B), in 50% of HER2 amplified tumours, and in 88% of basal-like carcinomas. The type of mutations changes according to the tumour subtype. Basallike tumours present higher frequency of deletions. Furthermore, the authors found that non inflammatory locally advanced BC with mutated P53 has a higher rate of response to dose-dense doxorubicin-cyclophosphamidechemotherapy than TP53-WT tumours. As recently reported[402], P53 is at the centre of the hallmarks of cancer, supporting genomic stability, exerting anti-angiogenic effects, controlling tumour inflammation and immune response, and repressing metastases. In BC, mutations inBRCA1 and BRCA2 result in protein truncations as consequence of small insertions, deletions or non- sensemutations. Although BRCA1 and BCRA2 mutations are hereditary, these genes would also be involved in the development of sporadic BC. Compared with normal breast epithelium, many BCs have shown low levels of the BRCA1mRNA[403][404], while BRCA2 has been found the target of frequent loss of heterozygosity (LOH) in BC[405][406].

Other omics data could be further integrated for a more inclusive analysis. Considering that proteins translate effects of CNAs into the biological functions of the cell, further studies could integrate protein-protein interactions networks with gene-gene co-expression networks. For example, by dissecting the protein-protein interaction network into disjoint sub networks, van den Akkerb *et al.*[407] found sub-population of genes by using pair wise GE correlation measures. The obtained genes were consistently found across different studies.

Also the DNA methylation could be integrated in a pathway analysis and could be combined with other biological data. Andrews *et al.*[408] integrated results from CNAs, GE profiling and methylation to identify differentially regulated pathways between a highly metastatic BC cell line and low metastatic parental cell line. Validation experiments confirmed that hypermethylated genes correlated with decreased expression in the metastatic, compared to the parental cell line.

Results generated from whole-genome analyses have been submitted in The Cancer Genome Atlas (TCGA) database, which includes CNAs, DNA methylation and GE profiles[409][410]. These data might be used for integrative analyses of results generated from a single technology platform[411].

232

4. Conclusions

Integrating genetics and epigenetics in BC may offer a powerful approach for the identification of biomarkers with diagnostic, prognostic and therapeutic potential. The experimental and computational methods presented in this review can be used to guide researchers for these integration studies.

5. Abbreviations

BC: Breast Cancer; CNA: Copy number alteration; GE: Gene expression; miRNA: microRNA; ER: Estrogen receptors; PR: Progesterone receptors;HER2: Human epidermal growth factor receptor-2; CN: Copy number; WT: Wild type; TSGs: Tumor suppressor genes; OGs: Oncogenes; LOH: Loss of heterozygosity; FISH: Fluorescence in situ hybridization technique; SNP: Single nucleotide polymorphism; NGS: Next generation sequencing; dChip: DNA-Chip analyzer; HMM: Hidden Markov model; CNAG: Copy number analyser for Gene Chip arrays; RMA: Robust multichip average; EGFR: Epidermal growth factor receptor; DE: Differentially expressed; RT-PCR: Real-time quantitative reverse transcription PCR.

Competing Interests

The authors declare that they have no competing interests.

Authors' Contributions

Conceived and designed the paper: CC, GB, IC. Performed the experiments: CC GB. Wrote the paper: CC, GB, IC. All authors read and approved the final manuscript.

Authors' Information

Not applicable.

Funding

This study was partially supported by INTEROMICS flagship project (http://www.interomics.eu/it/home), National Research Council CUPgrant B91J1 2000190001.

Availability of Data and Materials

Not applicable.

Source: Cava C, Bertoli G, Castiglioni I. Integrating genetics and epigenetics in breast cancer: biological insights, experimental, computational methods and therapeutic potential.[J]. Bmc Systems Biology, 2015, 9(1):641–650.

References

[1]   Polyak K. Heterogeneity in breast cancer. J Clin Invest. 2011; 10:3786–8.

[2]   Viale G. The current state of breast cancer classification. Ann Oncol. 2012; 23 Suppl 10:207–10.

[3]   Hsiao YH, Chou MC, Fowler C, Mason JT, Man YG. Breast cancer heterogeneity: mechanisms, proofs, and implications. J Cancer. 2010; 1(1):6–13.

[4]   Sotiriou C, Wirapati P, Loi S, Harris A, Fox S, Smeds J, *et al.* Gene expressionprofiling in breast cancer: understanding the molecular basis of histologicgrade to improve prognosis. J Natl Cancer Inst. 2006; 98(4):262–72.

[5]   Cava C, Bertoli G, Ripamonti M, Mauri G, Zoppis I, Della Rosa PA, *et al.*Integration of mRNA Expression Profile, Copy Number Alterations, andmicroRNA Expression Levels in Breast Cancer to Improve Grade Definition.PLoS One. 2014; 9(5):e97681.

[6]   Ivshina AV, George J, Senko O, Mow B, Putti TC, *et al.* Genetic reclassificationof histologic grade delineates new clinical subtypes of breast cancer.Cancer Res. 2006;66(21):10292–301.

[7]   Pinto R, De Summa S, Petriella D, Tudoran O, Danza K, Tommasi S. The value ofnew high-throughput technologies for diagnosis and prognosis in solid tumors.Cancer Biomark. 2014; 14(2–3):103–17.

[8]   Esteller M, Fraga MF, Guo M, Garcia-Foncillas J, Hedenfalk I, Godwin AK,*et al.* DNA methylation patterns in hereditary human cancers mimicsporadic tumorigenesis.

Hum Mol Genet. 2001; 10(26):3001–7.

[9]   Birgisdottir V, Stefansson OA, Bodvarsdottir SK, Hilmarsdottir H, Jonasson JG,Eyfjord JE. Epigenetic silencing and deletion of the BRCA1 gene in sporadic-breast cancer. Breast Cancer Res. 2006; 4:R38.

[10] Li Z, Chen B, Wu Y, Jin F, Xia Y, Liu X. Genetic and epigenetic silencing ofthe bec-lin 1 gene in sporadic breast tumors. BMC Cancer. 2010; 10:98.

[11] Yang Q, Nakamura M, Nakamura Y, Yoshimura G, Suzuma T, Umemura T, et al.Two-hit inactivation of FHIT by loss of heterozygosity and hypermethylation in-breast cancer. Clin Cancer Res. 2002; 9:2890–3.

[12] Feinberg AP, Ohlsson R, Henikoff S. The epigenetic progenitor origin ofhuman can-cer. Nat Rev Genet. 2006; 7(1):21–33.

[13] Gonzalez-Angulo AM, Hennessy BT, Mills GB. Future of personalizedmedicine in oncology: a systems biology approach. J Clin Oncol.2010; 28(16):2777–83.

[14] Beroukhim R, Mermel CH, Porter D, Wei G, Raychaudhuri S, Donovan J, et al.The landscape of somatic copy-number alteration across human cancers.Nature. 2010; 463(7283):899–905.

[15] Poplawski AB, Jankowski M, Erickson SW, Diaz de Stahl T, Partridge EC,Crasto C, et al. Frequent genetic differences between matched primary andmetastatic breast cancer provide an approach to identification ofbiomarkers for disease progression. Eur J Human Genet. 2010; 18:560–8.

[16] Slamon DJ, Clark GM, Wong SG, Levin WJ, Ullrich A, McGuire WL. Humanbreast cancer: correlation of relapse and survival with amplification of theHER-2/neu on-cogene. Science. 1987; 235:177–82.

[17] Staaf J, Jönsson G, Ringnér M, Vallon-Christersson J, Grabau D, Arason A, et al.Research article High-resolution genomic and expression analyses of copynumber alterations in HER2-amplified breast cancer. Breast Cancer Res.2010; 12:R25.

[18] Rizzolo P, Silvestri V, Falchetti M, Ottini L. Inherited and acquired alterationsin de-velopment of breast cancer. Appl Clin Genet. 2011; 4:145.

[19] Faivre EJ, Lange CA. Progesterone receptors upregulate Wnt-1 toinduceepidermal growth factor receptor transactivation and c-Src-dependentsustained activation of Erk1/2 mitogen-activated protein kinase in breast cancercells. Mol Cell Biol. 2007; 27(2):466–80.

[20] Tsutsui S, Ohno S, Murakami S, Hachitanda Y, Oda S. Prognostic value ofepidermal growth factor receptor (EGFR) and its relationship to theestrogen receptor status in 1029 patients with breast cancer. Breast CancerRes Treat. 2002; 71:67–75.

[21] Knoop AS, Knudsen H, Balslev E, et al. Retrospective analysis of topoisomerase IIaamplifications and deletions as predictive markers in primary breast cancerpa-tients randomly assigned to cyclophosphamide, methotrexate, and fluorouracilor cyclophosphamide, epirubicin, and fluorouracil:. Danish Breast CancerCooperative

Group. J Clin Oncol. 2005; 23:7483–90.

[22] O'Malley FP, Chia S, Tu D, *et al.* Topoisomerase II α and responsiveness ofbreast cancer to adjuvant chemotherapy. J Natl Cancer Inst. 2009; 101:644–50.

[23] Tanner M, Isola J, Wiklund T, *et al.* Topoisomerase IIα gene amplificationpredicts favorable treatment response to tailored and dose-escalatedanthracycline-based adjuvant chemotherapy in HER-2/neu–amplified breastcancer: Scandinavian Breast Group Trial 9401. J Clin Oncol. 2006; 24:2428–36.

[24] Gonzalez ‑ Angulo AM, Chen H, Karuturi MS, Chavez ‑ MacGregor M,Tsavachidis S, Meric ‑ Bernstam F, *et al.* Frequency of mesenchymal ‑ epithelialtransition factor gene (MET) and the catalytic subunit of phosphoinositide ‑ 3 ‑ kinase (PIK3CA) copy number elevation and correlation with outcome inpatients with early stage breast cancer. Cancer. 2013; 119(1):7–15.

[25] Xu J, Chen Y, Olopade OI. MYC and breast cancer. Gene Canc. 2010;1(6):629–40.

[26] Aulmann S, Bentz M, Sinn HP. C-myc oncogene amplification in ductalcarcinoma in situ of the breast. Breast Cancer Res Treat. 2002; 74:25–31.

[27] Robanus-Maandag EC, Bosch CA, Kristel PM, *et al.* Association of C-MYCamplification with progression from the in situ to the invasive stage inC-MYC-amplified breast carcinomas. J Pathol. 2003; 201:75–82.

[28] Aulmann S, Adler N, Rom J, Helmchen B, Schirmacher P, Sinn HP. c-myc amplifications in primary breast carcinomas and their local recurrences.J Clin Pathol. 2006; 59:424–8.

[29] Corzo C, Corominas JM, Tusquets I, *et al.* The MYC oncogene in breast cancerprogression: from benign epithelium to invasive carcinoma. Cancer GenetCytogenet. 2006; 165:151–6.

[30] Lundgren K, Brown M, Pineda S, Cuzick J, Salter J, Zabaglo L, *et al.* Effects of cyclinD1 gene amplification and protein expression on time to recurrence inpostmenopausal breast cancer patients treated with anastrozole or tamoxifen: aTransATAC study. Breast Cancer Res. 2012; 14(2):R57.

[31] Sherr CJ, Roberts JM. CDK inhibitors: positive and negative regulators ofG1-phase progression. Genes Dev. 1999; 13: 1501–12.

[32] Holst F, Stahl PR, Ruiz C, *et al.* Estrogen receptor alpha (ESR1) gene amplificationis frequent in breast cancer. Nat Genet. 2007; 39:655–60.

[33] Desouki MM, Liao S, Huang H, Conroy J, Nowak NJ, Shepherd L, *et al.* Identificationof metastasis-associated breast cancer genes using a high-resolution wholegenome profiling approach. J Cancer Res Clin Oncol. 2011; 137:795–809.

[34] Rodriguez C, Hughes-Davies L, Vallès H, *et al.* Amplification of the BRCA2pathway gene EMSY in sporadic breast cancer is related to negative outcome.Clin Cancer Res. 2004;10:5785–91.

[35] Wang C, Iakovlev VV, Wong V, Leung S, Warren K, Iakovleva G, *et al.* Genomical-terations in primary breast cancers compared with their sentinel and moredistal lymph node metastases: an aCGH study. Gene Chromosome Canc.2009; 48: 1091–101.

[36] Trapé AP, Gonzalez-Angulo AM. Breast cancer and metastasis: on the waytoward individualized therapy. Cancer Genomics-Proteomics.2012; 9(5):297–310.

[37] Imataka G, Arisaka O. Chromosome analysis using spectral karyotyping(SKY). Cell Biochem Biophys. 2012; 62(1):13–7.

[38] Salman M, Jhanwar SC, Ostrer H. Will the new cytogenetics replace the oldcytogenetics? Clin Genet. 2004; 66:265–75.

[39] Alkan C, Coe BP, Eichler EE. Genome structural variation discovery andgenotyping. Nat Rev Genet. 2011; 12(5):363–76.

[40] Park H *et al.* Discovery of common Asian copy number variants usingintegrated high-resolution array CGH and massively parallel DNAsequencing. Nat Genet. 2010; 42:400–5.

[41] Li W, Olivier M. Current analysis platforms and methods for detecting copynumber variation. Physiol Genomics. 2013; 45(1):1–16.

[42] Clevert DA, Mitterecker A, Mayr A, Klambauer G, Tuefferd M, De Bondt A, *et al.*cn. FARMS: a latent variable model to detect copy number variations inmicroarray data with a low false discovery rate. Nucleic Acids Res.2011; 39(12):e79–9.

[43] Huang J, Wei W, Zhang J, Liu G, Bignell GR, Stratton MR, *et al.* Whole genomeDNA copy number changes identified by high density oligonucleotide arrays.Hum Genomics. 2004; 1:287–99.

[44] Zhao X, Li C, Paez JG, Chin K, Janne PA, Chen TH, *et al.* An integrated viewof copy number and allelic alterations in the cancer genome using singlenucleotide polymorphism arrays. Cancer Res. 2004; 64(9):3060–71.

[45] Nannya Y, Sanada M, Nakazaki K, Hosoya N, Wang L, Hangaishi A, *et al.* Arobust algorithm for copy number detection using high-densityoligonucleotide single nucleotide polymorphism genotyping arrays. CancerRes. 2005;65(14):6071–9.

[46] Korn JM, Kuruvilla FG, McCarroll SA, Wysoker A, Nemesh J, Cawley S, *et al.*Integrated genotype calling and association analysis of SNPs, common copy-number polymorphisms and rare CNVs. Nat Genet. 2008; 40:1253–60.

[47] Bengtsson H, Irizarry R, Carvalho B, Speed TP. Estimation and assessmentof raw copy numbers at the single locus level. Bioinformatics.2008; 24:759–67.

[48] Gai X, Perin JC, Murphy K, O'Hara R, D'arcy M, Wenocur A, *et al.* CNVWorkshop: an integrated platform for high-throughput copy numbervariation discovery and clinical diagnostics. BMC Bioinformatics.2010; 11(1):74.

[49] Baross A, Delaney AD, Li HI, Nayar T, Flibotte S, Qian H, *et al.* Assessmentof algorithms for high throughput detection of genomic copy numbervariation in oligonuc-

leotide microarray data. BMC Bioinformatics.2007; 8:368.

[50] Eckel-Passow JE, Atkinson EJ, Maharjan S, Kardia SL, de Andrade M. Software-comparison for evaluating genomic copy number variation for Affymetrix 6.0 SNP array platform. BMC Bioinformatics. 2011; 12:220.

[51] Zhang D, Qian Y, Akula N, Alliey-Rodriguez N, Tang J, Gershon ES, *et al.*Accuracy of CNV detection from GWAS data. PLoS One. 2011; 6:e14511.

[52] Gordon DJ, Resio B, Pellman D. Causes and consequences of aneuploidy incancer. Nat Rev Genet. 2012; 13:189–203.

[53] Carling D. The AMP-activated protein kinase cascade—a unifyingsystem for energy control. Trends Biochem Sci. 2004; 29:18–24.

[54] Paez JG, Janne PA, Lee JC, Tracy S, Greulich H, Gabriel S, *et al.* EGFR mutationsin lung cancer: correlation with clinical response to gefitinib therapy. Science.2004; 304:1497–500.

[55] Shih J, Bashir B, Gustafson KS, Andrake M, Dunbrack RL, Goldstein LJ, *et al.*Cancer Signature Investigation: ERBB2 (HER2)-Activating Mutation andAmplification-Positive Breast Carcinoma Mimicking Lung Primary. J NatlCompr Canc Netw. 2015; 13(8):947–52.

[56] Baselga J, Norton L, Albanell J, Kim YM, Mendelsohn J. Recombinanthumanized anti-HER2 antibody (Herceptin) enhances the antitumor activityof paclitaxel and doxorubicin against HER2/neu overexpressing humanbreast cancer xenografts. Cancer Res. 1998; 58:2825–31.

[57] Baselga J, Cortés J, Kim SB, Im SA, Hegg R, Im YH, *et al.* Pertuzumab plustrastuzumab plus docetaxel for metastatic breast cancer. N Engl J Med.2012; 366 (2):109–19.

[58] Scheuer W, Friess T, Burtscher H, Bossenmaier B, Endl J, Hasmann M.Strongly enhanced antitumor activity of trastuzumab and pertuzumab combination treatment on HER2-positive human xenograft tumormodels. Cancer Res. 2009; 69:9330–6.

[59] Bird AP. CpG-rich islands and the function of DNA methylation. Nature.1986;321:209–13.

[60] Ehrlich M, Gama-Sosa MA, Huang LH, Midgett RM, Kuo KC, McCune RA,*et al.* Amount and distribution of 5-methylcytosine in human DNA from different types of tissues of cells. Nucleic Acids Res. 1982; 10:2709–21.

[61] Fullgrabe J, Kavanagh E, Joseph B. Histone onco-modifications. Oncogene.2011; 30:3391–403.

[62] Jones PA, Baylin SB. The epigenomics of cancer. Cell. 2007; 128:683–92.

[63] Stearns V, Zhou Q, Davidson NE. Epigenetic regulation as a newtarget for breast cancer therapy. Cancer Invest. 2007; 25:659–65.

[64] Lister R, Pelizzola M, Dowen RH, Hawkins RD, Hon G, Tonti-Filippini J,*et al*. Human DNA methylomes at base resolution show wide spread epigenomic differences. Nature. 2009; 462:315–22.

[65] Fackler MJ, McVeigh M, Mehrotra J, Blum MA, Lange J, Lapides A,*et al*. Quantitative multiplex methylation-specific PCR assay for the detection of promoter hypermethylation in multiple genes in breast cancer. Cancer Res. 2004; 13:4442–52.

[66] Jeronimo C, Monteiro P, Henrique R, Dinis-Ribeiro M, Costa I, Costa VL, *et al*.Quantitative hypermethylation of a small panel of genes augments the diagnostic accuracy in fine-needle aspirate washings of breast lesions.Breast Cancer Res Treat. 2008; 1:27–34.

[67] Radpour R, Kohler C, Haghighi MM, Fan AX, Holzgreve W, *et al*. Methylationprofiles of 22 candidate genes in breast cancer using high-throughput MALDI-TOF mass array. Oncogene. 2009; 28:2969–78.

[68] Nimmrich I, Sieuwerts AM, Meijer-van Gelder ME, Schwope I, Bolt-de Vries J,Harbeck N, *et al*. DNA hypermethylation of PITX2 is a marker of poor prognosis in untreated lymph node-negative hormone receptor-positivebreast cancer patients. Breast Cancer Res Treat. 2008; 3:429–37.

[69] Sunami E, Shinozaki M, Sim MS, Nguyen SL, Vu AT, Giuliano AE, *et al*.Estrogen receptor and HER2/neu status affect epigenetic differences oftumor-related genes in primary breast tumors. Breast Cancer Res.2008; 3:R46.

[70] Widschwendter M, Siegmund KD, Muller HM, Fiegl H, Marth C, Muller-Holzner E,*et al*. Association of breast cancer DNA methylation profiles with hormonereceptor status and response to tamoxifen. Cancer Res. 2004; 64:3807–13.

[71] Li L, Lee KM, Han W, Choi JY, Lee JY, Kang GH, *et al*. Estrogen and progesterone receptor status affect genome-wide DNA methylation profilein breast cancer. Hum Mol Genet. 2010; 21:4273–7.

[72] Fang F, Turcan S, Rimner A, Kaufman A, Giri D, Morris LG, *et al*. Breast cancermethylomes establish an epigenomic foundation for metastasis. Sci TranslMed. 2011; 3:75ra25.

[73] Leon SA, Shapiro B, Sklaroff DM, Yaros MJ. Free DNA in the serum of cancerpatients and the effect of therapy. Cancer Res. 1977; 37:646–50.

[74] Kloten V, Becker B, Winner K, Schrauder MG, Fasching PA, Anzeneder T, *et al*.Promoter hypermethylation of the tumor-suppressor genes ITIH5, DKK3, andRASSF1A as novel biomarkers for blood-based breast cancer screening. BreastCancer Res. 2013; 1:R4.

[75] Chimonidou M, Tzitzira A, Strati A, Sotiropoulou G, Sfikas C, Malamos N, etal. CST6 promoter methylation in circulating cell-free DNA of breast cancerpatients. Clin Biochem. 2013; 3:235–40.

[76] Chimonidou M, Strati A, Malamos N, Georgoulias V, Lianidou ES. SOX17promoter

methylation in circulating tumor cells and matched cell-freeDNA isolated from plasma of patients with breast cancer. Clin Chem. 2013; 1:270–9.

[77]   Guerrero-Preston R, Hadar T, Ostrow KL, Soudry E, Echenique M, Ili-GangasC, *et al*. Differential promoter methylation of kinesin family member 1a inplasma is associated with breast cancer and DNA repair capacity. OncolRep. 2014; 32:505–12.

[78]   Yang R, Pfütze K, Zucknick M, Sutter C, Wappenschmidt B, Marme F, *et al*.DNA methylation array analyses identified breast cancer associated HYAL2methylation in peripheral blood. Int J Cancer. 2015; 136:1845–55.

[79]   Elsheikh SE, Green AR, Rakha EA, Powe DG, Ahmed RA, Collins HM, *et al*.Global histone modifications in breast cancer correlate with tumor phenotypes, prognostic factors, and patient outcome. Cancer Res.2009; 9:3802–9.

[80]   Yokoyama Y, Matsumoto A, Hieda M, Shinchi Y, Ogihara E, Hamada M,*et al*. Loss of histone H4K20 trimethylation predicts poor prognosis in breast cancer and is associated with invasive activity. Breast Cancer Res.2014; 3:R66.

[81]   Dhingra T, Mittal K, Sarma GS. Analytical Techniques for DNA Methylation—An Overview. Curr Pharm Anal. 2014; 1:71–85.

[82]   Szyf M. DNA methylation signatures for breast cancer classification andprognosis. Genome Med. 2012; 3:26.

[83]   Gitan RS, Shi H, Chen CM, Yan PS, Huang TH. Methylation-specificoligonucleotide microarray: a new potential for high-throughput methylation analysis. Genome Res. 2002; 1:158–64.

[84]   Huang Y, Pastor WA, Shen Y, Tahiliani M, Liu DR, Rao A. The behaviour of5-hydroxymethylcytosine in bisulfite sequencing. PLoS ONE. 2010; 5:e8888.

[85]   Huang TH, Perry MR, Laux DE. Methylation profiling of CpG islands inhuman breast cancer cells. Hum Mol Genet. 1999; 3:459–70.

[86]   Yan PS, Chen CM, Shi H, Rahmatpanah F, Wei SH, Huang TH. Applications of CpG island microarrays for high-throughput analysis of DNA methylation.J Nutr. 2002; 132(8 Suppl):S2430–4.

[87]   Schumacher A, Kapranov P, Kaminsky Z, *et al*. Microarray-based DNA methylation profiling: technology and applications. Nucleic Acids Res.2006; 2:528–42.

[88]   Mohn F, Weber M, Schübeler D, Roloff TC. Methylated DNA immuno precipitation (MeDIP). Methods Mol Biol. 2009; 507:55–64.

[89]   Zhang B, Zhou Y, Lin N, Lowdon RF, Hong C, Nagarajan RP, *et al*. FunctionalDNA methylation differences between tissues, cell types, and across individuals discovered using the M&M algorithm. Genome Res. 2013; 23:1522–40.

[90]   Zhang M, Smith A. Challenges in understanding genome-wide DNAmethylation. J Comput Sci Technol. 2010; 1:26–34.

[91] Bhasin M, Zhang H, Reinherz E, Reche P. Prediction of methylated CpGs in DNA sequences using a support vector machine. FEBS Lett. 2005; 579:4302–8.

[92] Lu L, Lin K, Qian Z, Li H, Cai Y, Li Y. Predicting DNA methylation status using-word composition. J Biomedical Science and Engineering. 2010; 3:672–6.

[93] Ali I, Seker H. Detailed methylation prediction of CpG islands on humanchromosome 21. 10th WSEAS International Conference on Mathematics and Computers. In: Biology and Chemistry. 2009. p. 147–52.

[94] Fan S, Zhang M, Zhang X. Histone methylation marks play important rolesin predicting the methylation status of CpG islands. Biochem Biophys ResCommun. 2008; 374:559–64.

[95] Previti C, Harari O, Zwir I, del Val C. Profile analysis and prediction of tissuespecificCpG island methylation classes. BMC Bioinformatics. 2009; 10:116.

[96] Bell JT, Pai AA, Pickrell JK, Gaffney DJ, Pique-Regi R, Degner JF, et al. DNAmethylation patterns associate with genetic and gene expression variationin HapMap cell lines. Genome Biol. 2011; 12:R10.

[97] Eckhardt F, Lewin J, Cortese R, Rakyan VK, Attwood J, Burger M, et al. DNAmethylation profiling of human chromosomes 6, 20 and 22. Nat Genet. 2006; 38: 1378–85.

[98] Zhang W, Spector TD, Deloukas P, Bell JT, Engelhardt BE. Predicting genomewide DNA methylation using methylation marks, genomic position, and DNA regulatory elements. Genome Biol. 2015; 16:14.

[99] Du P, Bourgon R. methyAnalysis: DNA methylation data analysis and visualization.R package version 1.10.0. 2014.

[100] Barfield RT, Kilaru V, Smith AK, Conneely KN. CpGassoc: an R function foranalysis of DNA methylation microarray data. Bioinformatics. 2012; 9:1280–1.

[101] Assenov Y, Mueller F, Lutsik P, Walter J, Lengauer T, Bock C. Compehensive Analysis of DNA Methylation Data with RnBeads. Nat Methods. 2014; 11:1138–40.

[102] Wang D, Yan L, Hu Q, Sucheston LE, Higgins MJ, Ambrosone CB, et al. IMA: an R package for high-throughput analysis of Illumina's 450K Infinium methylation data. Bioinformatics. 2012; 5:729–30.

[103] Price EM, Cotton AM, Lam LL, Farré P, Emberly E, Brown CJ, et al. Additionalannotation enhances potential for biologically-relevant analysis of theil lumina infinium human methylation 450 beadchip array. EpigeneticsChromatin. 2013; 1:4.

[104] Aryee MJ, Jaffe AE, Corrada-Bravo H, Ladd-Acosta C, Feinberg AP. HansenKD and Irizarry RA Minfi: A flexible and comprehensive Bioconductor package for the analysis of Infinium DNA Methylation microarrays.Bioinformatics. 2014; 10:1363–9.

[105] Jaffe AE, Murakami P, Lee H, Leek JT, Fallin DM, Feinberg AP, et al. Bumphunting to identify differentially methylated regions in epigenetic epidemiology studies. Int J

Epidemiol. 2012; 1:200–9.

[106] Kanduri M, Cahill N, Göransson H, Enström C, Ryan F, Isaksson A, et al.Differential genome-wide array-based methylation profiles in prognostic subsets of chronic lymphocytic leukemia. Blood. 2010; 2:296–305.

[107] Wessely F, Emes RD. Identification of DNA methylation biomarkers from Infinium arrays. Front Genet. 2012; 3:161.

[108] Wilhelm-Benartzi CS, Koestler DC, Karagas MR, Flanagan JM, Christensen BC, Kelsey KT, et al. Review of processing and analysis methods for DNA methylation array data. Br J Cancer. 2013; 6:1394–402.

[109] Phipson B, Oshlack A. DiffVar: a new method for detecting differential variability with application to methylation in cancer and aging. GenomeBiol. 2014; 9:465.

[110] Goeman JJ, Bühlmann P. Analyzing gene expression data in terms of genesets: methodological issues. Bioinformatics. 2007; 23(8):980–7.

[111] Zhao N, Bell DA, Maity A, Staicu AM, Joubert BR, London SJ, et al. Globalanalysis of methylation profiles from high resolution CpG data. Genet Epidemiol. 2012;2: 53–64.

[112] Westfall PH, Stanley Young S. Resampling-Based Multiple Testing: Examplesand Methods for p-Value Adjustment. New York: Wiley-Interscience; 1993.

[113] Teng M, Wang Y, Kim S, Li L, Shen C, Wang G, et al. Empirical bayes modelcomparisons for differential methylation analysis. Comp Funct Genomics. 2012; 2012:376706.

[114] Li D, Xie Z, Pape ML, Dye T. An evaluation of statistical methods for DNAmethylation microarray data analysis. BMC Bioinformatics. 2015; 16:217.

[115] Subramaniam D, Thombre R, Dhar A, Anant S. DNA methyltransferases: anovel target for prevention and therapy. Front Oncol. 2014; 4:80.

[116] Appleton K, Mackay HJ, Judson I, Plumb JA, McCormick C, Strathdee G, et al.Phase I and pharmacodynamic trial of the DNA methyltransferase inhibitordecitabine and carboplatin in solid tumors. J Clin Oncol. 2007; 25:4603–9.

[117] Pouliot MC, Labrie Y, Diorio C, Durocher F. The Role of Methylation in Breast-Cancer Susceptibility and Treatment. Anticancer Res. 2015; 9:4569–74.

[118] Chen M, Shabashvili D, Nawab A, Yang SX, Dyer LM, Brown KD, et al. DNAmethyltransferase inhibitor, zebularine, delays tumor growth and induces apoptosis in a genetically engineered mouse model of breast cancer. MolCancer Ther. 2012; 11:370–82.

[119] Billam M, Sobolewski MD, Davidson NE. Effects of a novel DNA methyltransferaseinhibitor zebularine on human breast cancer cells. Breast Cancer Res Treat.2010; 120:581–92.

[120] Yoo CB, Jeong S, Egger G, Liang G, Phiasivongsa P, Tang C, et al. Delivery

of5-aza-2'-deoxycytidine to cells using oligodeoxynucleotides. Cancer Res.2007; 67:6400–8.

[121] Nie J, Liu L, Li X, Han W. Decitabine, a new star in epigenetic therapy: theclinical application and biological mechanism in solid tumors. Cancer Lett.2014; 354:12–20.

[122] Marson CM. Histone deacetylase inhibitors: design, structure-activity relationship-sand therapeutic implications for cancer. Anticancer Agents Med Chem.2009; 9:661–92.

[123] Munster PN, Thurn KT, Thomas S, Raha P, Lacevic M, Miller A, et al. Aphase II study of the histone deacetylase inhibitor vorinostat combined with tamoxifen for the treatment of patients with hormone therapy resistant breast cancer. Br J Cancer. 2011; 104:1828–35.

[124] Yardley DA, Ismail-Khan RR, Melichar B, Lichinitser M, Munster PN, Klein PM, et al.Randomized phase II, double-blind, placebo-controlled study of exemestane with or without entinostat in postmenopausal women with locally recurrent ormetastatic estrogen receptor-positive breast cancer progressing on treatment with a nonsteroidal aromatase inhibitor. J Clin Oncol. 2013; 17:2128–35.

[125] Bartel DP. MicroRNAs: genomics, biogenesis, mechanism, and function. Cell 2004; 116:281–97.

[126] Pasquinelli AE, Hunter S, Bracht J. MicroRNAs: a developing story. Curr OpinGenet Dev. 2005; 15:200–5.

[127] Iorio MV, Croce CM. MicroRNA dysregulation in cancer: diagnostics,monitoring and therapeutics. A comprehensive review. EMBO Mol Med.2012;4(3):143–59.

[128] Blenkiron C, Goldstein LD, Thorne NP, Spiteri I, Chin SF, Dunning MJ, et al.MicroRNA expression profiling of human breast cancer identifies newmarkers of tumor subtype. Genome Biol. 2007; 8: R214.

[129] Iorio MV, Ferracin M, Liu CG, Veronese A, Spizzo R, Sabbioni S, et al.MicroRNA gene expression deregulation in human breast cancer.Cancer Res. 2005;65:7065–70.

[130] Lowery AJ, Miller N, Devaney A, McNeill RE, Davoren PA, Lemetre C, etal. MicroRNA signatures predict oestrogen receptor, progester one receptor and HER2/neu receptor status in breast cancer. Breast CancerRes. 2009; 11:R27.

[131] Mattie MD, Benz CC, Bowers J, Sensinger K, Wong L, Scott GK, et al.Optimized high-throughput microRNA expression profiling provides novelbiomarker assessment of clinical prostate and breast cancer biopsies. Mol Cancer. 2006; 5:24.

[132] Gregory PA, Bracken CP, Bert AG, Goodall GJ. MicroRNAs as regulators ofepithelial–mesenchymal transition. Cell Cycle. 2008; 7:3112–8.

[133] Sempere LF, Christensen M, Silahtaroglu A, Bak M, Heath CV, Schwartz G, et al.Altered MicroRNA expression confined to specific epithelial cell subpopulations inbreast cancer. Cancer Res. 2007; 67:11612–20.

[134] Zhou M, Liu Z, Zhao Y, Ding Y, Liu H, Xi Y, *et al.* MicroRNA-125b confers the resistance of breast cancer cells to paclitaxel through suppression of pro-apoptotic Bcl-2 antagonist killer 1 (Bak1)expression. J Biol Chem. 2010; 285:21496–2507.

[135] Taylor MA, Sossey-Alaoui K, Thompson CL, Danielpour D, Schiemann WP. TGF-beta upregulates miR-181a expression to promote breast cancer metastasis. J Clin Invest. 2013; 123:150–63.

[136] Smith AL, Iwanaga R, Drasin DJ, *et al.* The miR-106b-25 cluster targetsSmad7, activates TGF-beta signaling, and induces EMT and tumor initiatingcell characteristics downstream of Six1 in human breast cancer. Oncogene.2012; 31:5162–71.

[137] de Souza Rocha Simonini P, Breiling A, Gupta N, *et al.* Epigenetically deregulated microRNA-375 is involved in a positive feedback loopwith estrogen receptor alpha in breast cancer cells. Cancer Res.2010; 70:9175–84.

[138] Reddy SD, Ohshiro K, Rayala SK, Kumar R. MicroRNA-7, a homeobox D10target, inhibits p21-activated kinase 1 and regulates its functions. Cancer Res. 2008; 68: 8195–200.

[139] Webster RJ, Giles KM, Price KJ, Zhang PM, Mattick JS, Leedman PJ. Regulationof epidermal growth factor receptor signaling in human cancer cells bymicroRNA-7. J Biol Chem. 2009; 284:5731–41.

[140] Yu Z, Willmarth NE, Zhou J, Katiyar S, Wang M, Liu Y, *et al.* microRNA 17/20 inhibits cellular invasion and tumor metastasis in breast cancer by heterotypic signaling. Proc Natl Acad Sci U S A. 2010; 107:8231–6.

[141] Yu Z, Wang C, Wang M, Li Z, Casimiro MC, Liu M, *et al.* A cyclin D1/microRNA 17/20 regulatory feed-back loop in control of breast cancer cellproliferation. J Cell Biol. 2008; 182:509–17.

[142] Xu D, Takeshita F, Hino Y, Fukunaga S, Kudo Y, Tamaki A, *et al.* miR-22represses cancer progres-sion by inducing cellular senescence. J Cell Biol.2011; 193:409–24.

[143] Patel JB, Appaiah HN, Burnett RM, Bhat-Nakshatri P, Wang G, Mehta R, *et al.*Control of EVI-1 oncogene expression in metastatic breast cancer cells through microRNA miR-22. Oncogene. 2011; 30:1290–301.

[144] Pandey DP, Picard D. miR-22 inhibits estrogen signaling by directly targetingthe estrogen receptor alpha mRNA. Mol Cell Biol. 2009; 29:3783–90.

[145] Wu F, Zhu S, Ding Y, Beck WT, Mo YY. MicroRNA-mediated regulation of Ubc9 expression in cancer cells. Clin Cancer Res. 2009; 15:1550–7.

[146] Yu F, Deng H, Yao H, Liu Q, Su F, Song E. Mir-30 reduction maintains selfrenewal and inhibits apoptosis in breast tumor-initiating cells. Oncogene.2010; 29:4194–204.

[147] Valastyan S, Reinhardt F, Benaich N, Calogrias D, Szász AM, Wang ZC, *et al.* Apleiotropically acting microRNA, miR-31, inhibits breast cancer metastasis.Cell. 2009; 137:1032–46.

[148] Valastyan S, Chang A, Benaich N, Reinhardt F, Weinberg RA. Concurrent suppression of integrin alpha5, radixin, and RhoA phenocopies the effectsof miR-31 on metastasis. Cancer Res. 2010; 70:5147–54.

[149] Valastyan S, Benaich N, Chang A, Reinhardt F, Weinberg RA. Concomitant suppression of three target genes can explain the impact of a microRNA on metastasis. Genes Dev. 2009; 23:2592–7.

[150] Harris TA, Yamakuchi M, Ferlito M, Mendell JT, Lowenstein CJ. MicroRNA-126regulates endothelial expression of vascular cell adhesion molecule 1. ProcNatl Acad Sci U S A. 2008; 105:1516–21.

[151] Sachdeva M, Zhu S, Wu F, Wu H, Walia V, Kumar S, *et al*. p53 repressesc-Myc through induction of the tumor suppressor miR-145. Proc Natl AcadSci U S A. 2009;106: 3207–12.

[152] Hurst DR, Edmonds MD, Scott GK, Benz CC, Vaidya KS, Welch DR. Breastcancer metastasis suppressor 1 up-regulates miR-146, which suppresses breast cancer metastasis. Cancer Res. 2009; 69:1279–83.

[153] Li XF, Yan PJ, Shao ZM. Downregulation of miR-193b contributes to enhanceurokinase-type plasminogen activator (uPA) expression and tumor progression and invasion in human breast cancer. Oncogene. 2009; 28:3937–48.

[154] Wu H, Zhu S, Mo YY. Suppression of cell growth and invasion by miR-205 inbreast cancer. Cell Res. 2009; 19:439–48.

[155] Song G, Zhang Y, Wang L. MicroRNA-206 targets notch3, activates apoptosis, and inhibits tumor cell migration and focus formation. J Biol Chem. 2009; 284:31921–7.

[156] Edmonds MD, Hurst DR, Vaidya KS, Stafford LJ, Chen D, Welch DR. Breastcancer metastasis suppressor 1 coordinately regulates metastasis-associatedmicroRNA expression. Int J Cancer. 2009; 125:1778–85.

[157] Li QQ, Chen ZQ, Cao XX, Xu JD, Xu JW, Chen YY, *et al*. Involvement of NF-κB/miR-448 regulatory feedback loop in chemotherapy-induced epithelia lmesenchymal transition of breast cancer cells. Cell Death Differ. 2011; 18:16–25.

[158] Reddy SD, Pakala SB, Ohshiro K, Rayala SK, Kumar R. MicroRNA-661,a c/EBPalpha target, inhibits metastatic tumor antigen 1 and regulatesits functions. Cancer Res. 2009; 69:5639–42.

[159] Yu F, Yao H, Zhu P, Zhang X, Pan Q, Gong C, *et al*. let-7 regulatesself renewal and tumorigenicity of breast cancer cells. Cell.2007; 131:1109–23.

[160] Mitchell PS, Parkin RK, Kroh EM, Fritz BR, Wyman SK, Pogosova-Agadjanyan EL,*et al*. Circulating microRNAs as stable blood-based markers for cancer detection. Proc Natl Acad Sci U S A. 2008; 105:10513–8.

[161] Taylor DD, Gercel-Taylor C. MicroRNA signatures of tumor-derivedexosomes as diagnostic biomarkers of ovarian cancer. Gynecol Oncol.2008; 110:13–21.

[162] Michael A, Bajracharya SD, Yuen PS, Zhou H, Star RA, Illei GG, et al. Exosome-sfrom human saliva as a source of microRNA biomarkers. Oral Dis. 2010; 16:34–8.

[163] Park NJ, Zhou H, Elashoff D, Henson BS, Kastratovic DA, Abemayor E, et al.Salivary microRNA: discovery, characterization, and clinical utility for oral cancer detection. Clin Cancer Res. 2009; 15:5473–7.

[164] Xie Y, Todd NW, Liu Z, Zhan M, Fang H, Peng H, et al. Altered miRNA expression in sputum for diagnosis of nonsmall cell lung cancer. LungCancer. 2010; 67:170–6.

[165] Yu L, Todd NW, Xing L, Xie Y, Zhang H, Liu Z, et al. Early detection of lungadeno-carcinoma in sputum by a panel of microRNA markers. Int J Cancer.2010; 127:2870–8.

[166] Lodes MJ, Caraballo M, Suciu D, Munro S, Kumar A, Anderson B. Detectionof cancer with serum miRNAs on an oligonucleotide microarray. PLoS One. 2009; 4:e6229.

[167] Madhavan D, Cuk K, Burwinkel B, Yang R. Cancer diagnosis and prognosis decoded by blood-based circulating microRNA signatures. Front Genet.2013; 4:116.

[168] Si H, Sun X, Chen Y, Cao Y, Chen S, Wang H, et al. Circulating microRNA-92aand microRNA-21 as novel minimally invasive biomarkers for primary breast cancer. J Cancer Res Clin Oncol. 2013; 139:223–9.

[169] Mar-Aguilar F, Mendoza-Ramirez JA, Malagon-Santiago I, Espino-Silva PK,Santuario-Facio SK, Ruiz-Flores P, et al. Serum circulating microRNA profi-lingfor identification of potential breast cancer biomarkers. Dis Markers.2013; 34:163–9.

[170] Zeng RC, Zhang W, Yan XQ, Ye ZQ, Chen ED, Huang DP, et al. Down regulation of miRNA-30a in human plasma is a novel marker for breast cancer. Med Oncol. 2013; 30:477.

[171] Madhavan D, Zucknick M, Wallwiener M, Cuk K, Modugno C, Scharpff M, et al.Circulating miRNAs as surrogate markers for circulating tumor cells and prognos-tic markers in metastatic breast cancer. Clin Cancer Res. 2012; 18:5972–82.

[172] Chen W, Cai F, Zhang B, Barekati Z, Zhong XY. The level of circulating miR-NA-10b and miRNA-373 in detecting lymph node metastasis of breast cancer: po-tential biomarkers. Tumour Biol. 2012; 34:455–62.

[173] Wang H, Tan G, Dong L, Cheng L, Li K, Wang Z, et al. Circulating MiR-125b as a marker predicting chemoresistance in breast cancer. PLoS ONE.2012; 7:e34210.

[174] Sun Y, Wang M, Lin G, Sun S, Li X, Qi J, et al. Serum microRNA-155 as apotential biomarker to track disease in breast cancer. PLoS ONE.2012; 7:e47003.

[175] Thompson RC, Deo M, Turner DL. Analysis of microRNA expression by insitu hy-bridization with RNA oligonucleotide probes. Methods.2007; 43(2):153–61.

[176] Stark MS, Tyagi DJ, Nancarrow GM, Boyle AL, Cook DC, Whiteman PG, et

*al.*Characterization of the Melanoma miRNA ome by Deep Sequencing. PLoSOne. 2010; 5(3):e9685.

[177] Farazi TA, Horlings HM, Ten Hoeve JJ, Mihailovic A, Halfwerk H, Morozov P,*et al.* MicroRNA sequence and expression analysis in breast tumors by deep sequencing. Cancer Res. 2011; 71:4443–53.

[178] Wu Q, Lu Z, Li H, Lu J, Guo L, Ge Q. Next-generation sequencing of microRNAs for breast cancer detection. J Biomed Biotechnol.2011; 2011:597145.

[179] Hu Z, Chen X, Zhao Y, Tian T, Jin G, Shu Y, *et al.* Serum microRNA signaturesidentified in a genome-wide serum microRNA expression profiling predict survival of non-small-cell lung cancer. J Clin Oncol Off J Am Soc Clin Oncol.2010; 28:1721–6.

[180] Xu JZ, Wong CW. Hunting for robust gene signature from cancer profiling data: sources of variability, different interpretations, and recent methodological developments. Cancer Lett. 2010; 296:9–16.

[181] Peltier HJ, Latham GJ. Normalization of microRNA expression levels inquantitative RT-PCR assays: identification of suitable reference RNAtargets in normal and cancerous human solid tissues. RNA.2008; 14:844–52.

[182] Maire G, Martin JW, Yoshimoto M, Chilton-MacNeill S, Zielenska M, SquireJA. Analysis of miRNA-gene expression-genomic profiles reveals complex mechanisms of microRNA deregulation in osteosarcoma. Cancer Genetics.2011; 204(3):138–46.

[183] Wang C, Su Z, Sanai N, *et al.* microRNA expression profile and differentiallyexpressedgenes in prolactinomas following bromocriptine treatment.Oncol Rep. 2012;27(5):1312–20.

[184] Lai EC, Wiel C, Rubin GM. Complementary miRNA pairs suggest a regulatoryrole for miRNA: miRNA duplexes. RNA. 2004; 10(2):171–5.

[185] Yu J, Liu F, Yin P, *et al.* Integrating miRNA and mRNA expression profiles inresponse to heat stress-induced injury in rat small intestine. Funct Integr Genomics. 2011; 11(2):203–13.

[186] Liu B, Liu L, Tsykin A, *et al.* Identifying functional miRNA mRNA regulatory modules with correspondence latent dirichlet allocation. Bioinformatics.2010; 26(24): 3105–3111.

[187] Nielsen JA, Lau P, Maric D, Barker JL, Hudson LD. Integrating microRNA and mRNA expression profiles of neuronal progenitors to identify regulatory networks underlying the onset of cortical neurogenesis. BMC Neurosci.2009; 10:98.

[188] Li L, Xu J, Yang D, Tan X, Wang H. Computational approaches for microRNAstudies: a review. Mamm Genome. 2010; 21(1–2):1–12.

[189] Grad Y, Aach J, Hayes GD, Reinhart BJ, Church GM, Ruvkun G, *et al.*Computational and experimental identification of C. elegans microRNAs.Mol. Cell. 2003; 11:1253–63.

[190] Lim LP, Lau NC, Weinstein EG, Abdelhakim A, Yekta S, Rhoades MW, *et al.*The microRNAs of Caenorhabditis elegans. Genes Dev. 2003; 17:991–1008.

[191] Lai EC, Tomancak P, Williams RW, Rubin GM. Computational identification of Drosophila microRNA genes. Genome Biol. 2003; 4:R42.

[192] Lee RC, Ambros V. An extensive class of small RNAs in Caenor habditis elegans. Science. 2001; 294:862–4.

[193] Berezikov E, Guryev V, Van DE, Belt J, Wienholds E, Plasterk RH, *et al.* Phylogenetic shadowing and computational identification of human microRNA genes. Cell. 2005; 120:21–4.

[194] Bentwich I, Avniel A, Karov Y, Aharonov R, Gilad S, *et al.* Identification of hundreds of conserved and nonconserved human microRNAs. Nat Genet.2005; 37: 766–70.

[195] Hofacker IL, Fontana W, Stadler PF, Bonhoeffer LS, Tacker M, Schus-Ter P.Fast folding and comparison of RNA secondary structures. Monatshefte fÄurChemie/Chemial Monthly. 1994; 125(2):167–88.

[196] Lindow M, Gorodkin J. Principles and limitations of computational microRNA gene and target finding. DNA Cell Biol. 2007; 26:339–51.

[197] Allmer J, Yousef M. Computational methods for ab initio detection of microRNAs. Front Genet. 2012; 3:209.

[198] Wang C, Ding C, Meraz RF, Holbrook SR. PSoL: a positive sample only learning algorithm for finding non-coding RNA genes. Bioinformatics.2006; 22:2590–6.

[199] Yousef M, Jung S, Showe LC, Showe MK. Learning from positive examples when the negative class is undetermined–microRNA gene identification.Algorithms Mol Biol. 2008;3:2.

[200] Hertel J, Stadler PF. Hairpins in a Haystack: recognizing microRNA precursors in comparative genomics data. Bioinformatics. 2006; 22:e197–202.

[201] Huang TH, Fan B, Rothschild MF, Hu ZL, Li K, Zhao SH. MiRFinder: an improved approach and software implementation for genome-wide fast microRNA precursor scans. BMC Bioinformatics. 2007; 8:341.

[202] Nam JW, Shin KR, Han J, Lee Y, Kim VN, Zhang BT. Human microRNA prediction through a probabilistic co-learning model of sequence and structure. Nucleic Acids Res. 2005; 33:3570–81.

[203] Terai G, Komori T, Asai K, Kin T. miRRim: a novel system to find conserved miR-NAs with high sensitivity and specificity. RNA.2007; 13:2081–90.

[204] Oulas A, Boutla A, Gkirtzou K, Reczko M, Kalantidis K, Poirazi P. Prediction ofnovel microRNA genes in cancer-associated genomic regions – a combined computational and experimental approach. Nucleic Acids Res.2009; 37:3276–87.

[205] Kadri S, Hinman V, Benos PV. HHMMiR: efficient de novo prediction of micro-

RNAs using hierarchical hidden Markov models. BMC Bioinformatics.2009; 10 Suppl 1:S35.

[206] Yousef M, Nebozhyn M, Shatkay H, Kanterakis S, Showe LC, Showe MK.Combining multi-species genomic data for microRNA identification using a Naive Bayes classifier. Bioinformatics. 2006; 22:1325–34.

[207] Bentwich I. Prediction and validation of microRNAs and their targets. FEBSLett. 2005; 579:5904–10.

[208] Xue C, Li F, He T, Liu GP, Li Y, Zhang X. Classification of real and pseudo micro-RNA precursors using local structure-sequence features and supportvector machine. BMC Bioinformatics. 2005; 6:310.

[209] Ng KL, Mishra SK. De novo SVM classification of precursor microRNAs fromgenomic pseudo hairpins using global and intrinsic folding measures.Bioinformatics. 2007; 23:1321–30.

[210] Sewer A, Paul N, Landgraf P, Aravin A, Pfeffer S, Brownstein MJ, *et al*.Identification of clustered microRNAs using an ab initio prediction method.BMC Bioinformatics. 2005; 6:267.

[211] Zhao X, Pan F, Holt CM, Lewis AL, Lu JR. Controlled delivery of antisenseoligo-nucleotides: a brief review of current strategies. Expert Opin DrugDeliv. 2009; 6:673–86.

[212] Dias N, Stein CA. Antisense oligonucleotides: basic concepts and mechanisms.Mol Cancer Ther. 2002; 1:347–55.

[213] Samantarrai D, Dash S, Chhetri B, Mallick B. Genomic and epigenomic cross talks in the regulatory landscape of miRNAs in breast cancer. Mol CancerRes. 2013; 11(4):315–28.

[214] Zoon CK, Starker EQ, Wilson AM, Emmert-Buck MR, Libutti SK, Tangrea MA.Current molecular diagnostics of breast cancer and the potential in corporation of microRNA. Expert Rev Mol Diagn. 2009; 9(5):455–67.

[215] Van't Veer LJ, Dai H, van de Vijver MJ, He YD, Hart AA, Mao M, *et al*. Geneex-pression profiling predicts clinical outcome of breast cancer. Nature. 2002; 415(6871):530–6.

[216] van de Vijver MJ, He YD, van't Veer LJ, Dai H, Hart AA, Voskuil DW, *et al*. Agene-expression signature as a predictor of survival in breast cancer. N EnglJ Med. 2002; 347(25):1999–2009.

[217] Buyse M, Loi S, van't Veer L, Viale G, Delorenzi M, Glas AM, *et al*. TRANSBIG-Consortium. Validation and clinical utility of a 70-gene prognostic signature forwo-men with node-negative breast cancer. J Natl Cancer Inst. 2006; 98(17):1183–92.

[218] Bueno-de-Mesquita JM, van Harten WH, Retel VP, van't Veer LJ, van Dam FS,Karsenberg K, *et al*. Use of 70-gene signature to predict prognosis of patients with node-negative breast cancer: a prospective community-based feasibility study

(RASTER). Lancet Oncol. 2007; 8(12):1079–87.

[219] Bueno-de-Mesquita JM, Linn SC, Keijzer R, Wesseling J, Nuyten DS, van Krimpen C, *et al*. Validation of 70-gene prognosis signature in node-negative breast cancer. Breast Cancer Res Treat. 2009; 117(3):483–95.

[220] Wittner BS, Sgroi DC, Ryan PD, Bruinsma TJ, Glas AM, Male A, *et al*. Analysis of the Mamma Print breast cancer assay in a predominantly postmenopausal cohort. Clin Cancer Res. 2008; 14(10):2988–93.

[221] Paik S, Shak S, Tang G, Kim C, Baker J, Cronin M, *et al*. A multigene assay topredict recurrence of tamoxifen-treated, node-negative breast cancer. NEngl J Med. 2004; 351(27):2817–26.

[222] Paik S, Shak S, Tang G, Kim C, Baker J, Cronin M, *et al*. Multi-gene RT-PCR assay for predicting recurrence in node negative breast cancer patients —NSABP studies B-20 and B-14. Breast Cancer Res Treat. 2003; 82:A16.

[223] Parker JS, Mullins M, Cheang MC, Leung S, Voduc D, Vickery T, *et al*.Supervised risk predictor of breast cancer based on intrinsic subtypes. J ClinOncol. 2009; 27(8):1160–7.

[224] Desmedt C, Giobbie-Hurder A, Neven P, Paridaens R, Christiaens MR, Smeets A, *et al*. The Gene expression Grade Index: a potential predictor of relapse for endocrine-treated breast cancer patients in the BIG 1–98 trial. BMC Med Genomics. 2009; 2:40.

[225] Bartlett JM, Thomas J, Ross DT, Seitz RS, Ring BZ, Beck RA, *et al*. Mammostrat as a tool to stratify breast cancer patients at risk of recurrence during endocrine therapy. Breast Cancer Res. 2010; 12(4):R47.

[226] Ring BZ, Seitz RS, Beck R, Shasteen WJ, Tarr SM, Cheang MC, *et al*. Novelprognostic immunohistochemical biomarker panel for estrogen receptor positive breast cancer. J Clin Oncol. 2006; 24(19):3039–47.

[227] Streit S, Michalski CW, Erkan M, Kleeff J, Friess H. Northern blot analysis for detection and quantification of RNA in pancreatic cancer cells and tissues.Nat Protoc. 2009; 4(1):37–43.

[228] Bustin SA. Absolute quantification of mRNA using real-time reverse transcription polymerase chain reaction assays. J Mol Endocrinol.2000; 25(2):169–93.

[229] Valasek MA, Repa JJ. The power of real-time PCR. Adv Physiol Educ.2005; 29(3):151–9.

[230] Costa C, Giménez-Capitán A, Karachaliou N, Rosell R. Comprehensive molecular screening: from the RT-PCR to the RNA-seq. Trans Lung CancerRes. 2013; 2(2):87–91.

[231] Taniguchi M, Miura K, Iwao H, Yamanaka S. Quantitative assessment of DNAmicroarrays—comparison with Northern blot analyses. Genomics.2001; 71(1):34–9.

[232] Alwine JC, Kemp DJ, Stark GR. Method for detection of specific RNAs inagarose gels by transfer to diazobenzyloxymethyl-paper and hybridization with DNA probes. Proc Natl Acad Sci USA. 1977; 74(12):5350–4.

[233] Pollock JD. Gene expression profiling: methodological challenges, results, and prospects for addiction research. Chem Phys Lipids.2002; 121(1–2):241–56.

[234] Wang Z, Gerstein M, Snyder M. RNA-Seq: a revolutionary tool for transcriptomics. Nat Rev Genet. 2009; 10(1):57–63.

[235] Velculescu VE, Zhang L, Vogelstein B, Kinzler KW. Serial analysis of gene expression. Science. 1995; 270(5235):484–7.

[236] Kodzius R, Kojima M, Nishiyori H, Nakamura M, Fukuda S, Tagami M, et al.CAGE: cap analysis of gene expression. Nat Methods. 2006; 3(3):211–22.

[237] Brenner S, Johnson M, Bridgham J, Golda G, Lloyd DH, Johnson D, et al.Gene expression analysis by massively parallel signature sequencing (MPSS)on microbead arrays. Nat Biotechnol. 2000; 18(6):630–4.

[238] Medvedev P, Stanciu M, Brudno M. Computational methods for discovering structural variation with next-generation sequencing. Nat Methods. 2009; 6(11 Suppl): S13–20.

[239] Van de Wiel MA, Picard F, van Wieringen WN, Ylstra B. Preprocessing anddownstream analysis of microarray DNA copy number profiles. Brief Bioinform. 2011; 12(1):10–21.

[240] Saeys Y, Inza I, Larrañaga P. A review of feature selection techniques in bioinformatics. Bioinformatics. 2007; 23(19):2507–17.

[241] Golub TR, Slonim DK, Tamayo P, Huard C, Gaasenbeek M, Mesirov JP, et al.Molecular classification of cancer: class discovery and class prediction by gene expression monitoring. Science. 1999; 286(5439):531–7.

[242] Bolón-Canedo V, Sánchez-Maroño N, Alonso-Betanzos A, Benítez JM, HerreraF. A review of microarray datasets and applied feature selection methods.Inf Sci. 2014; 282:111–35.

[243] Kumar AP, Valsala P. Feature Selection for high Dimensional DNA Micro array data using hybrid approaches. Bioinformation. 2013; 9(16):824–8.

[244] Chuang LY, Yang CS, Wu KC, Yang CH. Correlation-based gene selectionand classification using Taguchi-BPSO. Methods Inf Med. 2010; 49(3):254–68.

[245] Jafari P, Azuaje F. An assessment of recently published gene expression data analyses: reporting experimental design and statistical factors. BMCMed Inform Decis Mak. 2006; 6:27.

[246] Battiti R. Using mutual information for selecting features in supervised neural net learning. IEEE Trans Neural Netw. 1994; 5(4):537–50.

[247] Liu X, Krishnan A, Mondry A. An entropy-based gene selection method forcancer classification using microarray data. BMC Bioinformatics. 2005; 6:76.

[248] Tusher VG, Tibshirani R, Chu G. Significance analysis of micro arrays applied to the ionizing radiation response. Proc Natl Acad Sci U S A.2001; 98(9):5116–21.

[249] Oh IS, Lee JS, Moon BR. Hybrid genetic algorithms for feature selection. IEEETrans Pattern Anal Mach Intell. 2004; 26(11):1424–37.

[250] Chuang LY, Chang HW, Tu CJ, Yang CH. Improved binary PSO for feature selection using gene expression data. Comput Biol Chem.2008; 32(1):29–37.

[251] Sharma A, Imoto S, Miyano S. A top-r feature selection algorithm for micro array gene expression data. IEEE/ACM Trans Comput Biol Bioinform.2012; 9(3):754–64.

[252] Wanderley M, Gardeux V, Natowicz R, Braga A. Ga-kde-bayes: an evolutionary-wrapper method based on non-parametric density estimation applied to bioinformatics problems. In: 21st European Symposium on Artificial Neural Networks-ESANN. 2013. p. 155–60.

[253] Ambroise C, McLachlan GJ. Selection bias in gene extraction on the basis ofmicroarray gene-expression data. Proc Natl Acad Sci U S A. 2002; 99(10):6562–6.

[254] Goverdhana S, Puntel M, Xiong W, Zirger JM, Barcia C, Curtin JF, et al.Regulatable gene expression systems for gene therapy applications:progress and future challenges. Mol Ther. 2005; 12(2):189–211.

[255] Hallahan DE, Mauceri HJ, Seung LP, Dunphy EJ, Wayne JD, Hanna NN, et al.Spatial and temporal control of gene therapy using ionizing radiation. NatMed. 1995; 1(8):786–91.

[256] Kan O, Griffiths L, Baban D, Iqball S, Uden M, Spearman H, et al. Direct retroviral delivery of human cytochrome P450 2B6 for gene-directedenzyme prodrug therapy of cancer. Cancer Gene Ther. 2001; 8(7):473–82.

[257] Walther W, Siegel R, Kobelt D, Knösel T, Dietel M, Bembenek A, et al.Novel jet-injection technology for nonviral intratumoral gene transferin patients with melanoma and breast cancer. Clin Cancer Res.2008; 14(22):7545–53.

[258] Henrichsen CN, Vinckenbosch N, Zöllner S, Chaignat E, Pradervand S, Schütz F,et al. Segmental copy number variation shapes tissue transcriptomes. NatGenet. 2009; 41:424–9.

[259] Stranger BE, Forrest MS, Dunning M, Ingle CE, Beazley C, Thorne N, et al.Relative impact of nucleotide and copy number variation on gene expression phenotypes. Science. 2007; 315:848–53.

[260] Futcher B, Carbon J. Toxic effects of excess cloned centromeres. Mol CellBiol. 1986; 6:2213–22.

[261] Veitia RA. Exploring the etiology of haploinsufficiency. Bioessays.2002; 24:175–84.

[262] Pollack J, Srlie T, Perou C, Rees C, Jeffrey S, Lonning P, *et al*. Microarray analysis reveals a major direct role of DNA copy number alteration in the transcriptional program of human breast tumors. Proc Natl Acad Sci U S A.2002; 99:12963–8.

[263] Huang N, Shah PK, Li C. Lessons from a decade of integrating cancer copy number alterations with gene expression profiles. Brief Bioinform.2012; 13(3):305–16.

[264] Phillips JL, Hayward SW, Wang Y, *et al*. The consequences of chromosomal aneuploidy on gene expression profiles in a cell line model for prostate carcinogenesis. Cancer Res. 2001; 61:8143–9.

[265] Wolf M, Mousses S, Hautaniemi S, *et al*. High-resolution analysis of gene copy-number alterations in human prostate cancer using CGH on cDNA microarrays: impact of copy number on gene expression. Neoplasia. 2004; 6:240–7.

[266] Masayesva BG, Ha P, Garrett-Mayer E, *et al*. Gene expression alterations over large chromosomal regions in cancers include multiple genesunrelated to malignant progression. Proc Natl Acad Sci U S A.2004; 101:8715–20.

[267] National Cancer Institute. The Cancer Genome Atlas Homepage.http://cancergenome. nih.gov.

[268] Cava C, Zoppis I, Gariboldi M, Castiglioni I, Mauri G, Antoniotti M. Combined analysis of chromosomal instabilities and gene expression for colon cancer progression inference. J Clinical Bioinformatics. 2014; 4:2.

[269] Cava C, Zoppis I, Mauri G, Ripamonti M, Gallivanone F, Salvatore C, *et al*.Combination of gene expression and genome copy number alteration hasa prognostic value for breast cancer. In: Engineering in Medicine and Biology Society (EMBC), 2013 35th Annual International Conference of the IEEE. 2013. p. 608–11.

[270] Lee H, Kong SW, Park PJ. Integrative analysis reveals the direct and indirect interactions between DNA copy number aberrations and gene expression changes. Bioinformatics. 2008; 24:889–96.

[271] Monni O, Barlund M, Mousses S, *et al*. Comprehensive copy number andgene expression profiling of the 17q23 amplicon in human breast cancer.Proc Natl Acad Sci U S A. 2001; 98:5711–16.

[272] Chen W, Salto‐Tellez M, Palanisamy N, Ganesan K, Hou Q, Tan LK, *et al*.Targets of genome copy number reduction in primary breast cancer sidentified by integrative genomics. Genes Chromosom Cancer.2007; 46(3):288–301.

[273] Zhang Y, Martens JW, Yu JX, *et al*. Copy number alterations that predict metastatic capability of human breast cancer. Cancer Res. 2009; 69:3795–801.

[274] Andre F, Job B, Dessen P, *et al*. Molecular characterization of breast cancer with high-resolution oligonucleotide comparative genomic hybridization array. Clin Cancer Res. 2009; 15:441–51.

[275] Hyman E, Kauraniemi P, Hautaniemi S, Wolf M, Mousses S, Rozenblum E, etal. Impact of DNA amplification on gene expression patterns in breast cancer. Cancer

Res. 2002; 62:6240–5.

[276] Orsetti B, Nugoli M, Cervera N, *et al*. Genetic profiling of chromosome 1 in breast cancer: mapping of regions of gains and losses and identification of candidate genes on 1q. Br J Cancer. 2006; 95:1439–47.

[277] Chin K, Devries S, Fridlyand J, *et al*. Genomic and transcriptional aberrations linked to breast cancer pathophysiologies. Cancer Cell.2006; 10:529–41.

[278] Chin SF, Teschendorff AE, Marioni JC, *et al*. High-resolution array-CGH and expression profiling identifies a novel genomic subtype of ER negative breast cancer. Genome Biol. 2007; 8:R215.

[279] Lahti L, Schäfer M, Klein H U, Bicciato S, Dugas M. Cancer gene prioritization by integrative analysis of mRNA expression and DNA copy number data: acomparative review. Briefings in bioinformatics. 2012; bbs005.

[280] Menezes R, Boetzer M, Sieswerda M, *et al*. Integrated analysis of DNA copy number and gene expression microarray analysis using gene sets. BMC Bioinformatics. 2009; 10:203.

[281] Lahti L, Schäfer M, Klein HU, Bicciato S, Dugas M. Cancer gene prioritization by integrative analysis of mRNA expression and DNA copy number data: acomparative review. Brief Bioinform. 2013; (14):27–35.

[282] Solvang H, Lingjaerde O, Frigessi A, *et al*. Linear and non-linear dependencies between copy number aberrations and mRNA expressionreveal distinct molecular pathways in breast cancer. BMC Bioinformatics.2011; 12:197.

[283] Mayer CD, Lorent J, Horgan GW. Exploratory analysis of multiple omics data sets using the adjusted RV coefficient. Stat Appl Genet Mol Biol.2011; 10:14.

[284] Tsafrir D, Bacolod M, Selvanayagam Z, Tsafrir I, Shia J, Zeng Z, *et al*.Relationship of gene expression and chromosomal abnormalities incolorectal cancer. Cancer Res. 2006; 66:2129–37.

[285] Salari K, Tibshirani R, Pollack J. DR-Integrator: a new analytic tool forintegrating DNA copy number and gene expression data. Bioinformatics.2010; 26:414–6.

[286] Ortiz-Estevez M, De Las Rivas J, Fontanillo C, *et al*. Segmentation of genomic and transcriptomic microarrays data reveals major correlation between DNA copy number aberrations and gene-loci expression.Genomics. 2011; 97:86–93.

[287] Schäfer M, Schwender H, Merk S, *et al*. Integrated analysis of copy number alterations and gene expression: a bivariate assessment of equally directed abnormalities. Bioinformatics. 2009; 25: 3228–35.

[288] Lipson D, Ben-Dor A, Dehan E, *et al*. Joint analysis of DNA copy numbers and gene expression levels. In: Jonassen I, Kim J, editors. Proc Algorithms in Bioinformatics: 4th International Workshop WABI 2004. Germany: Springer; 2004.

[289] Alter O, Brown PO, Botstein D. Singular Value Decomposition for Genome-Wide

Expression Data Processing and Modeling. Proc Natl Acad Sci U S A.2000; 97:10. 101–10 106.

[290] Hastie T, Tibshirani R, Eisen MB, Alizadeh A, Levy R, Staudt L, *et al.* 'Geneshaving' as a method for identifying distinct sets of genes with similar expression patterns. Genome Biol. 2000; 1(3):1–20.

[291] Berger JA, Hautaniemi S, Mitra SK, Astola J. Jointly Analyzing Genes Expression and Copy Number Data in Breast Cancer using Data Reduction models. IEEE Trans Comput Biol Bioinform. 2006; 3(1):2–16.

[292] Soneson C, Lilljebjorn H, Fioretos T, Fontes M. Integrative analysis of gene expression and copy number alterations using canonical correlation analysis. BMC Bioinformatics. 2010; 11:191.

[293] Gonzalez I, DeJean S, Martin P, *et al.* Highlighting relationships between heterogeneous biological data through graphical displays based on regularized canonical correlation analysis. J Biol Syst. 2008; 17:173–99.

[294] Shen R, Olshen AB, Ladanyi M. Integrative clustering of multiple genomicdata types using a joint latent variable model with application to breast and lung cancer subtype analysis. Bioinformatics. 2009; 25:2906–12.

[295] Wieringen WN, Belien JA, Vosse SJ, and *et al.* ACE-it: a tool for genome-wide integration of gene dosage and RNA expression data. Bioinformatics. 2006; 22:1919–20.

[296] Kingsley CB, Kuo WL, Polikoff D, *et al.* Magellan: a web based system for the integrated analysis of heterogeneous biological data and annotations; application to DNA copy number and expression data in ovarian cancer.Cancer Inform. 2007; 2:10–21.

[297] Bicciato S, Spinelli R, Zampieri M, *et al.* A computational procedure toidentify significant overlap of differentially expressed and genomicim balanced regions in cancer datasets. Nucleic Acids Res.2009; 37:5057–70.

[298] Louhimo R, Hautaniemi S. CNAmet: an R package for integrating copy number, methylation and expression data. Bioinformatics. 2011; 27:887–8.

[299] Akavia UD, Litvin O, Kim J, *et al.* An integrated approach to uncover driversof cancer. Cell. 2010; 143:1005–17.

[300] Hervouet E, Cartron PF, Jouvenot M, Delage-Mourroux R. Epigenetic regulation of estrogen signaling in breast cancer. Epigenetics. 2013; 8:237–45.

[301] Sarkar S, Goldgar S, Byler S, Rosenthal S, Heerboth S. Demethylation and re-expression of epigenetically silenced tumor suppressor genes: sensitization of cancer cells by combination therapy. Epigenomics. 2013; 1:87–94.

[302] Chen K-C, Liao Y-C, Hsieh IC, Wang Y-S, Hu C-Y, Juo S-HH. OxLDLcauses both epigenetic modification and signaling regulation on themicroRNA-29b gene: novel mechanisms for cardiovascular diseases.J Mol Cell Cardiol. 2012; 52:587–95.

[303] Li Y, Kong D, Ahmad A, Bao B, Dyson G, Sarkar FH. Epigenetic deregulation of

miR-29a and miR-1256 by isoflavone contributes to the inhibition of prostate cancer cell growth and invasion. Epigenetics. 2012; 7:940–9.

[304] Li Q, Zhu F, Chen P. miR-7 and miR-218 epigenetically control tumor suppressor genes RASSF1A and Claudin-6 by targeting HoxB3 in breast cancer. Biochem Biophys Res Commun. 2012; 424:28–33.

[305] van Iterson M, Bervoets S, de Meijer EJ, Buermans HP, AC't Hoen P, Menezes RX,*et al.* Integrated analysis of microRNA and mRNA expression: adding biologicalsignificance to microRNA target predictions. Nucleic Acids Res. 2013; 41(15): e146.

[306] Zhong L, Zhu K, Jin N, *et al.* A Systematic Analysis of miRNA-mRNA Paired Variations Reveals Widespread miRNA Misregulation in Breast Cancer. BioMed Research International. 2014; 2014:291280.

[307] Cascione L, Gasparini P, Lovat F, Carasi S, Pulvirenti A, Ferro A, *et al.* IntegratedmicroRNA and mRNA signatures associated with survival in triple negative breast cancer. PLoS One. 2013; 8(2):e55910.

[308] Volinia S, Croce CM. Prognostic microRNA/mRNA signature from the integrated analysis of patients with invasive breast cancer. Proc Natl Acad Sci.2013; 110(18):7413–7.

[309] Buffa FM, Camps C, Winchester L, Snell CE, Gee HE, Sheldon H, *et al.* microRNA associated progression pathways and potential therapeutic targets identified byintegrated mRNA and microRNA expression profiling in breast cancer. Cancer Res. 2011; 71(17):5635–45.

[310] Van der Auwera I, Limame R, Van Dam P, Vermeulen PB, Dirix LY, Van Laere SJ.Integrated miRNA and mRNA expression profiling of the inflammatory breast cancer subtype. Br J Cancer. 2010; 103(4):532–41.

[311] Enerly E, Steinfeld I, Kleivi K, Leivonen SK, Aure MR, Russnes HG, *et al.* miRNA mRNA integrated analysis reveals roles for miRNAs in primary breast tumors.PLoS One. 2011; 6(2):e16915.

[312] Hannafon BN, Sebastiani P, De Las Morenas A, Lu J, Rosenberg CL. Expression ofmicroRNA and their gene targets are dysregulated in preinvasive breast cancer.Breast Cancer Res. 2011;13(2): R24.

[313] Luo D, Wilson JM, Harvel N, Liu J, Pei L, Huang S, *et al.* A systematic evaluation of miRNA: mRNA interactions involved in the migration and invasion of breast cancer cells. J Transl Med. 2013; 11:57.

[314] Rosenfeld N *et al.* MicroRNAs accurately identify cancer tissue origin. Nat Biotechnol. 2008; 26(4):462–9.

[315] Bertoli G, Cava C, Castiglioni I. MicroRNAs: New Biomarkers for Diagnosis, Prognosis, Therapy Prediction and Therapeutic Tools for Breast Cancer.Theranostics. 2015; 5(10):1122–43.

[316] O'Day E, Lal A. MicroRNAs and their target gene networks in breast cancer.Breast Cancer Res. 2010;12(2):201.

[317] Yan LX, Huang XF, Shao Q, Huang MY, Deng L, Wu QL, *et al*. MicroRNA miR-21overexpression in human breast cancer is associated with advanced clinicalstage, lymph node metastasis and patient poor prognosis. RNA. 2008; 14:2348–60.

[318] Bornachea O *et al*. EMT and induction of miR-21 mediate metastasisdevelopment in Trp53-deficient tumours. Sci Rep. 2012; 2:434.

[319] Si ML *et al*. miR-21-mediated tumor growth. Oncogene. 2007; 26(19):2799–803.

[320] Ma L, Teruya-Feldstein J, Weinberg RA. Tumour invasion and metastasisinitiated by microRNA-10b in breast cancer. Nature. 2007; 449:682–8.

[321] Ma L *et al*. Therapeutic silencing of miR-10b inhibits metastasis in a mousemammary tumor model. Nat Biotechnol. 2010; 28:341–7.

[322] Mayr C, Hemann MT, Bartel DP. Disrupting the pairing between let-7 andHmga2 enhances oncogenic transformation. Science. 2007; 315:1576–9.

[323] Yun J *et al*. Signalling pathway for RKIP and Let-7 regulates and predictsmetastatic breast cancer. EMBO J. 2011; 30:4500–14.

[324] Gregory PA, Bert AG, Paterson EL, Barry SC, Tsykin A, Farshid G, *et al*. ThemiR-200 family and miR-205 regulate epithelial to mesenchymal transitionby targeting ZEB1 and SIP1. Nat Cell Biol. 2008; 10:593–601.

[325] Korpal M *et al*. Direct targeting of Sec23a by miR-200s influences cancer cellsecretome and promotes metastatic colonization. Nat Med. 2011; 17:1101–8.

[326] Oskarsson T *et al*. Breast cancer cells produce tenascin C as a metastaticniche component to colonize the lungs. Nat Med. 2011; 17:867–74.

[327] Zhang J *et al*. SOX4 induces epithelial-mesenchymal transition andcontributes to breast cancer progression. Cancer Res. 2012; 72:4597–608.

[328] Png KJ *et al*. MicroRNA-335 inhibits tumor reinitiation and is silencedthrough genetic and epigenetic mechanisms in human breast cancer.Genes Dev. 2011; 25:226–31.

[329] Muniategui A, Pey J, Planes FJ, Rubio A. Joint analysis of miRNA and mRNAexpression data. Brief Bioinform. 2013; 14(3):263–78.

[330] Thomson DW, Bracken CP, Goodall GJ. Experimental strategies formicroRNA target identification. Nucleic Acids Res. 2011; 39(16):6845–53.

[331] Tsai KW, Liao YL, Wu CW, *et al*. Aberrant hypermethylation of miR-9 genesin gastric cancer. Epigenetics. 2011; 6(10):1189–97.

[332] Dudziec E, Gogol-Doring A, Cookson V, Chen W, Catto J. Integratedepigenome profiling of repressive histone modifications, DNA methylationand gene expression in normal and malignant urothelial cells. PLoS ONE.2012; 7(3):e32750.

[333] Bossel Ben-Moshe N, Avraham R, Kedmi M, Zeisel A, Yitzhaky A, Yarden Y, etal. Context-specific microRNA analysis: identification of functionalmicroRNAs and their mRNA targets. Nucleic Acids Res. 2012; 40:10614–27.

[334] Engelmann JC, Spang R. A least angle regression model for the predictionof canonical and non-canonical miRNA mRNA interactions. PLoS One.2012; 7:e40634.

[335] Vasudevan S, Tong Y, Steitz JA. Switching from repression to activation: micro-RNAs can up-regulate translation. Science. 2007; 318(5858):1931–4.

[336] Xiao F, Zuo Z, Cai G, et al. miRecords: an integrated resource for microRNA–target interactions. Nucleic Acids Res. 2009; 37:D105–10.

[337] Hsu S-D, Lin F-M, Wu W-Y, et al. miRTarBase: a database curatesexperimentally validated microRNA–target interactions. Nucleic Acids Res.2011; 39:D163–9.

[338] Beck D, Ayers S, Wen J, et al. Integrative analysis of next generationsequencing for small non-coding RNAs and transcriptional regulation inMyelodysplastic syndromes. BMC Med Genomics. 2011; 4:19.

[339] Ritchie W, Rajasekhar M, Flamant S, et al. Conserved expression patternspredict microRNA targets. PLoS Computat Biol. 2009; 5:8.

[340] Jayaswal V, Lutherborrow M, Ma DDF, et al. Identification of microRNAs withregulatory potential using a matched microRNA-mRNA time-course data.Nucleic Acids Res. 2009;37:e60.

[341] Ragan C, Zuker M, Ragan MA. Quantitative Prediction of miR-NA-mRNAInteraction Based on Equilibrium Concentrations. PLoS Computat Biol. 2011; 7:11.

[342] Nogales-Cadenas R, Carmona-Saez P, Vazquez M, et al. GeneCodis: interpreting gene lists through enrichment analysis and integration ofdiverse biological information. Nucleic Acids Res. 2009; 37:W317–22.

[343] Subramanian A, Tamayo P, Mootha VK, et al. Gene set enrichment analysis:a knowledge-based approach for interpreting genome-wide expressionprofiles. Proc Natl Acad Sci U S A. 2005; 102:15545–50.

[344] Mootha VK, Lindgren CM, Eriksson K-F, et al. PGC-1alpha-responsive genesinvolved in oxidative phosphorylation are coordinately downregulated inhuman diabetes. Nat Genet. 2003; 34:267–73.

[345] Goeman JJ, van de Geer SA, de Kort F, van Houwelingen HC. A global testfor groups of genes: testing association with a clinical outcome.Bioinformatics. 2004; 20:93–9.

[346] Liu H, Brannon AR, Reddy AR, et al. Identifying mRNA targets of microRNAdysregulated in cancer: with application to clear cell Renal Cell Carcinoma. BMC Syst Biol. 2010; 4:51.

[347] Gennarino VA, Sardiello M, Mutarelli M, et al. HOCTAR database: a unique re-

source for microRNA target prediction. Gene. 2011; 480:51–8.

[348] Sales G, Coppe A, Bisognin A, *et al.* MAGIA, a web-based tool for miRNA and genes integrated analysis. Nucleic Acids Res. 2010; 38:W352–9.

[349] Ritchie W, Flamant S, Rasko JEJ. mimiRNA: a microRNA expression profiler and classification resource designed to identify functional correlations between micro-RNAs and their targets. Bioinformatics. 2010; 26:223–7.

[350] Cho S, Jun Y, Lee S, *et al.* miRGator v2.0: an integrated system for functional investigation of microRNAs. Nucleic Acids Res. 2011; 39:D158–62.

[351] Li X, Gill R, Cooper NGF, *et al.* Modeling microRNA-mRNA interactions using PLS regression in human colon cancer. BMC Med Genomics. 2011; 4:44.

[352] Huang JC, Babak T, Corson TW, *et al.* Using expression profiling data toidentify human microRNA targets. Nat Methods. 2007; 4:1045–9.

[353] Stingo FC, Chen YA, Vannucci M, *et al.* A Bayesian graphical modeling approach to microRNA regulatory network inference. Ann Appl Stat.2011; 4:2024–48.

[354] Su N, Wang Y, Qian M, *et al.* Predicting MicroRNA targets by integrating sequence and expression data in cancer. IEEE Int Conf Syst Biol. 2011.

[355] Tavazoie SF, Alarcon C, Oskarsson T, *et al.* Endogenous human microRNAs that suppress breast cancer metastasis. Nature. 2008; 451(7175):147–52.

[356] Su N, Wang Y, Qian M, Deng M. Predicting MicroRNA targets by integratingsequence and expression data in cancer. In Systems Biology (ISB), 2011 IEEEInternational Conference. Zhuhai; 2011;219-24

[357] Scott GK, Goga A, Bhaumik D, Berger CE, Sullivan CS, Benz CC. Coordinatesuppression of ERBB2 and ERBB3 by enforced expression of micro-RNA miR-125a or miR-125b. J Biol Chem. 2007; 282:1479–86.

[358] Wang S, Huang J, Lyu H, Lee CK, Tan J, Wang J, *et al.* Functional cooperation of miR-125a, miR-125b, and miR-205 in entinostat-induced downregulation of erbB2/erbB3 and apoptosis in breast cancer cells. CellDeath Dis. 2013; 4(3):e556.

[359] Li L, Xie X, Luo J, Liu M, Xi S, Guo J, *et al.* Targeted expression of miR-34a using the T-VISA system suppresses breast cancer cell growth and invasion. Mol Ther. 2012; 20(12):2326–34.

[360] He L, He Z, Lim LP. A microRNA component of the p53 tumour suppressor network. Nature. 2007; 447:1130–5.

[361] Weidhaas JB, Babar I, Nallur SM, Trang P, Roush S, Boehm M, *et al.*MicroRNAs as potential agents to alter resistance to cytotoxic anticancertherapy. Cancer Res. 2007; 67(23):11111–6.

[362] Neilsen PM, Noll JE, Mattiske S, Bracken CP, Gregory PA, Schulz RB, *et al.*Mutant p53 drives invasion in breast tumors through up-regulation of miR-155. Oncogene.

2012; 32(24):2992–3000.

[363] Babar IA, Cheng CJ, Booth CJ, Liang X, Weidhaas JB, Saltzman WM, et al.Nanoparticle-based therapy in an in vivo microRNA-155 (miR-155)-dependent-mouse model of lymphoma Proc. Natl Acad Sci USA. 2012; 109:E1695–704.

[364] Calin GA, Sevignani C, Dumitru CD, Hyslop T, Noch E, Yendamuri S, et al.Human microRNA genes are frequently located at fragile sites and genomic regions involved in cancers. Proc Natl Acad Sci U S A.2004; 101:2999–3004.

[365] Zhang L, Huang J, Yang N, Greshock J, Megraw MS, Giannakakis A, et al.microRNAs exhibit high frequency genomic alterations in human cancer.Proc Natl Acad Sci U S A. 2006; 103:9136–41.

[366] Dvinge H, Git A, Gräf S, Salmon-Divon M, Curtis C, Sottoriva A, et al. Theshaping and functional consequences of the microRNA landscape in breast cancer. Nature. 2013; 497(7449):378–82.

[367] Hammond SM. MicroRNAs as oncogenes. Curr Opin Genet Dev. 2006; 16:4–9.

[368] Volinia S, Calin GA, Liu CG, Ambs S, Cimmino A, Petrocca F, et al. AmicroRNA expression signature of human solid tumors defines cancer gene targets. Proc Natl Acad Sci U S A. 2006; 103:2257–61.

[369] Inomata M, Tagawa H, Guo YM, Kameoka Y, Takahashi N, Sawada K.MicroRNA-17-92 down-regulates expression of distinct targets in different Bcel-llymphoma subtypes. Blood. 2009; 113:396–402.

[370] Calin GA, Croce CM. MicroRNAs and chromosomal abnormalities in cancer cells. Oncogene. 2006; 25(46):6202–10.

[371] Bergamaschi A, Kim YH, Wang P, Sørlie T, Hernandez-Boussard T, Lonning PE, et al. Distinct patterns of DNA copy number alteration are associated with different cli-nicopathological features and gene-expression subtypes ofbreast cancer. Genes Chromosomes Cancer. 2006; 45:1033–40.

[372] Aure MR, Leivonen SK, Fleischer T, Zhu Q, Overgaard J, Alsner J, et al. Indivi-dualand combined effects of DNA methylation and copy number alterations on-miRNA expression in breast tumors. Genome Biol. 2013; 14(11):R126.

[373] Negrini M, Rasio D, Hampton GM, Sabbioni S, Rattan S, Carter SL, et al.Definition and refinement of chromosome 11 regions of loss of heterozygosity in breast cancer: identification of a new region at 11q23.3. Cancer Res. 1995; 55:3003–7.

[374] Muller HM, Fiegl H, Goebel G, Hubalek MM, Widschwendter A, Muller-Holzner E,et al. MeCP2 and MBD2 expression in human neoplastic and non-neoplastic breast tissue and its association with oestrogen receptor status. Br J Cancer.2003; 89: 1934–1939.

[375] Chen D, Sun Y, Yuan Y, Han Z, Zhang P, Zhang J, et al. miR-100 InducesEpitheli-al-Mesenchymal Transition but Suppresses Tumorigenesis, Migration and Invasion. PLoS Genet. 2014; 10(2):e1004177.

[376] Nagai H, Negrini M, Carter SL, Gillum DR, Rosenberg AL, *et al*. Detection and cloning of a common region of loss of heterozygosity at chromosome 1pin breast cancer. Cancer Res. 1995; 55:1752–7.

[377] Tarasov V, Jung P, Verdoodt B, Lodygin D, Epanchintsev A, *et al*. Differential regulation of microRNAs by p53 revealed by massively parallel sequencing: miR-34a is a p53 target that induces apoptosis and G1-arrest. Cell Cycle.2007; 6:1586–93.

[378] Wang Y, Hu X, Greshock J, Shen L, Yang X, Shao Z, *et al*. Genomic DNAcopy-number alterations of the let-7 family in human cancers. PLoS One. 2012; 7(9):e44399.

[379] Meng F, Henson R, Lang M, Wehbe H, Maheshwari S, Mendell JT, *et al*.Involvement of human micro-RNA in growth and response to chemotherapy in-human cholangiocarcinoma cell lines. Gastroenterology. 2006; 130(7):2113–29.

[380] de Rinaldis E, Gazinska P, Mera A, Modrusan Z, Fedorowicz GM, Burford B, etal. Integrated genomic analysis of triple-negative breast cancers revealsnovel micro-RNAs associated with clinical and molecular phenotypes and sheds light on the pathways they control. BMC Genomics. 2013; 14(1):643.

[381] Srivastava N, Manvati S, Srivastava A, Pal R, Kalaiarasan P, Chattopadhyay S,*et al*. miR-24-2 controls H2AFX expression regardless of gene copy number alteration and induces apoptosis by targeting antiapoptotic gene BCL-2: apotential for therapeutic intervention. Breast Cancer Res. 2011; 13(2):R39.

[382] Fearon ER, Vogelstein B. A genetic model for colorectal tumorigenesis. Cell.1990; 61:759–67.

[383] Hanahan D, Weinberg RA. Hallmarks of cancer: the next generation. Cell. 2011; 5:646–74.

[384] Vogelstein B, Kinzler KW. Cancer genes and the pathways they control. Nat Med. 2004; 8:789–99.

[385] Tam WL, Weinberg RA. The epigenetics of epithelial-mesenchymal plasticity in cancer. Nat Med. 2013; 19:1438–49.

[386] Heerboth S, Housman G, Leary M, Longacre M, Byler S, Lapinska K, *et al*.EMT and Tumor Metastasis. Clinical and Translational Medicine. 2015; 1:1–13.

[387] Sarkar S, Horn G, Moulton K, Oza A, Byler S, Kokolus S, *et al*. Cancer development, progression, and therapy: an epigenetic overview. Int J Mol Sci.2013; 10:21087–113.

[388] Knudson AG. Two genetic hits (more or less) to cancer. Nat Rev Cancer.2001; 1:157–62.

[389] Meric-Bernstam F. Heterogenic loss of BRCA in breast cancer: the "two-hit" hypothesis takes a hit. Ann Surg Oncol. 2007; 14(9):2428–9.

[390] Konishi H, Mohseni M, Tamaki A, *et al*. Mutation of a single allele of the cancer susceptibility gene BRCA1 leads to genomic instability in human breast epithelial

cells. Proc Natl Acad Sci U S A. 2011; 108(43):17773–8.

[391] Eo HS, Heo JY, Choi Y, Hwang Y, Choi HS. A pathway-based classification of breast cancer integrating data on differentially expressed genes, copy number variations and MicroRNA target genes. Molecules and Cells.2012; 34(4):393–8.

[392] Cancer Genome Atlas Network. Comprehensive molecular portraits of human breast tumours. Nature. 2012; 490(7418):61–70.

[393] Kristensen VN, Vaske CJ, Ursini-Siegel J, Van Loo P, Nordgard SH, et al.Integrated molecular profiles of invasive breast tumors and ductal carcinoma in situ (DCIS) reveal differential vascular and interleukin signaling.Proc Natl Acad Sci. 2012;109(8):2802–7.

[394] Vaske CJ et al. Inference of patient-specific pathway activities from multi dimensional cancer genomics data using PARADIGM. Bioinformatics.2010; 26:i237–45.

[395] Yamamoto Y, Yoshioka Y, Minoura K, Takahashi RU, Takeshita F, Taya T, et al.An integrative genomic analysis revealed the relevance of microRNA and gene expression for drug-resistance in human breast cancer cells. MolCancer. 2011; 10:135.

[396] Kristensen VN, Lingjærde OC, Russnes HG, Vollan HKM, Frigessi A, Børresen-Dale AL. Principles and methods of integrative genomic analyses in cancer.Nat Rev Cancer. 2014; 14(5):299–313.

[397] Stephens PJ, Tarpey PS, Davies H, Van Loo P, Greenman C, Wedge DC, et al.The landscape of cancer genes and mutational processes in breast cancer. Nature. 2012; 7403:400–4.

[398] Malkin D, Li FP, Strong LC, Fraumeni Jr JF, Nelson CE, Kim DH, et al. Germline p53 mutations in a familial syndrome of breast cancer, sarcomas, and other neoplasms. Science. 1990; 250(4985):1233–8.

[399] Herceg Z, Hainaut P. Genetic and epigenetic alterations as biomarkers for cancer detection, diagnosis and prognosis. Mol Oncol. 2007; 1(1):26–41.

[400] Berchuck A, Heron KA, Carney ME, et al. Frequency of germline and somaticBRCA1 mutations in ovarian cancer. Clin Cancer Res. 1998; 4(10):2433–7.

[401] Bertheau P, Lehmann-Che J, Varna M, Dumay A, Poirot B, Porcher R, etal. p53 in breast cancer subtypes and new insights into response tochemotherapy. Breast. 2013; 22 Suppl 2:S27–9.

[402] Hainaut. TP53: coordinator of the processes that underlie the hallmarks of cancer p53 in the clinics. Springer. 2013; 1–23

[403] Thompson ME, Jensen RA, Obermiller PS, et al. Decreased expression of BRCA1 accelerates growth and is often present during sporadic breast cancer progression. Nat Genet. 1995; 9(4):444–50.

[404] Dobrovic A, Simpfendorfer D. Methylation of the BRCA1 gene in sporadic breast cancer. Cancer Res. 1997; 57(16):3347–50.

[405] Cleton-Jansen AM, Collins N, Lakhani SR, *et al*. Loss of heterozygosity in sporadic-breast tumours at the BRCA2 locus on chromosome 13q12-q13. Br J Cancer.1995; 72(5):1241–4.

[406] Hamann U, Herbold C, Costa S, *et al*. Allelic imbalance on chromosome 13q: evidence for the involvement of BRCA2 and RB1 in sporadic breast cancer. Cancer Res. 1996; 56(9):1988–90.

[407] van den Akker EB, Verbruggen B, Heijmans BT, Beekman M, Kok JN, Slagboom PE,*et al*. Integrating protein-protein interaction networks with gene-gene co-expression networks improves gene signatures for classifying breast cancer metastasis. J Integr Bioinformatics. 2011; 8:188.

[408] Andrews J, Kennette W, Pilon J, Hodgson A, Tuck AB, Chambers AF,*et al*. Multi-platform whole-genome microarray analyses refine the epigenetic signature of breast cancer metastasis with gene expression and copy number. PLoS One. 2010; 5:e8665.

[409] Chin L, Hahn WC, Getz G, Meyerson M. Making sense of cancer genomic data. Genes Dev. 2011; 25:534–55.

[410] Colaprico A, Silva TC, Olsen C, Garofano L, Cava C, Garolini D, Sabedot T,Malta T, Pagnotta SM, Castiglioni I, Ceccarelli M, Noushmehr H and Bontempi G (2015). TCGAbiolinks: An R/Bioconductor package for integrative analysis with TCGA data. Manuscript in preparation.

[411] Colaprico A, Cava C, Bertoli G, Bontempi G, Castiglioni I. Integrative analysis with Monte Carlo cross-validation reveals miRNAs regulating pathways cross-talk in aggressive breast cancer. Biomed Res Int. 2015; 2015:831314.

Chapter 9

A Joint Analysis of Metabolomics and Genetics of Breast Cancer

Xiaohu Tang[1,2], Chao-Chieh Lin[1,2], Ivan Spasojevic[3], Edwin S Iversen[4], Jen-Tsan Chi[1,2], Jeffrey R Marks[5]

[1]Department of Molecular Genetics and Microbiology, Duke University, 268 CARL Building, Research Drive, Durham, NC 27708, USA

[2]Duke Center for Genomic and Computational Biology, Duke University, 101 Science Drive, Durham, NC 27708, USA

[3]Department of Medicine, Duke University, 201 Trent Drive, Durham, NC 27710, USA

[4]Department of Statistical Science, Duke University, 214A Old Chemistry Building, Durham, NC27710, USA

[5]Department of Surgery, Division of Surgical Sciences, Duke University, 103 Research Drive, Durham, NC 27710, USA.

Abstract: Introduction: Remodeling of cellular metabolism appears to be a consequence and possibly a cause of oncogenic transformation in human cancers. Specific aspects of altered tumor metabolism may be amenable to therapeutic intervention and could be coordinated with other targeted therapies. In breast cancer, the genetic landscape has been defined most comprehensively in efforts such as The Cancer Genome Atlas (TCGA). However, little is known about how alterations of tumor metabolism correlate with this landscape. Methods: In total 25 cancers (23 fully analyzed by TCGA) and 5 normal breast specimens were analyzed by gas chromatography/mass spectrometry and liquid chromatography/mass spectrometry, quantitating 399 identifiable metabolites. Results: We found strong differences correlated with hormone receptor status with 18% of the metabolites elevated in estrogen receptor negative (ER−) cancers compared to estrogen receptor positive (ER+) including many glycolytic and glycogenolytic intermediates consistent with increased Warburg effects. Glutathione (GSH) pathway components were also elevated in ER- tumors consistent with an increased requirement for handling higher levels of oxidative stress. Additionally, ER− tumors had high levels of the oncometabolite 2-hydroxyglutarate (2-HG) and the immunomodulatory tryptophan metabolite kynurenine. Kynurenine levels were correlated with the expression of tryptophan-degrading enzyme (IDO1). However, high levels of 2-HG were not associated with somatic mutations or expression levels of IDH1 or IDH2. BRCA1 mRNA levels were positively associated with coenzyme A, acetyl coenzyme A, and GSH and negatively associated with multiple lipid species, supporting the regulation of ACC1 and NRF2 by BRCA1. Different driver mutations were associated with distinct patterns of specific metabolites, such as lower levels of several lipid-glycerophosphocholines in tumors with mutated TP53. A strong metabolomic signature associated with proliferation rate was also observed; the metabolites in this signature overlap broadly with metabolites that define ER status as receptor status and proliferation rate were correlated. Conclusions: The addition of metabolomic profiles to the public domain TCGA dataset provides an important new tool for discovery and hypothesis testing of the genetic regulation of tumor metabolism. Particular sets of metabolites may reveal insights into the metabolic dysregulation that underlie the heterogeneity of breast cancer.

1. Introduction

It is now well established that significant heterogeneity exists among human breast cancers. This heterogeneity is observable at every level of examination from the macroscopic to the molecular. Recent large-scale efforts to measure and describe human breast tumor heterogeneity include The Cancer Genome Atlas (TCGA) where a number of high-throughput "omic" technologies were systemically applied to hundreds of primary cancer specimens[1]. Mutation, germ line polymorphisms, DNA copy number, RNA expression, DNA methylation, and protein expression analyses were performed in parallel on a large and carefully curated set of breast cancer specimens to produce the most comprehensive molecular portrait of the disease to date.

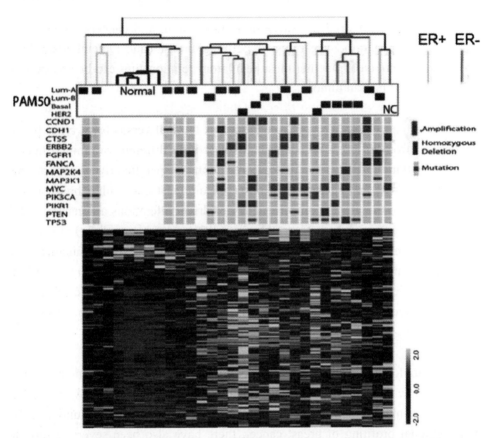

Figure 1. Breast cancers (n = 25) and normal breast tissues (n = 5) were grouped by unsupervised hierarchical clustering of metabolite levels and overlaid with intrinsic subtype and status of the somatic mutations of genetic drivers. Normalized metabolite levels were mean-centered, selected based on at least two-fold changes in two samples and arranged by hierarchical clustering. The estrogen receptor (ER) status, intrinsic subtypes, and identified somatic mutations in the indicated genes are shown for 23 tumors which were characterized by The Cancer Genome Atlas (TCGA).

One significant metric that was not included in TGCA was an unbiased analysis of tumor metabolism. While metabolic flux cannot be measured in fixed or frozen specimens, steady-state levels of numerous key metabolites may provide insight into these fundamental phenotypic traits. A number of studies in cancer have uncovered relationships between genetic abnormalities and various metabolic reprogramming suggesting that key metabolic process can be altered as a result of specific transformation events[2]–[6]. Relatively nonspecific cancer-related events such as increased proliferation may also underlie some of the inferred/observed metabolic remodeling. Glucose uptake, serine and glutamine

267

auxotrophy, mitochondrial oxidative phosphorylation, and cancer-associated fibroblasts all appear to have roles in defining breast cancer metabolism[7]–[11]. However, it is not clear whether these regulatory relationships can be observed in all or subsets of human tumors.

Breast cancers are broadly categorized as luminal versus basal types possibly derived from different precursor cells or at least different committed lineages[12]–[14]. Within these broad categories, alterations in specific driver genes are believed to produce the heterogeneity observed amongst and within breast tumor subtypes. While the identity and frequency of driver alterations are generally different in basal and luminal cancers, there is still considerable overlap. For example, TP53 mutations are very common in basal tumors and PI3KCA mutations are common in luminal cancer but neither is subtype exclusive. In contrast, MYC (8q24) amplification is common in both types[1]. Each of these genetic drivers has been associated with specific changes in cellular metabolism and therefore may have dominant effects that can be observed across tumor types.

Metabolomic profiling via mass spectrometry or nuclear magnetic resonance (NMR) is now an established approach that has been employed in several studies to analyze primary human breast tissues (normal and cancer)[15][16]. Building upon transcriptional profiling of breast cancer, there have also been several efforts to integrate steady-state metabolite levels with specific breast cancer subtypes defined by mRNA expression. Expression subtypes are dominated by estrogen receptor and ERBB2 status and thus, metabolic profiling was performed to seek an additional level of information to refine these existing classifications. These analyses identified a subclassification of luminal A-type cancers based on metabolite levels and found higher levels of Warburg-associated metabolites in more aggressive cancer types[9][17]. A separate study of breast cancer lipidomic identified the association between palmitate-containing phosphatidylcholines with estrogen receptor negative and cancer progression and patient survival[18]. However, none of these studies established associations of particular metabolites or metabolic pathways with specific somatic mutations or expression levels that have been extensively characterized in TCGA.

In order to more fully explore the relationship between genetics, tumor type, and metabolic state, we took advantage of our participation in the breast cancer

TCGA to perform joint analyses of metabolomics and genetics in a series of primary cancers. From the current study, we were able to identify several genetic determinants of the metabolic heterogeneity of human breast tumors that confirm and extend prior in vitro and in vivo observations.

2. Methods

2.1. Specimen Selection and Handling

Breast tissues were collected, stored and used under Duke University Medical Center Institutional Review Board (IRB) approved protocols (Pro00012025 and Pro00021284). A waiver of consent was obtained from the Duke IRB to conduct the study (Pro00021284) and subjects were not reconsented for participation. Twenty-five breast cancers (diagnosed and treated from 1989 to 1998) were selected for the current study based on their inclusion in The Cancer Genome Atlas (TCGA). Specifically, we selected cases that were either estrogen receptor (ER) positive or negative for both estrogen and progesterone receptors (PR) based on the clinical assay performed at the time of initial diagnosis (clinical and demographic information is provided in Table S1 in Additional file 1). Two of the ER + positive cancers were classified as PR negative by the clinical assay. In addition to the cancers, we selected five breast specimens obtained from reduction mammoplasties containing substantial amounts of normal epithelium. Each block of tissue was cryostat sectioned to analyze tumor epithelial content based on microscopic examination with a cutoff of 70% tumor nuclei for inclusion. Additional sections were also taken and stored desiccated at −80°C for future use. The remainder of the tissue block was submitted frozen to Metabolon Inc. (Durham, NC, USA) for extraction and metabolomic analysis. After trimming away the cryogenic-embedding compound (OCT), the weight of each sample (27mg to 115mg) was determined and used to normalize the extraction reagent volume.

2.2. Proliferation Analysis

Thin sections were fixed in acetone and then stained with MIB-1 antibody (Dako, Glostrup, Denmark) that recognizes the Ki-67 proliferation antigen. The mouse monoclonal antibody was used at a final concentration of 200μg/ml and detected with a biotinylated goat anti-mouse secondary antibody. Following chromogenic detection, each section was scored for the percentage of nuclear-stained epithelial cells. Two hundred epithelial cells were counted in each section spanning at least two high-powered (40X) fields. The proliferation rate was expressed as a percentage of the epithelial cells exhibiting nuclear staining.

2.3. Metabolomic Profiling

The sample preparation process at Metabolon was carried out using an automated MicroLab STAR™ system from the Hamilton Company (Reno, NV, USA). Recovery standards were added prior to the first step in the extraction process for quality control purposes. Sample preparation was conducted using a proprietary (Metabolon, Inc.) series of organic and aqueous extractions to remove the protein fraction while allowing maximum recovery of small molecules. The resulting extract was divided into two fractions; one for analysis by liquid chromatography (LC) and one for analysis by gas chromatography (GC). Samples were placed briefly on a Zymark TurboVap (Phoenix Equipment, Inc., Rochester, NY, USA) to remove the organic solvent. Each sample was then frozen and dried under vacuum. Samples were then prepared for the appropriate instrument, either LC/mass spectrometry (MS) or GC/MS.

The LC/MS portion of the platform is based on a Waters ACQUITY UPLC (Waters, Milford, MA, USA) and a Thermo-Finnigan LTQ mass spectrometer (Thermo Fisher Scientific, Waltham, MA, USA), which consists of an electrospray ionization (ESI) source and linear ion trap (LIT) mass analyzer. The sample extract was split into two aliquots, dried, then reconstituted in acidic or basic LC-compatible solvents, each of which contained 11 or more injection standards at fixed concentrations. One aliquot was analyzed using acidic positive ion optimized conditions and the other using basic negative ion optimized conditions in two independent injections using separate dedicated columns. Extracts reconstituted in acidic conditions were gradient eluted using water and methanol both containing 0.1% formic acid, while the basic extracts, which also used water/methanol, contained 6.5mm ammonium bicarbonate. The MS analysis alternated between MS and data-dependent MS^2 scans using dynamic exclusion.

The samples destined for GC/MS analysis were redried under vacuum desiccation for aminimum of 24 hrs prior to being derivatized under nitrogen using bis (trimethylsilyl) triflouroacetamide (BSTFA). The GC column was 5% phenyl and the temperature ramp was from 40° to 300°C in a 16min period. Samples were analyzed on a Thermo-Finnigan Trace DSQ fast-scanning single-quadrupole mass spectrometer using electron impact ionization (Thermo Fisher Scientific). The instrument was tuned and calibrated for mass resolution and mass accuracy on a daily basis. The information output from the raw data files was automatically extracted as discussed below.

For ions with counts greater than 2 million, an accurate mass measurement could be performed. Accurate mass measurements could be made on the parent ion as well as fragments. The typical mass error was less than 5 ppm. Fragmentation spectra (MS/MS) were typically generated in a data-dependent manner, but if necessary, targeted MS/MS was employed, such as in the case of lower level signals.

Identification of known chemical entities was based on comparison to metabolomic library entries of purified standards. More than 1,000 commercially available purified standard compounds have been registered into a database for distribution to both the LC and GC platforms for determination of their analytical characteristics. The combination of chromatographic properties and mass spectra gave an indication of a match to the specific compound or an isobaric entity.

2.4. Measurement of 2-Hydroxyglutarate

Quantification of L/D-2-hydroxyglutarate (2-HG) in biological media/tissues was performed by LC-ESI-MS/MS as described[19] with modifications to accommodate different sample matrices involved in the study. The method utilizes a chiral derivatization agent to produce diastereoisomers with L- and D-isomers of 2-HG, which can be separated by conventional reverse-phase LC. D-2-HG, L-2-HG, and diacetyl-L-tartaric anhydride (DATAN) were from Sigma-Aldrich (St Louis, MO, USA). Racemic mixtures of L- and D-2-HG-d4 were prepared by mixing 1mg of α-ketoglutarate-d6 (Sigma-Aldrich/Isotec) with 1mg of NaBH4 (Sigma-Aldrich) in 0.2mL anhydrous MeOH (Sigma-Aldrich) followed by 30min incubation at 60°C. Tissue or cell line homogenates, 200μL of deionized water, 1 mL of chloroform, and 4mm ceramic beads were vigorously mixed for 45 sec at speed 4 in FastPrep 120 'bead-beater' instrument (Thermo Savant, Holbrook, NY,

USA). After centrifugation (5min at 16,100×g), 200µL of the aqueous (upper) layer was transferred into 1.5-mL glass vial and dried (50°C, 60min). The dry residue was treated with 50mg/mL of freshly prepared DATAN in dichloromethane/glacial acetic acid (4/1 by volume) and heated at 75°C for 30min. After drying (50°C, 15min) the residue was dissolved in 100µL LC mobile phase A (see below) for analysis by LC/MS/MS with an Agilent 1200 series HPLC (Agilent Technologies, St Clara, CA, USA) and Sciex/Applied Biosystems API 3200 QTrap (Applied Biosystems, Foster City, CA, USA). Mobile phase A: water, 3% acetonitrile, 280µL ammonium hydroxide (approximately 25%), pH adjusted to 3.6 by formic acid (approximately 98%). Mobile phase B: methanol. Analytical column: Kinetex C18, 150×4.6mm, 2.6µm, and SafeGuard C18 4×3mm guard-column from Phenomenex (Torrance, CA, USA). Column temperature: 45°C. Elution gradient at 1 mL/min flow rate: 0 to 1min 0% B, 1 to 2min 0 to 100% B, 2 to 3.5min 100% B, 3.5 to 4min 100 to 0% B, 4 to 10min 0% B. Injection volume: 10µL. The Q1/Q3 (m/z) transitions monitored: 363/147 (2-HG) and 367/151 (2-HG-d4). A set of calibrator samples in corresponding matrix were prepared for calibration by adding appropriate amounts of pure D-2-HG at the following concentration levels: 0, 0.16, 0.54, 1.8, 6, and 20ug/mL. These samples were analyzed alongside the experimental samples.

2.5. Data Analysis

For pairwise comparison of metabolites from different sample categories (normal, ER+, ER−), we used Welch's t test. The false discovery rate was estimated using the q value[20].

The data were subjected to hierarchical clustering using Cluster 3.0 and displayed using TreeView[21]. The significance analysis of microarray (SAM) analyses were performed as described using indicated selection criteria[22]. For specific metabolite associations with genetic events, data were analyzed in GraphPad Prism (GraphPad Software, San Diego, CA, USA) for correlation and significance.

Genetic mutation and copy number, RNA expression data, and designation of tumor intrinsic subtype were all derived from the publically available TCGA data sets. Primary data were downloaded from the TCGA data portal[23] or analyzed using the online cBioPortal suite of tools[24]. For the cBioPortal, some analyses were performed on the "TCGA Nature 2012" data set and others on the 'TCGA Provisional' data set.

For analysis of the correlation between each pair of metabolites, Pearson correlations of the level of each pair of metabolites (log2 normalized value) among 399 metabolites from 25 tumors and 5 normal breast tissues were generated. The correlation coefficients were hierarchically clustered by Cluster 3.0 to produce the heat-map plot. For analysis of correlation between individual metabolite and proliferation rate, Pearson correlations between the level of individual metabolite (log2 normalized value) and Ki-67% (log2 value) were calculated. The supervised cluster plot was generated based on the correlation between individual metabolite levels and proliferation rate (Ki-67%) and displayed by TreeView.

For combined analysis of receptor status and proliferation, normalized metabolic data were natural log transformed yielding a symmetric distribution of the data about the mean. We used normal theory linear regression to assess the extent to which the metabolic assay data could be predicted by one, the other or both of the tumor's receptor status and proliferation rate (Ki-67%). We analyzed each metabolite separately and fit four models for each: (1) the model with intercept only; (2) the model with intercept and receptor status; (3) the model with intercept and log2 proliferation rate; and (4) the model with intercept, receptor status and log2 proliferation rate. We calculated analysis of variance tables for the two nested progressions of models: (1, 2, 4) and (1, 3, 4). We report the P values based on the associated F tests for (a) models 2 over 1, (b) 4 over 2, (c) 3 over 1 and (d) 4 over 3. The P values in (a) and (c) are for the regression of abundance of the metabolite on receptor status and for the regression of abundance of the metabolite on proliferation rate, respectively. The P values in (b) and (d) are for the regression of abundance of the metabolite on receptor status while adjusting for proliferation rate and for the regression of abundance of the metabolite on the proliferation rate while adjusting for receptor status, respectively.

3. Results

To date, over 900 primary breast cancers have been profiled by the TCGA initiative over a four-year period using an evolving set of molecular analyses. For this reason, not all cancers were analyzed by all techniques. For the current meta-bolomic study, we chose 25 cancers that had passed quality control and were accepted for analysis by TCGA: 16 ER positive (all but two were also PR positive) and 9 cancers that were both ER and PR negative, determined by standard immunopathologic analysis after cytoreductive surgery. Of these, 23 cancers (15 ER+ and 8 ER−) were eventually subjected to comprehensive genetic analysis by TCGA. In addition to the cancers, we selected 5 samples of normal breast tissue (from reduction mammoplasties not associated with cancer) that contained a substantial amount of epithelium based on histologic staining. We cut 20 sections from each block for in situ analyses before extraction for the quantitative profiling of small molecules (<1,000 Da) that was performed in a single batch on the Metabolon platform generating data on 399 identifiable metabolites (Table S2 in Additional file 2 contains the primary data on metabolites).

Primary tissues in this study were distributed into three main categories: (1) normal breast from reduction mammoplasties, (2) ER positive primary breast cancers, and (3) estrogen and PR negative primary cancers. Of the 25 cancers, all were accepted for TCGA study but only 23 were actually subjected to genetic analysis. The cancers are representative of the major subtypes of the disease based on the PAM50 classification[25] including basal, HER2, luminal A and luminal B. One sample was designated as 'not-classified' (NC). None of the tumors were classified as the relatively uncommon 'claudin low' subtype.

Hierarchical clustering of the samples based on these metabolites demonstrated that the 5 normal breast samples were tightly clustered together while the ER+ tumors exhibited significant heterogeneity: 6 of the ER+ tumors grouped with the 5 normal breast samples while the remaining 10 ER+ tumors clustered with the 9 ER− tumors (**Figure 1**). This relative heterogeneity of ER+ tumors is consistent with previous classification based on gene expression[12][26]. Pictured below the hierarchical clustering dendrogram for 23 of the cancers is TCGA data for the most common gene-based abnormalities (mutation, amplification, homozygous deletion) found in breast cancer, most of which are considered to be driver alterations. Also shown is the PAM50 intrinsic subtype classifier (based on gene expression) of the TCGA analyzed cancers (23 tumors) as well as the not- classified (NC) tumor. From this analysis, it is apparent that intrinsic expression tumor subtypes do not define the classification of the tumors by metabolite levels.

This composite diagram (**Figure 1**) demonstrates several aspects of breast cancer observed across many studies: (1) hormone receptor expression tracks closely with intrinsic subtype; (2) TP53 mutations are very frequent in basal-type cancers; and (3) PIK3CA mutations are common in luminal types. The metabolite-based clustering of these specimens places a group of luminal A cancers with the normal breast specimens and most of the basal cancers together in a single branch. A middle branch contains a combination of mostly luminal A and B cancers. HER2 cancers, as assigned by expression subtype (n = 2) or genomic copy number (n = 4) also tend to cluster in this middle branch. Overall, the cancers in the study appear to have a distribution of receptor status, intrinsic subtype, and genetic alterations typical of an unselected case series.

3.1. Estrogen Receptor Status Reflects a Broad Metabolic Division in Breast Cancer

Our next step in the analysis was to compare metabolite levels in the cancers based on ER status (ER+ versus ER−), the most consistent division in breast cancer from both a biologic and therapeutic perspective [**Figure 2(A)**]. Overall, ER status was a very strong divisor in metabolic space. The identity of the metabolites that vary by ER status supports a series of systematic differences in bioenergetics and biosynthetic pathways. Of the 399 named metabolites quantified in this study, 75 exhibited a statistically significant difference between ER+ and ER− tumors (Table S3 in Additional file 3, unadjusted t tests comparing levels between the three groups of samples, ER+, ER−, and normal breast). Of these, only 8 metabolites were increased in ER+ tumors including 3 carnitine derivatives, suggesting an increase in fatty acid transportation in hormone receptor positive cancers. Short and medium-chain fatty acids were also elevated in ER+ tumors whereas long-chain fatty acids and monoacylgly-cerols tended to be higher in ER- tumors indicating that systematic differences in lipolysis and fatty acid oxidation correlate with hormone receptor status.

ER− tumors had higher levels of glycogenolytic [maltopentose, maltotetraose, maltotriose and maltose, **Figure 2(B)** and pathways in **Figure 2(C)**] and glycolytic metabolites (glucose-6-phosphate, fructose-6-phosphate, fructose-1,6-bisphosphate, and lactate) [**Figure 2(D)**]. In contrast, there was a lower level of glucose in the tumors, especially ER- tumors [**Figure 2(D)**]. Warburg metabolism

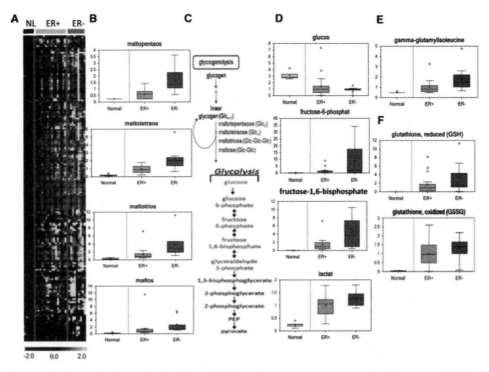

Figure 2. Supervised analysis of metabolites by estrogen receptor (ER) status. (A) Tumor-specific metabolites were zero-transformed against the mean of the five normal breast tumors, filtered and arranged by hierarchical clustering based on 16 ER + and 9 ER- tumors. (B-D) Significantly higher levels of metabolites in the glycogenolysis (B) and glycolysis (D) pathways, as shown in (C), were found in the ER- compared to ER + tumors. The names of elevated (labeled in red) and reduced (labeled in green) metabolites in the glycolysis (B) and glycogenolysis (D) pathways are shown in the metabolism diagram (C). Increased levels of gamma-glutamyl-isoleucine (E) and reduced (GSH) and oxidized (GSSG) glutathione (F) were also found. Primary data and P values for these comparisons can be found in Table S2 in Additional file 2 and Table S3 in Additional file 3.

is a means for rapidly dividing cells, such as cancer cells, to accelerate energy production through increased glycolysis and lactate production, bypassing the normal oxidation of pyruvate in the mitochondria. Thus, the metabolic profile of ER− tumors is consistent with an elevated Warburg effect.

To validate our results, we compared our data to recently published data on breast cancers collected using the same metabolomic platform[27]. Among the significant metabolites that tracked with hormone receptor status in our data, 57 of these were found in the Terunuma dataset and exhibited broadly similar differences between ER+ and ER− cancers (27 reaching significance in both data sets, Figure S1 in Additional file 4 and Table S4 in Additional file 5). Therefore, these identified subtype-specific metabolites can be validated using an independent dataset.

3.2. Reduced Glutathione (GSH) and Gamma-Glutamyl Amino Acids in ER– Tumors

ER– cancers also had higher levels of gamma-glutamyl amino acids coupled with increased glutathione synthesis [**Figure 2(E)**, Figure S2 in Additional file 4]. Gamma-glutamyl amino acids result from the transpeptidase-mediated catalytic reaction of amino acids with glutathione (Figure S2 in Additional file 4). These amino acid-glutathione conjugates traverse the cell membrane and release the amino acid intra-cellularly to regenerate glutathione[28]. Elevated levels of these gamma-glutamyl conjugates indicate an increased uptake of amino acids in ER-tumors. This may point to a potential shift in fuel substrates for energy production that favors amino acid catabolism. It is interesting to note that the most elevated gamma-glutamyl amino acids were the branched-chain amino acid (BCAA) conjugates of valine, leucine and isoleucine. Additionally, ER– tumors had increased glutathione (reduced, GSH) and oxidized glutathi-one (GSSG) [**Figure 2(F)**] indicating a trend toward increased glutathione synthesis, presumably to cope with the higher levels of oxidative stress.

3.3. Metabolite Correlations in Breast Cancers

We postulated that the level of multiple metabolites derived from the same and different metabolic pathway might be coordinated and serve as a better indicator of metabolic activity than any single compound alone. Pearson correlations were calculated for all pairwise comparisons between each of the 399 metabolites for all samples (Table S5 in Additional file 6). The resulting correlation coefficients were then used to group the 399 metabolites into distinct groups by hierarchical clustering (cluster 3.0) and then displayed with TreeView (**Figure 3**). We found that multiple groups of metabolites were highly clustered and correlated. These groups include many metabolites that are known to be in the same metabolic pathways as well as unexpected correlation between metabolites in different metabolic pathways. Metabolites from different pathways clustered in the same

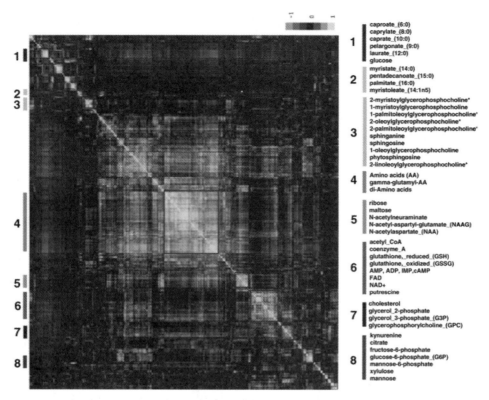

Figure 3. Hierarchical clustering of metabolites based on correlation coefficients. The correlation coefficients were calculated using Pearson product-moment of each pair of metabolites (log base 2 normalized) among 399 metabolites from 25 breast cancers and 5 normal breast tissues. Eight clusters of highly correlated metabolites are highlighted on the right panel.

groups might indicate two different metabolic pathways are coordinated by the same genetic alteration or affected similarly by the metabolic reprogramming. For example, we found a cluster of metabolites comprising many intermediates of various lipids associated with glycerophosphocholines (**Figure 3**, cluster 3). We also noted two separate clusters of amino acids and di-amino acids (glycine-proline, glutamate-leucine, alanine-tyrosine) (**Figure 3**, cluster 4) and N-acetyl-amino acids (N-acetyl-aspartate, N-acetyl-ornithine, N-acetyl-aspartyl-glutamate) (**Figure 3**, cluster 5). Both clusters may indicate products of protein degradation and catabolism and can be used to identify tumors with higher protein catabolism.

Another prominent cluster is composed of acetyl-CoA, CoA, FAD, AMP as well as GSH and GSSH (**Figure 3**, cluster 6). The co-cluster of these metabolites suggests a high degree of correlation between these energy metabolites and anti-oxidative capacity among the tumor tissues. We also noted connected clusters of metabolites related to glycolysis (fructose, glucose-6-phosphate, fructose-6-phosphate) and glycogenolysis (malto-triose, maltotetraose, malto-pentose) (**Figure 3**, cluster 8), both were elevated in ER- cancers (**Figure 2**).

3.4. Metabolites Associated with Specific Genetic Events

A novel and unexpected finding was the level of the oncometabolite 2-HG, elevated over 20-fold in ER+ tumors compared with normal tissue and over 200-fold in ER− tumors [**Figure 4(A)**]. A single ER− tumor exhibited 10-fold higher levels of 2-HG compared to any other sample (unscaled data). We further confirmed the levels of 2-HG in a subset of the breast cancer extracts using an independent assay based on MS performed at Duke and found a very high correlation between the results from these two independent platforms (Figure S3A in Additional file 4). Using this targeted assay, we also measured 2-HG in a series of breast cancer cell lines and found that two basal lines (Hs578T and BT20) had the highest levels, consistent with data from the primary cancers [**Figure 4(B)**]. A high level of 2-HG has been associated with missense mutations in IDH1 or IDH2 in glioma and several other tumor types[29] and may be an effector of tumor cell dedifferentiation[30]. Within the TCGA breast data set, two cancers (<0.5%) were found to harbor missense mutations in IDH1 that have a high probability of affecting the function of the enzyme (R132C, Y235C). Since these data were based on whole genome sequencing that could overlook specific mutations, we performed targeted sequencing in the tumor (TCGA-B6-A1KF) with very high levels of 2-HG to look for the recurrent mutations found in other tumors in IDH1 and IDH2. This tumor was wild type for both genes in these regions (Figure S3B in Additional file 4) suggesting an alternative mechanism leading to 2-HG production, such as the recently reported activation of the myc pathway[27]. Levels of IDH1 and IDH2 mRNA in these specimens also did not show a significant correlation with 2-HG levels.

A number of reports indicate that alterations in specific genes or genetic pathways can result in detectable metabolic changes in cancer. Our study with both detailed gene expression and metabolomic data provided a powerful means to test these associations and discover new ones. One of the least complex of such

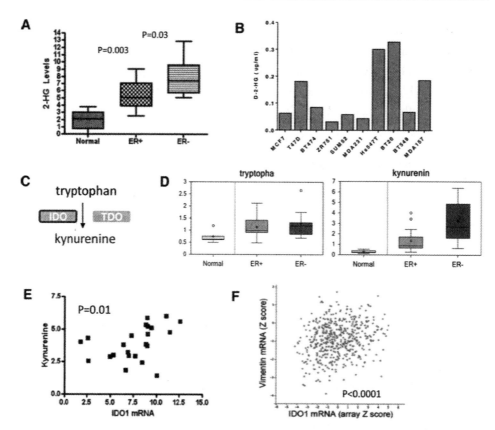

Figure 4. Specific metabolic/genetic associations. (A) The mean level of 2-hydroxyglutarate (2-HG) in 5 normal tissues, 16 estrogen receptor (ER) + and 9 ER− tumors. (B) The level of 2-HG in breast cancer cell lines (4 luminal type and 5 basal type cells). (C) Kynurenine is derived from tryptophan by indoleamine 2,3-dioxygenase (IDO) or tryptophan 2,3-dioxygenase (TDO) enzymatic activity. (D) The level of tryptophan and kynurenine in 5 normal tissues, 16 ER + and 9 ER− tumors. (E) The correlation between the level of kynurenine and IDO1 gene expression measured by RNAseq in 23 tumors analyzed by The Cancer Genome Atlas (TCGA). (F) The correlation between RNA expression of the mesenchymal/basal marker vimentin and IDO1 in TCGA breast cancers.

relationships is the link between the level of the tryptophan-degrading enzyme indoleamine 2,3-dioxygenase (IDO1) and levels of the immunomodulatory metabolite, kynurenine [**Figure 4(C)**]. Whereas the precursor molecule tryptophan did not vary between ER+ and ER− cancers, median levels of kynurenine were significantly elevated in ER− tumors [**Figure 4(D)**]. From RNAseq data of the 23 cancers in our study, we found a significant correlation between IDO1 expression and kynurenine levels [**Figure 3(E)**, $r = 0.55$, $P = 0.01$]. Comparing levels of IDO1 mRNA within the TCGA data set ($n = 748$) revealed a significant positive correlation of IDO1 mRNA levels with vimentin expression (a hallmark of basal cancers). This finding suggests that kynurenine accumulation commonly occurs in basal cancers and could lead to reduced immunosurveillance in this tumor type.

BRCA1 has been implicated in a number of metabolic processes including fatty acid synthesis and response to oxidative stress. Using the available RNAseq data, we correlated expression of BRCA1 with metabolite levels in the 23 TCGA cancers (Table S6 in Additional file 7). There was evidence of strong association between high levels of BRCA1 mRNA and elevated acetyl CoA, CoA, 3' dephospho-CoA, and several acylcarnitines all indicative of higher levels of fatty acid β-oxidation (**Figure 5**). This is consistent with the reported ability of BRCA1 to inhibit acetyl-coenzyme A carboxylase 1 (ACC1/ACACA) leading to reduced fatty acid synthesis and increased fatty acid β-oxidation resulting in the accumulation of acetyl-CoA and CoA[31]. In contrast, there were strong inverse correlations between BRCA1 levels and membrane components, long-chain fatty acids, and amino acids further supporting the role of BRCA1 in regulating the balance between fatty acid synthesis and oxidation (**Figure 5**)[32]. In addition, GSH and

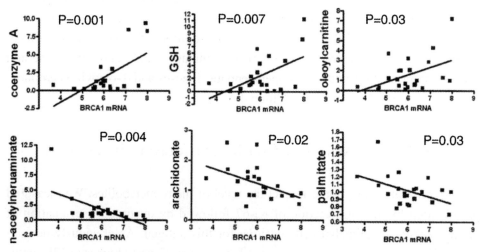

Figure 5. Correlation between selected metabolite levels and BRCA1 mRNA expression. Three representative metabolites (coenzyme A (CoA), reduced glutathione (GSH) and oleoyl-carnitine) that are positively and three (N-acetylneuraminate, arachidonate and palmitate) that are inversely correlated with BRCA1 mRNA levels from The Cancer Genome Atlas (TCGA) RNAseq data on 23 cancers are shown. The full list of metabolites correlated with BRCA1 is provided in Table S6 in Additional file 7 showing listing both normalized metabolite levels and metabolite levels with an additional log2 transformation to reduce the impact of outliers.

another antioxidant, 3-(4-hydroxyphenyl)lactate were also positively correlated with BRCA1 mRNA levels, supporting its role in activating NRF2, the master regulator of the oxidative stress response and GSH synthesis[33]-[35]. BRCA1 mRNA levels did not correlate with proliferation or ER status indicating that this is an independent set of variables. Furthermore, the BRCA1 mRNA did not correlate with the mRNA levels of genes in the fatty acid biosynthesis pathways; consistent with posttranscriptional regulation (Figure S4 in Additional file 4).

To further explore associations with the most common genetic events in breast cancer, we performed SAM analyses (Table S7 in Additional file 8) to identify metabolites associated with the somatic driver alterations (shown in **Figure 1**, used as categorical variables that is, mutant versus wild type, amplified/deleted versus diploid). Many of the genetic events are loosely associated with specific tumor subtypes (for example, PIK3CA mutations were not found in basal cancers) such that metabolite correlations with specific genetic features may be confounded by higher level associations. With this inmind, the results do support several relationships between metabolite profiles and tumor genetics. Most notably, compared to tumors with wild-type p53, cancers with TP53 alterations show a very specific pattern of decreased lipid glycerophosphocho-lines that is not apparent when classifying the cancers by ER status, (Figure S5 in Additional file 4). Other significant associations were observed between PIK3CA mutation and malonylcarnitine and ERBB2 amplification with docosapentaenoate, fucose, and 1-oleoylglycerophosphoethanolamine (Figure S6 in Additional file 4).

3.5. Metabolites Associated with Proliferation in Tumors

Proliferation rate could impact the level of many metabolites. We measured proliferation by in situ detection of Ki-67 followed by quantitative evaluation of the percentage of epithelial cells positive for this antigen. As previously demonstrated in many studies, proliferation tends to be significantly higher in ER− compared to ER+ tumors (mean of 32% versus 14%, P = 0.009 in our cohort) and epithelial cells in normal breast tissue have a very low rate of proliferation [**Figure 6(C)**]. Supervised clustering and correlation analysis of the metabolites with proliferation rate demonstrated sets of metabolites that were positively and inversely correlated with proliferation [**Figure 6(A)** and **Figure 6(B)**, and Table S8 in Additional file 9]. Predictably, the level of glucose was lower in rapidly proliferating

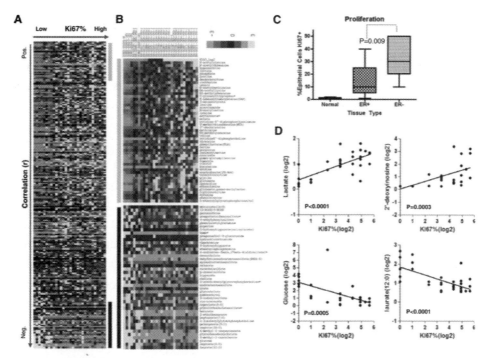

Figure 6. Proliferation rate is correlated with the level of many metabolites. (A) Supervised clustering of normalized metabolite levels as ordered by the proliferation rate (Ki-67%) (from low (left) to high (right)). (B) Zoomed views of the metabolites that are most positively (orange bar) or negatively (blue bar) correlated with proliferation. (C) Proliferation associated with receptor status and cancer status from the 30 samples in this study. (D) The correlation of representative metabolites positively or negatively associated with proliferation rate.

cancers whereas lactate was positively correlated with proliferation [**Figure 6(D)**]. N-acetyl amino acids and 2′-deoxyinosine were highly enriched in rapidly proliferating tumors. The biological roles of N-acetyl amino acids are largely unknown. However, aminoacylase-1 (encoded by ACY1), which is responsible for the degradation of these N-acetyl amino acids, has been found to be inactivated in several tumor types[36][37]. High levels of 2′-deoxyinosine (dI) may be an indication of misincorporation of dI into the DNA of ER- tumor cells, a lesion capable of generating A−> G transitions in DNA[38].

ER status was highly correlated with proliferation and therefore many of the same metabolites were associated with both of these parameters. We further analyzed the data to determine whether these two parameters had any degree of independence, and if so, for which sets of metabolites. Linear regression analyses show that, while correlated with one another, ER and proliferation status act as complementary explanatory factors for many of the metabolites (Figure S7 in Additional file 4). A relatively small number of metabolites were highly correlated with one parameter but not the other, most notably 2-HG with ER status but not proliferation (Table S9 in Additional file 10).

4. Discussion

Links between cancer genetics and altered metabolism have been established primarily in model and experimental systems but have rarely been tested in primary human cancers. The current study makes use of the comprehensive genetic data from TCGA on breast cancer[1] to test reported relationships and discover new and unexpected associations between genetics and metabolism. TCGA data provides an excellent platform in this regard for three reasons: (1) the tissues were subjected to stringent quality control criteria including tumor nuclei exceeding 70% and the absence of significant necrosis, (2) multiple analytes were measured in parallel on the same cancers including DNA sequence for mutations, DNA copy number assessment, RNA expression including RNAseq and microarray analysis, methylation, and protein and phosphoprotein levels, and (3) the data are in the public domain in easily accessible formats with standardized specimen identifiers that can be directly linked and co-analyzed with other types of newly generated data such as the metabolite levels that we measured in the current study. We include the primary data on these samples so that anyone can perform their own joint analysis on metabolites and genes of interest.

The frozen tissues were analyzed on a metabolomics platform that has been used in other cancer-related studies[39]–[41] and at the time of the analysis, included identification and quantitation of 399 named biochemicals (Mr < 1,000 Da). Unsupervised clustering by metabolite levels revealed two major categories, one containing the normal breast tissues and a subset of the ER+ cancers, and the other containing all of the ER− cancers and the remaining ER+ ones. Overlaying the TCGA data on these clusters revealed that all of the cancers clustering with normal breast were of the luminal A intrinsic subtype. The remaining luminal A and all of the luminal B cancers fell in the other major cluster along with all of the basal cancers and the two cancers designated as HER2 by PAM50. That the luminal A cancers do not all cluster together is consistent with a metabolomic study employing high resolution magic angle spinning magnetic resonance spectroscopy of predominantly luminal cancers[17]. In this study, three distinct categories of luminal A cancers were described by hierarchical clustering driven primarily by varying levels of glycolytic activity. Widely different proliferation rates in the ER+ cancers may at least partially underlie these luminal sub-clusters.

The basal subtype, a subset of the ER- cancers, demonstrated significant homogeneity with 4 of the 5 PAM50 basal cancers clustering on one sub-branch of the metabolomic hierarchical tree. A HER2 cancer was the only other member of this sub-branch but this cancer does share the common basal trait of having a TP53 mutation. Overlaying the most common genetic driver alterations in breast cancer on this cluster diagram allowed a visual assessment of whether branches may also be driven by specific oncogenic events. TP53 mutations and basal cancer status are nearly coincident and as described, the basal cancers are tightly clustered. Therefore, it is difficult to disentangle genetics from intrinsic subtype in this instance. Other not-able groupings that may be associated with a specific genetic driver include MYC amplification and PIK3CA mutation. PIK3CA mutations are tightly linked to the luminal subtypes whereas MYC amplification is common in both basal and luminal cancers. It may be noteworthy that none of the MYC amplified tumors clustered with the normal breast tissue.

Supervised classification and t tests based on the three categories of specimens (ER+, ER/PR-, normal) exhibited significant signals for many metabolites. Over half of the 399 identified metabolites were different between normal and cancer. Moreover, >18% of the metabolites varied significantly between ER+ and ER- cancers. These dramatic differences are consistent with previous reports showing strong remodeling of central metabolism between normal breast tissue and breast cancer[16] and between tumor subtypes[9]. Notably, glycolytic and glycogenolytic-associated metabolites including lactate were higher in ER- cancers with the prominent exception of low tumor glucose. The increased lactate production from ER- cancer may be caused by increased glycolysis and confirm our previous finding of a strong hypoxia program and the high 'Warburg' phenotype previously described in other studies of ER- cancer[7][9][16][27].

From TCGA data (for 23 of 25 of the cancers), we were able to confirm or identify known and unexpected associations between metabolite levels and various genetic events. Proof of principle for this approach was demonstrated by the correlation between kynurenine and the mRNA of its synthetic enzyme, IDO1. IDO1 expression was also found to correlate with the basal phenotype common to ER-cancers and the high levels of kynurenine produced could result in reduced immunosurveillance of these cancers[42]. Increased serum kynurenine/tryptophan ratio has been noted during the progression of several tumor types[43][44]. Our findings support a connection between high IDO levels and kynurenine in ER-tumors. Other a priori associations that were tested included PKM2 exon 9 versus 10 splice variant levels with proliferation and metabolite levels[45], IDH1 and 2 mRNA and mutations with 2-hydroxyglutarate levels[29], and levels of GGT1 mRNA and the gamma-glutamyl amino acids[46]. Of these, the strongest association was between GGT1 and a subset of the conjugated amino acids including leucine and isoleucine (Figure S8 in Additional file 10). GGT1 expression has been associated with a subset of basal cancers and our data indicating elevated levels of gamma-glutamyl amino acids in ER- cancers provides functional support for this genetic link.

A number of driver mutational events have been implicated in breast cancer development including amplification of ERBB2, CCND1 and MYC, loss of PTEN and CDH1, and missense mutations in TP53 and PIK3CA. Some of these events have been associated with changes in central metabolism in tumors and experimental systems[4][5][47]–[49]. Using these genetic alterations as categorical variables, we analyzed our data for signs of metabolic signatures associated with the most common genetic lesions. The co-existence of TP53 mutation and reduced levels of a series of lipid glycerophosphocholines was the most significant association detected. Altered choline metabolism in the form of decreased glycerophos- phocholine (GPC) was reported for several tumor types, consistent with an association with p53 status[50][51]. A specific connection between p53 and phospholipid metabolism was demonstrated previously with indication of feedback regulation between phospholipid turnover and p53 activity[52]–[55]. In our data, 8 different long-chain fatty acid glycerophosphocholines were strongly reduced in p53 mutant tumors suggesting an underlying regulatory relationship for this consistent association. An important caveat for this finding is the fact that p53 mutation status is associated with the basal intrinsic subtype in breast cancer. In our data set, all five of the basal cancers harbored p53 mutations and only one of the nonbasal cancers (HER2) had a mutation. Therefore, the strong association we observed between

TP53 status and the levels of these phospholipids may be confounded by intrinsic subtype something that cannot be distinguished in the current study. Another interesting metabolite-genetic association is the higher level of fucose in ERBB2+ tumors. Fucose is a simple sugar that is used to modify proteins and shown to be necessary for key functions of neoplastic progression of breast cancer cells[56]. The higher level of fucose may suggest that such glycoprotein modifications play a particular important role in ERBB2+ tumors.

Our findings with respect to BRCA1 further highlight the potential of these joint analyses. Germ line BRCA1 mutations typically lead to triple-negative cancers, but broad variation in mRNA expression is also observed outside of the context of the hereditary syndrome. High levels of BRCA1 mRNA were positively correlated with a group of metabolites indicative of elevated fatty acid β-oxidation and increased anti-stress response and inversely correlated with medium- and long-chain fatty acids and membrane components. BRCA1 protein via its BRCT domain was shown to bind to ACC1/ACACA preventing its dephosphorylation, keeping it in a phosphorylated and inactive form, thus inhibiting fatty acid synthesis and promoting fatty acid β-oxidation[31]. We found a number of metabolites that fit this mechanism. BRCA1 has also been implicated in redox homeostasis[33], potentially through an interaction with NRF2 that prevents its degradation and promotes its nuclear accumulation[35] and we found multiple metabolites that also fit this activity. These BRCA1 expression-metabolite associations are entirely consistent with in vitro mechanistic studies implicating BRCA1 in these processes and as such, constitute direct support for the physiologic relevance of these pathway connections in breast cancer.

Rate of proliferation is a key phenotypic property of breast cancers that can be used as an independent prognostic factor[57]. Gene expression indicative of proliferation constitutes a major component of the Oncotype Dx multi-gene recurrence score[58]. We measured proliferation in our specimens by scoring Ki-67 staining as a continuous variable and correlated this metric with metabolite levels. As anticipated, a number of strong correlations with proliferative rate were found including high levels of lactate and low levels of glucose consistent with glucose-consumption patterns in rapidly growing cells. Overall, many of the same metabolites correlated with both receptor status and proliferation. While proliferation did correlate with ER status in our study (and others), there were ER+ cancers with high proliferation rates and ER− cancers with relatively low proliferation rates in our sample set. We compared the relative contribution of these two factors (proliferation and receptor status) to metabolite levels through statistical analysis and found that a number of analytes were strongly associated with one parameter but not the other suggesting that there is some degree of independence. However, these results further highlight the potential confounding classification issue in breast cancer as receptor status, intrinsic subtype, and genetic and phenotypic properties are all correlated. The admixture of cancers we analyzed in the current study reinforces these relationships indicating that this data set is highly representative of the landscape of the disease. The inclusion of metabolite profiles as an additional dimension in the TCGA database provides a new level of resolution to this important public resource. Indexing our metabolite data to the rigorously curated, comprehensive, and standardized TCGA platform offers the opportunity for additional hypothesis testing and discovery based upon metabolic signatures and could produce novel insights for detection, prognostic, predictive, or therapeutic benefit.

5. Conclusions

We have identified categorical differences in the metabolic profile of ER− vs. ER+ breast tumors that may directly impact tumor behavior and clinical phenotypes. We found notable differences in energy needs, redox potential, protein uptake and catabolism which in the ER− samples correlated with increases in glutathione biosynthesis, NAD+ production, and proliferative signaling. The data are consistent with high Warburg metabolism in the ER- tumors, as several biochemical intermediates of the glycolytic pathway including lactate were found to be increased in these cancers. Joint analysis with genetic alterations further identified several gene-metabolite correlations validating the physiologic relevance of reported in vitro associations and providing indications of novel regulatory relationships between tumor genetics and metabolism. The addition of metabolomic data to the public domain TCGA dataset provides an important new tool for the discovery and hypothesis testing of the genetic regulatory of tumor metabolism.

Additional Files

Additional file 1: Table S1. Demographic and clinical data for the breast cancer subjects from which the tissues for this study were derived.

Additional file 2: Table S2. Metabolite levels (normalized and imputed) of the breast samples with genetic driver alterations indicated.

Additional file 3: Table S3. t tests comparing metabolite levels between the three groups of specimens; normal breast, estrogen receptor (ER) + cancers, and ER- cancers.

Additional file 4: Figure S1. Metabolomic comparison between our dataset and Terunuma *et al.*'s dataset. Lipid-containing metabolites are highlighted in blue typeface. Figure S2. Significantly higher levels ofseveral metabolites in the cysteine and glutathione homeostasis and amino acid cycle were found in estrogen receptor (ER)− compared to ER+ tumors. Figure S3. (A) Highly correlated 2-hydroxyglutarate (2-HG)level measured by two different laboratories and methods. On the y-axis arethe values from Metabolon and the x-axis are the same samples analyzed in the Duke Cancer Pharmacology Laboratory. The right hand plot normalizes the scales for each set of measurements to spread out the points.(B) Absence of IDH1 and IDH2 mutations in very high 2-HG sample(TCGA-B6-A1KF). For comparison, the IDH1 R132C mutation is shown from HT1080 cells. Figure S4. Heatmap of expression of BRCA1 and genes in fatty acid biosynthesis pathway based on The Cancer Genome Atlas (TCGA) mRNA data. Figure S5. A series of lipid glycerophosphocholines significantly reduced in cancers with TP53 mutations. Figure S6. Examples of metabolites significantly higher in tumors with mutant PIK3CA or ERBB2amplified tumors. Figure S7. Scatter plots of the associations of each metabolite with log proliferation versus the same for receptor status given that log proliferation status is already accounted for in themodel (and vice versa). Each point corresponds to a metabolite and the color corresponds to the overall strength of association between receptor and proliferation and the metabolite. The dashed red linescorrespond to $P = 0.05$. Note that two of the four metabolites (in each analysis) most highly associated with proliferation or receptor statusshow significant additional explanatory ability for receptor status (red dots); these m etab olites repr esent t he strong est o verall associations.

Figure S8. Correlation between GGT1 mRNA levels and selected gamma-glutamyl amino acids.

Additional file 5: Table S4. Comparison with the Terunuma *et al.*'s (JCI 2014) dataset for discrimination of estrogen receptor (ER)+ and ER− cancers.

Additional file 6: Table S5. Pearson's correlations between all metabolites in the study.

Additional file 7: Table S6. Pearson's correlations between BRCA1 mRNA levels and metabolites for 23 cancers comparing normalized metabolite levels and then log2 transformed normalized metabolite levels with RNAseq expression data from The Cancer Genome Atlas (TCGA). The metabolites that are significantly associated with BRCA1 mRNA levels are labeled in red (positive correlation) or green (negative correlation).

Additional file 8: Table S7. Significance of microarray (SAM) analysis of metabolites using each genetic driver alteration as a separate binary condition.

Additional file 9: Table S8. Pearson's correlations between KI-67 (proliferation rate) and metabolite levels.

Additional file 10: Table S9. Linear regression analyses of proliferation (KI-67), estrogen receptor (ER) status, and metabolite levels.

Abbreviations

2-HG: 2-hydroxyglutarate; ACC1: acetyl-coenzyme A carboxylase 1, encoded by ACACA (acetyl-CoA carboxylase alpha); ER: estrogen receptor; GC/MS: gas chromatography/mass spectrometry; GSH: glutathione, reduced; GSSG: glutathione, oxidized; HER2: amplified ERBB2 oncogene; IDO: indoleamine 2,3-dioxygenase; LC/MS: liquid chromatography/mass spectrometry; NMR: nuclear magnetic resonance; NFE2L2: NFE2-related factor 2; PAM50: 50 gene expression signature separating breast cancers into 5 intrinsic subtypes; PR: progesterone receptor; TCGA: The Cancer Genome Atlas.

Competing Interests

The authors declare that they have no competing interests.

Authors' Contributions

XT, CCL, JTC and JRM designed and performed sample preparation, analysis, and molecular biological experiments. IS performed the mass spectrometry to quantitate 2-HG in breast cancers and cell lines. ESI performed statistical analysis. XT, JTC and JRM designed the overall experimental focus, analyzed data, and wrote the manuscript. All authors read and approved the manuscript.

Acknowledgements

We wish to acknowledge the generous financial support from the NIH (CA084955 to JRM, CA125618, and CA106520 to JTC) and Department of Defense (W81XWH-12-1-0148 to JTC). We are also grateful to James Koh for critical discussions and editing of the manuscript.

Source: Tang X, Lin C C, Spasojevic I, *et al*. A joint analysis of metabolomics and genetics of breast cancer[J]. Breast Cancer Research Bcr, 2014, 16(4):1–15.

References

[1] Cancer Genome Atlas Network: Comprehensive molecular portraits of human breast tumours. Nature 2012, 490:61–70.

[2] Levine AJ, Puzio-Kuter AM: The control of the metabolic switch in cancers by oncogenes and tumor suppressor genes. Science 2010, 330:1340–1344.

[3] Reitman ZJ, Jin G, Karoly ED, Spasojevic I, Yang J, Kinzler KW, He Y, Bigner DD, Vogelstein B, Yan H: Profiling the effects of isocitrate dehydrogenase 1 and 2 mutations on the cellular metabolome. Proc Natl Acad Sci U S A 2011, 108:3270–3275.

[4] Yuneva MO, Fan TW, Allen TD, Higashi RM, Ferraris DV, Tsukamoto T, Mates JM, Alonso FJ, Wang C, Seo Y, Chen X, Bishop JM: The metabolic profile of tumors depends on both the responsible genetic lesion and tissue type. Cell Metab 2012, 15:157–170.

[5] Maddocks OD, Berkers CR, Mason SM, Zheng L, Blyth K, Gottlieb E, Vousden KH: Serine starvation induces stress and p53-dependent metabolic remodelling in cancer cells. Nature 2013, 493:542–546.

[6] Garcia-Cao I, Song MS, Hobbs RM, Laurent G, Giorgi C, de Boer VC, Anastasiou D,

Ito K, Sasaki AT, Rameh L, Carracedo A, Vander Heidenmg, Cantley LC, Pinton P, Haigis MC, Pandolfi PP: Systemic elevation of PTEN induces a tumor-suppressive metabolic state. Cell 2012, 149:49–62.

[7] Gatza ML, Kung HN, Blackwell KL, Dewhirst MW, Marks JR, Chi JT: Analysis of tumor environmental response and oncogenic pathway activation identifies distinct basal and luminal features in HER2-related breast tumor subtypes. Breast Cancer Res 2011, 13:R62.

[8] Palaskas N, Larson SM, Schultz N, Komisopoulou E, Wong J, Rohle D, Campos C, Yannuzzi N, Osborne JR, Linkov I, Kastenhuber ER, Taschereau R, Plaisier SB, Tran C, Heguy A, Wu H, Sander C, Phelps ME, Brennan C, Port E, Huse JT, Graeber TG, Mellinghoff IK: 18 F-fluorodeoxy-glucose positron emission tomography marks MYC-overexpressing human basal-like breast cancers. Cancer Res 2011, 71:5164–5174.

[9] Brauer HA, Makowski L, Hoadley KA, Casbas-Hernandez P, Lang LJ, Roman-Perez E, D'Arcy M, Freemerman AJ, Peroucm, Troester MA: Impact of tumor microenvironment and epithelial phenotypes on metabolism in breast cancer. Clin Cancer Res 2013, 19:571–585.

[10] Jerby L, Wolf L, Denkert C, Stein GY, Hilvo M, Oresic M, Geiger T, Ruppin E: Metabolic associations of reduced proliferation and oxidative stress in advanced breast cancer. Cancer Res 2012, 72:5712–5720.

[11] Kung HN, Marks JR, Chi JT: Glutamine synthetase is a genetic determinant of cell type-specific glutamine independence in breast epithelia. PLoS Genet 2011, 7:e1002229.

[12] Peroucm, Sorlie T, Eisen MB, van de Rijn M, Jeffrey SS, Rees CA, Pollack JR, Ross DT, Johnsen H, Aksien LA, Fluge O, Pergamenschikov A, Williams C, Zhu SX, Lonning PE, Borresen-Dale AL, Brown PO, Botstein D: Molecular portraits of human breast tumours. Nature 2000, 406:747–752.

[13] Lim E, Vaillant F, Wu D, Forrest NC, Pal B, Hart AH, Asselin-Labat ML, Gyorki DE, Ward T, Partanen A, Feleppa F, Huschtscha LI, Thorne HJ, kConFab, Fox SB, Yan M, French JD, Brown MA, Smyth GK, Visvader JE, Lindeman GJ: Aberrant luminal progenitors as the candidate target population for basal tumor development in BRCA1 mutation carriers. Nat Med 2009, 15:907–913.

[14] Shipitsin M, Campbell LL, Argani P, Weremowicz S, Bloushtain-Qimron N, Yao J, Nikolskaya T, Serebryiskaya T, Beroukhim R, Hu M, Halushka MK, Sukumar S, Parker LM, Anderson KS, Harris LN, Garber JE, Richardson AL, Schnitt SJ, Nikolsky Y, Gelman RS, Polyak K: Molecular definition of breast tumor heterogeneity. Cancer Cell 2007, 11:259–273.

[15] Sitter B, Lundgren S, Bathen TF, Halgunset J, Fjosne HE, Gribbestad IS: Comparison of HR MAS MR spectroscopic profiles of breast cancer tissue with clinical parameters. NMR Biomed 2006, 19:30–40.

[16] Budczies J, Denkert C, Muller BM, Brockmoller SF, Klauschen F, Gyorffy B, Dietel

M, Richter-Ehrenstein C, Marten U, Salek RM, Griffin JL, Hilvo M, Oresic M, Wohlgemuth G, Fiehn O: Remodeling of central metabolism in invasive breast cancer compared to normal breast tissue a GC-TOFMS based metabolomics study. BMC Genomics 2012, 13:334.

[17] Borgan E, Sitter B, Lingjaerde OC, Johnsen H, Lundgren S, Bathen TF, Sorlie T, Borresen-Dale AL, Gribbestad IS: Merging transcriptomics and metabolomics– advances in breast cancer profiling. BMC Cancer 2010, 10:628.

[18] Hilvo M, Denkert C, Lehtinen L, Muller B, Brockmoller S, Seppanen-Laakso T, Budczies J, Bucher E, Yetukuri L, Castillo S, Berg E, Nygren H, Sysi-Aho M, Griffin JL, Fiehn O, Loibl S, Richter-Ehrenstein C, Radke C, Hyotylainen T, Kallioniemi O, Iljin K, Oresic M: Novel theranostic opportunities offered by characterization of altered membrane lipid metabolism in breast cancer progression. Cancer Res 2011, 71:3236–3245.

[19] Struys EA, Jansen EE, Verhoeven NM, Jakobs C: Measurement of urinary D- and L-2-hydroxyglutarate enantiomers by stable-isotope-dilution liquid chromatography-tandem mass spectrometry after derivatization with diacetyl-L-tartaric anhydride. Clin Chem 2004, 50:1391–1395.

[20] Storey JD, Tibshirani R: Statistical significance for genomewide studies. Proc Natl Acad Sci U S A 2003, 100:9440–9445.

[21] Eisen MB, Spellman PT, Brown PO, Botstein D: Cluster analysis and display of genome-wide expression patterns. Proc Natl Acad Sci U S A 1998, 95:14863–14868.

[22] Tusher VG, Tibshirani R, Chu G: Significance analysis of microarrays applied to the ionizing radiation response. Proc Natl Acad Sci U S A 2001, 98:5116–5121.

[23] The Cancer Genome Atlas-data portal. [https://tcga-data.nci.nih.gov/tcga/]

[24] cBioPortal for Cancer Genomics. [http://www.cbioportal.org/public-portal/]

[25] Chia SK, Bramwell VH, Tu D, Shepherd LE, Jiang S, Vickery T, Mardis E, Leung S, Ung K, Pritchard KI, Parker JS, Bernard PS, Peroucm, Ellis MJ, Nielsen TO: A 50-gene intrinsic subtype classifier for prognosis and prediction of benefit from adjuvant tamoxifen. Clin Cancer Res 2012, 18:4465–4472.

[26] Sorlie T, Peroucm, Tibshirani R, Aas T, Geisler S, Johnsen H, Hastie T, Eisen MB, van de Rijn M, Jeffrey SS, Thorsen T, Quist H, Matese JC, Brown PO, Botstein D, Eystein Lonning P, Borresen-Dale AL: Gene expression patterns of breast carcinomas distinguish tumor subclasses with clinical implications. Proc Natl Acad Sci U S A 2001, 98:10869–10874.

[27] Terunuma A, Putluri N, Mishra P, Mathe EA, Dorsey TH, Yi M, Wallace TA, Issaq HJ, Zhou M, Killian JK, Stevenson HS, Karoly ED, Chan K, Samanta S, Prieto D, Hsu TY, Kurley SJ, Putluri V, Sonavane R, Edelman DC, Wulff J, Starks AM, Yang Y, Kittles RA, Yfantis HG, Lee DH, Ioffe OB, Schiff R, Stephens RM, Meltzer PS, *et al*: MYC-driven accumulation of 2-hydroxyglutarate is associated with breast cancer prognosis. J Clin Invest 2014, 124:398–412.

[28] Griffith OW, Bridges RJ, Meister A: Transport of gamma-glutamyl amino acids: role of glutathione and gamma-glutamyl transpeptidase. Proc Natl Acad Sci U S A 1979, 76:6319–6322.

[29] Dang L, White DW, Gross S, Bennett BD, Bittinger MA, Driggers EM, Fantin VR, Jang HG, Jin S, Keenan MC, Marks KM, Prins RM, Ward PS, Yen KE, Liau LM, Rabinowitz JD, Cantley LC, Thompson CB, Vander Heidenmg, Su SM: Cancer-associated IDH1 mutations produce 2-hydroxyglutarate. Nature 2009, 462:739–744.

[30] Rohle D, Popovici-Muller J, Palaskas N, Turcan S, Grommes C, Campos C, Tsoi J, Clark O, Oldrini B, Komisopoulou E, Kunii K, Pedraza A, Schalm S, Silverman L, Miller A, Wang F, Yang H, Chen Y, Kernytsky A, Rosenblum MK, Liu W, Biller SA, Su SM, Brennan CW, Chan TA, Graeber TG, Yen KE, Mellinghoff IK: An inhibitor of mutant IDH1 delays growth and promotes differentiation of glioma cells. Science 2013, 340:626–630.

[31] Moreau K, Dizin E, Ray H, Luquain C, Lefai E, Foufelle F, Billaud M, Lenoir GM, Venezia ND: BRCA1 affects lipid synthesis through its interaction with acetyl-CoA carboxylase. J Biol Chem 2006, 281:3172–3181.

[32] Singh KK, Shukla PC, Yanagawa B, Quan A, Lovren F, Pan Y, Wagg CS, Teoh H, Lopaschuk GD, Verma S: Regulating cardiac energy metabolism and bioenergetics by targeting the DNA damage repair protein BRCA1. J Thorac Cardiovasc Surg 2013, 146:702–709.

[33] Bae I, Fan S, Meng Q, Rih JK, Kim HJ, Kang HJ, Xu J, Goldberg ID, Jaiswal AK, Rosen EM: BRCA1 induces antioxidant gene expression and resistance to oxidative stress. Cancer Res 2004, 64:7893–7909.

[34] Fan S, Meng Q, Saha T, Sarkar FH, Rosen EM: Low concentrations of diindolylmethane, a metabolite of indole-3-carbinol, protect against oxidative stress in a BRCA1-dependent manner. Cancer Res 2009, 69:6083–6091.

[35] Gorrini C, Baniasadi PS, Harris IS, Silvester J, Inoue S, Snow B, Joshi PA, Wakeham A, Molyneux SD, Martin B, Bouwman P, Cescon DW, Elia AJ, Winterton-Perks Z, Cruickshank J, Brenner D, Tseng A, Musgrave M, Berman HK, Khokha R, Jonkers J, Mak TW, Gauthier ML: BRCA1 interacts with Nrf2 to regulate antioxidant signaling and cell survival. J Exp Med 2013, 210:1529–1544.

[36] Cook RM, Franklin WA, Moore MD, Johnson BE, Miller YE: Mutational inactivation of aminoacylase-I in a small cell lung cancer cell line. Genes Chromosomes Cancer 1998, 21:320–325.

[37] Zhong Y, Onuki J, Yamasaki T, Ogawa O, Akatsuka S, Toyokuni S: Genome-wide analysis identifies a tumor suppressor role for aminoacylase 1 in iron-induced rat renal cell carcinoma. Carcinogenesis 2009, 30:158–164.

[38] Yasui M, Suenaga E, Koyama N, Masutani C, Hanaoka F, Gruz P, Shibutani S, Nohmi T, Hayashi M, Honma M: Miscoding properties of 2'-deoxyinosine, a nitric oxide-derived DNA Adduct, during translesion synthesis catalyzed by human DNA

polymerases. J Mol Biol 2008, 377:1015–1023.

[39] Sreekumar A, Poisson LM, Rajendiran TM, Khan AP, Cao Q, Yu J, Laxman B, Mehra R, Lonigro RJ, Li Y, Nyati MK, Ahsan A, Kalyana-Sundaram S, Han B, Cao X, Byun J, Omenn GS, Ghosh D, Pennathur S, Alexander DC, Berger A, Shuster JR, Wei JT, Varambally S, Beecher C, Chinnaiyan AM: Metabolomic profiles delineate potential role for sarcosine in prostate cancer progression. Nature 2009, 457:910–914.

[40] Chinnaiyan P, Kensicki E, Bloom G, Prabhu A, Sarcar B, Kahali S, Eschrich S, Qu X, Forsyth P, Gillies R: The metabolomic signature of malignant glioma reflects accelerated anabolic metabolism. Cancer Res 2012, 72:5878–5888.

[41] Hitosugi T, Zhou L, Elf S, Fan J, Kang HB, Seo JH, Shan C, Dai Q, Zhang L, Xie J, Gu TL, Jin P, Aleckovic M, LeRoy G, Kang Y, Sudderth JA, DeBerardinis RJ, Luan CH, Chen GZ, Muller S, Shin DM, Owonikoko TK, Lonial S, Arellano ML, Khoury HJ, Khuri FR, Lee BH, Ye K, Boggon TJ, Kang S, et al: Phosphoglycerate mutase 1 coordinates glycolysis and biosynthesis to promote tumor growth. Cancer Cell 2012, 22:585–600.

[42] Platten M, Wick W, Van den Eynde BJ: Tryptophan catabolism in cancer: beyond IDO and tryptophan depletion. Cancer Res 2012, 72:5435–5440.

[43] Suzuki Y, Suda T, Furuhashi K, Suzuki M, Fujie M, Hahimoto D, Nakamura Y, Inui N, Nakamura H, Chida K: Increased serum kynurenine/tryptophan ratio correlates with disease progression in lung cancer. Lung Cancer 2010, 67:361–365.

[44] Lyon DE, Walter JM, Starkweather AR, Schubertcm, McCain NL: Tryptophan degradation in women with breast cancer: a pilot study. BMC Res Notes 2011, 4:156.

[45] Wang Z, Chatterjee D, Jeon HY, Akerman M, Vander Heidenmg, Cantley LC, Krainer AR: Exon-centric regulation of pyruvate kinase M alternative splicing via mutually exclusive exons. J Mol Cell Biol 2012, 4:79–87.

[46] Kim S, Kim Do H, Jung WH, Koo JS: Metabolic phenotypes in triple-negative breast cancer. Tumour Biol 2013, 34:1699–1712.

[47] Dang CV: MYC, metabolism, cell growth, and tumorigenesis. Cold Spring Harb Perspect Med 2013, 3:1–15.

[48] Freed-Pastor WA, Mizuno H, Zhao X, Langerod A, Moon SH, Rodriguez-Barrueco R, Barsotti A, Chicas A, Li W, Polotskaia A, Bissell MJ, Osborne TF, Tian B, Lowe SW, Silva JM, Borresen-Dale AL, Levine AJ, Bargonetti J, Prives C: Mutant p53 disrupts mammary tissue architecture via the mevalonate pathway. Cell 2012, 148:244–258.

[49] Foster R, Griffin S, Grooby S, Feltell R, Christopherson C, Chang M, Sninsky J, Kwok S, Torrance C: Multiple metabolic alterations exist in mutant PI3K cancers, but only glucose is essential as a nutrient source. PLoS One 2012, 7:e45061.

[50] Aboagye EO, Bhujwalla ZM: Malignant transformation alters membrane choline

phospholipid metabolism of human mammary epithelial cells. Cancer Res 1999, 59:80–84.

[51] Iorio E, Mezzanzanica D, Alberti P, Spadaro F, Ramoni C, D'Ascenzo S, Millimaggi D, Pavan A, Dolo V, Canevari S, Podo F: Alterations of choline phospholipid metabolism in ovarian tumor progression. Cancer Res 2005, 65:9369–9376.

[52] Zhang XH, Zhao C, Seleznev K, Song K, Manfredi JJ, Ma ZA: Disruption of G1-phase phospholipid turnover by inhibition of Ca2 + –independent phospholipase A2 induces a p53-dependent cell-cycle arrest in G1 phase. J Cell Sci 2006, 119:1005–1015.

[53] Goldstein I, Rotter V: Regulation of lipid metabolism by p53-fighting two villains with one sword. Trends Endocrinol Metab 2012, 23:567–575.

[54] Li CH, Cheng YW, Liao PL, Kang JJ: Translocation of p53 to mitochondria is regulated by its lipid binding property to anionic phospholipids and it participates in cell death control. Neoplasia 2010, 12:150–160.

[55] He H, Conrad CA, Nilsson CL, Ji Y, Schaub TM, Marshall AG, Emmett MR: Method for lipidomic analysis: p53 expression modulation of sulfatide, ganglioside, and phospholipid composition of U87mg glioblastoma cells. Anal Chem 2007, 79:8423–8430.

[56] Listinsky JJ, Siegal GP, Listinskycm: The emerging importance of alpha-L- fucose in human breast cancer: a review. Am J Transl Res 2011, 3:292–322.

[57] Luporsi E, Andre F, Spyratos F, Martin PM, Jacquemier J, Penault-Llorca F, Tubiana-Mathieu N, Sigal-Zafrani B, Arnould L, Gompel A, Egele C, Poulet B, Clough KB, Crouet H, Fourquet A, Lefranc JP, Mathelin C, Rouyer N, Serin D, Spielmann M, Haugh M, Chenard MP, Brain E, de Cremoux P, Bellocq JP: Ki-67: level of evidence and methodological considerations for its role in the clinical management of breast cancer: analytical and critical review. Breast Cancer Res Treat 2012, 132:895–915.

[58] Paik S, Shak S, Tang G, Kim C, Baker J, Cronin M, Baehner FL, Walkermg, Watson D, Park T, Hiller W, Fisher ER, Wickerham DL, Bryant J, Wolmark N: A multigene assay to predict recurrence of tamoxifen-treated, node-negative breast cancer. N Engl J Med 2004, 351:2817–2826.

Chapter 10

Aberrant PTPRO Methylation in Tumor Tissues as a Potential Biomarker That Predicts Clinical Outcomes in Breast Cancer Patients

Shao-ying Li[1,2], Rong Li[2], Yu-li Chen[3], Li-kuang Xiong[4],hui-lin Wang[4], Lei Rong[5], Rong-cheng Luo[2]

[1]Department of Breast Surgery, Bao'an Maternal and Child health hospital, Shenzhen, China
[2]TCM-Integrated Cancer Center of Southern Medical University, 510515guangzhou, China
[3]Department of Women's health, Bao'an Maternal and Child health hospital, Shenzhen, China
[4]Central Lab, Bao'an Maternal and Child health hospital, Shenzhen, China
[5]Department of Breast Surgery, ShenZhen Maternal and Child health hospital, Shenzhen, China

Abstract: Background: Aberrant hypermethylation of gene promoter regions is a primary mechanism by which tumor suppressor genes become inactivated in breast cancer. Epigenetic inactivation of the protein tyrosine phosphatase receptor-type Ogene (PTPRO) has been described in several types of cancer. Results: We screened primary breast cancer tissues for PTPRO promoterhy permethylation and assessed potential associations with pathological features and patient outcome. We also evaluated its potential as a breast cancer biomarker. PTPRO methylation was observed in 53 of 98 (54%) breast cancer tissues but not in adjacent normal tissue. Among matched peripheral blood samples from breast cancer patients, 33 of 98 (34%) exhibited methylated PTPRO in plasma. In contrast, no methylated PTPRO was observed in normal peripheral blood from 30healthy individuals. PTPRO methylation was positively associated with lymph node involvement (P = 0.014), poorly differentiatedhistology (P = 0.037), depth of invasion (P = 0.004), andhER2 amplification (P = 0.001). Multivariate analysis indicated that aberrant PTPRO methylation could serve as an independent predictor for overall survival hazard ratio (HR): 2.7; 95% CI: 1.1–6.2; P = 0.023), especially for patients with-hER2-positive (hazard ratio (HR): 7.5; 95% CI: 1.8–31.3; P = 0.006), but not in ER+ and PR+ subpopulation. In addition, demethylation induced by 5-azacytidine led togene reactivation in PTPRO-methylated and silenced breast cancer cell lines. Conclusions: here, we report that tumor PTPRO methylation is a strong prognostic factor in breast cancer. Methylation of PTPRO silences its expression and plays an important role in breast carcinogenesis. The data we present here may provide insight into the development of novel therapies for breast cancer treatment. Additionally, detection of PTPRO methylation in peripheral blood of breast cancer patients may provide a noninvasive means to diagnose and also monitor the disease.

Keywords: Protein Tyrosine Phosphatase Receptor-Type O (PTPRO), Methylation, Breast Cancer, Clinical Outcome, Biomarker

1. Background

Breast cancer is one of the most common cancers among women worldwide, and its incidence, unfortunately, continues to rise. Breast tumor is aheterogeneous disease derived from different molecular subtypes and displaying varied clinical behavior[1]. Considerable efforts have been made to improve survival via early diagnosis and treatment with targeted therapies[2].however, the limited success of current therapeutic modalitieshas led to calls for new prognostic tools and for the development of additional targeted therapies[3].

Promoterhy permethylation is a type of epigenetic alteration associated with gene silencing. In cancer, many tumor suppressor genes are inactivated in this way hypermethylation of key tumor suppressors is a key contributor to breast tumorigenesis and acts in concert withgenetic alterations to drive disease progression[4]. Epigenetic modifications of tumor DNA may have prognostic significance for breast cancer patients and provide targets for treatment because they are potentially reversible. Epigenetic changes may also serve as markers for early detection of the disease. As an example, screening for RASSF1Ahypermethylation in serum has been proposed as a form of surveillance to detect early stage breast cancer[5].

In recent years, there has been considerable interest in better understanding the role of tyrosine phosphorylation in cancer[6]–[11], especially since this post-translational modification helps regulate diverse cellular processes, including proliferation, differentiation, metabolism, cell-to-cell communication, transcription, and survival[12]. Phosphorylation is a dynamic process that is positively regulated by protein tyrosine kinases (PTKs) and negatively regulated by protein tyrosine phosphatases (PTPs). More than 80% of oncogenes encode PTKs[13]; in contrast, many PTPshave been described to function as tumor suppressors[14]. For example, the tyrosine phosphatase PTPN2 activates TP53 and induces apoptosis inhuman tumor cells[15]. Another phosphatase, PTP1B, negatively regulates insulin signaling via dephosphorylation of insulin receptor kinase[16]. Computational analysis of the human genome identified 38 classical PTPgenes, 19 of which mapped to regions frequently deleted inhuman cancers. Thirty of these protein phosphataseshave been implicated in tumorigenesis[17], further demonstrating their potential roles as tumor suppressors.

Protein tyrosine phosphatase receptor-type O (PTPRO) is classified as a receptor-type PTP of the R3 subtype[18] and exhibits characteristics of a tumor suppressor in multiple cancers[19]. Several PTPRO variant shave been described due to use of distinct transcriptional start sites and to alternative splicing; while many lymphoid-derived cells express a truncated PTPRO is of orm, most epithelial tissues, including the breast, express the full-length form[19]. Previous studieshave reported methylation-mediated down-regulation of PTPRO expression in breast cancer and other tumor types, such as rathepatocellular carcinoma,human chronic lymphocytic leukemia,human lung cancer, esophageal carcinoma[6]–[11][20] hypermethylation of PTPRO occurs frequently in esophageal carcinoma and may be a potential biomarker of the disease[20]. A recent study also revealed that acute lymphoblastic leukemia patients with PTPRO methylation showed increased rates of relapse and chemoresistance[9].

More recently, a tumor suppressive role for PTPRO in breast cancerhas emerged. Tumor-specific PTPRO promoter methylation was documented in primary human breast cancer cases[10]. The authors of this study also found that PTPRO expression was reduced upon treatment with estrogen but increased by treatment with the anti-estrogen Tamoxifen. Furthermore, ectopic expression of PTPRO in non-expressing MCF-7 cells sensitized them to the growth suppressive effects of Tamoxifen. PTPRO methylationhas been further confirmed to be clinically relevant in breast cancer, particularly inhER2-amplified patients. huang *et al.* showed that overall survival is significantly worse inhER2-positive patients with methylated PTPRO compared to tumors lacking methylation of this promoter region[21]. Another study found that low expression of PTPRO correlated with reduced survival forhER2-positive breast cancer patients[11]. It is possible that the pronounced impact of PTPRO specifically inhER2-positive disease could be due to the fact thathER2 itself is a direct substrate of PTPRO phosphatase activity[11]; specifically, loss of PTPRO was shown to increasehER2 phosphorylation andhER2-induced proliferation and transformation of breast cancer cell lines. Taken together, these data support a role for PTPRO as a tumor suppressor in breast cancer and suggest that its methylation and expression may have prognostic significance in the disease.

In the current study we investigated the methylation status of PTPRO in primary human breast cancer from fresh frozen specimens with the aim of defining the frequency of this epigenetic aberration in the disease. We examined the methylation status of PTPRO in primary breast tumors and matched peripheral blood samples and determined if promoter methylation was associated with decreasedgene expression in breast cancer cell lines. We also examined associations between PTPRO methylation and several clinic opathological parameters, including patient outcome.

2. Methods

2.1. Tumor Samples

Between 2006 and 2009, we obtained 98 tumor samples and matched preoperative peripheral blood samples from women undergoing surgery for primary invasive breast carcinoma at ShenZhen Maternal and Child health hospital, an affiliate of Southern Medical University in China. None of the patients had received any pre-operative treatment, including chemotherapy or radiotherapy. This is a well-characterized series of patients under the age of 74 years (median, 46 years). The median follow-up time of patients in the study was 60 months (range 43 - 70 months). All patients were treated uniformly at a single institution.

Pathologic characteristics, including histological grade, histological tumor type, tumor size, and lymph node involvement were routinely assessed; several patient characteristics, including age and family history of cancer and menopause, were also recorded. Survival data were maintained prospectively. At the end of the study period, 39 (40%) patients had died because of disease recurrence. In total, 98% of node-positive and 82% of node-negative patients received adjuvant systemic therapy consisting of either hormone therapy alone or hormone therapy plus chemotherapy.

Tumor samples were immediately frozen in liquid nitrogen and stored at −80°C until use. All tumors were confirmed histopathologically and their clinical features were classified based on the TNM system of the International Union Against Cancer[22]. Corresponding adjacent non-cancerous tissues were also obtained from surgical resections. Peripheral venous blood samples from breast tumor patients were collected in EDTA-containing tubes and immediately centrifuged at 2500g for 15min to prepare plasma. The plasma samples were stored at −80°C until further processing. Peripheral blood samples from an additional 30healthy volunteers were used as normal controls. Estrogen receptor (ER), progesterone receptor (PgR), and human epidermal growth factor receptor 2 (HER2) immune histochemistry was performed on TMA sections as previously described[23].

Approval for the use of human tissues and clinical information was obtained from the Committee for Ethical Review of Research involving human Subjects at Southern Medical University. All patients provided written informed consent for sample collection prior to surgery.

2.2. Cell Culture and Treatment

Human breast cancer cell lines MCF-7, MDA-MB-231, andhs578t (provided by Dr. Qi T. Yan, Southern Medical University, guangzhou, China), were maintained in DMEM supplemented with 5% fetal bovine serum and 1mM non-essential amino acids in a 5% CO_2 incubator. Normalhuman mammary epithelial cells (HMEC 48R; provided by Dr. Qi T. Yan, Southern Medical University,guangzhou, China) were maintained in MEGM (Cambrex Corp., USA) as previously described[10]. To confirm that methylation of the PTPRO promoter in breast cancer cell lines was responsible for its suppression, MCF-7 and MDA-MB-231 cells were treated with 5-azacytidine (5-AzaC, Sigma Chemical Co.,hK), a DNA-hypomethylating agent, according to the following conditions: 1μmol/L for 72h for MCF-7 cells, and 2.5μmol/L for 96h for MDA-MB-231 cells. The response of different cell lines to demethylating agents probably varies due to different drug sensitivities as well as different kinetics of association/ dissociation of chromatin remodelers with specificgenes. All cells used in this study were between passages 8 and 11.

2.3. DNA Extraction and Bisulfite Modification

Genomic DNA from primary tumors and plasma was extracted using a QIAamp DNAmini Kit (Qiagen, Germany) and QIAamp DNA bloodmini Kit (Qiagen, Germany).gene methylation status was evaluated using sodium bisulfite modification of DNA and subsequent methylation-specific PCR (MSP), essentially as previously described[24]–[26]. DNA (1 - 2μg) from each sample was subjected to bisulfite modification using EpiTect 96 Bisulfite Kits according to the manufacturer's instructions (Qiagen, Germany). Bisulfite-modified DNA was typically immediately used for PCR.

2.4. Methylation-Specific PCR Analysis

Primer sequences for PCR amplification of methylated and unmethylated alleles of PTPRO were previously published[10] and are listed in **Table 1**. Primers were synthesized by Shenggong (Shenggong Biotech, Shanghai, China). Primers were designed to amplify 170bp (methylated) or 201bp (unmethylated) regions of the CpG island within the PTPRO promoter[8]. For each reaction, 3μl of sodium bisulfite-converted DNA was added to a total volume of 50μl of PCR mix (EpiTect MSP Kits, Qiagen, Germany) according to the manufacturer's instructions.

Table 1. PCR primer sequences for methylation analysis of PTPRO.

Primers	Sequences	Product size
PTPRO-forward	5'-CTCCACCCAAATCACTCTTCGCAG-3'	268bp
PTPRO-reverse	5'-ACCATTGTTGAGACGGCTATGAACG-3'	
18 s rRNA-forward	5'-TCAAGAACGAAAGTCGGAGG-3'	110bp
18 s rRNA-reverse	5'-GGACATCTAAGGGCATCACA-3'	
MSP-methylated-forward	5'-CGTTTTTGGAGGATTTCGGGC-3'	170bp
MSP-methylated-reverse	5'-AAAACACGACTACGCTAACG-3'	
MSP-unmethylated-forward	5'-ATGTTTTTGGAGGATTTTGGGT-3'	201bp
MSP-unmethylated-reverse	5'-ATACCCCATCACTACACAAACA-3'	

Briefly, samples were initially incubated at 95°C for 10min. This was followed by 35 cycles of denaturation at 95°C for 15 s, annealing at 55°C for 30 s, and extension at 72°C for 30 s; finally, there was one round of extension at 72°C for 10min. An additional 15 cycles of denaturing (30 s at 94°C), annealing (15 s at 50.4°C), and extension (30 s at 72°C) were required for blood samples. PCR products were analyzed by electrophoresis on 2% agarosegels. Primers for unmethylated PTPRO (**Table 1**) were used to confirm the presence of DNA in each sample following bisulfite modification. This control was run for each sample on the same day that MSP analysis was carried out for the PTPRO gene. Breast tumor samples previously identified as DNA hypermethylated were used as positive controls. For each PCR assay, experimental reactions were accompanied by a black reaction (no DNA), a negative control reaction (blood DNA), and a positive control reaction (breast cancer DNA).

2.5. Bisulfitegenomic Sequencing

Bisulfite-converted DNA was used to PCR amplify the PTPRO CpG island from −208bp to +236bp with respect to the transcription start site as described earlier; ref.[7][8][19]. The PCR product was purified using agel extraction kit (Qiagen,

Germany). The purified PCR product was used for bisulfite sequencing and was cloned into the pDrive vector according to the instructions of the PCR cloning kit (Qiagen, Germany). Ten randomly selected clones were subjected to automated sequencing. Direct sequencing was performed using the Thermo Sequenase Radiolabeled terminator cycle sequencing kit (Qiagen, Germany) with the primerhGlepp1-BS-F3 (5'-TAGGGGgATTGGAAAGGTAG-3') following the manufacturer's protocol.

2.6. RNA Isolation and Reverse Transcription PCR Analysis

Total RNA was isolated using the RNeasymini kit (Qiagen, Germany). Reverse transcription of deoxyribonuclease-treated RNA (1 μg) was carried out according to instructions provided with the QuantiTect Reverse Transcription kit (Qiagen, Germany). Semi-quantitative PCR for PTPRO expression was performed. 0.2 mM of each primer was added to a 25 μl PCR reaction mixture. Cycling conditions were as follows: denaturation at 94°C, annealing at 54.5°C (for PTPRO) or 65°C (for 18S rRNA), and extension at 72°C. For PTPRO, a total of 32 cycles were run, and for18S rRNA, 25 cycles were used. The PCR products were separated on 2% agarose, stained with ethidium bromide, and imaged under UV light using Bio-rad Quantity One software. 18S rRNA transcripts in each sample were also amplified as internal controls for normalization. gene-specific primers used for amplification of PTPRO and 18S rRNA are listed in **Table 1**.

2.7. Statistical Analysis

The $\chi 2$ test was used to determine associations between methylation of PTPRO and various phenotypic or molecular features of breast cancer. Fisher's exact test was used when individual cell numbers were less than 5. All P values were derived from two-tailed statistical tests and significance was assumed at $P < 0.05$. Kaplan-Meier analysis was used to assess cumulative survival probabilities, and differences were evaluated using the log-rank test. Multinominal logistic regression analyses were used to assess the hazard model for the survival of breast cancer patients. All analyses were performed using the SPSS 19.0 (Chicago, IL, US) statistical software package.

3. Results

3.1. Frequent Methylation of PTPRO in Primary Tumors and Peripheral Blood Samples

Methylation of the PTPRO promoterhas been demonstrated in different tumor types, including breast cancer[7][8][10]. These observations, along with thegrowth- suppressive properties not only of PTPRO[7][8] but of PTPs ingeneral[27], prompted us to further investigate PTPRO methylation status in a large series of human breast tumors.genomic DNA isolated from tumor tissue, surrounding normal tissue, and matched peripheral blood samples ($n = 98$) was subjected to MSP analysis. Among the 98 primary breast tumor specimens investigated, 53 (54%) showedhypermethylation of PTPRO. Methylation of thisgene was not observed in any adjacent normal tissues. 33 of 98 (34%) patients exhibited detectable levels of methylated PTPRO in matched plasma. No methylated PTPRO was observed in normal peripheral blood samples from 30healthy individuals. The $\chi2$ test revealed that PTPRO methylation in plasma was significantly correlated to that in tumor tissue ($r = 0.435$; $P < 0.0001$, **Table 2**). Representative MSP results from primary tumors are shown in **Figure 1(a)**, **Figure 1(b)**.

3.2. Clinicopathological Significance of PTPRO Methylation in Breast Tumors and Peripheral Blood Samples

Associations between PTPRO methylation and clinico-pathological and molecular features of breast tumors in this study are shown in **Table 3**. The strongest correlation was between PTPRO methylation andhER2 amplification

Table 2. Association of methylation of PTPROgene between tumor tissues and plasma.

Tumor tissues	Plasma		
	M	U	Total
M	29	24	53
U	4	41	45
Total	33	65	98

M: Methylated; U: Unmethylated.

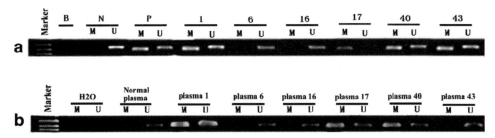

Figure 1. Representative MSP results for methylation of the PTPROgene. (a) primary breast tumors; (b) matched peripheral blood samples. Numbers indicate the sample number. B, blank (no DNA); N, negative control; P, positive control; M, methylated; U, unmethylated.

(P = 0.001). PTPRO methylation was also significantly more frequent in node positive (P = 0.014), poorly differentiated (P = 0.037), and stage III (P = 0.004) tumors. Thehighest frequency of PTPRO methylation (84%) was seen in late stage tumors. Trends were also observed for more frequent PTPRO methylation in ER- and PR-negative tumors but no associations were apparent with patient age, tumor size,histological tumor type, or TP53 mutation. Methylation of PTPRO in plasma was more frequent in those withhHER2 amplification (P = 0.018). For all other clinical and pathological parameters, there was no statistically significant correlation associated with methylation of PTPRO in plasma (**Table 3**).

3.3. Prognostic Significance of Tumor Tissue and Plasma PTPRO Methylation

Univariate analysis examined clinic opathologic parameters including PTPRO methylation and their association with overall survival end points. The results showed that survival was significantly worse in patients with lymph node involvement (P = 0.0001), late stage tumors (P = 0.0001), poorly differentiated tumors (P = 0.033), larger tumors (P = 0.019), positive hER2 amplification (P = 0.022), TP53 mutation (P = 0.012) and PTPRO methylation (hazard ratio (HR): 3.8; 95% CI: 1.9–7.5; P = 0.0001; **Table 4**). We then stratified all patients into subpopulations according to ER, PR andhER2 status. In ER- positive, PR- positive andhER2-positive patients, the methylated PTPROgroup show significantly worse overall survival compared to those of unmethylated PTPRO (P = 0.001, P = 0.012 and P = 0.010, respectively, **Table 4**). Kaplan-Meier curves for overall tumor group and the above subgroups according to PTPRO methylation are shown

Table 3. Associations between PTPRO methylation and clinicopathological features of breast cancer.

Characteristics	No.	PTPRO methylation					
		Tumor tissue (%)	χ2	P value	plasma (%)	χ2	P value
Total	98	53 (54)			33 (34)		
Age							
<45 years	45	22 (49)			16 (36)		
≥45 years	53	31 (59)	0.903	0.417	17 (32)	0.132	0.716
Nodal involvement							
Negative	61	27 (44)			18 (30)		
Positive	37	26 (70)	6.273	0.014	15 (40)	0.935	0.334
Stage							
I/II	79	37 (47)			24 (30)		
III	19	16 (84)	8.616	0.004	9 (47)	1.979	0.159
Histological type							
Non-ductal	23	12 (52)			7 (30)		
Ductal	75	41 (55)	1.000	0.510	26 (35)	0.141	0.707
Tumour size							
≤20 mm	47	26 (55)			12 (26)		
>20 mm	51	27 (53)	0.056	0.842	21 (40)	2.234	0.135
Histologicalgrade							
Well/mod diff.	60	27 (45)			18 (30)		
Poorly diff.	38	26 (68)	5.139	0.037	15 (40)	0.935	0.334
ER status							
Negative	24	16 (67)			10 (42)		
Positive	74	37 (50)	2.027	0.167	23 (31)	0.909	0.340
PR status							
Negative	29	20 (69)			10 (35)		
Positive	69	33 (48)	3.674	0.076	23 (33)	0.012	0.912
HER2 status							
Normal	51	19 (37)			12 (24)		
Amplified	47	34 (72)	12.124	0.001	21 (46)	5.570	0.018
TP53 status							
Normal	59	30 (51)			17 (29)		
Mutant	39	23 (59)	0.624	0.535	16 (41)	1.568	0.211

Table 4. Univariate and multivariate cox proportionalhazard model for the survival of breast cancer patients.

Variable	Univariate analysis			Multivariate analysis		
	Hazard ratio	95% CI	P	Hazard ratio	95% CI	P
Tumor size (large vs small)	2.4	1.2-4.9	0.019			
Lymph node status (pos. vs neg.)	4.9	2.4-9.8	0.0001	4.0	1.6-9.9	0.003
Histologicalgrade (poor vs well)	2.1	1.1-4.0	0.033			
Stage (III vs I/II)	3.2	1.7-5.9	0.0001			
HER2 status (amp. vs wildtype)	2.2	1.1-4.2	0.022			
TP53 (mutant vs wildtype)	2.3	1.2-4.3	0.012			
Tumor tissue PTPRO methylation (yes vs no)	3.8	1.9-7.5	0.0001	2.7	1.1-6.2	0.023
ER +group tumor tissue PTPRO methylation (yes vs no)	3.9	1.7-8.7	0.001	2.8	1.0-8.4	0.060
PR +group tumor tissue PTPRO methylation (yes vs no)	3.1	1.2-7.4	0.012	3.2	0.8-11.9	0.091
HER2+group tumor tissue PTPRO methylation(yes vs no)	5.0	1.8-16.8	0.010	7.5	1.8-31.3	0.006

in **Figure 2**. As shown, tumor tissue PTPRO methylation was associated with significantly worse cancer-specific survival in the overall tumorgroup [log-rank test P = 0.0001; **Figure 2(a)**]. Subgroup analysis revealed that PTPRO methylation also showed significant prognostic value within the ER + (P = 0.0001), PR + (P = 0.007), andhER2-amplified (P = 0.003) patientgroups [**Figure 2(b)-2(d)**, respectively].

To confirm the significance of this finding, we performed multivariate analysis, treating methylated-PTPRO as a factor with tumor size, lymph node metastasis,histologicalgrade, stage,hER2 status and TP53 status for their impact on overall survival. After adjustment for these convariates, methylated-PTPRO was identified as an independent predictor for overall survival in all tumorgroup (hazard ratio (HR): 2.7; 95% CI: 1.1 - 6.2; P = 0.023) andhER2+ subpopulation (hazard ratio (HR): 7.5; 95% CI: 1.8 - 31.3; P = 0.006), but not in ER + and PR + subpopulation. Similarly, lymph node metastasis alsohad an independent association with overall survival in this patient series. We also analyzed the potential prognostic value of plasma PTPRO methylation but no significant data were obtained.

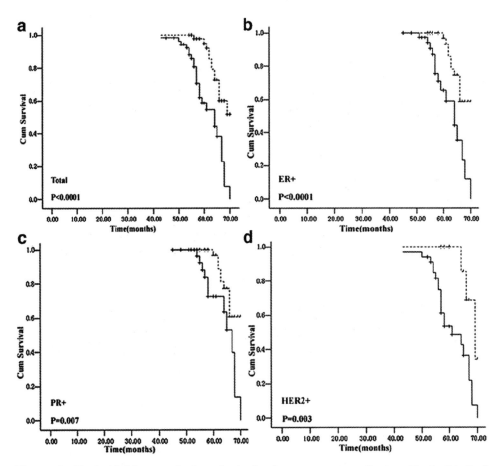

Figure 2. Kaplan-Meier survival analysis for breast cancer patients with (solid line) PTPRO tumor methylation or without (dotted line). (a) overallgroup; (b) ER+; (c) PR+; (d)hER2-amplified subgroup.

3.4. PTPRO Expression Is Inversely Correlated with Methylation Status

We next sought to determine the relationship between PTPRO methylation andgene expression in a panel of breast cancer cell lines (MCF-7, MDA-MB-231, andhs578t) and in normalhuman mammary epithelial cells (HMEC, 48R). In normal mammary epithelial cells, PTPRO is expressed at appreciable levels and its promoter region is not methylated; in contrast, PTPRO expression was relatively low in two (MCF-7, MDA-MB-231) of the three breast cancer cell lines examined and its promoter was methylated [**Figure 3(a)**, **Figure 3(b)**].

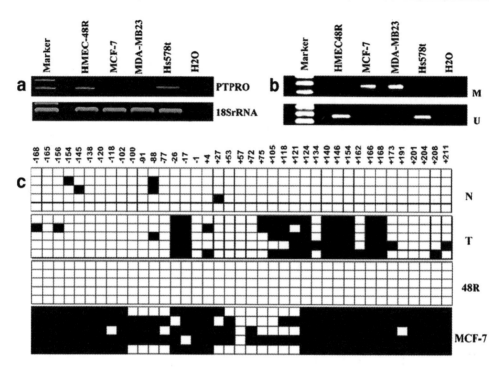

Figure 3. PTPRO is methylated in breast cancer cell lines but not in normal breast epithelial cells. (a) Expression of PTPRO in normalhuman mammary epithelial cells (48R) andhuman breast cancer cell lineshs578t, MCF-7, and MDA-MB-231. Total RNA isolated from cell lines was subjected to RT-PCR analysis using PTPRO-specific primers. 18S rRNA was used as an internal loading control. (b) MSP analysis of PTPRO methylation status in breast cancer cell lines.hMESC48R was used as a normal control. M, methylated; U, unmethylated. (c) PTPRO CpG island from randomly selected breast tumor tissue and its matched normal tissue; also shown arehMEC 48R and MCF-7 cells, all of which were subjected to BSgenomic sequencing. Each solid square represents a methylated cytosine and an open square represents unmethylated cytosine in a CpG dinucleotide. Each row corresponds to a single clone. N, normal corresponding adjacent non-cancerous tissue; T, tumor tissue.

We performed bisulfitegenomic sequencing from ten pairs of breast tumor tissue and matched normal tissue, one representativehMEC (48R), and one breast cancer cell line (MCF-7) to determine if the CpG Island located in the promoter of PTPRO was differentially methylated. Complete bisulfite conversion was confirmed by the presence of substituted thymine for all cytosine residues at non-CpG sites. We detectedhypermethylation of CpGs in both PTPRO-silenced tumors and in MCF-7 cells. In contrast, the PTPRO-expressing cell linehMEC 48R and matched normal breast tissue exhibited low levels or no methylation of the PTPRO promoter—strongly supporting the MSP results [**Figure 3(c)**].

To confirm thathypermethylation of the PTPRO promoter was responsible for its suppression, both MCF-7 and MDA-MB-231 cells (hypermethylated PTPRO promoter; silenced mRNA expression) were treated with 5-AzaC at a final concentration of 1μM for MCF-7 cells and 2.5μM for MDA-MB-231 cells. Re-expression of PTPRO in both cell lines was observed after exposure to this demethylating agent for 72h and 96h, respectively [**Figure 4(a)**]. Moreover, the MSP result showed that unmethylated PTPRO alleles increased after 5-AzaC treatment [**Figure 4(b)**]. These data further support the notion that methylation of the PTPRO CpG island plays an important role ingene silencing.

4. Discussion

Although protein tyrosine kinaseshave long been recognized as key players in oncogenesis, the role of protein tyrosine phosphatases in the initiation and progression of cancer is only nowgaining increased attention[27]–[29]. In this study, the breast cancer series investigatedhere for DNA methylation is well characterized and conventional pathological indicators, including nodal involvement,

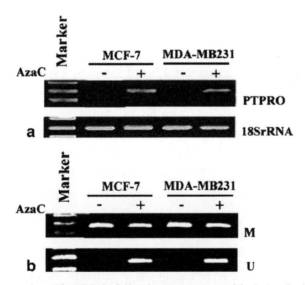

Figure 4. Re-expression of PTPRO following treatment with 5-AzaC. (a) Breast cancer cell lines MCF-7 and MDA-MB-231 were treated with 1μM 5-AzaC for 72h and 2.5μM 5-AzaC for 96h, respectively. Total RNA from cells was subjected to RT-PCR to amplify PTPRO mRNA. 18S rRNA was used for normalization; (b) MSP analysis of PTPRO methylation status in breast cancer cell lines with or without 5-AzaC treatment. M, methylated; U, unmethylated.

311

histologicalgrade, tumor size, and stage, all show the expected prognostic significance. PTPRO methylation was detected in two of three breast cancer cell lines and in 53 of 98 (54%) primary human breast cancer specimens; however, no PTPRO methylation was observed in adjacent normal tissue. This result is within the range (52% to 81%) reported in previous studies of human cancers[7]–[10][20][30]. The rather high frequency of methylation suggests that PTPRO is a common target for epigenetic silencing in breast tumors and that it may contribute to the development of this tumor type. As reported previously, demethylation of the PTPRO promoter resulted ingene re-expression[31]. These observations demonstrate growth-suppressor characteristics of PTPRO that are typical of a classical tumor suppressor gene.

Aberrant hypermethylation of tumor suppressor genes is an important epigenetic event in the development and progression of many human cancers and may serve as a biomarker for disease detection at early stages[32]–[34]. In this study, we detected PTPRO methylation in the plasma of 34% (33/98) of patients; this value was significantly correlated with PTPRO methylation detected in tumor tissue. Such a high correlation confirmed that peripheral blood samples could potentially be used to assist the detection and diagnosis of breast cancer. Moreover, this assay appears to be robust and highly specific; no methylated PTPRO was detected in plasma from breast cancer patients without primary tumor methylation or from normal healthy control peripheral blood samples. These findings are consistent with results published by huang et al.[21] who also examined PTPRO methylation in peripheral blood samples from breast cancer cases. Among 24 matched plasma samples, PTPRO was aberrantly methylated in 11 (45.8%) cases. Importantly and consistent with our findings, no methylation was observed in normal control plasma samples from 10healthy individuals. These data help confirm that PTPRO methylation in plasma samples may provide a robust, specific, noninvasive means for early detection of breast cancer. however, the frequency of PTPRO methylation detected in plasma was lower than in cancer tissues and less association of methylation were found in plasma with clnicopathological data. This might due to fewer tumors DNA releasing in the circulation, or poor quality of DNA when extracted from peripheral blood, whose impact factors include acquisition condition, storage time, human factor, etc. Our method of detecting PTPRO methylation from plasma may not be extremely robust. The more standard conditions and a larger series of breast cancer patients should be involved for more understanding the molecular mechanism and clinical behavior of these tumors, as well as provide targets for better diagnosis and therapy. For sure, a more robust method must be used if this is translated to clinical application.

In agreement with You et al.[20], we found a strong correlation between PTPRO methylation and tumor stage (**Table 2**), with 84% of stage III tumors found to be methylated. Similar to huang et al.[21], PTPRO methylation correlated with higher histological grade. The current study is the first to report an association between PTPRO methylation and positive lymph node status andhER2 amplification in breast cancer. We also observed more frequent PTPRO methylation in ER-negative and PR-negative patient groups, possibly due to the association between these features and poor prognosis. Interestingly, Ramaswamy et al.[10] found that positive PTPRO expression was associated with improved response to tamoxifen; these results are consistent with previous reports of protein tyrosine phosphatasegene (PTPG)[35][36]. Therefore, estrogen-mediated suppression of PTPRO and the methylation of this gene may play important roles in estrogen-induced tumorigenesis. While interesting, each of the above associations with PTPRO methylation requires confirmation in larger studies. Moreover, it remains to be established whether the characteristic aggressive phenotype is linked to methylation via silencing of gene expression or through other mechanisms.

The significant associations between PTPRO methylation and nodal involvement, poorly differentiated histology, stage III tumors, andhER2 amplification suggest that PTPRO expression may be involved in breast tumor invasion. given these aforementioned correlations, it is not surprising that PTPRO methylation served as a prognostic indicator of worse outcome. Although PTPRO methylation was weakly associated with ER− and PR− status, these factors had no prognostic value in the current tumor series (data not shown). Similar tohuang et al.[21], unmethylated PTPRO was significantly associated with favorable outcome in ER + and PR + subgroups, as well as in patients withhER2 amplification. As reported, activation of ER results in multiple downstream effects[37]. Recent studies indicate that ERβ expression is decreased inhuman neoplastic breast tissue, suggesting that ERβ may be an inhibitor of tumorigenesis[38]–[40]. For clinically apparent tumors, the proposed tumor-associated factors mayhelp protect against tumor progression. Thus, according to prior studies, inactive PTPRO might be a stimulating factor during tumorigenesis, explain the ineffection of endocrine therapy and more precise subpopulations could be stratified to decide whether the patients with ER-positive need a regimen containing tamoxifen.

In a univariate model including strong prognostic factors such as nodal status, histological grade, tumor size, stage,hER2 amplification, and TP53 mutation status, PTPRO methylation of overall tumors, ER+, PR + andhER2+group was found to be predictive of poorer outcome for breast cancer. Multivariate analysis identified methylated-PTPRO as an independent predictor for overall survival (P = 0.023), expecially inhER2+ subpopulation (P = 0.006). In contrast to our findings, huang *et al.* reported that PTPRO methylation only correlated with higher histologicalgrade but not with any other clinical parameters assessed[21]. This could be due to differences in sample size or to differences in sample processing. For example, while we used fresh tumor tissue, huang *et al.* made use of formalin- fixed paraffin-embedded samples. Despite this, the trend is still in the same direction. That is, PTPRO methylation and low expression are associated with worse prognostic features, especially forhER2-positive patients. Further supporting our claim is work from another group showing that the receptor tyrosine kinase ErbB2/HER2 is a direct substrate of PTPRO, and low levels of PTPRO expression correlated with reduced survival ofhER2-positive breast cancer patients[11]. This may also help explain why plasma PTPRO methylation was only significantly associated withhER2 amplification. The data we present here, in conjunction with earlier work, establish PTPRO as a likely tumor suppressor in breast cancer. Moreover, PTPRO methylation status might predict response to anti-HER-targeted therapies inhER2-positive patients, even provide extensive survival benefits or improve the efficiency of targeted drugs due to active PTPRO. To further study, patients who receive targeted therapy are required.

5. Conclusion

In summary, our results confirm that PTPRO methylation is detected at a high frequency in breast cancer, occurring at a higher rate than either TP53 mutation orhER2 amplification. Positive associations with nodal involvement, poorly differentiated histology, and hER2 amplification indicate that PTPRO methylation may contribute to an aggressive breast tumor phenotype. This was particularly evident for ER+, PR+, andhER2-amplified breast cancer subgroups, which all showed that PTPRO methylation in tumor tissues was a strong prognostic factor.

Methylated- PTPRO could serve as an independent predictor for overall survival, expecially inhER2-positive breast cancer patients. Changes in protein tyrosine phosphatase activity likely play an important role in breast carcinogenesis and may provide a useful target for the development of novel therapies.

Competing Interests

The authors declare that they have no competing interests.

Authors' Contributions

SL and RL developed the study and drafted the manuscript. YC and LR participated in sample collection and data analysis. LX and hW carried out the molecular genetic studies and participated in sequence alignment. *RL participated in the design of the study and its coordination and helped draft the manuscript. All authors read and approved the manuscript.

Acknowledgements

We thank Professor Barry Iacopetta from the School of Surgery, University of Western Australia for his critical reading of the manuscript. We also thank Dr. Qi T. Yan for his gracious gift of cell lines. The authors are grateful to Professor Tasneem Motiwala for information on primer sequences. This work was supported by the Science and Technology Planning Project of Shenzhen China grant 201103049 (SY Li).

Source: Li S Y, Li R, Chen Y L, *et al*. Aberrant PTPRO methylation in tumor tissues as a potential biomarker that predicts clinical outcomes in breast cancer patients[J]. Bmcgenetics, 2014, 15(1):1–10.

References

[1]   Simpson PT, Reis-Filho JS, gale T, Lakhani SR: Molecular evolution of breast cancer.

J Pathol 2005, 205:248–254.

[2]   Curiglianog, Spitalerig, Dettori M, Locatelli M, Scarano E,goldhirsch A: Vaccine immunotherapy in breast cancer treatment: Promising, but still early. Expert Rev Anticancer Ther 2007, 7:1225–1241.

[3]   Emens LA, Reilly RT, Jaffee EM: Augmenting the potency of breast cancer vaccines: Combined modality immunotherapy. Breast Dis 2004, 20:13–24.

[4]   Dworkin AM,huang TH, Toland AE: Epigenetic alterations in the breast: Implications for breast cancer detection, prognosis and treatment. Semin Cancer Biol 2009, 19:165–171.

[5]   Hesson LB, Cooper WN, Latif F: The role of RASSF1A methylation in cancer. Dis Markers 2007, 23:73–87.

[6]   Motiwala T,ghoshal K, Das A, Majumder S, Weichenhan D, Wu YZ,holman K, James SJ, Jacob ST, Plass C: Suppression of the protein tyrosine phosphatase receptor type Ogene (PTPRO) by methylation in hepatocellular carcinomas. Oncogene 2003, 22:6319–6331.

[7]   Motiwala T, Majumder S, Kutayh, Smith DS, Neuberg DS, Lucas DM, Byrd JC,grever M, Jacob ST: Methylation and silencing of protein tyrosine phosphatase receptor type O in chronic lymphocytic leukemia. Clin Cancer Res 2007, 13:3174–3181.

[8]   Motiwala T, Kutayh,ghoshal K, Bai S, Seimiyah, Tsuruo T, Suster S, Morrison C, Jacob ST: Protein tyrosine phosphatase receptor-type O (PTPRO) exhibits characteristics of a candidate tumor suppressor inhuman lung cancer. Proc Natl Acad Sci U S A 2004, 101:13844–13849.

[9]   Hogan LE, Meyer JA, Yang J, Wang J, Wong N, Yang W, Condosg,hunger SP, Raetz E, Saffery R, Relling MV, Bhojwani D, Morrison DJ, Carroll WL: Integrated genomic analysis of relapsed childhood acute lymphoblastic leukemia reveals therapeutic strategies. Blood 2011, 118:5218–5226.

[10]   Ramaswamy B, Majumder S, Roy S, Wang J, Wong N, Yang W, Condosg,hunger SP, Raetz E, Saffery R, Relling MV, Bhojwani D, Morrison DJ, Carroll WL: Estrogen-mediated suppression of thegene encoding protein tyrosine phosphatase PTPRO inhuman breast cancer: mechanism and role in tamoxifen sensitivity. Mol Endocrinol 2009, 23:176–187.

[11]   Yu M, Ling, Arshadi N, Kalatskaya I, Xue B,haider S, Nguyen F, Boutros PC, Elson A, Muthuswamy LB, Tonks NK, Muthuswamy SK: Expression profiling during mammary epithelial cell three-dimensional morphogenesis identifies PTPRO as a novel regulator of morphogenesis and ErbB2-mediated transformation. Mol Cell Biol 2012, 32:3913–3924.

[12]   Hunter T: Signaling-2000 and beyond. Cell 2000, 100:113–127.

[13]   Fischer EH: Cell signaling by protein tyrosine phosphorylation. Adv Enzyme Regul

1999, 39:359–369.

[14] Laczmanska I, Sasiadek MM: Tyrosine phosphatases as a super family of tumor suppressors in colorectal cancer. Acta Biochim Pol 2011, V58N4:467–470.

[15] Gupta S, Radha V, Sudhakar C, Swarupg: A nuclear protein tyrosine phosphatase activates p53 and induces caspase-1-dependent apoptosis. FEBS Lett 2002, 532:61–66.

[16] Salmeen A, Andersen JN, Myers MP, Tonks NK, Barford D: Molecular basis for the dephosphorylation of the activation segment of the insulin receptor by protein tyrosine phosphatase 1B. Mol Cell 2000, 6:1401–1412.

[17] Alonso A, Sasin J, Bottini N, Friedberg I, Friedberg I, Osterman A, godzik A, hunter T, Dixon J, Mustelin T: Protein tyrosine phosphatases in the human genome. Cell 2004, 117:699–711.

[18] Andersen JN, Mortensen OH, PetersgH, Drake PG, Iversen LF, Olsen OH, Jansen PG, AndersenhS, Tonks NK, Møller NP: Structural and evolutionary relationships among protein tyrosine phosphatase domains. Mol Cell Biol 2001, 21:7117–7136.

[19] Jacob ST, Motiwala T: Epigenetic regulation of protein tyrosine phosphatases: potential molecular targets for cancer therapy. Cancergene Ther 2005, 12:665–672.

[20] You YJ, Chen YP, Zheng XX, Meltzer SJ, Zhangh: Aberrant methylation of the PTPROgene in peripheral blood as a potential biomarker in esophageal squamous cell carcinoma patients. Cancer Lett 2012, 315:138–144.

[21] Huang YT LIFF, Ke C, Li Z, Li ZT, Zou XF, Zheng XX, Chen YP, Zhangh: PTPRO promoter methylation is predictive of poorer outcome forhER2- positive breast cancer: indication for personalized therapy. J Transl Med 2013, 11:245.

[22] Sobin LH, Wittekind C: International Union Against Cancer (UICC), 5th ed., TNM classification of malignant tumors. Baltimore (MD): Wiley-Liss; 1997:54–58.

[23] Abd El-Rehim DM, Balg, Pinder SE, Rakha E, Paish C, Robertson JF, Macmillan D, Blamey RW, Ellis IO:high-throughput protein expression analysis using tissue microarray technology of a large well-characterised series identifies biologically distinct classes of breast cancer confirming recent cDNA expression analyses. Int J Cancer 2005, 116:340–350.

[24] Li SY, Rong MN, Iacopetta B: DNA hypermethylation in breast cancer and its association with clinic opathological features. Cancer Lett 2006, 237:272–280.

[25] Herman JG,graff JR, Myohanen S, Nelkin BD, Baylin SB: Methylation-specific PCR: a novel PCR assay for methylation status of CpG islands. Proc Natl Acad Sci U S A 1996, 93:9821–9826.

[26] Paulin R, Grigg G, Davey MW, Piper AA: Urea improves efficiency of bisulphate-mediated sequencing of 50-methylcytosine ingenomic DNA. Nucleic Acids Res 1998, 26:5009–5010.

[27] Motiwala T, Jacob ST: Role of protein tyrosine phosphatases in cancer. Prog Nucleic Acid Res Mol Biol 2006, 81:297–329.

[28] Tonks NK: Protein tyrosine phosphatases: fromgenes, to function, to disease. Nat Rev Mol Cell Biol 2006, 7:833–846.

[29] Ostman A, hellberg Cand Bohmer FD: Protein-tyrosine phosphatases and cancer. Nat Rev Cancer 2006, 6:307–320.

[30] Hsu SH, Motiwala T, Roy S, Claus R, Mustafa M, Plass C, Freitas MA,ghoshal K, Jacob ST: Methylation of the PTPROgene in human hepatocellular carcinoma and identification of VCP as its substrate. J Cell Biochem 2013, 114:1810–1818.

[31] Motiwala T, Majumder S,ghoshal K, Kutayh, Datta J, Roy S, Lucas DM, Jacob ST: PTPROt inactivates the oncogenic fusion protein BCR/ABL and suppresses trans-formation of K562 cells. J Biol Chem 2009, 284:455–464.

[32] Jin Z, Cheng Y, Olaru A, Kan T, Yang J, Paun B, Ito T,hamilton JP, David S, Agarwal R, Selaru FM, Sato F, Abraham JM, Beer DG, Mori Y, Shimada Y, Meltzer SJ: Pro-moterhyper methylation of CDH13 is a common, early event inhuman esophageal adeno carcinogenesis and correlates with clinical risk factors. Int J Cancer 2008, 123:2331–2336.

[33] Jin Z, hamilton JP, Yang J, Mori Y, Olaru A, Sato F, Ito T, Kan T, Cheng Y, Paun B, David S, Beer DG, Agarwal R, Abraham JM, Meltzer SJ: hypermethylation of the AKAP12 promoter is a biomarker of Barrett's associated esophageal neoplastic pro-gression. Cancer Epidemiol Biomarkers Prev 2008, 17:111–117.

[34] Jin Z, Olaru A, Yang J, Sato F, Cheng Y, Kan T, Mori Y, Mantzur C, Paun B, hamil-ton JP, Ito T, Wang S, David S, Agarwal R, Beer DG, Abraham JM, Meltzer SJ: hypermethylation of tachykinin-1 is a potential biomarker inhuman esophageal can-cer. Clin Cancer Res 2007, 13:6293–6300.

[35] Liu S, Sugimoto Y, Sorio C, Tecchio C, Lin YC: Function analysis of estrogenically regulated protein tyrosine phosphatase (PTPs) inhuman breast cancer cell line MCF-7. Oncogene 2004, 23:1256–1262.

[36] Zheng J, Kulp SK, Zhang Y, Sugimoto Y, Dayton MA, govindan MV, Brueggemeier RW, Lin YC: 17-Estradiol-regulated expression of protein tyrosine phosphatasegene in cultured human normal breast and breast cancer cells. Anticancer Res 2000, 20:11–19.

[37] Henderson BE, FeigelsonhS: hormonal carcinogenesis. Carcinogenesis 2000, 21: 427–433.

[38] Dotzlawh, Leygue E, Watson PH, Murphy LC: Estrogen receptor messenger RNA expression inhuman breast tumor biopsies: relationship to steroid receptor status and regulation by progestins. Cancer Res 1999, 59:529–532.

[39] Iwao K, Miyoshi Y, Egawa C, Ikeda N, Noguchi S: Quantitative analysis of estro-gen receptor-β mRNA and its variants inhuman breast cancers. Int J Cancer 2000,

88:733–736.

[40] Roger P, Sahla ME, Makela S,gustafsson JA, Baldet P, Rocheforth: Decreased ex-
      pression of estrogen receptor-β protein in proliferative preinvasive mammary tumors.
      Cancer Res 2001, 61:2537–2541.

Chapter 11

New Concepts in Breast Cancer Genomics and Genetics

Rodrigo Goncalves[1,2,3], Wayne A Warner[1,2,3,4], Jingqin Luo[2,3,5], Matthew J Ellis[1,2,3]

[1]Breast Cancer Program, Department of Medical Oncology, Washington University School of Medicine, 660 S. Euclid Ave, St Louis, MO 63110, USA

[2]Siteman Cancer Center, Washington University School of Medicine, 660S. Euclid Ave, St Louis, MO 63110, USA

[3]Lester and Sue Smith Breast Center, Baylor College of Medicine, One Baylor Plaza, 320A Cullen MS600, Houston, TX 77030, USA

[4]Department of Cell Biology and Physiology, Washington University, 660 S. Euclid Ave, St Louis, MO63110, USA

[5]Division of Biostatistics, Washington University School of Medicine, 660 S. Euclid Ave, St Louis, MO 63110, USA

Abstract: Massively parallel DNA and RNA sequencing approaches have generated data on thousands of breast cancer genomes. In this review, we consider progress largely from the perspective of new concepts and hypotheses raised so far. These include challenges to the multistep model of breast carcinogenesis and the discovery of new defects in DNA repair through sequence analysis. Issues for functional genomics include the development of strategies to differentiate between mutations that are likely to drive carcinogenesis and bystander background mutations, as well as the importance of mechanistic studies that examine the role of mutations in genes with roles in splicing, histone methylation, and long non-coding

RNA function. The application of genome-annotated patient-derived breast cancer xenografts as a potentially more reliable preclinical model is also discussed. Finally, we address the challenge of extracting medical value from genomic data. A weakness of many datasets is inadequate clinical annotation, which hampers the establishment of links between the mutation spectra and the efficacy of drugs or disease phenotypes.Tools such as dGene and the DGIdb are being developed to identify possible druggable mutations, but these programs are a work in progress since extensive molecular pharmacology is required to develop successful "genome-forward" clinical trials. Examples are emerging, however, including targeting HER2 in HER2 mutant breast cancer and mutant ESR1 in ESR1 endocrine refractory luminal-type breast cancer. Finally, the integration of DNA- and RNA- based sequencing studies with mass spectrometry-based peptide sequencing and an unbiased determination of post-translational modifications promises a more complete view of the biochemistry of breast cancer cells and points toward a new discovery horizon in our understanding of the pathophysiology of this complex disease.

1. Introduction

A decade after the first version of the human genome was published[1], annotation efforts continue, bringing us to the 19th revision, which is the current research standard. Analysis of protein-coding genes and their regulatory sequences is nearing completion, but these functions are served by only a small fraction of the genome. The rest is more functional than once thought, encoding, for example, many non-protein coding RNA genes with emerging regulatory and catalytic roles in cellular physiology and cancer[2]. Furthermore, mass spectrometry-based peptide sequencing is rapidly maturing, promoting studies that provide an unbiased analysis of information flowing from DNA to mRNA to protein to post-translational modification without the need for probes or antibodies at the individual gene or protein level[3]. Finally, deregulation of histone function and DNA methylation is readily evident in many tumor types and is a further consideration in cancer pathogenesis[4]. There is a growing chasm between our understanding of the breast cancer genome and our ability to translate these insights into improved patient outcomes. In this review, we present some of the most recent findings in the genomics field, from the biological discoveries emanating from genome sequencing studies to the clinical implications of those findings and finally to the future areas of potential research in the field.

2. Recent Biologically Relevant Findings in the Genomics Field

2.1. Significantly Mutated Genes Versus Background Mutations in Breast Cancer

Sequencing of DNA and RNA from tumors by using massively parallel sequencing with a capture or other sequence selection approach (exomes or candidate genes) or unbiased "whole genome" approach has become a standard research tool now that the technology has been extensively commercialized[5]-[7]. One objective of cancer sequencing studies is to identify genes that have undergone somatic mutations, which contribute to malignant transformation. Genes that accumulate somatic mutations at a higher than stochastic rate are referred to as "significantly mutated genes" (SMGs) and are considered likely drivers of malignant progression. In breast cancer, there is a dramatic difference in the SMG list between luminal-type breast cancer and basal-like breast cancer. In The Cancer Genome Atlas (TCGA) breast cancer data, at least 20 SMGs were observed in luminaltype A, eight in luminal-type B, but only three in basal-like breast cancer (**Table 1**). This is not because luminal breast cancer genomes are more complex than those of basal-like breast cancer; in fact, the opposite is true. Basal-like breast cancer genomes are often so complex that it has proven difficult to identify the causal events by using mutation recurrence statistics. Furthermore, structural rearrangements (large-scale chromosomal deletions, amplifications, inversions, and translocations) are likely to play a particularly critical role in basal-like breast cancer, and the complete delineation of these events requires whole genome sequencing, which is technically demanding and expensive[8].

Detection of SMGs is complicated by the presence of a large number of likely irrelevant mutations referred to as "background mutations"[9]-[11]. These occur not only in genes irrelevant to transformation but even within the SMGs themselves; that is, a missense mutation in a large tumor suppressor gene cannot be assumed to be always inactivating or cause dysfunction in the encoded protein.

Table 1. Significantly mutated genes based on all luminal versus basal-like breast cancers in The Cancer Genome Atlas dataset.

Gene	Luminal A (n = 225)			Luminal B (n = 126)			Basal-like (n = 93)		
	Number of cases	LRT	CT	Number of cases	LRT	CT	Number of cases	LRT	CT
TP53	28	0	0	39	0	0	74	0	0
PIK3CA	105	0	0	40	0	0	8	4.0×10^{-6}	3.4×10^{-7}
GATA3	32	0	0	19	0	0	2	NA	NA
MAP3K1	30	0	0	6	1.7×10^{-8}	4.7×10^{-7}	0	NA	NA
MLL3	19	1.5×10^{-10}	1.7×10^{-11}	7	NA	NA	6	NA	NA
CDH1	23	0	0	6	3.6×10^{-3}	6.6×10^{-3}	0	NA	NA
MAP2K4	16	0	0	3	NA	NA	0	NA	NA
RUNX1	13	0	0	3	NA	NA	0	NA	NA
PTEN	9	4.3×10^{-9}	1.3×10^{-11}	6	3.7×10^{-6}	1.9×10^{-7}	1	NA	NA
TBX3	6	1.0×10^{-6}	2.7×10^{-5}	6	9.4×10^{-5}	1.4×10^{-4}	1	NA	NA
PIK3R1	4	NA	NA	4	NA	NA	2	NA	NA
AKT1	8	1.4×10^{-11}	3.2×10^{-9}	3	NA	NA	0	NA	NA
CBFB	5	4.2×10^{-5}	2.7×10^{-5}	2	NA	NA	0	NA	NA
TBL1XR1	5	2.9×10^{-2}	1.2×10^{-3}	1	NA	NA	0	NA	NA
NCOR1	12	3.8×10^{-8}	6.8×10^{-9}	3	NA	NA	2	NA	NA
CTCF	9	8.8×10^{-4}	3.0×10^{-6}	2	NA	NA	1	NA	NA
ZFP36L1	2	NA	NA	4	1.3×10^{-2}	1.7×10^{-2}	1	NA	NA
GPS2	4	1.2×10^{-3}	6.0×10^{-3}	1	NA	NA	1	NA	NA
SF3B1	7	1.1×10^{-6}	5.3×10^{-5}	0	NA	NA	1	NA	NA
CDKN1B	3	5.4×10^{-3}	1.9×10^{-2}	1	NA	NA	0	NA	NA
USH2A	7	NA	NA	4	NA	NA	10	NA	NA
RPGR	2	NA	NA	2	NA	NA	4	NA	NA
RB1	1	NA	NA	4	NA	NA	4	2.5×10^{-2}	4.8×10^{-2}
AFF2	3	NA	NA	3	NA	NA	4	NA	NA

NF1	6	NA	NA	5	NA	NA	2	NA	NA
PTPN22	1	NA	NA	3	NA	NA	0	NA	NA
RYR2	6	NA	NA	10	NA	NA	2	NA	NA
PTPRD	4	NA	NA	5	NA	NA	1	NA	NA
OR6A2	2	NA	NA	1	NA	NA	0	NA	NA
HIST1H2BC	1	NA	NA	1	NA	NA	1	NA	NA
GPR32	3	8.9×10^{-3}	4.3×10^{-2}	1	NA	NA	1	NA	NA
CLEC19A	0	NA	NA	1	NA	NA	0	NA	NA
CCND3	2	1.5×10^{-4}	1.1×10^{-3}	0	NA	NA	0	NA	NA
SEPT13	2	NA	NA	0	NA	NA	1	NA	NA
DCAF4L2	1	NA	NA	3	NA	NA	1	NA	NA

CT, chemotherapy; LRT, loco-regional treatment; NA, mutations observed were not considered statistically significant.

Mutant allele expression determined by RNA sequencing (RNA seq) is one starting point for disambiguating biologically relevant mutations on SMGs versus irrelevant ones. Many mutations detected at the DNA level are not expressed at the RNA level and thus, at least from the gain-of-function perspective, are unlikely to be major players in the carcinogenesis process[12]. Although there are challenges left to functionalize many of the SMGs as drivers of carcinogenesis, some progress has been made. RNA seq is widely used for the nomination and validation of expressed fusion genes and was recently used to define an endocrine therapy resistance-associated ESR1 translocation[12]. Ultimately, functional studies are critical for resolving the role of mutations in certain SMGs versus background mutations, since the large number of mutations requiring annotation creates an extreme challenge, if this is done in an unbiased way[13]. An alternative approach is to be selective and initially study those associated with a therapeutic hypothesis. Another priority consists of the SMGs themselves, as the biology served by many of these, particularly those involved in mechanisms such as histone methylation, splicing, transcription, and long non-coding (lnc) RNA function is unclear. For example, whole genome analysis revealed clustered mutations in MALAT1, suggesting a gain-of-function role for this poorly understood and abundant lncRNA in breast cancer[14]. The functions of luminal SMGs have particularly striking similarities to drivers in hematopoietic malignancies[14], a link also emphasized by a recent study on the role of estradiol in hematopoiesis[15]. A particularly vexing problem is the functional resolution of mutated genes that drive pathogenesis in just a few patients or even in only one patient. A significant number of cases of luminal-type breast cancer in the TCGA analysis did not harbor a single SMG[16], suggesting that current genomic approaches would potentially benefit from additional refinement.

2.2. The Genomic Structure of Breast Cancer Reveals Underlying DNA Repair Defects

Aside from the focus on the identification of individual genes that are repetitively disrupted in breast cancer, a more broad-based analysis of breast cancer genome structures has led to a paradigm shift in the way we view pathogenesis. The standard multistep model of carcinogenesis postulates that mutations accumulate gradually, one at a time, in a process of Darwinian selection in which individual mutant-bearing clones effectively compete with normal cells and other clones within the tumor through the acquisition of the ability to transform, invade, metastasize, and evade drug treatment[17]. However, it was recently demonstrated that multiple mutations can arise over a very short period wherein multiple chromosomal breaks that occurred during a single catastrophic cell division event are (rarely) viably repaired, reshuffling the genome in a way that rapidly triggers transformation though the simultaneous oncogene amplifications and tumor suppressor gene deletions in the vicinity of the multiple translocations that ensue (chromothripsis)[18] (**Figure 1**). The reported frequency of chromothripsis in breast cancer varies from 2% to 11.06%[18][19]. Since chromothripsis and interval breast cancer are both marked by the suddenness of their appearance, we hypothesize that chromothripsis might explain the development of rapidly progressing, so-called "interval", breast cancers that arise suddenly between screening visits. For this class of tumors, screening could never be effective as the time span of tumor development is too short. The genomic structure of interval breast cancers should be pursued aggressively as these tumors carry a high mortality burden. As more patients are included in clinical trials that include longitudinal genome sequencing of tumor samples, this hypothesis will be tested in the near future.

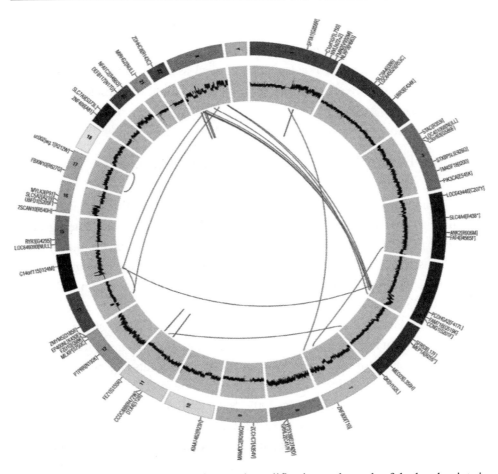

Figure 1. The presence of translocations and amplification at the ends of the breakpoints is evidence of chromothripsis in this Circos plot from a breast cancer sample. Chromothripsis scars the genome when localized chromosome shattering and repair occur in a one-off catastrophe.

In another conceptual breakthrough, investigators at the Sanger Institute demonstrated that there are more than 20 different patterns of somatic mutation in cancer based on copy number aberrations and nucleotide substitution patterns, with a subset of these recurrently observed in breast cancer (APOBEC, BRCA1/2, Signature B)[20]. Overexpression of cytidine deaminase APOBEC family members, in particular, has come into sharp focus. Clustered mutations characteristic of APOBEC activity have been particularly observed in and around chromosomal breakpoints, suggesting that single-stranded DNA generated during aberrant DNA repair is a substrate for APOBEC enzymatic activity[21]. Differences in DNA repair defects explain the striking finding that some breast cancers display many more

327

mutations than others[20][22]. Thus, even in the absence of a known SMG, it is possible to classify breast cancers on the basis of DNA repair defects and this could be clinically relevant. For example, clinical assays in development aim to identify tumors with defects in homologous recombination, which sensitize tumors to cytotoxic chemotherapy[23].

2.3. Intra-Tumor Heterogeneity in Breast Cancer

Chromothripsis, multistep progression, and defects in DNA repair combine to produce astonishing levels of both intra-tumoral and inter-tumoral heterogeneity in breast cancer. This complexity is an obvious explanation for the difficulty in curing breast cancer, particularly when advanced. As the tumor progresses and disseminates, the repertoire of biological possibilities encoded within billions of malignant cells, each subtly genetically different, means that resistance to targeted or more traditional cytotoxic therapy is almost inevitable. There is still not enough genomic data from multiple cancer samples from the same patient to track somatic mutation patterns from the primary through to metastatic disease and subsequent drug resistance. Longitudinal studies of this type, however, have been conducted successfully in individual cases. In 2009, Shah and colleagues[24] described the mutational evolution of a lobular breast carcinoma by using next-generation sequencing. Out of the 32 somatic, protein-coding mutations present in the metastasis, 19 could not be detected in the primary, five were prevalent in the primary, and six were present in the primary with a lower frequency. The Washington University group investigated the progression of a breast cancer to the brain at the whole genome level and found that the primary tumor and metastasis harbored approximately 48 somatic, protein-coding mutations[8]. In the metastatic sample, there were few de novo mutations, but higher variant allele frequencies and a few much lower, supporting a "clonal remodeling" hypothesis for metastatic spread. At the single cell level of the tumor, various techniques have been used to directly visualize and quantify chromosomal aberrations, including duplications, deletions, and other distinctive chromosomal rearrangements. These studies show that breast cancers routinely exhibit genetic heterogeneity at preferred loci[25]–[29].

Evidence for marked tumor heterogeneity can be found in studies of other cancer types. For example, in a study of a renal cancer with metastasis to the lung and in the chest wall, sequencing of the metastases and nine different areas within the primary tumor found that only a third of mutations were common to all samples[30]. Based on these data, we can infer that heterogeneity and different subclones develop within the primary tumor, not all of which have the same metastatic potential. Metastases can develop early or late in each cancer's evolutionary history and are products of ongoing clonal evolution, which can be slow or very rapid. The ability to sequence individual cancer cells[31] will further illuminate this issue, although the complexity of the data analysis remains a considerable challenge.

3. Clinical Implications of Genomic Discoveries

3.1. Clinical Translation of Massively Parallel Sequencing of DNA in Breast Cancer

The sequencing of cancer with data return to the patient and physician is being piloted through "genomic tumor boards"[32]. However, the complexity of the breast cancer genome has slowed progress, as has the relative paucity of obvious drug mutation matches[33]. Unlike drug therapy matched somatic mutations to melanoma and non-small cell lung cancer, drug therapy matched to the presence of a somatic mutation has yet to be robustly established as a standard approach in breast cancer. A number of strategies to increase the productivity and "translatability" of DNA, RNA, and peptide sequencing studies in breast cancer should be considered. The initial set of sequencing-based studies in breast cancer revealed that this is one of the most heterogeneous forms of cancer, with the four commonly accepted subtypes (luminal-type A, luminal-type B, HER2-enriched, and basal-like) displaying distinct somatic mutation, gene copy, and epigenetic profiles[16]. Within the next few years, tens of thousands of primary breast cancers will likely be sequenced but often through clinical sequencing programs without a current systematic and broad based plan to integrate the data with clinical endpoints. These studies risk following the course of the TCGA breast cancer study. While a technical tour de force, TCGA was largely a cross-platform genome-cataloging exercise and not a systematic clinical research addressing a particular problem in oncology[16]. Thus, it will not be possible to link the TCGA data to important clinical phenotypes such as drug response. Since poly-pharmacy is the rule in breast cancer treatment, establishing a link between mutational events and the efficacy of individual drugs is impossible unless a dedicated study is conducted. The neoadjuvant treatment setting allows ethical treatment plans with single agents as well as the acquisition of serial samples to assess the effect of treatment on breast cancer somatic genomes another subject in its infancy in breast cancer. Thus, a systematic approach linking high-quality sample acquisition, uniform neoadjuvant therapy regimens, and integrated "omics" should be a high priority for clinical investigators. An example is provided by an integrated analysis of whole genome, exome-based somatic mutation detection, gene-expression, and gene copy profiles that identified molecular correlates of aromatase inhibitor-resistant proliferation by using samples from a neoadjuvant study[14]. Mutations in TP53 were associated with endocrine therapy resistance, poor prognosis luminal-type B features, mutations in the stress kinase MAP3K1 with low proliferation and luminal-type A features, and mutations in GATA3 with increased responsiveness to aromatase inhibition. A current research focus is to confirm these findings and to conduct additional studies with large sample sizes to link other breast cancer SMGs to clinical outcomes.

3.2. The Druggable Breast Cancer Genome

A major obstacle to the translation of newly defined genetic alterations into clinical benefit for patients lies in the identification of biologically relevant druggable aberrations that can be used as therapeutic targets[34]. To address this goal, programs such as dGene[35] and DGIdb[36] have been developed. The dGene program is an updated version of the druggable genome concept introduced in 2002 by Hopkins and Groom[37]. The druggable genome refers to a subset of genes that are known or predicted to interact with drugs. The software stratifies mutations from any database containing gene symbols into 10 different gene classes that are both potentially druggable and clinically relevant to cancer biology. An annotation and filtering tool is used to prioritize mutations for consideration. The analysis of a recent breast cancer genomic study[14] highlights the potential utility of this approach. From a total of 2,622 single-nucleotide variants identified in the neoadjuvant aromatase inhibitor discussed above, dGene identified 368 mutations out of 2,622 single-nucleotide variants as occurring in 255 druggable genes. When filtered for recurrence, that number was narrowed to 37 potentially druggable mutated genes present in at least two patients (**Table 2**). Despite its utility, dGene does not provide information on the type of mutation or guarantee clinical

Table 2. Categorization of single-nucleotide variants in 77 breast cancer tumors using dGene: 37 dGene entries present in at least 2 out of 77 samples, organized by class and patients affected.

NCBI symbol	Full name	dGene class	Patients affected
CASR	Calcium-sensing receptor	G protein-coupled receptor	3
GPR112	G protein-coupled receptor 112	G protein-coupled receptor	3
AGTR2	Angiotensin II receptor, type 2	G protein-coupled receptor	2
MC5R	Melanocortin 5 receptor	G protein-coupled receptor	2
OR2L2	Olfactory receptor, family 2, subfamily L, member 2	G protein-coupled receptor	2
OR51B5	Olfactory receptor, family 51, subfamily B, member 5	G protein-coupled receptor	2
PIK3CA	Phosphoinositide-3-kinase, catalytic, alpha polypeptide	PI3K	37
BIRC6	Baculoviral IAP repeat containing 6	Proteinase inhibitor	4
CPAMD8	C3 and PZP-like, α-2-macroglobulin domain containing 8	Proteinase inhibitor	3
COL28A1	Collagen, type XXVIII, alpha 1	Proteinase inhibitor	2
COL6A3	Collagen, type VI, alpha 3	Proteinase inhibitor	2
AGBL1	ATP/GTP binding protein-like 1	Protease	2
CPVL	Carboxypeptidase, vitellogenic-like	Protease	2
PCSK5	Proprotein convertase subtilisin/kexin type 5	Protease	2
RELN	Reelin	Protease	2
SENP7	SUMO1/sentrin specific peptidase 7	Protease	2
USP9X	Ubiquitin specific peptidase 9, X-linked	Protease	2
PTPRF	Protein tyrosine phosphatase, eceptor type, F	Phosphatase	2
PTPRU	Protein tyrosine phosphatase, receptor type, U	Phosphatase	2
SSH3	Slingshot homolog 3 (Drosophila)	Phosohatase	2
MAP3K1	Mitogen-activated protein kinase kinase kinase 1	Serine theonine kinase	9
TTN	Titin	Serine theonine kinase	6

ATR	Ataxia telangiectasia and Rad3 related	Serine theonine kinase	5
OBSCN	Obscurin	Serine theonine kinase	3
SMG1	Smg-1 homolog	Serine theonine kinase	3
ALPK2	Alpha-kinase 2	Serine theonine kinase	2
BRAF	V-raf murine sarcoma viral oncogene homolog B1	Serine theonine kinase	2
DCLK3	Doublecortin-like kinase 3	Serine theonine kinase	2
LRRK2	Leucine-rich repeat kinase 2	Serine theonine kinase	2
MAP2K4	Mitogen-activated protein kinase kinase 4	Serine theonine kinase	2
TAF1L	TATA box binding protein (TBP)-associated factor	Serine theonine kinase	2
TBK1	TANK-binding kinase 1	Serine theonine kinase	2
ULK4	Unc-51-like kinase 4	Serine theonine kinase	2
INSRR	Insulin receptor-related receptor	Tyrosine kinase	3
KIT	C-kit	Tyrosine kinase	2
PDGFRA	Platelet-derived growth factor receptor	Tyrosine kinase	2
TEX14	Testis expressed 14	Tyrosine kinase	2

NCBI, National Center for Biotechnology Information.

pertinence of mutations associated with any specific gene. This underscores the critical need to functionally test these and other genomic results.

A similar tool is DGIdb[36]. The concept behind the DGIdb is to classify gene mutations into two classes: genes that are known to have drug interactions and genes that are potentially druggable according to their gene category. DGIdb was developed by integrating data from 13 different sources and contains over 14,000 drug-gene interactions. It also includes 6,761 genes that belong to one or more of 39 potentially druggable gene categories. The utility of DGIdb was demonstrated by analyzing a cohort of 1,273 patients who were included in whole-genome or exome sequencing studies[16][38]–[41]. The software identified 6 of 31 genes (AKT1, CDH1, LRP2, PIK3CA, RYR2, and TP53) that were recurrently mutated in at least 2.5% of patients and also have known drug-gene interactions. With the addition of the top 1% of recurring mutations, the number of genes increased to 315. Six sources DrugBank, MyCan-cerGenome, the Pharmacogenetics Knowledge Base (PharmGKB), Trends in the Exploitation of Novel Drug Targets

(TEND), Targeted Agents in Lung Cancer (TALC), and Therapeutic Target Database (TTD) were interrogated by DGldb to identify a total of 354 possible druggable gene interactions among the 315 genes. There was limited overlap between the sources, and only one drug-gene interaction was present in all six sources simultaneously [**Figure 2(a)**]. The nature and extent of curation as well as the overall methodologies employed by each source are different [**Figure 2(a)**], which explains the limited overlap between the different sources. Some of the 315 genes are in potentially druggable categories (dGene), and others represent opportunities for drug discovery [**Figure 2(b)**].

This analysis serves to emphasize that these druggable genome approaches remain unvalidated by clinical trials and the pre-existing pharmacopeia is obviously inadequate, although "drug repurposing" the concept of redirecting US Food and Drug Administration-approved drugs to new secondary indications is clearly an opportunity. Thus, in their current form, these computational approaches are mostly hypothesis-generating tools that are intended to accelerate medical research, not tools for clinical action (at least not yet). The next logical step after using such tools is to design functional studies to test the related drugs and find a more reliable answer as to whether such mutations are drivers of carcinogenesis or just background mutations.

3.3. HER2 and ESR1 Mutations as Examples of Novel Druggable Targets

The utility of detailed preclinical work on potentially druggable genes is nicely illustrated by the study of HER2 mutations in breast cancer. Data from eight breast cancer genome-sequencing studies identified 25 patients with HER2 somatic mutations without HER2 amplification[14][16][24][38]–[42]. Thirteen HER2 mutations were functionally characterized by using in vitro kinase assays, protein structure analysis, cell culture, and xenograft experiments[43]. The results showed that the investigational drug neratinib, an irreversible HER2 inhibitor, rather than lapatinib, an approved HER2 kinase inhibitor, was a better approach for clinical studies since some of the recurrent mutations were naturally lapatinib-resistant. This is a result that simple drug somatic mutation matching software would not have revealed. Currently, patients with advanced HER2 mutation-positive tumors

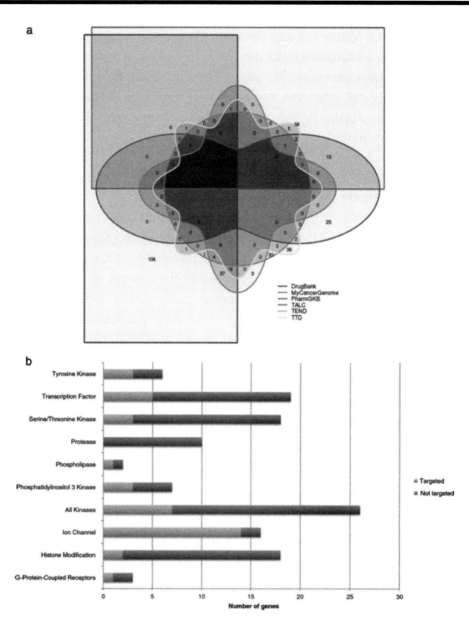

Figure 2. Druggability of significantly mutated gene (SMG) in breast cancer. (a) Overlap between six sources that generated a list of 354 possible drug-gene interactions among 315 genes recurrently mutated in breast cancer patients and analyzed by DGIdb. One hundred and seventy-six drug-gene interactions were identified by DrugBank, 87 by MyCancerGenome, 77 by Therapeutic Target Database (TTD), 71 by Trends in the Exploitation of Novel Drug Targets (TEND), 49 by Targeted Agents in Lung Cancer (TALC), and 44 by the Pharmacogenetics Knowledge Base (PharmGKB). (b) Distribution of 315 genes in potentially druggable categories (from dGene) and the numbers of genes in these categories that are targeted by a known drug.

are being enrolled into a single-agent study of neratinib (NCT01670877). Point mutations in the estradiol-binding domain of the estrogen receptor gene (ESR1) are emerging as a potent cause of acquired endocrine therapy resistance. Although there are no drugs that specifically target these mutations, alternative endocrine therapies may be effective in this setting[44][45] and this possibility will soon be addressed in clinical trials.

3.4. Patient-Derived Xenografts as Genomic Models for Breast Cancer

A major criticism of standard cell lines as a model for human breast cancer is that they are essentially disconnected from the individuals from whom they were derived. Without knowledge of the progenitor tumor genome as a reference point and no knowledge of the clinical characteristics of the patient who donated the tissue, it is uncertain what the cell lines actually model from an individual patient perspective and to what degree genetic drift has occurred after prolonged in vitro culture. These limitations likely contribute to the poor predictive utility of cell line panels in drug development[46]–[48]. An alternative preclinical model for drug optimization and target validation is the patient-derived xenograft (PDX) approach. Detailed information covering the continuum from specimen acquisition to development of patient-derived xenografts has been presented and reviewed elsewhere[8][49]–[52]. In brief, a biopsy-sized sample of primary or metastatic tumor is transferred directly into an immunodeficient mouse by orthotopic or subcutaneous implantation. Once tumor engraftment has occurred, RNA and DNA sequencing or chip-based analysis is employed to compare the patient tumor to the PDX. PDXs maintain fidelity to the patient tumor based on molecular subtypes, mutational spectrum, copy number variations, gene expression profiles, and histopathology[50][53]–[56]. PDX models faithfully recapitulate the intra-tumor heterogeneity and response to chemotherapy[53]. This close resemblance between the PDXs and the patient tumor makes it a suitable predictive preclinical model. The deployment of PDXs therefore can be considered a "test bed" for personalized precision medicine in which genome-forward hypotheses can be assessed preclinically. However, despite the great promise and utility of PDXs, there are some drawbacks that need to be resolved to ensure wider adoption and improved utility. The limitations are the higher comparative cost, high level of technical expertise needed, the lack of an immune system, the effect of differences between the mouse and human microenvironment, and the degree of genetic drift and how this affects conclusions regarding biological and pharmacological findings.

Even with the mentioned limitations, the PDX model has great utility in breast cancer research. Through the genome sequencing of different PDX lines, Li and colleagues[12] identified new ESR1 point mutations and translocations. These gene mutations and the ESR1-YAP1 gene fusion were further investigated through functional studies that directly implicated them in resistance to treatment. Not coincidentally, the patients from whom these PDXs were derived presented with endocrine treatment resistance during their course of treatment.

4. Future Areas of Research

Proteomics as the Next Step in the Annotation of the Breast Cancer Genome

A fundamental problem in the study of cancer genomics at the level of DNA and RNA is that conclusions regarding pathway activation are indirect since proteins, not nucleic acids, execute these functions. Thus, when signaling and biology are discussed, it is through inference from signal transduction databases that may or may not have been conducted in the relevant biological context and that may or may not be correct. Informatics approaches generate hypotheses, not conclusions[57][58]. The reverse phase protein array (RPPA) is one answer to the problem of efficiently tracking protein levels and phosphorylation events[59]. Here, tumor protein extracts from many tumors are spotted into slides and probed with highly quality-controlled antibodies. Unfortunately, the generation of RPPA-quality antibodies is technically challenging; in particular, the number of phosphosite-specific antibodies is very limited. Therefore, mass spectrometry is being developed to examine the protein biochemistry of the cancer cells in less biased ways by direct protein sequencing and mass analysis to determine post-translational modifications[3]. Next-generation proteomic technologies are poised to provide deep information on tumor proteomes and on post-translational modifications of all types. When combined with genomic data, proteomics may enable a deeper understanding of complex mechanisms that regulate gene function and dysfunction in cancer.

These objectives are being realized by the National Cancer Institute Clinical Pro-teomic Tumor Analysis Consortium, which is applying standardized proteome analysis platforms to analyze tumor tissues from the TCGA program as well as unique cell and xenograft models and other tissue collections, all of which are ac-companied by rich genomic datasets[60].

5. Conclusions

The expansion of knowledge in genomics is already having a profound ef-fect on breast cancer research and increasingly on treatment. It is clear, however, that genome-sequencing studies have still not been adequately designed to address specific questions in breast cancer oncology. This is essential to translate the com-prehensive catalog of recurrent mutations in breast cancer to a functionally and pharmacologically annotated treatment road map. Through the sequencing of tu-mors in different time-points, we will be able to identify cellular pathways and targets for drug development and use this information for the development of clin-ically testable hypotheses. Integrated approaches that not only account for DNA and RNA aberrations but also document protein function and biochemistry are clearly the next technical horizon[60].

6. Abbreviations

AKT1: v-akt murine thymoma viral oncogene homolog1; APOBEC: Apoli-poprotein B mRNA editing enzyme, catalytic polypeptide-like; BRCA1: Breast cancer 1, early onset; BRCA2: Breast cancer 2, early onset; CDH1: Cadherin 1, type 1, E-cadherin (epithelial); ESR1: Estrogen receptor 1; GATA3: GATA binding protein 3; HER2: Human epidermal growth factor receptor 2; lnc: Long non-coding; LRP2: Low density lipoprotein receptor-related protein 2; MALAT1: Metastasis associated lung adenocarcinoma transcript 1; MAP3K1: Mitogen-activated protein kinase kinase kinase 1, E3 ubiquitin protein ligase; PDX: Patientderived xenograft; PIK3CA: Phosphatidylinositol-4,5-bisphosphate 3-kinase, catalytic subunit alpha; RNA seq: RNA sequencing; RPPA: Reverse phase protein array; RYR2: Ryano-dine receptor 2 (cardiac); SMG: Significantly mutated gene; TCGA: The cancer genome Atlas; TP53: Tumor protein p53.

Competing Interests

MJE declares patent and royalty income from BioClassifier LLC (St Louis, MO, USA) through a license on the PAM50 patents to Nanostring (Seattle, WA, USA) for the intrinsic subtype test "Prosigna". The other authors declare that they have no competing interests.

Authors' Contributions

All the authors made substantial contributions to the conception and design of this article, participated in drafting the article or revising it critically for important intellectual content, and gave final approval of the version submitted.

Acknowledgements

RG was supported by a grant from the AVON Foundation for Women. WAW was supported by Washington University School of Medicine, Graduate School of Arts & Sciences/CGFP Fund 94028C. JL was supported by a Siteman Cancer Center Support Grant (P30CA091842). MJE was supported by Susan G. Komen for the Cure (PG12220321), the Clinical Proteomic Tumor Analysis Consortium (U24 CA160035 and R01 CA095614), the AVON Foundation for Women, a Siteman Cancer Center Support Grant (P30CA091842), and the Breast Cancer Research Foundation.

Source: Goncalves R, Warner W A, Luo J, et al. New concepts in breast cancer genomics and genetics[J]. Breast Cancer Research, 2014, 16(16):1–11.

References

[1]   Lander ES, Linton LM, Birren B, Nusbaum C, Zody MC, Baldwin J, Devon K, Dewar K, Doyle M, FitzHugh W, Funke R, Gage D, Harris K, Heaford A, Howland J, Kann L, Lehoczky J, LeVine R, McEwan P, McKernan K, Meldrim J, Mesirov JP, Miranda C, Morris W, Naylor J, Raymond C, Rosetti M, Santos R, Sheridan A, Sougnez C, Stange-Thomann N, et al: Initial sequencing and analysis of the human

genome. Nature 2001, 409:860–921.

[2] ENCODE Project Consortium: The ENCODE (ENCyclopedia Of DNA Elements) Project. Science 2004, 306:636–640.

[3] Ellis MJ, Perou CM: The genomic landscape of breast cancer as a therapeutic roadmap. Cancer Discov 2013, 3:27–34.

[4] Tsai HC, Baylin SB: Cancer epigenetics: linking basic biology to clinical medicine. Cell Res 2011, 21:502–517.

[5] Mardis ER: Genome sequencing and cancer. Curr Opin Genet Dev 2012, 22:245–250.

[6] Koboldt DC, Steinberg KM, Larson DE, Wilson RK, Mardis ER: The next-generation sequencing revolution and its impact on genomics. Cell 2013, 155:27–38.

[7] Mutz KO, Heilkenbrinker A, Lönne M, Walter JG, Stahl F: Transcriptome analysis using next-generation sequencing. Curr Opin Biotechnol 2013, 24:22–30.

[8] Ding L, Ellis MJ, Li S, Larson DE, Chen K, Wallis JW, Harris CC, McLellan MD, Fulton RS, Fulton LL, Abbott RM, Hoog J, Dooling DJ, Koboldt DC, Schmidt H, Kalicki J, Zhang Q, Chen L, Lin L, Wendl MC, McMichael JF, Magrini VJ, Cook L, McGrath SD, Vickery TL, Appelbaum E, Deschryver K, Davies S, Guintoli T, Lin L, et al: Genome remodelling in a basal-like breast cancer metastasis and xenograft. Nature 2010, 464:999–1005.

[9] Vogelstein B, Papadopoulos N, Velculescu VE, Zhou S, Diaz LA Jr, Kinzler KW: Cancer genome landscapes. Science 2013, 339:1546–1558.

[10] Kalari S, Pfeifer GP: Identification of driver and passenger DNA methylation in cancer by epigenomic analysis. Adv Genet 2010, 70:277–308.

[11] Bignell GR, Greenman CD, Davies H, Butler AP, Edkins S, Andrews JM, Buck G, Chen L, Beare D, Latimer C, Widaa S, Hinton J, Fahey C, Fu B, Swamy S, Dalgliesh GL, Teh BT, Deloukas P, Yang F, Campbell PJ, Futreal PA, Stratton MR: Signatures of mutation and selection in the cancer genome. Nature 2010, 463:893–898.

[12] Li S, Shen D, Shao J, Crowder R, Liu W, Prat A, He X, Liu S, Hoog J, Lu C, Ding L, Griffith OL, Miller C, Larson D, Fulton RS, Harrison M, Mooney T, McMichael JF, Luo J, Tao Y, Goncalves R, Schlosberg C, Hiken JF, Saied L, Sanchez C, Giuntoli T, Bumb C, Cooper C, Kitchens RT, Lin A, et al: Endocrine-therapy-resistant ESR1 variants revealed by genomic characterization of breast-cancer-derived xenografts. Cell Rep 2013, 4:1116–1130.

[13] Liu ET: Functional genomics of cancer. Curr Opin Genet Dev 2008, 18:251–256.

[14] Ellis MJ, Ding L, Shen D, Luo J, Suman VJ, Wallis JW, Van Tine BA, Hoog J, Goiffon RJ, Goldstein TC, Ng S, Lin L, Crowder R, Snider J, Ballman K, Weber J, Chen K, Koboldt DC, Kandoth C, Schierding WS, McMichael JF, Miller CA, Lu C, Harris CC, McLellan MD, Wendl MC, DeSchryver K, Allred DC, Esserman L, Unzeitig G, et al: Whole-genome analysis informs breast cancer response to aromatase inhibition.

Nature 2012, 486:353–360.

[15] Nakada D, Oguro H, Levi BP, Ryan N, Kitano A, Saitoh Y, Takeichi M, Wendt GR, Morrison SJ: Oestrogen increases haematopoietic stem-cell self-renewal in females and during pregnancy. Nature 2014, 505:555–558.

[16] Network CGA: Comprehensive molecular portraits of human breast tumours. Nature 2012, 490:61–70.

[17] Nowell PC: The clonal evolution of tumor cell populations. Science 1976, 194:23–28.

[18] Stephens PJ, Greenman CD, Fu B, Yang F, Bignell GR, Mudie LJ, Pleasance ED, Lau KW, Beare D, Stebbings LA, McLaren S, Lin ML, McBride DJ, Varela I, Nik-Zainal S, Leroy C, Jia M, Menzies A, Butler AP, Teague JW, Quail MA, Burton J, Swerdlow H, Carter NP, Morsberger LA, Iacobuzio-Donahue C, Follows GA, Green AR, Flanagan AM, Stratton MR, et al: Massive genomic rearrangement acquired in a single catastrophic event during cancer development. Cell 2011, 144:27–40.

[19] Cai H, Kumar N, Bagheri HC, von Mering C, Robinson MD, Baudis M: Chromothripsis-like patterns are recurring but heterogeneously distributed features in a survey of 22,347 cancer genome screens. BMC Genomics 2014, 15:82.

[20] Nik-Zainal S, Alexandrov LB, Wedge DC, Van Loo P, Greenman CD, Raine K, Jones D, Hinton J, Marshall J, Stebbings LA, Menzies A, Martin S, Leung K, Chen L, Leroy C, Ramakrishna M, Rance R, Lau KW, Mudie LJ, Varela I, McBride DJ, Bignell GR, Cooke SL, Shlien A, Gamble J, Whitmore I, Maddison M, Tarpey PS, Davies HR, Papaemmanuil E, et al: Mutational processes molding the genomes of 21 breast cancers. Cell 2012, 149:979–993.

[21] Roberts SA, Lawrence MS, Klimczak LJ, Grimm SA, Fargo D, Stojanov P, Kiezun A, Kryukov GV, Carter SL, Saksena G, Harris S, Shah RR, Resnick MA, Getz G, Gordenin DA: An APOBEC cytidine deaminase mutagenesis pattern is widespread in human cancers. Nat Genet 2013, 45:970–976.

[22] Greenman C, Stephens P, Smith R, Dalgliesh GL, Hunter C, Bignell G, Davies H, Teague J, Butler A, Stevens C, Edkins S, O'Meara S, Vastrik I, Schmidt EE, Avis T, Barthorpe S, Bhamra G, Buck G, Choudhury B, Clements J, Cole J, Dicks E, Forbes S, Gray K, Halliday K, Harrison R, Hills K, Hinton J, Jenkinson A, Jones D, et al: Patterns of somatic mutation in human cancer genomes. Nature 2007, 446:153–158.

[23] Yap TA, Sandhu SK, Carden CP, de Bono JS: Poly(ADP-ribose) polymerase (PARP) inhibitors: exploiting a synthetic lethal strategy in the clinic. CA Cancer J Clin 2011, 61:31–49.

[24] Shah SP, Morin RD, Khattra J, Prentice L, Pugh T, Burleigh A, Delaney A, Gelmon K, Guliany R, Senz J, Steidl C, Holt RA, Jones S, Sun M, Leung G, Moore R, Severson T, Taylor GA, Teschendorff AE, Tse K, Turashvili G, Varhol R, Warren RL, Watson P, Zhao Y, Caldas C, Huntsman D, Hirst M, Marra MA, Aparicio S: Mutational evolution in a lobular breast tumour profiled at single nucleotide resolution. Nature 2009, 461:809–813.

[25] Roka S, Fiegl M, Zojer N, Filipits M, Schuster R, Steiner B, Jakesz R, Huber H, Drach J: Aneuploidy of chromosome 8 as detected by interphase fluorescence in situ hybridization is a recurrent finding in primary and metastatic breast cancer. Breast Cancer Res Treat 1998, 48:125–133.

[26] Park SY, Lee HE, Li H, Shipitsin M, Gelman R, Polyak K: Heterogeneity for stem cell-related markers according to tumor subtype and histologic stage in breast cancer. Clin Cancer Res 2010, 16:876–887.

[27] Farabegoli F, Santini D, Ceccarelli C, Taffurelli M, Marrano D, Baldini N: Clone heterogeneity in diploid and aneuploid breast carcinomas as detected by FISH. Cytometry 2001, 46:50–56.

[28] Teixeira MR, Pandis N, Bardi G, Andersen JA, Heim S: Karyotypic comparisons of multiple tumorous and macroscopically normal surrounding tissue samples from patients with breast cancer. Cancer Res 1996, 56:855–859.

[29] Teixeira MR, Pandis N, Bardi G, Andersen JA, Mitelman F, Heim S: Clonal heterogeneity in breast cancer: karyotypic comparisons of multiple intra- and extra-tumorous samples from 3 patients. Int J Cancer 1995, 63:63–68.

[30] Gerlinger M, Rowan AJ, Horswell S, Larkin J, Endesfelder D, Gronroos E, Martinez P, Matthews N, Stewart A, Tarpey P, Varela I, Phillimore B, Begum S, McDonald NQ, Butler A, Jones D, Raine K, Latimer C, Santos CR, Nohadani M, Eklund AC, Spencer-Dene B, Clark G, Pickering L, Stamp G, Gore M, Szallasi Z, Downward J, Futreal PA, Swanton C: Intratumor heterogeneity and branched evolution revealed by multiregion sequencing. N Engl J Med 2012, 366:883–892.

[31] Navin N, Kendall J, Troge J, Andrews P, Rodgers L, McIndoo J, Cook K, Stepansky A, Levy D, Esposito D, Muthuswamy L, Krasnitz A, McCombie WR, Hicks J, Wigler M: Tumour evolution inferred by single-cell sequencing. Nature 2011, 472:90–94.

[32] Roychowdhury S, Iyer MK, Robinson DR, Lonigro RJ, Wu YM, Cao X, Kalyana-Sundaram S, Sam L, Balbin OA, Quist MJ, Barrette T, Everett J, Siddiqui J, Kunju LP, Navone N, Araujo JC, Troncoso P, Logothetis CJ, Innis JW, Smith DC, Lao CD, Kim SY, Roberts JS, Gruber SB, Pienta KJ, Talpaz M, Chinnaiyan AM: Personalized oncology through integrative high-throughput sequencing: a pilot study. Sci Transl Med 2011, 3:111ra121.

[33] Simon R, Roychowdhury S: Implementing personalized cancer genomics in clinical trials. Nat Rev Drug Discov 2013, 12:358–369.

[34] Natrajan R, Wilkerson P: From integrative genomics to therapeutic targets. Cancer Res 2013, 73:3483–3488.

[35] Kumar RD, Chang LW, Ellis MJ, Bose R: Prioritizing potentially drug gable mutations with Gene: an annotation tool for cancer genome sequencing data. PLoS One 2013, 8:e67980.

[36] Griffith M, Griffith OL, Coffman AC, Weible JV, McMichael JF, Spies NC, Koval J, Das I, Callaway MB, Eldred JM, Miller CA, Subramanian J, Govindan R, Kumar

RD, Bose R, Ding L, Walker JR, Larson DE, Dooling DJ, Smith SM, Ley TJ, Mardis ER, Wilson RK: DGIdb: mining the druggable genome. Nat Methods 2013, 10:1209–1210.

[37] Hopkins AL, Groom CR: The druggable genome. Nat Rev Drug Discov 2002, 1:727–730.

[38] Banerji S, Cibulskis K, Rangel-Escareno C, Brown KK, Carter SL, Frederick AM, Lawrence MS, Sivachenko AY, Sougnez C, Zou L, Cortes ML, Fernandez-Lopez JC, Peng S, Ardlie KG, Auclair D, Bautista-Piña V, Duke F, Francis J, Jung J, Maffuz-Aziz A, Onofrio RC, Parkin M, Pho NH, Quintanar-Jurado V, Ramos AH, Rebollar-Vega R, Rodriguez-Cuevas S, Romero-Cordoba SL, Schumacher SE, Stransky N, et al: Sequence analysis of mutations and translocations across breast cancer subtypes. Nature 2012, 486:405–409.

[39] Kan Z, Jaiswal BS, Stinson J, Janakiraman V, Bhatt D, Stern HM, Yue P, Haverty PM, Bourgon R, Zheng J, Moorhead M, Chaudhuri S, Tomsho LP, Peters BA, Pujara K, Cordes S, Davis DP, Carlton VE, Yuan W, Li L, Wang W, Eigenbrot C, Kaminker JS, Eberhard DA, Waring P, Schuster SC, Modrusan Z, Zhang Z, Stokoe D, de Sauvage FJ, et al: Diverse somatic mutation patterns and pathway alterations in human cancers. Nature 2010, 466:869–873.

[40] Shah SP, Roth A, Goya R, Oloumi A, Ha G, Zhao Y, Turashvili G, Ding J, Tse K, Haffari G, Bashashati A, Prentice LM, Khattra J, Burleigh A, Yap D, Bernard V, McPherson A, Shumansky K, Crisan A, Giuliany R, Heravi-Moussavi A, Rosner J, Lai D, Birol I, Varhol R, Tam A, Dhalla N, Zeng T, Ma K, Chan SK, et al: The clonal and mutational evolution spectrum of primary triple-negative breast cancers. Nature 2012, 486:395–399.

[41] Stephens PJ, Tarpey PS, Davies H, Van Loo P, Greenman C, Wedge DC, Nik-Zainal S, Martin S, Varela I, Bignell GR, Yates LR, Papaemmanuil E, Beare D, Butler A, Cheverton A, Gamble J, Hinton J, Jia M, Jayakumar A, Jones D, Latimer C, Lau KW, McLaren S, McBride DJ, Menzies A, Mudie L, Raine K, Rad R, Chapman MS, Teague J, et al: The landscape of cancer genes and mutational processes in breast cancer. Nature 2012, 486:400–404.

[42] Lee JW, Soung YH, Seo SH, Kim SY, Park CH, Wang YP, Park K, Nam SW, Park WS, Kim SH, Lee JY, Yoo NJ, Lee SH: Somatic mutations of ERBB2 kinase domain in gastric, colorectal, and breast carcinomas. Clin Cancer Res 2006, 12:57–61.

[43] Bose R, Kavuri SM, Searleman AC, Shen W, Shen D, Koboldt DC, Monsey J, Goel N, Aronson AB, Li S, Ma CX, Ding L, Mardis ER, Ellis MJ: Activating HER2 mutations in HER2 gene amplification negative breast cancer. Cancer Discov 2013, 3:224–237.

[44] Toy W, Shen Y, Won H, Green B, Sakr RA, Will M, Li Z, Gala K, Fanning S, King TA, Hudis C, Chen D, Taran T, Hortobagyi G, Greene G, Berger M, Baselga J, Chandarlapaty S: ESR1 ligand-binding domain mutations in hormone-resistant breast cancer. Nat Genet 2013, 45:1439–1445.

[45] Robinson DR, Wu YM, Vats P, Su F, Lonigro RJ, Cao X, Kalyana-Sundaram S, Wang R, Ning Y, Hodges L, Gursky A, Siddiqui J, Tomlins SA, Roychowdhury S, Pienta KJ, Kim SY, Roberts JS, Rae JM, Van Poznak CH, Hayes DF, Chugh R, Kunju LP, Talpaz M, Schott AF, Chinnaiyan AM: Activating ESR1 mutations in hormone-resistant metastatic breast cancer. Nat Genet 2013, 45:1446–1451.

[46] Ellis LM, Fidler IJ: Finding the tumor copycat. Therapy fails, patients don't. Nat Med 2010, 16:974–975.

[47] Johnson JI, Decker S, Zaharevitz D, Rubinstein LV, Venditti JM, Schepartz S, Kalyandrug S, Christian M, Arbuck S, Hollingshead M, Sausville EA: Relationships between drug activity in NCI preclinical in vitro and in vivo models and early clinical trials. Br J Cancer 2001, 84:1424–1431.

[48] Voskoglou-Nomikos T, Pater JL, Seymour L: Clinical predictive value of the in vitro cell line, human xenograft, and mouse allograft preclinical cancer models. Clin Cancer Res 2003, 9:4227–4239.

[49] Jin K, Teng L, Shen Y, He K, Xu Z, Li G: Patient-derived human tumour tissue xenografts in immunodeficient mice: a systematic review. Clin Transl Oncol 2010, 12:473–480.

[50] Morton CL, Houghton PJ: Establishment of human tumor xenografts in immunodeficient mice. Nat Protoc 2007, 2:247–250.

[51] Rubio-Viqueira B, Hidalgo M: Direct in vivo xenograft tumor model for predicting chemotherapeutic drug response in cancer patients. Clin Pharmacol Ther 2009, 85:217–221.

[52] Sausville EA, Burger AM: Contributions of human tumor xenografts to anticancer drug development. Cancer Res 2006, 66:3351-3354.

[53] DeRose YS, Wang G, Lin YC, Bernard PS, Buys SS, Ebbert MT, Factor R, Matsen C, Milash BA, Nelson E, Neumayer L, Randall RL, Stijleman IJ, Welm BE, Welm AL: Tumor grafts derived from women with breast cancer authentically reflect tumor pathology, growth, metastasis and disease outcomes. Nat Med 2011, 17:1514–1520.

[54] McEvoy J, Ulyanov A, Brennan R, Wu G, Pounds S, Zhang J, Dyer MA: Analysis of MDM2 and MDM4 single nucleotide polymorphisms, mRNA splicing and protein expression in retinoblastoma. PLoS One 2012, 7:e42739.

[55] Reyal F, Guyader C, Decraene C, Lucchesi C, Auger N, Assayag F, De Plater L, Gentien D, Poupon MF, Cottu P, De Cremoux P, Gestraud P, Vincent-Salomon A, Fontaine JJ, Roman-Roman S, Delattre O, Decaudin D, Marangoni E: Molecular profiling of patient-derived breast cancer xenografts. Breast Cancer Res 2012, 14:R11.

[56] Zhao X, Liu Z, Yu L, Zhang Y, Baxter P, Voicu H, Gurusiddappa S, Luan J, Su JM, Leung HC, Li XN: Global gene expression profiling confirms the molecular fidelity of primary tumor-based orthotopic xenograft mouse models of medulloblastoma. Neuro Oncol 2012, 14:574–583.

[57] Ng S, Collisson EA, Sokolov A, Goldstein T, Gonzalez-Perez A, Lopez-Bigas N, Benz C, Haussler D, Stuart JM: PARADIGM-SHIFT predicts the function of mutations in multiple cancers using pathway impact analysis. Bioinformatics 2012, 28:i640–i646.

[58] Vaske CJ, Benz SC, Sanborn JZ, Earl D, Szeto C, Zhu J, Haussler D, Stuart JM: Inference of patient-specific pathway activities from multi-dimensional cancer genomics data using PARADIGM. Bioinformatics 2010, 26:i237–245.

[59] Tabchy A, Hennessy BT, Gonzalez-Angulo AM, Bernstam FM, Lu Y, Mills GB: Quantitative proteomic analysis in breast cancer. Drugs Today (Barc) 2011, 47:169–182.

[60] Ellis MJ, Gillette M, Carr SA, Paulovich AG, Smith RD, Rodland KK, Townsend RR, Kinsinger C, Mesri M, Rodriguez H, Liebler DC, Clinical Proteomic Tumor Analysis Consortium (CPTAC): Connecting genomic alterations to cancer biology with proteomics: the NCI Clinical Proteomic Tumor Analysis Consortium. Cancer Discov 2013, 3:1108–1112.

Chapter 12

Obtaining Informed Consent for Clinical Tumor and Germline Exome Sequencing of Newly Diagnosed Childhood Cancer Patients

Sarah Scollon[1,2], Katie Bergstrom[1,2], Robin A Kerstein[1,2], Tao Wang[3], Susan G Hilsenbeck[3], Uma Ramamurthy[4], Richard A Gibbs[5,6], Christine M Eng[6], Murali M Chintagumpala[1,2,3], Stacey L Berg[1,2,3], Laurence B McCullough[7], Amy L McGuire[3,5,7], Sharon E Plon[1,2,3,5,6], D Williams Parsons[1,2,3,5,6]

[1]Texas Children's Cancer Center, 6701 Fannin Street #1400, Houston, TX 77030, USA

[2]Department of Pediatrics, Baylor College of Medicine, One Baylor Plaza, Houston, TX 77030, USA

[3]Dan L. Duncan Cancer Center, Baylor College of Medicine, One Baylor Plaza, Houston, TX 77030, USA

[4]Dan L. Duncan Institute for Clinical and Translational Research, Baylor College of Medicine, One Baylor Plaza, Houston, TX 77030, USA

[5]Human Genome Sequencing Center, Baylor College of Medicine, One Baylor Plaza, Houston, TX 77030, USA

[6]Department of Molecular and Human Genetics, Baylor College of Medicine, One

Baylor Plaza, Houston, TX 77030, USA

[7]Center for Medical Ethics and Health Policy, Baylor College of Medicine, One Baylor Plaza, Houston, TX 77030, USA.

Abstract: Background: Effectively educating families about the risks and benefits of genomic tests such as whole exome sequencing (WES) offers numerous challenges, including the complexity of test results and potential loss of privacy. Research on best practices for obtaining informed consent (IC) in a variety of clinical settings is needed. The BASIC3 study of clinical tumor and germline WES in an ethnically diverse cohort of newly diagnosed pediatric cancer patients offers the opportunity to study the IC process in the setting of critical illness. We report on our experience for the first 100 families enrolled, including study participation rates, reasons for declining enrollment, assessment of clinical and demographic factors that might impact study enrollment, and preferences of parents for participation in optional genomics study procedures. **Methods:** A specifically trained IC team offered study enrollment to parents of eligible children for procedures including clinical tumor and germline WES with results deposited in the medical record and disclosure of both diagnostic and incidental results to the family. Optional study procedures were also offered, such as receiving recessive carrier status and deposition of data into research databases. Stated reasons for declining participation were recorded. Clinical and demographic data were collected and comparisons made between enrolled and non-enrolled patients. **Results:** Over 15 months, 100 of 121 (83%) eligible families elected to enroll in the study. No significant differences in enrollment were detected based on factors such as race, ethnicity, use of Spanish interpreters and Spanish consent forms, and tumor features (central nervous system versus non-central nervous system, availability of tumor for WES). The most common reason provided for declining enrollment (10% of families) was being overwhelmed by the new cancer diagnosis. Risks specific to clinical genomics, such as privacy concerns, were less commonly reported (5.5%). More than 85% of parents consented to each of the optional study procedures. **Conclusions:** An IC process was developed that utilizes a specialized IC team, active communication with the oncology team, and an emphasis on scheduling flexibility. Most parents were willing to participate in a clinical germline and tumor WES study as well as optional procedures such as genomic data sharing independent of race, ethnicity or language spoken.

346

1. Background

The process of obtaining informed consent for subject participation in clinical research protocols is multifaceted and includes the researcher and subject or guardian reviewing the study purpose, procedures and informed consent document. Previous studies investigating parental and young adult preferences for informed consent in clinical trials in pediatric oncology settings have demonstrated that participants generally prefer: (1) to receive more information but risk feeling overwhelmed with the quantity or pace of information provided; (2) that the information be presented in a stepwise and organized manner; and (3) to be given sufficient time to process the information, especially in the context of their emotional state, before making a decision[1][2]. The presentation of additional audio or visual learning materials is also suggested[1]. These studies emphasize that, while there are essential aspects of informed consent, details need to be adapted to fit the needs and questions of the individual or family.

The challenge of successfully informing potential participants without overwhelming them with content can be particularly daunting for research involving genome-scale tests, given the amount and complexity of the information to be conveyed and the differential informational priorities and preferences of the parties involved (patients, parents, clinicians)[3]. It is critical that the participant understand the purpose of the research, the type of test(s) to be performed, the various types of results that they will receive (and not receive) through participation and in which situations they have a choice about receipt of results in these categories, as well as the potential risks and benefits of participation. Studies have shown that, although the public is familiar with the terminology of genetics and its association with disease, there are still significant gaps in conceptual knowledge[4]-[7]. Although there is limited research looking specifically at public knowledge of concepts in the setting of whole exome sequencing (WES) and whole genome sequencing (WGS), early studies have illustrated such gaps exist but are improved by the informed consent process[8]. In addition, the long-term risks of the inclusion of genomic information in the medical record and research databases remain unknown, although some level of protective legislation is in place (through the Genetic Information Nondiscrimination Act of 2008, GINA)[9]. Thus, specific considerations for the informed consent process in studies utilizing WES/WGS include the higher likelihood of obtaining unanticipated results and the risk of identifiability or loss of privacy through data sharing[10]. As is true for other types of research, traditional barriers such as language and education level can also factor into the challenges of obtaining informed consent for WES/WGS studies. Previous studies have suggested a differential enthusiasm for participation in medical research among racial and ethnic groups[11]-[13], but further evaluation in the specific context of clinical genomic research is needed.

Patient understanding of genomic testing in cancer patients may also be complicated by confusion over the conceptual differences between germline mutations and tumor or somatic mutations. Interview studies assessing attitudes among adults diagnosed with cancer toward personalized medicine revealed that a majority of participants expressed understanding of the difference between germline and somatic genetic testing based on descriptions provided to them. However, when asked about specific benefits and risks of somatic testing some participants described examples typically associated with germline genetic testing, such as learning about familial risk or insurance discrimination, suggesting the distinction still may have remained unclear[14].

As WES and WGS are transitioned from the laboratory to the clinic, there is a need for additional research to provide insight into the best practices for obtaining informed consent for these tests in a variety of clinical settings. The BASIC3 (Baylor Advancing Sequencing in Childhood Cancer Care) study seeks to integrate information from clinical germline and tumor WES into the care of newly diagnosed solid tumor patients at Texas Children's Cancer Center (TCCC) and evaluate the impact of these exome data on the patients' families and oncologists as part of the National Human Genome Research Institute Clinical Sequencing Exploratory Research (CSER) program[15]. This study offers a unique opportunity to investigate the informed consent process for clinical germline and tumor WES in the pediatric oncology setting. The TCCC serves a racially and ethnically diverse patient population, including a large number of families of Hispanic ethnicity and frequently utilizing Spanish-speaking interpreters and Spanish consent forms for both clinical care and enrollment on research studies, facilitating evaluation of the role of such factors in the informed consent process. The goals of this manuscript are to describe the informed consent process utilized for BASIC3 and to report on our experience for the first 100 families enrolled, including (1) the proportion of parents who decline enrollment of their child on this clinical WES study and their reasons for doing so, (2) a comparison of clinical and demographic factors (such as race and ethnicity) between patients whose parents agree to or decline study enrollment, and (3) the preferences of parents for participation in optional genomics study procedures such as inclusion of recessive carrier data in WES reports and deposition of patient data into research databases.

2. Methods

2.1. Study Design

The BASIC3 study was approved by the institutional review board (IRB) of Baylor College of Medicine (BCM), which is also the IRB for Texas Children's Hospital (TCH), the study clinical site. The study conformed to the Declaration of Helsinki. Study enrollment is offered for all patients with newly diagnosed solid tumors (including central nervous system (CNS) tumors) under the age of 18 years who undergo their initial tumor surgery and have ongoing oncologic treatment at TCCC and have at least one parent who speaks English or Spanish. Enrollment for parent-specific study procedures is separately offered to the parents of the patients. All study documents, education aids and consent forms have been fully translated into Spanish and medically trained Spanish interpreters are utilized as needed. The primary oncologists caring for the BASIC3 patients are separately consented to participate in study procedures, including oncologist interviews and surveys, but that process is not described in detail here.

Patient-participants are enrolled in the study within 60 days of completion of the pathology report from their diagnostic cancer surgery (**Figure 1**). Newly diagnosed solid tumor patients are identified by the study team in cooperation with the TCH surgical and neurosurgical services, TCCC Solid Tumor and Neuro-Oncology clinical teams, and TCH pathology. Potential eligibility is confirmed through a review of the medical record and in consultation with the primary oncologist.

In brief, the study procedures are as follows (**Figure 1**). After informed consent for study enrollment (described in detail below) has been obtained, patient blood and tumor samples are sent to the Clinical Laboratory Improvement Amendments-certified and College of American Pathologists-certified Whole Genome

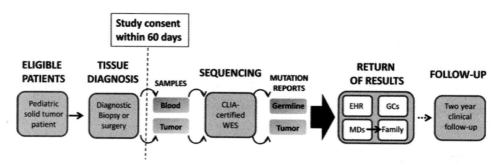

Figure 1. BASIC3 clinical study design. CLIA, Clinical Laboratory Improvement Amendments; EHR, electronic health record; GCs, genetic counselors; MDs, pediatric oncologists; WES, whole exome sequencing.

and Cancer Genetics Laboratories of the Medical Genetics Laboratories of BCM for germline (including the mitochondrial DNA) and tumor WES. If tumor sample is not available for research, patients remain eligible for the study but only germline WES is performed. Blood samples are obtained from both biological parents when available and utilized by the laboratory to interpret the inheritance of germline variants identified by WES in the patient-participant as previously described[16]; of note, these parental samples are not subjected to clinical WES. After the germline and tumor WES reports are generated (turnaround time of 3 to 4 months), they are placed into the electronic health record and reviewed with the patient's primary oncologist by the BASIC3 principal investigators and genetic counselor(s).

The focused germline WES reports, as previously described[16], include all variants identified in four categories (**Figure 2**): (1) deleterious mutations in disease genes related to cancer susceptibility or other patient phenotype; (2) variants of uncertain significance in those same phenotype-associated disease genes; (3) medically actionable mutations in disease genes unrelated to cancer susceptibility; and (4) limited panel of pharmacogenomic variant alleles. In addition, at the time of study enrollment parents [or the child's legal guardian (s), hereafter referred to as parents] are given the option to have the report include their child's carrier status results for recessive disease. The germline reports utilized for this study do not include other disease-associated mutations, including those associated with adult-onset conditions unrelated to cancer. The tumor WES reports (**Figure 2**) comprise an annotated listing of all somatic (tumor-specific) mutations identified in the patient's tumor, prioritized based upon potential clinical relevance for the patient-participant.

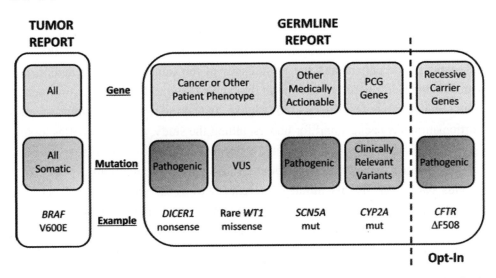

Figure 2. Categories of whole exome sequencing results returned to BASIC3 study families. PCG, pharmacogenetic; VUS, variant of uncertain significance.

After the parents have been notified that their child's WES results are available, an appointment is scheduled for a "disclosure visit" to review the results with their primary oncologist and a study genetic counselor in the TCCC clinic or inpatient oncology unit. A hard copy of the WES report(s) and a genetic counseling letter are provided to the family at this visit, which is audiore-corded. The longitudinal aims of this study include one parent per family being asked to complete surveys and a subset being interviewed at three time points: after study enrollment, after receipt of WES results, and one year after receipt of WES results.

2.2. Informed Consent Process

The study team actively involved in the enrollment process includes SEP, study PI and clinical geneticist; DWP, study PI and pediatric oncologist; SS and KB, study genetic counselors; RK, study coordinator. The patient's primary pediatric oncologist advises the study team on when an appropriate time to meet with the family might be, given the clinical status of the patient and the emotional state of the family. Once this "green light" has been given by the oncologist, one or more members of the study team approaches the family about the study. First, a brief (<10 minutes) overview of the study is provided by the BASIC3 team and a study brochure is provided. For families who express interest after the study overview, a more detailed explanation of the study is provided, referred to here as the consent conference. The setting for the consent conference is dictated by the clinical status of the patient and the preferences of the family. The information provided includes a full description of study events (**Figure 1**), the types of potential tumor and germline results reported (**Figure 2**), and the risks and benefits of study participation. As background for understanding the study, a brief "genetics lesson" is provided for the families, including concepts such as how cancers develop and the distinctions between tumor (somatic) and germline mutations. Ideally, both parents participate in this initial conference; however, often only one parent is available and the ultimate decision about study enrollment is delayed until the family can discuss the study at home and/or a follow-up conference with the second parent is held.

Several printed visual aids (in English or Spanish) are used to complement the informed consent document and verbal overview. First, as noted above, a study brochure is provided to parents either by the oncologist or during the consent conference which includes a brief introduction to the study goals and procedures, an overview of the relevance of germline and somatic mutations to cancer development (with two diagrams), and a listing of the types of potential results that may be received during the study. Second, bulleted printed summaries of the types of results that may be received in both the tumor and germline reports are provided to emphasize this important information. Finally, aids are used to explain the concepts of carrier status for recessive and X-linked conditions. These consist of publicly available diagrams published by the US National Library of Medicine[17][18] as well as key facts (developed by the study staff) regarding each mode of inheritance, including what it means to be a carrier, how this information applies directly to the participant and other family members, and reproductive risk.

2.3. Study Consent Forms

Separate consent forms are used for the enrollment of patients and their parents in the study. The Patient Consent Form (Additional file 1) on which the parent consents to the enrollment of their child in the study describes all key study-related events (**Figure 1**), including the study samples to be obtained and the details of the germline and tumor WES tests. The purpose of the study is explained as learning "how to best report and use the clinical exome sequencing test results for childhood cancer patients." Specific examples of the types of potential clinically relevant tumor WES results and the likelihood of such an event are described, such as "rare" cases in which tumor findings might include mutations that "are normally found in a different type of tumor from what your child was diagnosed with" (for example, mutations of potential diagnostic utility) and "very rare" cases in which the mutations "make your doctor think your child's tumor will respond better or worse to a particular cancer treatment" (for example, mutations of potential therapeutic utility). Similarly, categories and examples of potential clinically relevant germline WES results are provided (**Figure 2**), including "inherited mutations that cause your child to have an increased risk of developing other cancers... [and] may also provide information about the risk of cancer in close family members" (for example, cancer susceptibility mutations), "inherited mutations that are unrelated to cancer but provide information about a different medical condition for which treatment is available and recommended as standard medical care" (for example, medically actionable incidental findings), and "inherited mutations that might affect how your child's body responds to certain medicines" (for example, pharmacogenomic variants).

In addition to the required study procedures, the Patient Consent Form also includes a number of optional elements to which parents may separately consent or decline, including the option to include or exclude the child's recessive carrier mutations in the germline WES report. Other choices relate to additional research procedures, such as the analysis of patient samples using other non-clinical genomic methods and the release of the child's genetic and clinical information into scientific databases (**Table 1**).

Several potential risks of study enrollment are included in the consent form, including the physical risks of obtaining a blood sample, the risk of anxiety related to disclosure of genetic results, and the potential disclosure of non-paternity through genetic testing. The risk of loss of privacy of genetic information is discussed in relation to the collection and storage of research data as well as the inclusion of genetic information in the medical record, for example, "Health insurance companies may also have access to this information. There are laws to protect against the use of this information in making decisions about health insurance and employment. However, you may be asked to provide medical record information when your child applies for life insurance or disability insurance". It is stated that

Table 1. Optional BASIC3 study events listed in patient and parent consent forms.

Participant	Study event
Patient	Inclusion of carrier status results in germline exome report
Patient	Use of diagnostic tumor sample for additional genomic research
Patient	Use of blood sample for additional genomic research
Patient	Use of future tumor samples for additional genomic research
Patient	Release of blood/tumor samples and genetic/clinical information to other researchers
Patient	Release of genetic and clinical information into scientific databases
Parent	Use of blood sample for additional genomic research
Parent	Release of blood sample and genetic/clinical information to other researchers
Parent	Release of genetic/clinical information into scientific databases
Both	Permission for future re-contact

there are "additional risks of loss of privacy" if parents consent to the optional study procedures of sharing genetic and clinical data with other BCM investigators or the deidentified release of genetic information into scientific databases.

The possibility of identifying either tumor or germline data that may impact the care of the patient and/or other family members is listed as a potential benefit; however, it is stated that "we do not think that the mutations that are found are likely to change the planned cancer treatment for most children" and that in that circumstance the benefit is more to society than the individual. The probability of a tumor mutation being identified that has implications for treatment is estimated to be "very rare". It is clarified that there are no study costs for patients and that families will be reimbursed a nominal amount ($25) for participation in study surveys and interviews.

For parents who decline participation for their children we record the answer to an open-ended question: "Would you please tell us why you decided to not participate", patient tumor type, age at diagnosis, language used during the consent conference (English or Spanish), use of an interpreter for consent conference, and race/ethnicity as listed in the electronic health record at the time of initial hospital admission.

The Parent Consent Form (Additional file 1) on which the parent consents to their own enrollment in the study utilizes similar structure and language to the Patient Consent Form, including identical Background and Purpose sections as well as a description of potential WES results and study risks and benefits. Information about required and optional study samples and procedures for the patient is replaced by a description of optional parental blood samples that may be provided for interpretation of variants identified in the patient's germline WES report and additional research procedures. No parental blood samples are required for study participation.

2.4. Child Assent for Study Enrollment

As per BCM and TCCC guidelines, assent was obtained for each child who was judged "capable of providing assent based on age maturity and psychologic state", and documented by the parent on the Patient Consent Form document using the standard BCM/TCCC language (Additional file 1). TCCC standard operating procedures for obtaining informed consent for research studies recommends that assent be obtained from subjects greater than 6 years of age and under 18 years of age. The extent of child participation in the consent process is guided by each child and their parents. The consent conference(s) is conducted with the child in the room and the child is encouraged to participate to the extent of their interest and understanding. In only one case did the parents specifically request to have their child not be present for part of the discussion: a 12 year old girl with a CNS tumor and developmental delay who was present for most of the conference but became bothered by the lengthy discussion of the study.

2.5. Data Collection and Analysis

A password-protected web accessible study database was created to track all study events and procedures and collect clinical data for enrolled subjects, including subject age, gender, race, ethnicity, tumor diagnosis, grade, stage, the presence of metastatic disease at diagnosis, and whether chemotherapy and/or radiation therapy was planned.

Subjects' characteristics were summarized descriptively. Comparisons were made between enrolled and non-enrolled patients for the following variables: patient age, gender, ethnicity, race, tumor location (CNS or non-CNS), whether an interpreter and Spanish consent form were used, whether tumor was available for WES, and the time from surgery to the decision about study enrollment. Two sample rank sum tests were used to compare the continuous data and Fisher's exact tests were used for the categorical data. The P-value for ethnicity was calculated with "not reported" subjects excluded. For race, the comparison made was between "white" subjects and all others with "not reported" subjects excluded.

3. Results

The study staff began approaching all families of potentially eligible newly diagnosed solid tumor patients on 1 August 2012 and the one-hundredth subject was enrolled on 3 September 2013. Over this time period, 121 families met eligibility criteria and were offered enrollment in the study. Twenty-one families declined enrollment, resulting in a rate of study enrollment of 83% (100/121, 95% confidence interval 75% to 88%). Due to the complexity of the study and the potential implications of study enrollment for other family members, the study consent conference is generally conducted as a multi-step process rather than a single meeting, with most occurring in the patient room on the inpatient oncology floor (if the child is hospitalized) or in the outpatient TCCC clinic, often while patients are having chemotherapy infusions. The interval from date of initial tumor surgery to parental decision about study enrollment ranged from 5 to 63 days (median 36 days) for patients enrolled in the study. Enrolled patients were diagnosed with a diverse representation of pediatric solid tumors. Tumor was available for WES in 84% of subjects. Further tumor-directed treatment (chemotherapy and/or radiation therapy) was planned for 82% of subjects. Initial evaluation revealed that 34% of tumors were metastatic at the time of diagnosis.

Forty-five percent of enrolled subjects were female (**Table 2**). Ages ranged between 1 month and 17 years (median of 5.1 years) at the time of tumor surgery. Forty-three percent self-identified as being of Hispanic ethnicity and 56% as white race. A Spanish-speaking interpreter and Spanish consent form were utilized for 15% of subjects. Fourteen different oncologists had patients enrolled in the study, with the number of enrolled patients per oncologist ranging between 1 and 22 (median

Table 2. Characteristics of patients enrolled and not enrolled in the study.

Characteristic	Enrolled (n = 100)	Declined (n = 21)	P-value
Median age in years (range)	5.1 (0.1 - 17.0)	4.0 (0.1 - 14.2)	0.73
Female gender	45 (45%)	5 (24%)	0.09
Ethnicity			1a
Hispanic	43 (43%)	10 (48%)	
Non-Hispanic	51 (51%)	11 (52%)	
Not reported	6 (6%)	-	
Race			0.17b
White	56 (56%)	18 (85%)	
Black or African American	12 (12%)	1 (5%)	
Asian	4 (4%)	1 (5%)	
American Indian or Alaska Native	4 (4%)	1 (5%)	
Multiple	6 (6%)	-	
Not reported	18 (18%)	-	
Tumor location			0.22
CNS	33 (33%)	10 (48%)	
Non-CNS	67 (67%)	11 (52%)	
Tumor metastatic at diagnosis	34 (34%)	ND	
Adjuvant tumor treatment planned	82 (82%)	ND	
Tumor available for WES	84 (84%)	14 (67%)	0.12
Interpreter and Spanish consent form used	15 (15%)	4 (19%)	0.74
Median days from surgery to study decision (range)	36 (5-63)	42 (20 - 61)	0.052

[a]P-value was calculated with "Not reported" subjects excluded. [b]Comparison was made between "White" versus others with "Not reported" subjects excluded. Two sample rank sum tests were used to compare the continuous data and Fisher's exact tests were used for the categorical data. CNS, central nervous system; ND, not determined; WES, whole exome sequencing.

4.5, mean 7.1) and the fraction of eligible patients per oncologist enrolling in the study ranging between 57% and 100% (**Figure 3**). There was no correlation between the number of patients approached per oncologist and the fraction enrolled (Spearman's rank correlation = −0.35, P = 0.21).

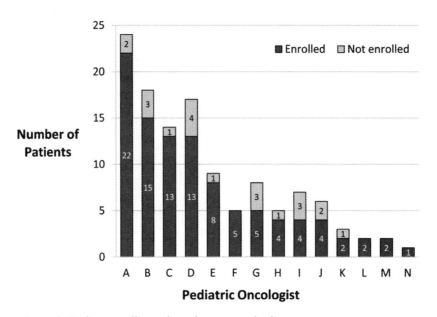

Figure 3. Patient enrollment by primary oncologist.

The most common reason provided by parents for choosing not to participate in the study was that they were overwhelmed by their child's new cancer diagnosis and did not wish to participate in an additional research study (10% of
families offered study enrollment; **Figure 4**). Other reasons reported included
concern about privacy risks (3%), anxiety about receiving genetic testing results
(2.5%), and a desire for no further blood to be obtained for research study procedures (2%).

No significant differences were detected when comparing the 100 enrolled
patients with the 21 patients who were not enrolled in the study for age, gender,
tumor location (CNS or non-CNS), whether tumor was available for WES, or the
time from surgery to the decision about study enrollment (**Table 2**). In addition, no
significant difference was observed in the proportion of children identified by
their parents as being of Hispanic ethnicity between those who enrolled in the
study (46% of patients with race reported) compared with those who declined
enrollment (48%). Similarly, a Spanish interpreter and Spanish consent forms were
used in a similar proportion of parents agreeing to (15%) or declining study
enrollment (19%). The proportion of patients identified as being of white race was
numerically but not significantly lower for children enrolled in the study (68%)
compared with those not enrolled (85%, P = 0.17).

We then examined decisions about optional patient-related study procedures made by the parents of the enrolled children (**Figure 5**). Notably, 88% of parents chose to have information about carrier status for recessive diseases included in their child's germline WES report. Parents also consented to the remaining optional study procedures at a very high rate, including use of the diagnostic tumor sample for additional research studies (94%), collection of tumor for research purposes

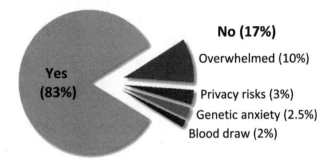

Figure 4. Proportion of patients enrolled in the study and stated reasons for parents declining enrollment.

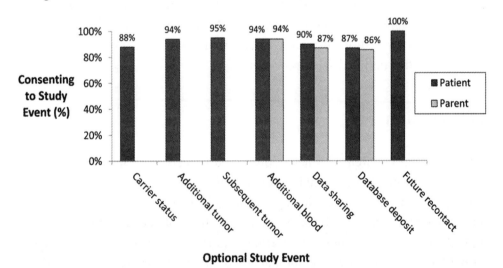

Figure 5. Consent for optional study events. Carrier status: reporting of germline carrier status for recessive diseases. Additional tumor: use of diagnostic tumor for additional research studies. Subsequent tumor: use of tumor from subsequent surgeries for additional research studies. Additional blood: collection of blood sample for additional research studies. Data sharing: sharing of study samples and/or de-identified genetic/clinical data with other investigators for IRB-approved studies. Database deposit: deposition of de-identified genetic/clinical data into scientific databases. Future re-contact: to obtain follow-up clinical information or request additional study samples.

from any subsequent tumor surgeries (95%), collection of an additional 1 to 2 teaspoon blood sample for research purposes (94%), sharing of de-identified genetic and clinical data with other BCM investigators with IRB-approved protocols (90%), and deposition of deidentified genetic and clinical data into scientific databases (87%). All parents allowed future re-contact by study investigators.

One hundred and forty-seven parents (1.5 parents/patient) chose to enroll in the study, resulting in 4 families with no parent enrolled, 45 with one parent enrolled, and 51 with two parents enrolled. Two enrolled parents were not biologically related to the enrolled child and were not asked to provide blood samples for the study. Most parents consented to the optional study procedures (**Figure 5**), including collection of an additional 2 teaspoon parental blood sample for research purposes (94%), sharing of de-identified genetic and clinical data with other BCM investigators with IRB-approved protocols (87%), and deposition of de-identified genetic and clinical data into scientific databases (87%). All enrolled parents allowed future re-contact by study investigators. With regard to actual phlebotomy data, blood samples for interpretation of their child's germline WES results have been obtained to date from 68% of enrolled parents; blood samples for additional research have been obtained from 67% of parents consenting to that optional study procedure.

4. Discussion

Parents of children with newly diagnosed cancers were found to have significant interest in a research study of clinical and tumor WES, with more than 80% agreeing to study enrollment. No significant differences were seen in the clinical and demographic factors analyzed between the cohorts of patients enrolled and not enrolled on the study, including race, ethnicity, the use of Spanish interpreters and consent forms and the type of tumor diagnosed. In this clinical setting it is perhaps unsurprising that parents would be eager to obtain any potentially clinically relevant information that might help guide treatment of their child's cancer, even if it is described as being of uncertain benefit by study investigators. This is consistent with previous studies which demonstrated that the majority of mothers of childhood cancer patients were willing to have their child undergo genetic testing for cancer susceptibility at a time when the benefits of such testing remained hypothetical[19]. However, two observations suggest that factors other than a desire for tumor WES results that could direct cancer therapy also play a role in the decision of parents to enroll in the BASIC3 study. First, most parents of patients for whom no tumor was available for WES still consented to study enrollment, albeit at a slightly decreased rate: 70% if no tumor compared with 86% if tumor available (P = 0.12). This could result from the fact that our study provided germline WES on study patients. Questions such as "why did this happen to my child?" and "will my other children also get cancer?" are a nearly universal component of initial diagnostic discussions between oncologists and families of newly diagnosed cancer patients. Germline WES of their child has the potential to provide insight into these questions by identifying pathogenic cancer susceptibility mutations. Perhaps equally importantly for families, it may help to provide reassurance that the patient's siblings are unlikely to develop a childhood cancer if no such mutations are found. Second, a very high proportion of parents of children enrolled in the study also agreed to optional study procedures that have both immediate risks (blood draws) and theoretical risks (privacy and insurability concerns) despite the fact that those procedures were not required to obtain either tumor and germline WES results, indicating that altruistic considerations were also likely relevant to decision-making by parents regarding enrollment in this study of clinical genomics.

Although not emphasized in discussions of genomic sequencing, the clinical context is very important to the consent process[20]. The period surrounding a new diagnosis of cancer or other life-threatening disease is one of remarkable stress for patients and their families, which can complicate the informed consent process[21][22]. Accordingly, we attempted to be sensitive to the specific clinical and social circumstances when approaching families about potential study enrollment, including close coordination with the primary oncologist and inpatient oncology team for determination of the timing and ideal setting (inpatient or outpatient) for this initial contact. For example, several months after the study opened, we extended the allowable window for study enrollment from 30 days to 60 days from definitive pathologic diagnosis in order to provide additional flexibility in the consent process. Despite these efforts, the reason provided by the majority of parents who chose not to enroll their child in the study was that they were overwhelmed by their child's new cancer diagnosis and treatment and did not wish to participate in any research study. Consequently, the observed 17% rate of families declining enrollment in the study may overestimate the proportion of parents who would decline WES in a clinical, non-study setting not requiring a long study consent process or additional research study procedures. Given that their child's illness was the most frequent explanation provided by parents for declining study enrollment, it is possible that the children whose parents declined were more severely ill than those who were enrolled in study. We did not obtain detailed clinical data on the non-enrolled children and cannot compare the clinical characteristics of the two groups; however, the diagnoses of the non-enrolled patients (including five pilocytic astrocytomas and three Wilms tumors, both tumor types with excellent survival rates) do not appear to carry an unusually poor prognosis. Parental reasons for declining enrollment related to the anticipated risks of clinical sequencing described in the consent form, such as the loss of privacy and potential anxiety about genetic test results, were in aggregate reported by only 5.5% of parents approached (for example, by 33% of parents declining study participation).

A majority of the time during study consent conferences was spent discussing the types of results that can be discovered by tumor and germline WES (and the potential clinical relevance of germline findings for other family members) and the risks of genomic research, with a particular emphasis on the implications of the loss of privacy of genomic data. It was stressed to parents that tumor and germline WES reports for patient-participants in the study would be incorporated into the electronic health record and that families should not participate in the study if they objected to that required study procedure. The finding that more than 80% of parents elected to enroll their children in the study suggests that the perceived risks of genomic research were outweighed for most families by the potential benefits of study participation. This concept has been previously described among parents offered genome scale research sequencing (where results did not appear in the medical record) in the setting of chronically ill children[23]. Overall, the clinical context of the genomic study appears to play a role in the potential subjects' willingness to participate despite potential concerns about obtaining genetic information. In the context of a child recently diagnosed with a life-threatening condition such as cancer, parents were generally very interested in participating in the study and only a small percentage viewed these potential "genetic privacy" risks as reason enough to decline participation. The observed rate of enrollment in this genomic study mirrors the high participation rates on therapeutic clinical trials for children with cancer[24].

Our study has several key limitations which offer opportunities for future research. First, the data reported do not include an assessment of parental understanding of the study procedures or the key concepts of genetics and genomic sequencing. The extent to which parents comprehend the complex issues inherent in clinical WES when they consent to their child's participation (and are not simply agreeing to participate in the hope that clinically relevant information can be obtained) and whether differences in understanding exist between the parents who agree or decline to have their child participate in the study remain unclear. Given previous research suggesting that participants in both cancer trials[25] and genomic studies[26] often have a poor understanding of relevant scientific concepts and study procedures, further study of this topic is needed. Data to be obtained through longitudinal surveys and interviews of BASIC3 study parents may provide relevant information regarding parental understanding of study procedures and level of satisfaction with study enrollment. Second, relatively little information (consisting of a brief explanation of reasons for declining study participation and limited clinical and demographic data) was collected from parents who declined participation on the study. A more extensive analysis of study "decliners" would have the potential to provide deeper insight into the factors behind this decision and could be useful for improving the informed consent process, although it would be potentially difficult to obtain since this group of parents stated that they were currently overwhelmed with their obligations. Finally, although the childhood cancer patients were present for the informed consent conferences and included (to the extent of their interest and capabilities) in study discussions, the current study does not provide data on the details of their involvement or their understanding of study procedures. Further research will be required to shed light on this critical aspect of clinical genomic studies involving pediatric patients.

5. Conclusions

Obtaining informed consent for clinical tumor and germ-line WES of children with newly diagnosed cancers offers many challenges, most fundamentally the difficulty of conveying complex genomic information in sufficient, but not excessive, detail to families who are immersed in a medically and personally critical situation. We have developed an informed consent process and document for clinical WES in the pediatric oncology clinic that utilize a dedicated informed consent team with specific genomics training and experience and rely upon active communication with the patient's clinical team regarding the clinical status of the patient and the emotional status of the family. As is the case when obtaining consent for treatment protocols for newly diagnosed patients, flexibility in all aspects of the informed consent process is critical at this unpredictable and stressful time for families[1][27], including the timing and location of the initial conference as well as the understanding that the "conference" is in reality most often a series of meetings involving multiple family members and significant repetition of information, consistent with the concept of informed consent as a process and not a single event[28]. Although we did not collect data on the duration of the consent conferences, we estimate that the typical time per family is approximately an hour, similar to that required to consent families to cancer treatment protocols[29][30]. Key points in our consent forms (Additional file 1) and the consent conference(s) include: an explanation of the multiple different types of potential tumor and germline WES results, with specific examples of mutations in each category provided; an emphasis on the fact that germline results have potential implications for other family members; and careful explanation of the known and unknown privacy risks of having genomic information in the medical record, including what is protected (and not protected) by GINA and full translation of all consent documents and educational aids for non-English speaking families.

Most parents of children with newly diagnosed cancers were willing to allow clinical tumor and germline WES to be performed, as well as optional research procedures without the possibility of direct benefit to the child or family. In this clinical setting, we did not observe that the willingness to participate in clinical genomics research was significantly impacted by patient-specific factors such as age, gender, race, or ethnicity. It is our impression that the parents of most children with newly diagnosed cancers are singularly focused on their child's diagnosis and clinical care and their assessment is that the potential benefit of identifying any clinically relevant information (even if unlikely) through WES outweighs risks of privacy loss and genetic anxiety. Follow-up study data, including ongoing analysis of semi-qualitative longitudinal interviews with study parents (before and after receipt of WES results as well as one year later), will help to shed light on this decision-making and differences in parental perspectives on clinical WES over time.

6. Additional File

Additional file 1: Patient and Parent Consent Forms for the BASIC3 study.

7. Abbreviations

BASIC3: Baylor Advancing Sequencing in Childhood Cancer Care; BCM: Baylor College of Medicine; CNS: central nervous system; GINA: Genetic Information Nondiscrimination Act; IRB: institutional review board; TCCC: Texas Children's Cancer center; TCH: Texas Children's Hospital; WES: whole exome sequencing; WGS: whole genome sequencing.

Competing Interests

The authors declare that they have no competing interests.

Authors' Contributions

SS, KB, RK, MC, SB, SP, WP, LM and AM participated in the study design, development of study consent forms and consent process. SS, KB, RK, WP and SP enrolled subjects and helped to draft the manuscript. TW and SH performed the statistical analysis. UR developed the study database. CE and RG developed the clinical exome sequencing test used in the study. WP and SP conceived of the study, participated in its design and coordination, and helped to draft the manuscript. All authors read and approved the final manuscript.

Acknowledgements

This study is a Clinical Sequencing Exploratory Research (CSER) program project supported by NHGRI/NCI 1U01HG006485. The authors are grateful to the solid tumor patients/families, pediatric oncologists, and clinical staff at Texas Children's Cancer Center for their participation in the study. The authors also thank Stephanie Gutierrez, study data manager, and Dr Ramamurthy's database development team: Medha Naik, Xingquan Lu, and Vivek Ramanathan.

Source: Scollon S, Bergstrom K, Kerstein R A, et al. Obtaining informed consent for clinical tumor and germline exome sequencing of newly diagnosed childhood cancer patients[J]. Genome Medicine, 2014, 6(9):1–11.

References

[1]   Baker JN, Leek AC, Salas HS, Drotar D, Noll R, Rheingold SR, Kodish ED: Suggestions from adolescents, young adults, and parents for improving informed consent in phase 1 pediatric oncology trials. Cancer 2013, 119:4154–4161.

[2]   Miller VA, Nelson RM: Factors related to voluntary parental decision-making in pediatric oncology. Pediatrics 2012, 129:903–909.

[3]   Levenseller BL, Soucier DJ, Miller VA, Harris D, Conway L, Bernhardt BA: Stakeholders' opinions on the implementation of pediatric whole exome sequencing: implications for informed consent. J Genet Couns 2013, 23:552–565.

[4]   Lea DH, Kaphingst KA, Bowen D, Lipkus I, Hadley DW: Communicating genetic and genomic information: health literacy and numeracy considerations. Public Health Genom 2011, 14:279–289.

[5]   Mesters I, Ausems A, De Vries H: General public's knowledge, interest and information needs related to genetic cancer: an exploratory study. Eur J Cancer Prev 2005, 14:69–75.

[6]   Lanie AD, Jayaratne TE, Sheldon JP, Kardia SL, Anderson ES, Feldbaum M, Petty EM: Exploring the public understanding of basic genetic concepts. J Genet Couns 2004, 13:305–320.

[7]   Molster C, Charles T, Samanek A, O'Leary P: Australian study on public knowledge of human genetics and health. Public Health Genom 2009, 12:84–91.

[8]   Kaphingst KA, Facio FM, Cheng MR, Brooks S, Eidem H, Linn A, Biesecker BB, Biesecker LG: Effects of informed consent for individual genome sequencing on relevant knowledge. Clin Genet 2012, 82:408–415.

[9]   The Genetic Information Nondiscrimination Act of 2008. [http://www.eeoc.gov/laws/statutes/gina.cfm].

[10]   Tabor HK, Berkman BE, Hull SC, Bamshad MJ: Genomics really gets personal: how exome and whole genome sequencing challenge the ethical framework of human genetics research. Am J Med Genet A 2011, 155A:2916–2924.

[11]   McGuire AL, Oliver JM, Slashinski MJ, Graves JL, Wang T, Kelly PA, Fisher W, Lau CC, Goss J, Okcu M, Treadwell-Deering D, Goldman AM, Noebels JL, Hilsen-

beck SG: To share or not to share: a randomized trial of consent for data sharing in genome research. Genet Med 2011, 13:948–955.

[12] Murthy VH, Krumholz HM, Gross CP: Participation in cancer clinical trials: race-, sex-, and age-based disparities. JAMA 2004, 291:2720–2726.

[13] Katz R, Kegeles S, Kressin N, Green B, James S: Willingness to participate in bio-medical research. African-Americans vs Whites. Ann Epidemiol 2000, 10:456-457.

[14] Gray SW, Hicks-Courant K, Lathan CS, Garraway L, Park ER, Weeks JC: Attitudes of patients with cancer about personalized medicine and somatic genetic testing. J Oncol Pract 2012, 8:329-335. 322 p following 335.

[15] Clinical Sequencing Exploratory Research (CSER) [https://cser-consortium.org/].

[16] Yang Y, Muzny DM, Reid JG, Bainbridge MN, Willis A, Ward PA, Braxton A, Beuten J, Xia F, Niu Z, Hardison M, Person R, Bekheirnia MR, Leduc MS, Kirby A, Pham P, Scull J, Wang M, Ding Y, Plon SE, Lupski JR, Beaudet AL, Gibbs RA, Eng CM: Clinical whole-exome sequencing for the diagnosis of mendelian disorders. N Engl J Med 2013, 369:1502–1511.

[17] National Library of Medicine (US): Genetics Home Reference: Autosomal recessive. [http://ghr.nlm.nih.gov/handbook/illustrations/autorecessive].

[18] National Library of Medicine (US): Genetics Home Reference: X-linked recessive (carrier mother).http://ghr.nlm.nih.gov/handbook/illustrations/xlinkrecessivemother.

[19] Patenaude AF, Basili L, Fairclough DL, Li FP: Attitudes of 47 mothers of pediatric oncology patients toward genetic testing for cancer predisposition. J Clin Oncol 1996, 14:415–421.

[20] Biesecker LG, Burke W, Kohane I, Plon SE, Zimmern R: Next-generation sequencing in the clinic: are we ready? Nat Rev Genet 2012, 13:818–824.

[21] Ruccione K, Kramer RF, Moore IK, Perin G: Informed consent for treatment of childhood cancer: factors affecting parents' decision making. J Pediatr Oncol Nurs1991, 8:112–121.

[22] Levi RB, Marsick R, Drotar D, Kodish ED: Diagnosis, disclosure, and informed consent: learning from parents of children with cancer. J Pediatr Hematol Oncol 2000, 22:3–12.

[23] Tabor HK, Stock J, Brazg T, McMillin MJ, Dent KM, Yu JH, Shendure J, Bamshad MJ: Informed consent for whole genome sequencing: a qualitative analysis of participant expectations and perceptions of risks, benefits, and harms. Am J Med Genet A 2012, 158A:1310–1319.

[24] Gurney JG, Davis S, Severson RK, Fang JY, Ross JA, Robison LL: Trends in cancer incidence among children in the U.S. Cancer 1996, 78:532–541.

[25] Joffe S, Cook EF, Cleary PD, Clark JW, Weeks JC: Quality of informed consent in cancer clinical trials: a cross-sectional survey. Lancet 2001, 358:1772–1777.

[26] Robinson JO, Slashinski MJ, Wang T, Hilsenbeck SG, McGuire AL: Participants' recall and understanding of genomic research and large-scale data sharing. J Empir Res Hum Res Ethics 2013, 8:42–52.

[27] Simon CM, Siminoff LA, Kodish ED, Burant C: Comparison of the informed consent process for randomized clinical trials in pediatric and adult oncology. J Clin Oncol 2004, 22:2708–2717.

[28] Lidz CW, Appelbaum PS, Meisel A: Two models of implementing informed consent. Arch Intern Med 1988, 148:1385–1389.

[29] Miller VA, Baker JN, Leek AC, Drotar D, Kodish E: Patient involvement in informed consent for Pediatric Phase I Cancer Research. J Pediatr Hematol Oncol 2014, [Epub ahead of print].

[30] Truong TH, Weeks JC, Cook EF, Joffe S: Outcomes of informed consent among parents of children in cancer clinical trials. Pediatr Blood Cancer 2011, 57:998–1004.

Chapter 13

Primer on Tumor Immunology and Cancer Immunotherapy

Timothy J. Harris[1], Charles G. Drake[2]

[1]Department of Radiation Oncology & Molecular Radiation Sciences, Johns Hopkins University School of Medicine and Sidney Kimmel Comprehensive Cancer Center, Baltimore, MD, USA

[2]Department of Oncology and Brady Urological Institute, Johns Hopkins University School of Medicine and Sidney Kimmel Comprehensive Cancer Center, 1650 Orleans St., CRB I #410, Baltimore, MD 21231, USA

Abstract: Individualized cancer therapy is a central goal of cancer biologists. Immunotherapy is a rational means to this end—because the immune system can recognize a virtually limitless number of antigens secondary to the biology of genetic recombination in B and T lymphocytes. The immune system is exquisitely structured to distinguish self from non-self, as demonstrated by anti-microbial immune responses. Moreover the immune system has the potential to recognize self from "altered-self", which is the case for cancer. However, the immune system has mechanisms in place to inhibit self-reactive responses, many of which are usurped by evolving tumors. Understanding the interaction of cancer with the immune system provides insights into mechanisms that can be exploited to disinhibit anti-tumor immune responses. Here, we summarize the 2012 SITC Primer, reviewing past, present, and emerging immunotherapeutic approaches for the treatment of cancer—including targeting innate versus adaptive immune components; targeting and/or utilizing dendritic cells and T cells; the role of the tumor microenvironment; and immune checkpoint blockade.

Keywords: Immunotherapy, Cancer Vaccine, Immune Checkpoint, Adoptive T Cell Therapy

1. Introduction

The immune system is able to distinguish self from non-self, and is able to vigorously attack non-self and infected self tissues. This is the basis for anti-microbial responses. The immuno-editing theory suggests that the immune system is able to recognize and eradicate subclinical tumors, but at some point equilibrium is reached and the tumor remains in situ, in a state of balance with a partially efficacious response[1]. Unfortunately, many tumors escape from this equilibrium state, and cancer becomes clinically apparent. The goal of the cancer immunotherapist is to understand the mechanisms by which cancer is able to escape the immune system and to therapeutically intervene at critical points to promote anti-tumor immune responses. Broadly, such interventions fall under the umbrella of "immunotherapy" and can include cancer vaccines, cytokine therapy, the administration of monoclonal antibodies to block immune checkpoints, and others. The Society for Immunotherapy of Cancer (SITC) organized a Primer on Tumor Immunology and Cancer Immunotherapy with the assistance of Willem W. Overwijk, PhD (Innate Immunity and Inflammation), Madhav Dhodapkar, MD (Dendritic Cells), Helen Chen, MD (Immunology of Antibodies as Therapy), Susan M. Kaech, PhD (Effector and Memory T Cell Differentiation), Thomas F. Gajewski, MD, PhD (Immunobiology of the Tumor Microenvironment), Jonathan Powell, MD, PhD (T Cell Intracellular Signaling), Pedro J. Romero, MD (Tumor Antigen and Immunogenicity), Charles G. Drake, MD, PhD (Coinhibition and Costimulation), and Cassian Yee, MD (Adoptive Cellular Therapy). Mario Sznol, MD and Charles Drake, MD, PhD served as co-organizers.

2. Review

2.1. Innate Immunity and Inflammation

The innate immune system recognizes pathogens based on repeated patterns and responds quickly with a variety of effector mechanisms. This is in contrast to the adaptive immune system, consisting of T and B cells, which responds more slowly, but which is more specific. An innate immune response is often evidenced by Inflammation: a local response to tissue injury—defined by the presence of Rubor (redness), Calor (heat), Dolor (pain), and Tumor (swelling). The innate immune response functions to eradicate invasive pathogen; limit the spread of infection; initiate adaptive immune responses involving T and B cells; and to initiate tissue repair. Immune responses and inflammation are generally advantageous for the host, and may include suppressing growth of smaller tumors. Interestingly however, inflammation can also promote neoplastic transformation and tumor progression. For example, in a genetically engineered lung cancer model using mice with a mutation in K-ras, cigarette smoke induced inflammation and tumor development through the activation of myeloid cells[2]. In a preclinical model of squamous cell carcinoma related to HPV E6/E7, chronic inflammation caused by lymphocytes and Fc Gamma Receptor signaling on myeloid cells was responsible for malignant transformation, and tumorigenesis could be abrogated via lymphocyte depletion or Fc Gamma Receptor blockade[3]. Mutations within tumors can play a role in this process; BRAF mutations drive tumor cells to produce proinflammatory cytokines like VEGF, IL-10, and IL-6, while at the same time decreasing expression of anti-tumor cytokines such as IL-12[4]. Mutated BRAF also promotes the secretion of IL-1α and IL-1β, innate inflammatory mediators which can drive tumor cells to protect themselves from immune attack by up-regulating molecules that inhibit the function of anti-tumor lymphocytes[5]. Another molecular mechanism linking chronic inflammation to cancer progression involves a transcription factor known as STAT3 (signal transducer and activator of transcription 3). In areas of chronic inflammation, tumors up-regulate activated (phosphorylated) STAT3, which, in addition to being anti-apoptotic, drives expression of cytokines that dysregulate anti-tumor immune responses[6]. Tumors can also cause systemic immunosuppression as noted in preclinical models demonstrating an increase in splenic myeloid suppressor cells, which are a specialized population of innate myeloid cells[7][8]. Taken together, these data provide examples of how the innate immune system can promote tumor progression, and suggest pathways for intervention.

2.2. Dendritic Cells

Dendritic cells (DC) link the innate immune system to the adaptive immune response. These cells dwell in the tissues, continually sampling the microenvironment and taking up antigens primarily through pinocytosis. When the innate immune system is activated in their vicinity, DCs sense this as "danger"[9], cease antigen uptake and travel to local lymph nodes, where their role is to present antigen to specific T lymphocytes. The microenvironment in which a DC acquires antigen determines whether the DC will have the capacity to activate an antigen-specific lymphocyte or to tolerize the lymphocyte. In addition to pinocytosis, immature DCs are also able to internalize antigen through Fc receptor-mediated endocytosis, a process in which Fc receptors on the DC bind antibody-bound antigen. Emerging data suggest that the subtype of Fc receptor involved in antigen internalization helps to determine whether the response to that antigen will be activating or inhibitory[10]. As introduced above, the ultimate outcome of the lymphocyte-DC interaction is based primarily on the state of the DC. DCs can produce distinct cytokine groups that can skew T lymphocytes toward divergent functions. Moreover, triggering distinct Toll-like receptors (TLRs) on DCs elicits different cytokine profiles and different immune responses. Signaling through TLRs 4, 5, or 11 results in DC production of IL-12, which in turn skews T-cells towards a TH1 phenotype capable of promoting anti-tumor immune responses[11]. Signaling through TLRs 1, 2, or 6 causes DCs to produce IL-10, which in turn promotes T-cell development towards regulatory or TH2 phenotypes incapable of promoting anti-tumor immune responses[11]. In mice, a subset of DCs that express CD8 is primarily responsible for priming anti-tumor immune responses[12]. Their human equivalent is thought to be CD141[+] DCs[13]–[16]. These subsets are known to produce IL-12 and cross-present antigens to lymphocytes.

How can our knowledge of DC biology be used to develop immunotherapy for patients? While it is clear that activation of these cells is desirable, there are two general approaches to achieve that end: ex vivo and in vivo activation. Ex vivo strategies for DC-based immunotherapies include generation of DCs from circulating monocytes via subsequent culture, as well as procedures in which DCs are derived from circulating CD34[+] hematopoetic stem cells (HSCs). In the U.S., an immunotherapy based on ex vivo activated DCs has been FDA-approved to treat patients with metastatic prostate cancer. This product, sipuleucel-T is generated by incubating a patient's monocytes with a fusion protein that links the target antigen (Prostatic Acid Phosphatase) to the cytokine GM-CSF; here GM-CSF serves to mature the monocytes toward DCs, and assists in internalization of the antigen.

After ex vivo incubation, the mixed cellular product, including maturing DCs, is re-infused into patients. In a randomized control trial for prostate cancer patients, this product resulted in a 4.1 month improvement in median survival compared to placebo (HR 0.78; P = 0.03)[17]. Another common strategy for DC-based immunotherapy involves maturation of immature monocytes into DCs by culturing them for several days in the presence of GM-CSF and IL-4. The DCs are then loaded with tumor-specific peptides or in some variation with whole protein antigens which they must subsequently process and present[18]. While ex vivo stimulation of DCs often results in quantifiable immune and clinical responses with no dose limiting toxicities, the overall clinical response rates to this therapeutic approach have remained somewhat low[19]. The other major strategy under study is to target antigens specifically to DCs in vivo. This routinely involves the use an adjuvant (e.g. TLR agonist) in combination with signaling antibodies (e.g. anti-CD40, anti-DC-SIGN, anti-MMR, anti-DEC-205) and tumor-specific antigen[20]. In summary, an evolving understanding of DC biology has led to the first commercially approved cellular immunotherapy for the treatment (not prevention) of a solid tumor, and further developments in this field are likely.

2.3. Antibodies as Therapy

Monoclonal antibodies are now widely utilized in the treatment of a number of tumor types; pertinent examples including trastuzumab (anti-Her-2) for the treatment of breast cancer, rituximab (anti-CD20) for the treatment of lymphoma, and the recently approved immunoconjugate T-DM1, which fuses trastuzumab to a highly potent chemotherapy, emtansine (DM1 [deacetyl maytansine]) to facilitate local delivery and minimize systemic toxicity[21]. Antibody-based immunotherapeutics can be exquisitely specific treatment tools, based on the diverse and nanomolar level affinity of the Fv region of the antibody for its target, as well as the ability of the Fc region to engage components of the host immune system. How do monoclonal antibodies work? The mechanisms of action of unconjugated monoclonal antibodies include blocking a pro-survival signal, as well as facilitating tumor cell destruction by the binding of the Fc portion of the antibody to Fc Receptors on natural killer (NK) cells—promoting the ability of NK cells to lyse their targets through a process known as antigen-dependent cytotoxicity (ADCC). Monoclonal antibodies can also mediate cytotoxicity by binding to complement receptors on effector cells, a process known as complement-dependent cytotoxicity

(CDCC). The Fc portion of a monoclonal antibody plays a major role in determining the immune mechanisms induced, with monoclonal antibodies of the human IgG4 isotype primarily functioning as "blockers". One interesting aspect involved in the development of monoclonal antibodies for the clinic involves their affinity, while higher antibody affinity results in increased target engagement and ADCC, higher affinities can also result in decreased tumor penetration and compromised efficacy[22]–[24].

Several recent clinical developments highlight the increasingly prominent role of antibody-based therapy in cancer. In an important recent result, Yu et al. showed an 11% absolute benefit in 2-year survival in patients with advanced neuroblastoma treated with a combination of IL-2, GM-CSF, and an antibody targeting GD2 (disialoganglioside 2) (P = 0.02)[25]. As discussed above, a great deal of recent interest involves conjugating monoclonal antibodies to either a cytotoxic agent, examples include brentuximab vedotin (anti-CD30-MMAE [monomethyl auristatin E]) for anaplastic large cell and Hodgkin lymphoma, trastuzumab emtansine (anti-HER2-DM1) for breast cancer, and glembatumumab vedotin (anti-GPNMB-MMAE) for breast cancer[21][26][27]. In addition, T cells can be re-engineered to express chimeric (antibody-based) antigen receptors (CARs) to target the powerful killing machinery of cytotoxic lymphocytes directly to tumor antigen[28]. CAR transformed T cells have been developed against a variety of antigens, including CEA, CAIX, EGFR, HER2, CD19, and CD20, but serious adverse events have been reported[29][30]. In a particularly relevant report, Porter et al. recently showed that a CAR specific for CD19 could mediate a major clinical response in a patient with chronic lymphocytic leukemia[29]. Another fascinating application of monoclonal antibody technology involves the engineering of bi- specific antibodies, in which one arm carries specificity for a tumor antigen, and the other arm is specific for the CD3 complex on T cells. The idea behind this technology is to physically co-localize lymphocytes to tumors, inducing anti-tumor T cell responses. Bi-specific antibodies against CD19 (blinatumomab) have shown promise in Phase I-II studies[31][32].

2.4. Tumor Microenvironment

In vivo, a tumor is significantly more complex than a simple group of clonogenic cells. The three-dimensional mass that is appreciated on imaging studies contains, in addition to tumor cells, extracelluar matrix components, supportive stromal cells (e.g. neovasculature, fibroblasts, and macrophages), and a number of inflammatory cells. In terms of mounting an anti-tumor immune response, there is further complexity involved, since the priming and effector phases of the immune response are separated by time and space. While priming occurs in lymph nodes, the effector functions must operate within the tumor mass. Potential barriers to anti-tumor responses encountered during the priming phase include a paucity of "danger" signals from innate immune cells, poor recruitment of DCs for cross-presentation, and inadequate expression of costimulatory ligands on tumor cells or APCs. Potential barriers to efficacy during the effector phase involve inadequate recruitment of activated effector T cells secondary to abnormal vascular endothelial cells and/or chemokines, the presence of dominant immune inhibitory mechanisms capable of abrogating T cell effector function (e.g. the inhibitory receptors PD-1 and CTLA-4), extrinsic suppressive cells (T_{REGs}, myeloid-derived suppressor cells), metabolic inhibitors (IDO, arginase), and inhibitory cytokines (IL-10, TGF-β)[33].

The genetic profile of the tumor microenvironment and its potential correlation with anti-tumor immune responses has become an area of increased study in recent years. In one preclinical study of metastatic melanoma, the expression of a subset of chemokines were associated with CD8$^+$ T cell infiltration[34]. In patients with metastatic melanoma, the expression of T cell markers and chemokines correlated with response to a DC-based vaccine[35]. Likewise, a pro-inflammatory gene expression profile within the tumor microenvironment was associated with survival following administration of a protein-based vaccine in patients with metastatic melanoma[36]. Response to CTLA-4 blockade in patients with metastatic melanoma was also correlated with expression of interferon inducible genes and T_H1 associated markers[37]. Finally, expression of T cell homing genes in the tumor vascular endothelium has also been implicated in mitigating lymphocyte infiltration[38]. Two important implications of these data include the potential for improved patient selection for administration of immunotherapeutics and identifying potential strategies for improved response to immunotherapies in patient populations that would otherwise respond poorly to immunologic interventions.

2.5. T Cell Intracellular Signaling

To understand how the adaptive arm of the immune system is engaged, a basic knowledge of T cell biology and activation can be helpful. T cells detect antigenbound to MHC molecules, with the CD4$^+$ T cell subset binding to MHC Class II primarily expressed on APCs while CD8$^+$ T cells are activated by binding to MHC Class I, which can be expressed by APCs as well as normal cells. Following initial APC-driven activation, CD8$^+$ T cells may later recognize target cells expressing their cognate antigen, resulting in cell-mediated cytotoxicity. For T cells to be fully activated, the APC must provideother signals in addition to the peptide/MHC (signal 1). The B7-CD28 interaction, with B7 expressed on the APC and CD28 on T cells, was one of the first co-stimulatory signaling pathways elucidated[39]. CD28 signaling is complex, but most likely functions in part by increasing T cell expression of anti-apoptotic proteins (e.g. Bcl-xL) and autocrine growth factors like IL-2[40][41]. Additional co-stimulatory interactions (APC: T-cell) include OX40L-OX40, CD70-CD27, CD137L-CD137, and B7RP1-ICOS[42]. Ultimately, an effective tumor vaccine requires activating APCs to express appropriate co-stimulatory molecules to promote durable anti-tumor immune responses through intracellular signaling cascades.

Following T cell engagement with appropriately activated APCs, intracellular signaling results in activation of three signaling cascades: NF-AT, NF-kB, and AP-1[43]. Of these, the NF-AT pathway is particularly interesting, since NF-AT signaling in the absence of AP-1 results in immune tolerance, whereas in vivo blockade of NF-AT decreases both T cell activation and limits tolerance[44][45]. Recent data showed that the Adenosine 2a Receptor (A2aR) is a component of the negative feedback loop for T cell activation that is upregulated during T cell activation, and blockade of A2aR has been shown to increase the efficacy of tumor vaccines in pre-clinical models[46].

T cell activation is clearly influenced by the spectrum of cytokines present during antigen recognition, and several cytokines exert their immunologic effects by modulating the function of STAT proteins during T cell activation. In that regard, STAT4 has thus far been demonstrated to be crucial to T cell mediated anti-tumor immune responses. IL-12 activates STAT4, which in turn skews T cells toward a TH1 phenotype and IFN-γ production[6]. Recent data show that, in addition to the canonical pathways such as NF-AT and AP-1, the mTOR (mammalian target of rapamycin) pathway also plays a critical role in T cell activation and function. mTOR is an evolutionarily conserved serine/threonine protein kinase central to integrating nutrient and hormone signaling pathways[47], which in turn regulates SGK1, a protein important in epithelial survival. In preclinical models, SGK1 knockout mice had increased response to tumor immunotherapy compared to mice with functional SGK1, suggesting that mTOR up-regulation dampens or inhibits anti-tumor immunity (unpublished data from Dr. Jonathan D. Powell, Johns Hopkins University). In summary, T cell activation is relatively complex, and is generally only partially understood, but plays a critical role in generating an adaptive anti-tumor immune response.

2.6. Memory T-Cells

Following initial activation, a minority (5%–10%) of T cells become long-lived memory cells with enhanced functional responses upon antigen re-encounter as compared to naïve T cells. For cancer immunotherapy the importance of generating functional memory cells is two-fold. First, the presence of memory cells could potentially decrease metastatic spread and prevent tumor re-growth after an initial response. Second, memory cells could limit de novo induction of a second malignancy. The importance of tumor infiltrating memory T cells is further illustrated with the novel Immunoscore, which has demonstrated prognostic and predictive value in colorectal cancer through the quantification of tumor infiltrating cytotoxic effector cells and memory T cells[48]. Current understanding of memory T cells is derived largely from the study of the immune response to microbes; however, in the absence of good models of memory induction in tumor bearing animals or humans, one can reasonably extrapolate these findings to anti-tumor responses. It was originally hypothesized that memory T cells were selected randomly from the naïve T cell pool during the expansion phase of an effector response; but it is now thought that some T cells are intrinsically more likely than others to persist after an initial response as memory cells[49]. Thus, cells more likely to become memory cells express the IL-7 Receptor alpha (IL-7Rα) chain, CD27 (Tumor Necrosis Factor Receptor Superfamily 7), BCL-2, and downregulate the effector molecule KLRG1 (Killer Cell Lectin-like Receptor Subfamily G1)[50]–[52]. However, this expression profile is not exclusive to memory cells, as there are short-lived IL-7Rα^+ cells that also have high expression of KLRG1[50]. Memory cells also can be divided into three relatively distinct subsets including: (1) "effector-memory" having more cytotoxic function; (2) "central-memory" cells, which likely represent the more classic quiescent memory cell with high proliferative capacity once re-stimulated; and (3) "tissue-resident-memory" associated with an organ-specific distribution in vivo[53].

Multiple models exist for T cell diversification and long-term cell fate. The Separate-Precursor model, which is less feasible compared to other models that will be discussed, states that cells are pre-programmed in the thymus for subsequent development into a memory cell or an effector cell[53]. The Decreasing- Potential model postulates that repetitive exposure to antigen and stimuli drives T cells away from a memory phenotype towards terminal effector differentiation[53]. The Signal-Strength model proposes that memory cell development is dependent on the overall strength of the signals received by the T cell through antigen (signal 1), costimulation (signal 2), and pro-inflammatory cytokines (signal 3)[53]. Finally, the Asymmetric-Cell-Fate model posits that when a T cell encounters an APC and divides while still bound to the APC, the daughter cell that remains attached to the DC (immunologic synapse) will receive greater signals through TCR and costimulation resulting in greater potential for terminal effector differentiation. Conversely, the daughter cell that is not adjacent to the immunologic synapse will have greater potential for memory cell differentiation[53].

Differential transcription factor expression is associated with the memory versus effector transcriptome. T-bet, BLIMP1, ID2, and STAT4 activity are associated with effector T cells[53][54]. Similarly, EOMES, BCL-6, and STAT3 activity are more associated with memory T cells[53][55]. Contemporary modeling supports a graded expression of these transcription factors resulting ultimately in the final lymphocyte phenotype. Additionally, there are metabolic differences between memory and effector T cells. Interestingly, memory cells—being more quiescent as compared to effector T cells—sustain ATP through fatty acid oxidation, whereas effector T cells utilize aerobic glycolysis and lipid synthesis[56]. In that regard, mTOR is at least partially responsible for the aerobic metabolism found in effector T cells[57].

When T cells are continually exposed to antigen, as is often the case for lymphocytes specific for tumor-associated antigens, there exists the potential for such T cells to become "exhausted". T cell exhaustion is characterized by loss of effector cytokine production (IL-2, TNF-α, and IFN-γ), impaired proliferation, and decreased cytotoxicity. Whereas memory T cells require IL-7 and IL-15 for maintenance, exhausted T cells appear to be maintained via continued exposure to antigen. Exhausted T cells also have a distinct transcriptome with upregulation of BLIMP1, EOMES, BATF and down-regulation of T-bet. Furthermore, exhausted lymphocytes express negative regulatory surface molecules including PD-1, LAG-3, TIM-3, 2B4, and CD160[58]. Exhaustion is clearly reversible in some cases, as PD-1 blockade in a viral model of exhaustion was able to rescue the T cells from their exhausted phenotype[59], and blocking these immune checkpoint molecules associated with exhaustion is showing promise in multiple clinical trials[60]. Taken together, these new insights into memory cell differentiation and function offer multiple novel avenues for intervention in terms of generating a productive anti-tumor response.

2.7. Tumor Antigens and Immunogenicity

T cells recognize antigen in the form of small peptides, derived from proteolysed substrates, and presented in the context of MHC molecules. MHC molecules are genetically diverse, and for each MHC variant, only specific peptide sequences from a given antigen are able to bind for presentation to T cells and subsequent induction of anti-tumor immune responses. Understanding the specific antigens recognized by the immune system and the specific peptide sequences presented on MHC can be important in improving immunotherapies directed against a specific antigen. Several approaches have been used to identify tumor specific antigens, including molecular cloning; sequencing of antigenic peptides; and computer algorithms, each of which has its relative benefits and deficiencies.

Multiple processing pathways exist for proteolysis of antigen through the proteosome and presentation in MHC molecules[61]. Determinants of a peptide's ability to induce an immune response (*i.e.* its "antigenicity") include its affinity to the MHC, as well as the affinity of the peptide/MHC complex for a given T Cell Receptor (TCR). A critical facet of this interaction is a set of amino acids which are integral to MHC binding, so-called MHC-anchor-residues. To induce more robust immune responses, it is possible to modify antigenic peptides in several ways. MHC variable peptides (MVP), for example, are peptides designed with amino acid point changes involving MHC-contact residues, usually optimized for improved MHC affinity. Conversely, altered peptide ligands (APL) are peptides with amino acid substitutions designed to optimize interactions with the T cell receptor. These altered peptides have been used in an attempt to augment immune response against a specific antigen[62]. MVPs/APLs have been used in both the preclinical and clinical setting resulting in improved immunogenicity for a number of tumor antigens, including gp100, CEA, and NY-ESO/LAGE-1[63]–[65]. Understanding the specific antigen/peptide associated with anti-tumor immune responses allows for monitoring of ongoing immunologic responses with ex vivo studies including enumeration via tetramer and functionality via IFN-γ production, ELISPOT, lytic activity, functional avidity, and replicative history assayed via enumerating telomere length.

The term "cancer vaccine" encompasses a variety of approaches sharing the common goal of activating and expanding a population of specific T cells to generate an anti-tumor response. A variety of vaccine approaches have been explored, including synthetic peptides, recombinant virus-like particles (VLP), naked/stabilized nucleic acids, recombinant viruses, recombinant bacteria, and dendritic cells. One notable facet of cancer vaccines is that they must provide antigen (signal 1) in addition to a second signal (signal 2) to elicit full effector function. The addition of an appropriate adjuvant to a vaccine (*i.e.* a "danger" signal[9]), can be important in providing Signal 2. Despite a great deal of work, only two cancer vaccines have been approved for clinical use, including Oncophage (Russia, 2008) and Provenge (sipuleucel-T) (USA, 2010). The PSA-targeting viral vaccine ProstVac VF is currently in phase III trials worldwide[17][66]. Although monitoring vaccine responses in peripheral blood is challenging, recent studies suggest that patients treated with sipuleucel-T do mount detectable antigen-specific T and B cells responses, which correlate to some degree with outcome[67]. Clinically, single agent efficacy of most cancer vaccines is less obvious, with objective clinical responses rarely detected[68]. Although multiple mechanisms may underlie this observation, data showing expression of immune checkpoint molecules like PD-1 and CTLA-4 on tumor-specific lymphocytes suggests that combining immune checkpoint blockade with vaccination might be one way to optimize a vaccine-initiated anti-tumor immune response[69].

2.8. Coinhibition and Costimulation in Cancer Immunotherapy

As discussed above, the T-cell/APC interaction involves engagement of the

TCR with the antigen-MHC complex; in addition, costimulation/coinhibition interactions also occur and these secondary receptor/ligand binding events ultimately affect downstream T cell responses. Classically, costimulation involves the interaction of B7-CD28-disruption of this interaction by CTLA-4 expression on T cells, with associated tight binding to B7 is referred to as co-inhibition[39][70]. Early preclinical studies demonstrated that blockade of CTLA-4 could mitigate inhibition of anti-tumor immune responses[71]. This finding was eventually confirmed clinically in Phase III trials in patients with metastatic melanoma[72]. In addition to CTLA-4, tumor infiltrating lymphocytes may express the negative regulatory receptors PD-1, LAG-3, TIM-3 and others[73]-[75]. Preclinical blockade of these pathways results in improved anti-tumor immunity[76]-[78]. Interestingly, a single tumor-infiltrating lymphocyte may express multiple immune checkpoint molecules simultaneously, so it is not surprising that combined blockade suggests improved efficacy in preclinical models[77]. The ligand for PD-1 is PD-L1, and expression of PD-L1 in tumors correlated with patient response to anti-PD-1 therapy[79]. These data would suggest that there could be potential biomarkers for checkpoint blockade therapy. Current preclinical studies are combining checkpoint blockade with tyrosine kinase inhibitors, radiation therapy and cancer vaccines.

2.9. Adoptive Cellular Therapy

Adoptive T cell therapy allows for ex vivo stimulation of lymphocytes in a non-tolerizing environment followed by re-infusion of activated T cells into patients. There are varying sources and types of T cells used for adoptive therapy, these include tumor infiltrating lymphocytes (TILs), T cells engineered to express a cancer-specific TCR, and T cells engineered to express a chimeric antigen receptor (CAR) that combines the extracellular portion of an antibody with the T cell receptor signaling machinery. Of these approaches, expanded TILs are the least labor intensive to produce, yet require an invasive procedure to obtain. Additionally, maintenance of TILs after adoptive transfer usually requires high dose IL-2, which results in significant toxicity. Clinical response rates in patients with metastatic melanoma treated with expanded TILs is impressive, approximately 50% in several studies[80]. Furthermore, pretreatment of patients with lymphodepletion can result in a greater proportion of clinical responses and more durable responses[81]. As previously discussed, host T cells can be re-engineered to express CAR in place of the TCR. The CAR expresses an antibody Fv region in place of the extracellular domain of the TCR allowing the T cell to recognize whole antigen as opposed to MHC-restricted antigen[82]. This approach is efficient and results in T cells with uniform specificity, but is limited to some degree by transduction efficiency and potential toxicity. Another approach to adoptive T cell therapy is the use of endogenous tumor-specific T cells. This approach involves pheresis of circulating tumor-specific T cells, in vitro expansion and activation, and lastly reintroduction into the host via adoptive transfer[83]. This approach is considered to be the most physiologic, but is most labor intensive as it involves multiple pheresis sessions and significant laboratory labor for the expansion and activa-tion steps. Given the recent high-profile success of chimeric antigen receptor modified T cells for patients with CLL, these approaches are attracting increasing attention and enthusiasm[29][84].

3. Conclusions

The immune system is exquisitely poised to recognize and distinguish self from non-self. Further, the immune system is able to recognize self from "altered-self", which is the case for cancer. Although clinically apparent malignancies have likely circumvented endogenous anti-tumor immune responses, immunotherapy has the potential to augment responses in order to mitigate tumor progression. As reviewed above, immune responses can be divided between innate and adaptive responses. Innate immune responses recognize general patterns of non-self (e.g. double-stranded RNA, single-stranded DNA, LPS) and are able to initiate pro-inflammatory responses which in turn can attract immune components leading to adaptive immunity. Adaptive immunity is defined by acquired immunity to specific antigens, and is mediated through B cells via antibody secretion and T cells through cell-mediated immunity. Dendritic cells are antigen presenting cells which function at the crossroads of innate and adaptive immunity and are able to cross-present antigen to, and activate, T cells. Dendritic cells are a target of various immunotherapeutic approaches either through the use of adjuvant cytokines which activate dendritic cells or more directly through the use of dendritic cell vaccines. Antibodies produced by B cells are highly specific for cognate antigen and have been engineered through various mechanisms to simultaneously target the tumor antigen and potentiate anti-tumor immune responses. T cells are ultimately responsible for cell-mediated immune responses, which are thought to be the most important mechanism of immune related tumor killing for solid malignancies. T cells can be activated through antibody blockade of inhibitory signaling, vaccination, or ex vivo stimulation followed by adoptive transfer into patients. A more complete understanding of the cellular and molecular components of the tumor-immune system interaction is crucial to the development of rational and efficacious immunotherapies in the future. This primer serves as a starting point for the cancer biologist and budding immunotherapist to better understand and appreciate the past, present, and future of immunotherapeutics.

Competing Interests

The authors declare that they have no competing interests.

Authors' Contributions

TH and CG contributed equally to the background research and writing of this review. Both authors read and approved the final manuscript.

Source: Harris T J, Drake C G. Primer on tumor immunology and cancer immunotherapy[J]. Journal for Immunotherapy of Cancer, 2013, 1(1):1–9.

References

[1]   Dunn GP, Bruce AT, Ikeda H, Old LJ, Schreiber RD: Cancer immunoediting: from immunosurveillance to tumor escape. Nat Immunol 2002, 3:991–998.

[2]   Takahashi H, Ogata H, Nishigaki R, Broide DH, Karin M: Tobacco smoke promotes lung tumorigenesis by triggering IKKbeta-and JNK1-dependent inflammation. Canc Cell 2010, 17:89–97.

[3]   Andreu P, Johansson M, Affara NI, Pucci F, Tan T, Junankar S, Korets L, Lam J, Tawfik D, DeNardo DG, Naldini L, de Visser KE, De Palma M, Coussens LM: FcRgamma activation regulates inflammation-associated squamous carcinogenesis. Canc Cell 2010, 17:121–134.

[4]   Sumimoto H, Imabayashi F, Iwata T, Kawakami Y: The BRAF-MAPK signaling pathway is essential for cancer-immune evasion in human melanoma cells. J Exp

Med 2006, 203:1651–1656.

[5]   Khalili JS, Liu S, Rodriguez-Cruz TG, Whittington M, Wardell S, Liu C, Zhang M, Cooper ZA, Frederick DT, Li Y, Joseph RW, Bernatchez C, Ekmekcioglu S, Grimm E, Radvanyi LG, Davis RE, Davies MA, Wargo JA, Hwu P, Lizee G: Oncogenic BRAF(V600E) promotes stromal cell-mediated immunosuppression via induction of interleukin-1 in melanoma. Clin Canc Res 2012, 18:5329–5340.

[6]   Yu H, Pardoll D, Jove R: STATs in cancer inflammation and immunity: a leading role for STAT3. Nat Rev Canc 2009, 9:798–809.

[7]   Bronte V, Chappell DB, Apolloni E, Cabrelle A, Wang M, Hwu P, Restifo NP: Unopposed production of granulocyte-macrophage colony-stimulating factor by tumors inhibits CD8+ T cell responses by dysregulating antigen-presenting cell maturation. J Immunol 1999, 162:5728–5737.

[8]   Ugel S, Delpozzo F, Desantis G, Papalini F, Simonato F, Sonda N, Zilio S, Bronte V: Therapeutic targeting of myeloid-derived suppressor cells. Curr Opin Pharmacol 2009, 9:470–481.

[9]   Fuchs EJ, Matzinger P: Is cancer dangerous to the immune system? Semin Immunol 1996, 8:271–280.

[10] Nimmerjahn F, Ravetch JV: Fcgamma receptors as regulators of immune responses. Nat Rev Immunol 2008, 8:34–47.

[11] Pulendran B, Ahmed R: Translating innate immunity into immunological memory: implications for vaccine development. Cell 2006, 124:849–863.

[12] Hashimoto D, Miller J, Merad M: Dendritic cell and macrophage heterogeneity in vivo. Immunity 2011, 35:323–335.

[13] Bachem A, Guttler S, Hartung E, Ebstein F, Schaefer M, Tannert A, Salama A, Movassaghi K, Opitz C, Mages HW, Henn V, Kloetzel PM, Gurka S, Kroczek RA: Superior antigen cross-presentation and XCR1 expression define human CD11c+ CD141+ cells as homologues of mouse CD8+ dendritic cells. J Exp Med 2010, 207:1273–1281.

[14] Crozat K, Guiton R, Contreras V, Feuillet V, Dutertre CA, Ventre E, Vu Manh TP, Baranek T, Storset AK, Marvel J, Boudinot P, Hosmalin A, Schwartz-Cornil I, Dalod M: The XC chemokine receptor 1 is a conserved selective marker of mammalian cells homologous to mouse CD8alpha+ dendritic cells. J Exp Med 2010, 207:1283–1292.

[15] Jongbloed SL, Kassianos AJ, McDonald KJ, Clark GJ, Ju X, Angel CE, Chen CJ, Dunbar PR, Wadley RB, Jeet V, Vulink AJ, Hart DN, Radford KJ: Human CD141+ (BDCA-3) + dendritic cells (DCs) represent a unique myeloid DC subset that cross-presents necrotic cell antigens. J Exp Med 2010, 207:1247–1260.

[16] Poulin LF, Salio M, Griessinger E, Anjos-Afonso F, Craciun L, Chen JL, Keller AM, Joffre O, Zelenay S, Nye E, Le Moine A, Faure F, Donckier V, Sancho D, Cerundolo

V, Bonnet D, Reis e Sousa C: Characterization of human DNGR-1+ BDCA3+ leukocytes as putative equivalents of mouse CD8alpha + dendritic cells. J Exp Med 2010, 207:1261–1271.

[17] Kantoff PW, Higano CS, Shore ND, Berger ER, Small EJ, Penson DF, Redfern CH, Ferrari AC, Dreicer R, Sims RB, Xu Y, Frohlich MW, Schellhammer PF: Sipuleu-cel-T immunotherapy for castration-resistant prostate cancer. N Engl J Med 2010, 363:411–422.

[18] Dhodapkar MV, Steinman RM, Sapp M, Desai H, Fossella C, Krasovsky J, Donahoe SM, Dunbar PR, Cerundolo V, Nixon DF, Bhardwaj N: Rapid generation of broad T-cell immunity in humans after a single injection of mature dendritic cells. J Clin Invest 1999, 104:173–180.

[19] Rosenberg SA, Yang JC, Restifo NP: Cancer immunotherapy: moving beyond current vaccines. Nat Med 2004, 10:909–915.

[20] Palucka K, Banchereau J, Mellman I: Designing vaccines based on biology of human dendritic cell subsets. Immunity 2010, 33:464–478.

[21] Verma S, Miles D, Gianni L, Krop IE, Welslau M, Baselga J, Pegram M, Oh DY, Dieras V, Guardino E, Fang L, Lu MW, Olsen S, Blackwell K: Trastuzumab emtan-sine for HER2-positive advanced breast cancer. N Engl J Med 2012, 367:1783–1791.

[22] Fujimori K, Covell DG, Fletcher JE, Weinstein JN: A modeling analysis of monoclonal antibody percolation through tumors: a binding-site barrier. J Nucl Med 1990, 31:1191–1198.

[23] Adams GP, Schier R, McCall AM, Simmons HH, Horak EM, Alpaugh RK, Marks JD, Weiner LM: High affinity restricts the localization and tumor penetration of single-chain fv antibody molecules. Canc Res 2001, 61:4750–4755.

[24] Rudnick SI, Lou J, Shaller CC, Tang Y, Klein-Szanto AJ, Weiner LM, Marks JD, Adams GP: Influence of affinity and antigen internalization on the uptake and penetration of Anti-HER2 antibodies in solid tumors. Canc Res 2011, 71:2250–2259.

[25] Yu AL, Gilman AL, Ozkaynak MF, London WB, Kreissman SG, Chen HX, Smith M, Anderson B, Villablanca JG, Matthay KK, Shimada H, Grupp SA, Seeger R, Reynolds CP, Buxton A, Reisfeld RA, Gillies SD, Cohn SL, Maris JM, Sondel PM: An-ti-GD2 antibody with GM-CSF, interleukin-2, and isotretinoin for neuroblastoma. N Engl J Med 2010, 363:1324–1334.

[26] Pro B, Advani R, Brice P, Bartlett NL, Rosenblatt JD, Illidge T, Matous J, Ramchandren R, Fanale M, Connors JM, Yang Y, Sievers EL, Kennedy DA, Shustov A: Brentuximab vedotin (SGN-35) in patients with relapsed or refractory systemic anaplastic large-cell lymphoma: results of a phase II study. J Clin Oncol 2012, 30:2190–2196.

[27] Rose AA, Grosset AA, Dong Z, Russo C, Macdonald PA, Bertos NR, St-Pierre Y, Simantov R, Hallett M, Park M, Gaboury L, Siegel PM: Glycoprotein nonmetastatic B is an independent prognostic indicator of recurrence and a novel therapeutic target

in breast cancer. Clin Canc Res 2010, 16:2147–2156.

[28] Sadelain M, Brentjens R, Riviere I: The promise and potential pitfalls of chimeric antigen receptors. Curr Opin Immunol 2009, 21:215–223.

[29] Porter DL, Levine BL, Kalos M, Bagg A, June CH: Chimeric antigen receptor-modified T cells in chronic lymphoid leukemia. N Engl J Med 2011, 365: 725–733.

[30] Morgan RA, Yang JC, Kitano M, Dudley ME, Laurencot CM, Rosenberg SA: Case report of a serious adverse event following the administration of T cells transduced with a chimeric antigen receptor recognizing ERBB2. Mol Ther 2010, 18:843–851.

[31] Bargou R, Leo E, Zugmaier G, Klinger M, Goebeler M, Knop S, Noppeney R, Viardot A, Hess G, Schuler M, Einsele H, Brandl C, Wolf A, Kirchinger P, Klappers P, Schmidt M, Riethmuller G, Reinhardt C, Baeuerle PA, Kufer P: Tumor regression in cancer patients by very low doses of a T cell-engaging antibody. Science 2008, 321:974–977.

[32] Topp MS, Gokbuget N, Zugmaier G, Degenhard E, Goebeler ME, Klinger M, Neumann SA, Horst HA, Raff T, Viardot A, Stelljes M, Schaich M, Kohne-Volland R, Bruggemann M, Ottmann OG, Burmeister T, Baeuerle PA, Nagorsen D, Schmidt M, Einsele H, Riethmuller G, Kneba M, Hoelzer D, Kufer P, Bargou RC: Long-term follow-up of hematologic relapse-free survival in a phase 2 study of blinatumomab in patients with MRD in B-lineage ALL. Blood 2012, 120:5185–5187.

[33] Gajewski TF, Fuertes M, Spaapen R, Zheng Y, Kline J: Molecular profiling to identify relevant immune resistance mechanisms in the tumor microenvironment. Curr Opin Immunol 2011, 23:286–292.

[34] Harlin H, Meng Y, Peterson AC, Zha Y, Tretiakova M, Slingluff C, McKee M, Gajewski TF: Chemokine expression in melanoma metastases associated with CD8+ T-cell recruitment. Canc Res 2009, 69:3077–3085.

[35] Gajewski T, Zha Y, Thurner B, Schuler G: Association of gene expression profile in metastatic melanoma and survival to a dendritic cell-based vaccine. J Clin Oncol 2009, 27:9002.

[36] Ulloa-Montoya F, Louahed J, Dizier B, Gruselle O, Spiessens B, Lehmann FF, Suciu S, Kruit WH, Eggermont AM, Vansteenkiste J, Brichard VG: Predictive Gene Signature in MAGE-A3 Antigen-Specific Cancer Immunotherapy. J Clin Oncol 2013, 31:2388–2395.

[37] Ji RR, Chasalow SD, Wang L, Hamid O, Schmidt H, Cogswell J, Alaparthy S, Berman D, Jure-Kunkel M, Siemers NO, Jackson JR, Shahabi V: An immune-active tumor microenvironment favors clinical response to ipilimumab. Canc Immunol Immunother 2012, 61:1019–1031.

[38] Buckanovich RJ, Facciabene A, Kim S, Benencia F, Sasaroli D, Balint K, Katsaros D, O'Brien-Jenkins A, Gimotty PA, Coukos G: Endothelin B receptor mediates the endothelial barrier to T cell homing to tumors and disables immune therapy. Nat Med

2008, 14:28–36.

[39] Azuma M, Cayabyab M, Buck D, Phillips JH, Lanier LL: CD28 interaction with B7 costimulates primary allogeneic proliferative responses and cytotoxicity mediated by small, resting T lymphocytes. J Exp Med 1992, 175:353–360.

[40] Yang SY, Denning SM, Mizuno S, Dupont B, Haynes BF: A novel activation pathway for mature thymocytes. Costimulation of CD2 (T, p50) and CD28 (T, p44) induces autocrine interleukin 2/interleukin 2 receptor-mediated cell proliferation. J Exp Med 1988, 168:1457–1468.

[41] Boise LH, Minn AJ, Noel PJ, June CH, Accavitti MA, Lindsten T, Thompson CB: CD28 costimulation can promote T cell survival by enhancing the expression of Bcl-XL. Immunity 1995, 3:87–98.

[42] Driessens G, Kline J, Gajewski TF: Costimulatory and coinhibitory receptors in anti-tumor immunity. Immunol Rev 2009, 229:126–144.

[43] Sieber M, Baumgrass R: Novel inhibitors of the calcineurin/NFATc hub - alternatives to CsA and FK506? Cell Commun Signal 2009, 7:25.

[44] Macian F, Garcia-Cozar F, Im SH, Horton HF, Byrne MC, Rao A: Transcriptional mechanisms underlying lymphocyte tolerance. Cell 2002, 109:719–731.

[45] Iannone R, Casella JF, Fuchs EJ, Chen AR, Jones RJ, Woolfrey A, Amylon M, Sullivan KM, Storb RF, Walters MC: Results of minimally toxic nonmyeloablative transplantation in patients with sickle cell anemia and beta-thalassemia. Biol Blood Marrow Transplant 2003, 9:519–528.

[46] Ohta A, Gorelik E, Prasad SJ, Ronchese F, Lukashev D, Wong MK, Huang X, Caldwell S, Liu K, Smith P, Chen JF, Jackson EK, Apasov S, Abrams S, Sitkovsky M: A2A adenosine receptor protects tumors from antitumor T cells. Proc Natl Acad Sci USA 2006, 103:13132–13137.

[47] Powell JD, Pollizzi KN, Heikamp EB, Horton MR: Regulation of immune responses by mTOR. Annu Rev Immunol 2012, 30:39–68.

[48] Angell H, Galon J: From the immune contexture to the Immunoscore: the role of prognostic and predictive immune markers in cancer. Curr Opin Immunol 2013, 25:261–267.

[49] Antia R, Ganusov VV, Ahmed R: The role of models in understanding CD8+ T-cell memory. Nat Rev Immunol 2005, 5:101–111.

[50] Sarkar S, Kalia V, Haining WN, Konieczny BT, Subramaniam S, Ahmed R: Functional and genomic profiling of effector CD8 T cell subsets with distinct memory fates. J Exp Med 2008, 205:625–640.

[51] Hendriks J, Gravestein LA, Tesselaar K, van Lier RA, Schumacher TN, Borst J: CD27 is required for generation and long-term maintenance of T cell immunity. Nat Immunol 2000, 1:433–440.

[52] Grayson JM, Zajac AJ, Altman JD, Ahmed R: Cutting edge: increased expression of Bcl-2 in antigen-specific memory CD8+ T cells. J Immunol 2000, 164:3950–3954.

[53] Kaech SM, Cui W: Transcriptional control of effector and memory CD8+ T cell differentiation. Nat Rev Immunol 2012, 12:749–761.

[54] Joshi NS, Cui W, Chandele A, Lee HK, Urso DR, Hagman J, Gapin L, Kaech SM: Inflammation directs memory precursor and short-lived effector CD8(+) T cell fates via the graded expression of T-bet transcription factor. Immunity 2007, 27:281–295.

[55] Banerjee A, Gordon SM, Intlekofer AM, Paley MA, Mooney EC, Lindsten T, Wherry EJ, Reiner SL: Cutting edge: The transcription factor eomesodermin enables CD8+ T cells to compete for the memory cell niche. J Immunol 2010, 185:4988–4992.

[56] Pearce EL: Metabolism in T cell activation and differentiation. Curr Opin Immunol 2010, 22:314–320.

[57] Chi H: Regulation and function of mTOR signalling in T cell fate decisions. Nat Rev Immunol 2012, 12:325–338.

[58] Wherry EJ: T cell exhaustion. Nat Immunol 2011, 12:492–499.

[59] Barber DL, Wherry EJ, Masopust D, Zhu B, Allison JP, Sharpe AH, Freeman GJ, Ahmed R: Restoring function in exhausted CD8 T cells during chronic viral infection. Nature 2006, 439:682–687.

[60] Pardoll DM: The blockade of immune checkpoints in cancer immunotherapy. Nat Rev Canc 2012, 12:252–264.

[61] Vigneron N, van den Eynde BJ: Insights into the processing of MHC class I ligands gained from the study of human tumor epitopes. Cell Mol Life Sci 2011, 68:1503–1520.

[62] Edwards LJ, Evavold BD: T cell recognition of weak ligands: roles of signaling, receptor number, and affinity. Immunol Res 2011, 50:39–48.

[63] Salgaller ML, Marincola FM, Cormier JN, Rosenberg SA: Immunization against epitopes in the human melanoma antigen gp100 following patient immunization with synthetic peptides. Canc Res 1996, 56:4749–4757.

[64] Iero M, Squarcina P, Romero P, Guillaume P, Scarselli E, Cerino R, Carrabba M, Toutirais O, Parmiani G, Rivoltini L: Low TCR avidity and lack of tumor cell recognition in CD8(+) T cells primed with the CEA-analogue CAP1-6D peptide. Canc Immunol Immunother 2007, 56:1979–1991.

[65] Valmori D, Dutoit V, Lienard D, Rimoldi D, Pittet MJ, Champagne P, Ellefsen K, Sahin U, Speiser D, Lejeune F, Cerottini JC, Romero P: Naturally occurring human lymphocyte antigen-A2 restricted CD8+ T-cell response to the cancer testis antigen NY-ESO-1 in melanoma patients. Canc Res 2000, 60:4499–4506.

[66] Kim JW, Gulley JL: Poxviral vectors for cancer immunotherapy. Expert Opin Biol Ther 2012, 12:463–478.

[67] Sheikh NA, Petrylak D, Kantoff PW, Dela Rosa C, Stewart FP, Kuan LY, Whitmore JB, Trager JB, Poehlein CH, Frohlich MW, Urdal DL: Sipuleucel-T immune parameters correlate with survival: an analysis of the randomized phase 3 clinical trials in men with castration-resistant prostate cancer. Canc Immunol Immunother 2013, 62:137–147.

[68] Wood C, Srivastava P, Bukowski R, Lacombe L, Gorelov AI, Gorelov S, Mulders P, Zielinski H, Hoos A, Teofilovici F, Isakov L, Flanigan R, Figlin R, Gupta R, Escudier B: An adjuvant autologous therapeutic vaccine (HSPPC-96; vitespen) versus observation alone for patients at high risk of recurrence after nephrectomy for renal cell carcinoma: a multicentre, open-label, randomised phase III trial. Lancet 2008, 372:145–154.

[69] Sierro SR, Donda A, Perret R, Guillaume P, Yagita H, Levy F, Romero P: Combination of lentivector immunization and low-dose chemotherapy or PD-1/PD-L1 blocking primes self-reactive T cells and induces anti-tumor immunity. Eur J Immunol 2011, 41:2217–2228.

[70] Tivol EA, Borriello F, Schweitzer AN, Lynch WP, Bluestone JA, Sharpe AH: Loss of CTLA-4 leads to massive lymphoproliferation and fatal multiorgan tissue destruction, revealing a critical negative regulatory role of CTLA-4. Immunity 1995, 3:541–547.

[71] Chambers CA, Kuhns MS, Egen JG, Allison JP: CTLA-4-mediated inhibition in regulation of T cell responses: mechanisms and manipulation in tumor immunotherapy. Annu Rev Immunol 2001, 19:565–594.

[72] Hodi FS, O'Day SJ, McDermott DF, Weber RW, Sosman JA, Haanen JB, Gonzalez R, Robert C, Schadendorf D, Hassel JC, Akerley W, van den Eertwegh AJ, Lutzky J, Lorigan P, Vaubel JM, Linette GP, Hogg D, Ottensmeier CH, Lebbe C, Peschel C, Quirt I, Clark JI, Wolchok JD, Weber JS, Tian J, Yellin MJ, Nichol GM, Hoos A, Urba WJ: Improved survival with ipilimumab in patients with metastatic melanoma. N Engl J Med 2010, 363:711–723.

[73] Sfanos KS, Bruno TC, Meeker AK, De Marzo AM, Isaacs WB, Drake CG: Human prostate-infiltrating CD8+ T lymphocytes are oligoclonal and PD-1+. Prostate 2009, 69:1694–1703.

[74] Matsuzaki J, Gnjatic S, Mhawech-Fauceglia P, Beck A, Miller A, Tsuji T, Eppolito C, Qian F, Lele S, Shrikant P, Old LJ, Odunsi K: Tumor-infiltrating NY-ESO-1-specific CD8+ T cells are negatively regulated by LAG-3 and PD-1 in human ovarian cancer. Proc Natl Acad Sci USA 2010, 107:7875–7880.

[75] Fourcade J, Sun Z, Benallaoua M, Guillaume P, Luescher IF, Sander C, Kirkwood JM, Kuchroo V, Zarour HM: Upregulation of Tim-3 and PD-1 expression is associated with tumor antigen-specific CD8+ T cell dysfunction in melanoma patients. J Exp Med 2010, 207:2175–2186.

[76] Iwai Y, Ishida M, Tanaka Y, Okazaki T, Honjo T, Minato N: Involvement of PD-L1 on tumor cells in the escape from host immune system and tumor immunotherapy by PD-L1 blockade. Proc Natl Acad Sci USA 2002, 99:12293–12297.

[77] Woo SR, Turnis ME, Goldberg MV, Bankoti J, Selby M, Nirschl CJ, Bettini ML, Gravano DM, Vogel P, Liu CL, Tangsombatvisit S, Grosso JF, Netto G, Smeltzer MP, Chaux A, Utz PJ, Workman CJ, Pardoll DM, Korman AJ, Drake CG, Vignali DA: Immune inhibitory molecules LAG-3 and PD-1 synergistically regulate T-cell function to promote tumoral immune escape. Canc Res 2012, 72:917–927.

[78] Ngiow SF, von Scheidt B, Akiba H, Yagita H, Teng MW, Smyth MJ: Anti-TIM3 antibody promotes T cell IFN-gamma-mediated antitumor immunity and suppresses established tumors. Canc Res 2011, 71:3540–3551.

[79] Topalian SL, Hodi FS, Brahmer JR, Gettinger SN, Smith DC, McDermott DF, Powderly JD, Carvajal RD, Sosman JA, Atkins MB, Leming PD, Spigel DR, Antonia SJ, Horn L, Drake CG, Pardoll DM, Chen L, Sharfman WH, Anders RA, Taube JM, McMiller TL, Xu H, Korman AJ, Jure-Kunkel M, Agrawal S, McDonald D, Kollia GD, Gupta A, Wigginton JM, Sznol M: Safety, activity, and immune correlates of anti-PD-1 antibody in cancer. N Engl J Med 2012, 366:2443–2454.

[80] Dudley ME, Wunderlich JR, Robbins PF, Yang JC, Hwu P, Schwartzentruber DJ, Topalian SL, Sherry R, Restifo NP, Hubicki AM, Robinson MR, Raffeld M, Duray P, Seipp CA, Rogers-Freezer L, Morton KE, Mavroukakis SA, White DE, Rosenberg SA: Cancer regression and autoimmunity in patients after clonal repopulation with antitumor lymphocytes. Science 2002, 298:850–854.

[81] Rosenberg SA, Yang JC, Sherry RM, Kammula US, Hughes MS, Phan GQ, Citrin DE, Restifo NP, Robbins PF, Wunderlich JR, Morton KE, Laurencot CM, Steinberg SM, White DE, Dudley ME: Durable complete responses in heavily pretreated patients with metastatic melanoma using T-cell transfer immunotherapy. Clin Canc Res 2011, 17:4550–4557.

[82] Ertl HC, Zaia J, Rosenberg SA, June CH, Dotti G, Kahn J, Cooper LJ, Corrigan-Curay J, Strome SE: Considerations for the clinical application of chimeric antigen receptor T cells: observations from a recombinant DNA Advisory Committee Symposium held June 15, 2010. Canc Res 2011, 71:3175–3181.

[83] Chapuis AG, Thompson JA, Margolin KA, Rodmyre R, Lai IP, Dowdy K, Farrar EA, Bhatia S, Sabath DE, Cao J, Li Y, Yee C: Transferred melanoma-specific CD8+ T cells persist, mediate tumor regression, and acquire central memory phenotype. Proc Natl Acad Sci USA 2012, 109:4592–4597.

[84] Kalos M, Levine BL, Porter DL, Katz S, Grupp SA, Bagg A, June CH: T cells with chimeric antigen receptors have potent antitumor effects and can establish memory in patients with advanced leukemia. Sci Transl Med 2011, 3:95ra73.

Chapter 14

Diagnosis and Treatment of Solid Pseudopapillary Tumor of the Pancreas: Experience of One Single Institution from Turkey

Ayşe Yagcı[1], Savas Yakan[2], Ali Coskun[2], Nazif Erkan[2], Mehmet Yıldırım[2], Evrim Yalcın[1], Hakan Postacı[1]

[1]Department of Pathology, M.D, SB Izmir Bozyaka Education and Research Hospital, Izmir, Turkey
[2]Department of Surgery, M.D, SB Izmir Bozyaka Education and Research Hospital, Izmir, Turkey

Abstract: Background: Solid pseudopapillary neoplasia (SPN) of the pancreas is an extremely rare epithelial tumor of low malignant potential. SPN accounts for less than 1% to 2% of exocrine pancreatic tumors. The aim of this study is to report our experience with SPN of the pancreas. It includes a summary of the current literature to provide a reference for the management of this rare clinical entity. Methods: A retrospective analysis was performed of all patients diagnosed and treated for SPN in our hospital over the past 15 years (1998 to 2013). A database of the characteristics of these patients was developed, including age, gender, tumor location and size, treatment, and histopathological and immunohistochemical features. Results: During this time period, 255 patients with pancreatic malignancy (which does not include ampulla vateri, distal choledocal and duodenal tumor) were admitted to our department, only 10 of whom were diagnosed as having SPN (2.5%). Nine patients were women (90%) and one patient was a man (10%). Their median age was 38.8 years (range 18 to 71). The most common symptoms were abdominal pain and dullness. Seven patients (70%) presented with abdominal pain or abdominal dullness and three patient (30%) were asymptomatic with the diagnosis made by an incidental finding on routine examination. Abdominal computed tomography and/or magnetic resonance imaging showed the typical features of solid pseudopapillary neoplasm in six (60%) of the patients. Four patients underwent distal pancreatectomy with splenectomy, one patient underwent a total mass excision, and one patient underwent total pancreatic resection. Two required extended distal pancreatectomy with splenectomy. Two underwent spleen-preserving distal pancreatectomy. Conclusions: SPN is a rare neoplasm that primarily affects young women. The prognosis is favorable even in the presence of distant metastasis. Although surgical resection is generally curative, a close follow-up is advised in order to diagnose a local recurrence or distant metastasis and choose the proper therapeutic option for the patient.

Keywords: Solid Pseudopapillary Neoplasia, Diagnosis, Treatment

1. Background

Solid pseudopapillary neoplasia (SPN) of the pancreas is an extremely rare epithelial tumor of low malignant potential. SPN accounts for less than 1% to 2% of exocrine pancreatic tumors[1]. Until it was defined by the World Health Organization (WHO) in 1996 as "solid pseudopapillary tumor" of the pancreas, this tumor was described by using various names including "solid cystic tumor", "papillary cystic tumor", "papillary epithelial neoplasia", "solid and papillary epithelial neoplasia", "papillary epithelial tumor" and "Frantz's tumor", "solid and papillary tumor", "solid-cysticpapillary epithelial neoplasm", "benign or malignant papillary tumor of the pancreas"[2]. These tumors typically occur in young women during the second to fourth decade of life and are histologically characterized by cystic areas and solid pseudopapillary arranged cells. The origin of these tumors is still a matter of controversy.

In this study, we report our experience with SPN of the pancreas and include a summary of the current literature to provide a reference for the management of this rare clinical entity.

2. Methods

A retrospective analysis was carried out of all patients diagnosed and treated for SPN in our hospital over the past 15 years (1998 to 2013). A database of the characteristics of these patients was developed, including age, gender, tumor location (data were derived from radiological investigations or surgical records) and size (data were derived from radiological investigations or surgical records and finally confirmed by pathology), treatment (data were derived from the medical records, including the types of surgery), and histopathological and immunohisto-chemical features. Pre-operative fine needle aspiration cytology FNAC) was performed in one patient. All the patients who underwent resection were followed up every six months. The investigations performed included routine blood studies, chest X-ray, CA-19-9 level and either an ultrasound or computed tomography (CT) scan of the abdomen.

This study was approved by the Local Institutional Review Board of Izmir Bozyaka Education and research hospital.

3. Results

During this time period, of 255 patients with pancreatic malignancy (which does not include ampulla vateri, distal choledocal and duodenal tumor) admitted to our department, only 10 were diagnosed as having SPN (2.5%). Nine patients were women (90%) and one patient was a man (10%). The patients had a median age of 38.8 years (range 18 to 71). The most common symptoms were abdominal pain and dullness. Seven patients (70%) presented with abdominal pain or abdominal dullness and three patients (30%) were asymptomatic with the diagnosis made by an incidental finding on routine examination. Abdominal CT and/or magnetic resonance imaging (MRI) showed the typical features of solid pseudopapillary neoplasm in six (60%) of the patients (**Figure 1**). Tumor markers (AFP, CEA, CA 19–9 and CA 125) were normal preoperatively in all patients. Usually, the tumors appeared as well-circumscribed lesions with a mixed cystic and solid component

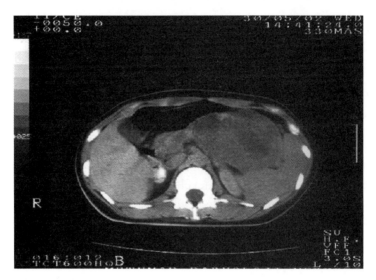

Figure 1. Magnetic resonance imaging shows that the tumor is a well-marginated, large, encapsulated, solid and cystic mass with areas of hemorrhagic degeneration, as revealed by high signal intensity.

but were almost entirely solid or else cystic with thick walls. In one patient the tumor was located in the pancreatic head (10%), in four patients in the body (40%) and in the remaining five patients in the tail (50%). Four patients underwent distal pancreatectomy with splenectomy, one patient underwent a total mass excision and one patient underwent total pancreatic resection. Two required extended distal pancreatectomy with splenectomy. Two underwent spleen-preserving distal pancreatectomy. The mean diameter of the tumor was 8 cm (range 3 to 13 cm). Patient characteristics are summarized in **Table 1**.

In eight cases lymph node dissection was done in a number between 4 and 14, whereas no dissection was needed for two patients. No lymph node metastasis was present in any patient. Macroscopically, there was diffuse hemorrhage and minimal necrosis between solid and cystic areas (**Figure 2**). At histopathological examination, tumor mass separated from pancreas with a fibrous capsule was seen. Pseudopapillary, cystic and solid growth patterns were seen in the tumor mass. Tumor cells had an ovally shaped, small and centrally localized nucleus and large eosinophilic cytoplasm. Tumors consisted of pseudo-papillary structures made of cells aligned around fine vessels, solid areas, hemorrhagic areas and cystic areas of different size (**Figure 3**). No mitosis was seen in five cases, whereas minimal mitosis was present in two cases (2/10 per high powered field) and multiple mitosis

Table 1. Patients characteristics.

	Patient 1	Patient 2	Patient 3	Patient 4	Patient 5	Patient 6	Patient 7	Patient 8	Patient 9	Patient 10
Age/Gender	30/F	18/F	21/F	18/F	62/F	50/F	40/F	33/F	71/F	45/M
Operation	Distal pancreatectomy + splenectomy	Distal pancreatectomy + splenectomy	Total mass exicion	Spleen preserving distal pancreatectomy	Distal pancreatectomy + splenectomy	Subtotal distal pancreatectomy + splenectomy	Total pancreatectomy	Distal pancreatectomy + splenectomy	Subtotal distal pancreatectomy + splenectomy	Spleen preserving distal pancreatectomy
Tumor location	Body	Tail	Head	Tail	Tail	Body + Tail	Head + Body	Tail	Body + Tail	Tail
Size (cm)	9 × 7 × 5	13 × 9 × 6.5	13 × 6 × 5.5	6.5 × 5.7 × 36	4.5 × 3.5 × 3.2	12.5 × 11 × 6	4.3 × 3 × 3	4 × 3 × 2	11 × 7 × 7	3 × 3 × 2
Invasion	(–)	Capsule and spleen	(–)	(–)	(–)	Capsule	(–)	(–)	Capsule	(–)
Nodal status	0/14	0/10	(–)	(–)	0/6	0/14	0/4	0/7	0/11	0/5
Follow-up	Healthy	Healthy	Healthy	Healthy	Healthy	7th month Liver and omental Metastasis 9th month exitus	29th day biliary and pancrea-tic fistula, 41th day exitus	Healthy	20th month Liver and omental Metastasis 24th month exitus	Healthy

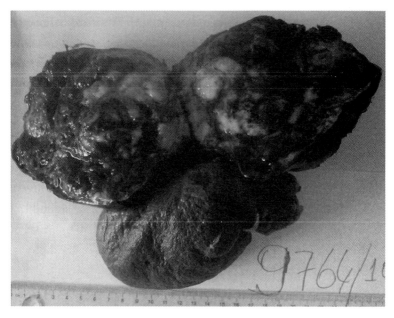

Figure 2. Macroscopic appearance of distal pancreatectomy + splenectomy specimen by SPN showing the solid and cystic component with hemorrhagic areas. SPN, solid pseudopapillary neoplasia.

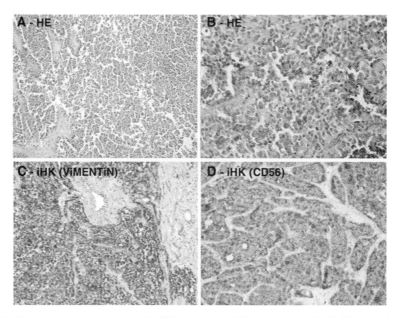

Figure 3. Histologic appearance of solid pseudopapillar tumors. (A) Solid pseudopapillar tumors exhibit a pseudopapillary pattern. (B) A portion of the tumor tissue shows a collection of hyaline globules. (C) Tumor cells typically show strong immunoreactivity for vimentin in the cytoplasm. (D) CD56 shows positive cytoplasmic membranous staining.

were present in two cases (20/10 per high powered field; case numbers 6 and 9) (**Table 2**). The immunohistochemistry profiles are summarized in **Table 3**. Capsular invasion was present in three cases (case numbers 2, 6 and 9), spleen invasion was also present in case number 2. Along with capsular invasion, mitosis, nuclear polymorphism and necrosis were also significant in case numbers 6 and 9 at the time of diagnosis. These two cases were considered as malignant SPN and treated with six courses of gemcitabine+ cis-platinum chemotherapy. Multiple liver and omentum metastases developed in case number 2 at the seventh postoperative month; this patient died at the ninth month. Multiple liver and omentum metastases developed in case number 9 at the 20th postoperative month and she died at the 24th month. The other eight cases have been followed up closely for an average of 7.9 years (between 1 and 16 years) and no recurrence or metastasis has been seen.

4. Discussion

SPN is very rare; in fact, they only constitute about 5% of cystic pancreatic tumors and about 1% to 2% of exocrine pancreatic neoplasms[3]. They present mainly in the second and third decades of life[4]. Our series presented with a median age of 38.8 years, which is significantly older than in the literature (median age of 26 years)[5][6]. The origin of solid pseudopapillary tumors still remains unclear. These neoplasms have been suggested to have a ductal epithelial, neuroendocrine, multipotent primordial cell, or even an extra-pancreatic genital ridge angle-related cell origin[7].

The clinical presentation of the tumor is usually non-specific. Abdominal discomfort or vague pain is the most common symptom, followed by a gradually enlarging mass and compression signs induced by the tumor. Some patients are completely asymptomatic, with the tumor detected incidentally by imaging studies or routine physical examination. Usually there is no evidence of pancreatic insufficiency, abnormal liver function tests, cholestasis, elevated pancreatic enzymes or an endocrine syndrome. Tumor markers are also generally unremarkable[4][8]. In our series, seven patients (70%) presented with abdominal pain or abdominal dullness, three patients (30%) were asymptomatic with the diagnosis made by an incidental finding on routine examination and preoperative tumor markers (AFP, CEA, CA 19-9 and CA 125) were within normal limits in all patients.

Table 2. Histopathologic features.

	Patient 1	Patient 2	Patient 3	Patient 4	Patient 5	Patient 6	Patient 7	Patient 8	Patient 9	Patient 10
Development pattern	Solid, cystic, papillary	Cystic, papillary	Cystic, solid, papillary	Cystic, papillary	Cystic, solid, papillary	Solid, cystic, papillary	Solid, cystic, papillary	Solid, cystic, papillary	Solid, cystic, papillary	Cystic + papillary
Necrosis	(−)	minimal	minimal	(−)	(−)	(+)	(−)	(−)	(+)	(−)
Mitosis	(−)	(−)	2/10 per HPF	2/10 per HPF	2/10 per HPF	20/10 per HPF	(−)	(−)	20/10 per HPF	(−)
Pleomorphism	minimal	(−)	minimal	minimal	minimal	manifest	minimal	(−)	manifest	(−)

Table 3. The immunohistochemistry study.

	Patient 1	Patient 2	Patient 3	Patient 4	Patient 5	Patient 6	Patient 7	Patient 8	Patient 9	Patient 10
Cytokeratin	Focal (+)	Focal (+)	Focal (+)	Focal (+)	Focal (+)	(−)	Focal (+)	(−)	(−)	(−)
CEA	(−)	(−)	(−)	(−)	(−)	(−)	(−)	(−)	(−)	(−)
Vimentin	(+)	(+)	(+)	(+)	(+)	Focal (+)	(+)	(+)	(+)	(+)
Chromogranin	(−)	(−)	(−)	(−)	Focal strong (+)	(−)	(−)	(−)	(−)	(−)
Neuron specific enolase	(+)	(+)	(+)	Focal slight (+)	(−)	(+)	(+)	(+)	(+)	(+)
CD10	(+)	Slight (+)	(+)	(+)	Focal (+)	(+)	(+)	(+)	(+)	(+)
CD56	Slight (+)	Slight (+)	(+)	(+)	(−)	(+)	(+)	(+)	(+)	(+)
Synaptophysin	Focal (+)	Focal (+)	Focal (+)	(−)	(+)	Slight focal (+)	Slight focal (+)	(−)	(−)	(−)
P53	Focal slight (+)	(−)	(−)	(−)	(−)	10% (+)	5% (+)	(−)	10% (+)	(−)
Ki67	(−)	(−)	(−)	(−)	Under 1% (+)	10% (+)	3% (+)	(−)	10% (+)	(−)
Progesterone	(−)	(+)	(+)	(−)	(+)	(−)	(+)	(+)	(−)	(+)
EMA	Rare (+)	Rare cells (+)	Rare cells (+)	Rare cells (+)	(−)	Rare cells (+)	(−)	(−)	(−)	(−)

SPN can occur in every part of the pancreas but they are slightly more common in the tail[3]. Grossly, it appears as a large and encapsulated mass, generally well-demarcated from the remaining pancreas. In fact, invasion of the adjacent organs, such as the spleen or the duodenal wall, is rare. Depending on the tumor position (head, body or tail of the pancreas), the differential diagnosis includes adrenal mass, pancreatic endocrine tumor, liver cyst or tumor, or a pseudocyst[9].

Abdominal ultrasound and CT show a well encapsulated, complex mass with both solid and cystic components and displacement of nearby structures. There may be calcifications at the periphery of the mass and intravenous contrast enhancement inside the mass suggesting hemorrhagic necrosis[10]. However, when compared with MR imaging, CT has inherent limitations in showing certain tissue characteristics, such as hemorrhage, cystic degeneration, or the presence of a capsule. These features may, as shown at pathology, be suggestive of specific lesions such as SPN of the pancreas. Therefore, MR imaging may further aid in showing these characteristics and in the differential diagnosis of complex cystic masses within the pancreas[11]. Despite the technological improvements, preoperative diagnosis is difficult because of the similarity of findings among cystic lesions. Some studies advocate preoperative endosonography guided fine-needle aspiration biopsy for preoperative detection of the tumor, but this may not be accepted by others because of the uncertainty in diagnosis and the possible tumor spread[12][13]. In our series, preoperative endosonography guided fine-needle aspiration biopsy was performed in one out of ten patients and histology confirmed SPN.

In approximately 85% of the patients, SPN is limited to the pancreas, while about 10% to 15% of tumors have already metastasized at the time of presentation[14]. The most common sites for metastasis are the liver, regional lymph nodes, mesentery, omentum and peritoneum.

Once the diagnosis of SPN is made, surgery is the first choice of treatment. SPN is usually surrounded by a pseudocapsule and exhibits benign or low-grade malignancy. Conservative resection with preservation of as much pancreatic tissue as possible is the treatment of choice. According to the location of the tumor, distal pancreatectomy with or without splenectomy, pylorous preserving pancreatoduodenectomy, Whipple operation or enucleation can be performed. In our series, four patients underwent distal pancreatectomy with splenectomy, one patient underwent a total mass excision and one patient underwent total pancreatic resection. Two required extended distal pancreatectomy with splenectomy. Two underwent spleen-preserving distal pancreatectomy. Many studies have demonstrated that less aggressive surgical procedures could be preferred for the treatment of SPN[15]. Extensive lymphatic dissection or more radical approaches are not indicated when the disease is localized. Local invasion and metastases are not contraindications for resection. Portal vein resection is advocated when there is evidence of tumor invasion. For the metastases, surgical debulking should be performed, in contrast to other pancreatic malignancies. Metastases can be removed with enucleations or lobectomies and some patients with unresectable SPN may also have a long term survival[14]. The overall five-year survival rate of patients with SPN is about 95%[8].

Malignant SPN, designated as a solid-pseudopapillary carcinoma, occurs in 15% of adult patients. According to the WHO classification system, these are: 1) solid-pseudopapillary neoplasms with borderline malignancy potential; and 2) solid-pseudopapillary carcinomas. Criteria which distinguish potentially malignant tumors and which are classified as 'SP carcinoma' are: 1) angioinvasion; 2) perineural invasion; and 3) deep invasion of the surrounding pancreatic parenchyma. A recent study showed that some histological features, such as extensive necrosis, nuclear atypia, high mitotic rate, immunohisto-chemistry findings of expression of Ki-67 and sarcomatoid areas may be associated with aggressive behavior[16].

Adjuvant therapy is used only in a small number of patients because of the high resectability of SPN. The role of chemotherapy or chemoradiotherapy in the treatment of SPN is also unclear. In some studies, adjuvant chemotherapy and radiotherapy are reported in some unresectable cases with good results[17][18]. Neoadjuvant chemotherapy or chemoradiotherapy is also reported to have been successful in a few cases[19]–[22].

In the light of previous studies, our two patients (patients number 6 and 9) had capsular invasion besides significant mitosis (20/10 per HPF), nuclear pleomorphism and necrosis at the time of diagnosis and Ki-67 index was 10% (+). These two patients were accepted as having malignant SPN. They were given gemcitabine+ cis-platinum chemotherapy. Multiple liver and omentum metastases developed in case number 2 at the seventh postoperative month; she died at the ninth postoperative month. Multiple liver and omentum metastases developed in case number 9 at the 20th postoperative month and she died at the 24th postoperative month.

5. Conclusions

SPN is a rare neoplasm that primarily affects young women. The prognosis is favorable even in the presence of distant metastasis. Although surgical resection is generally curative, a close follow-up is advised in order to diagnose a local recurrence or distant metastasis and choose the proper therapeutic option for the patient.

6. Abbreviations

SPN: Solid pseudopapillary neoplasia; HPF: High-power fields; CT: Abdominal computed tomography; MRI: Magnetic resonance imaging.

Competing Interests

The authors declare that they have no competing interests.

Authors' Contributions

AY and SY participated in the data acquisition, data analysis, literature review and drafted the manuscript of this article. AC, NE and MY planned the analysis, participated in data acquisition, data analysis, literature review, patient treatment, and drafting and critical revision of the manuscript. EY and HP participated in immunohistochemisty and data analysis. All authors read and approved the final manuscript.

Source: Yagcı A, Yakan S, Coskun A, et al. Diagnosis and treatment of solid pseudopapillary tumor of the pancreas: experience of one single institution from Turkey[J]. World Journal of Surgical Oncology, 2013, 11(1):1–7.

References

[1]   Martin RC, Klimstra DS, Brennan MF, Conlon KC: Solid pseudopapillary tumor of the pancreas: a surgical enigma? Ann Surg Oncol 2002, 9:35–40.

[2]   Kloppel G, Solcia E, Longnecker DS, Capella C, Sobin LH: Histological typing of tumors of the exocrine pancreas. In [World Health Organization International Histological Classification of Tumours]. 2nd edition. Berlin, Heidelberg, New York: Springer; 1996:8452/1. ISBN [ISBN 3-540-60280-1].

[3]   Klimstra DS, Wenig BM, Heffess CS: Solid pseudopapillary tumor of the pancreas: a typically cystic carcinoma of low malignant potential. Semin Diagn Pathol 2000, 17:66–80.

[4]   Yu PF, Hu ZH, Wang XB, Guo JM, Cheng XD, Zhang YL, Xu Q: Solid pseudopapillary tumor of the pancreas: a review of 553 cases in Chinese literature. World J Gastroenterol 2010, 16:1209–1214.

[5]   Lam KY, Lo CY, Fan ST: Pancreatic solid-cystic-papillary tumor: clinico pathologic features in eight patients from Hong Kong and review of the literature. World J Surg 1999, 23:1045–1050.

[6]   Nishihara K, Nagoshi M, Tsuneyoshi M, Yamaguchi K, Hayashi I: Papillary cystic tumor of the pancreas. Assessment of their malignant potential. Cancer 1993, 71:82–92.

[7]   Eder F, Schulz HU, Röcken C, Lippert H: Solid-pseudopapillary tumor of the pancreatic tail. World J Gastroenterol 2005, 11:4117–4119.

[8]   Papavramidis T, Papavramidis S: Solid pseudopapillary tumors of the pancreas: review of 718 patients reported in English literature. J Am Coll Surg 2005, 200:965–972.

[9]   Canzonieri V, Berretta M, Buonadonna A, Libra M, Vasquez E, Barbagallo E, Bearz A, Berretta S: Solid pseudopapillary tumour of the pancreas. Lancet Oncol 2003, 4:255–256.

[10] Dong PR, Lu DS, Degregario F, Fell SC, Au A, Kadell BM: Solid and papillary neoplasm of the pancreas: Radiological-pathological study of five cases and review of the literature. Clin Radiol 1996, 51:702–705.

[11] Cantisani V, Mortele KJ, Levy A, Glickman JN, Ricci P, Passariello R, Ros PR, Silverman SG: MR imaging features of solid pseudopapillary tumor of the pancreas in adult and pediatric patients. Am J Roentgenol 2003, 181:395–401.

[12] Bardales RH, Centeno B, Mallery JS, Lai R, Pochapin M, Guiter G, Stanley MW: Endoscopic ultrasound-guided fine-needle aspiration cytology diagnosis of solid-pseudopapillary tumor of the pancreas: a rare neoplasm of elusive origin but characteristic cytomorphologic features. Am J Clin Pathol 2004, 121:654–662.

[13] Raffel A, Cupisti K, Krausch M, Braunstein S, Trobs B, Goretzki PE, Willnow U: Therapeutic strategy of papillary cystic and solid neoplasm (PCSN): a rare non-endocrine tumor of pancreas in children. Surg Oncol 2004, 13:1–6.

[14] Mao C, Guvendi M, Domenico DR, Kim K, Thomford NR, Howard JM: Papillary cystic and solid tumors of the pancreas: A pancreatic embryonic tumor? Studies of three cases and cumulative review of the world's literature. Surgery 1995, 118:821–828.

[15] Zhang H, Liang TB, Wang WL, Shen Y, Ren GP, Zheng SS: Diagnosis and treatment of solid-pseudopapillary tumor of the pancreas. Hepatobiliary Pancreat Dis Int 2006, 5:454–458.

[16] Tang LH, Aydin H, Brennan MF, Klimstra DS: Clinically aggressive solid pseudopapillary tumor of the pancreas. A report of two cases with components of undifferentiated carcinoma and a comparative clinicopathologic analysis of 34 conventional cases. Am J Surg Pathol 2005, 29:512–519.

[17] Fried P, Cooper J, Balthazar E, Fazzini E, Newall J: A role for radiotherapy in the treatment of solid and papillary neoplasms of the pancreas. Cancer 1985, 56:2783–2785.

[18] Matsuda Y, Imai Y, Kawata S, Nishikawa M, Miyoshi S, Saito R, Minami Y, Tarui S: Papillary cystic neoplasm of the pancreas with multiple hepatic metastases: a case report. Gastroenterology Jpn 1987, 22:379–384.

[19] Strauss JF, Hirsch VJ, Rubey CN, Pollock M: Resection of a solid and papillary epithelial neoplasm of the pancreas following treatment with cisplatinum and 5-fluorouracil: a case report. Med Pediatr Oncol 1993, 21:365–367.

[20] Das G, Bhuyan C, Das BK, Sharma JD, Saikia BJ, Purkystha J: Spleen-preserving distal pancreatectomy following neoadjuvant chemotheraphy for papillary solid and cystic neoplasm of pancreas. Indian J Gastroenterol 2004, 23:188–189.

[21] Maffuz A, Bustamante FT, Silva JA, Torres-Vargas S: Preoperative gemcitabine for unresectable, solid pseudopapillary tumour of the pancreas. Lancet Oncol 2005, 6:185–186.

[22] Zauls JA, Dragun AE, Sharma AK: Intensity-modulated radiation therapy for unresectable solid pseudopapillary tumor of the pancreas. Am J Clin Oncol 2006, 29:639–640.

Chapter 15

Multiple Tumor Marker Protein Chip Detection System in Diagnosis of Pancreatic Cancer

Fangfeng Liu[1], Futian Du[2], Xiao Chen[1]

[1]Department of Hepatobiliary Surgery, Shandong Provincial Hospital Affiliated to Shandong University, 9677 Jingshi Road, Jinan 250021, Shandong Province, China
[2]Department of Hepatobiliary Surgery, People's Hospital of Weifang, Weifang 261041, Shandong Province, China

Abstract: Background: The clinical stage of the disease at diagnosis often determines the prognosis and survival rate of a patient with pancreatic cancer. Early symptoms of pancreatic cancer are often not obvious on imaging (ultrasound, computed tomography (CT), and so on), and when patients present with weight loss, jaundice and abdominal pain and other symptoms, they are usually already in the advanced stages of pancreatic cancer. However, the examination of combined tumor markers might improve their sensitivity or specificity in aiding diagnosis. Methods: Twelve tumor markers including AFP, CEA, NSE, CA125, CA15-3, CA242, CA19-9, PSA, f-PSA, FER, β-HCG and HGH were measured by the protein biochip detection in serum in 235 pancreatic cancer patients, 230 benign pancreatic disease patients and 240 healthy people. Results: Positive detection rates of tumor markers were: CA19-9 (49.3%), CA125 (45.1%), FER (44.2%), CA242 (42.5%), CEA (38.6%), CA15-3 (36.7%), β-HCG (29.6%), AFP (24.5%), NSE (18.2%), PSA (19.5%), f-PSA (9.4%) and HGH (8.7%) respectively. There was significant difference in CA19-9, NSE, CEA, CA242 and CA125 by multi-tumor marker protein biochip detection among patients with cancer, benign disease and healthy people (P < 0.05). The positive rate of 5 tumor markers was 94.9%, and this was much higher than that of any single marker. Conclusion: The detection of CA19-9, NSE, CEA, CA242 and CA125 in the multi-tumor marker protein bio-chip system is helpful in the diagnosis of pancreatic cancer.

Keywords: Tumor Marker, Protein Biochip, Pancreatic Cancer

1. Background

Early detection of cancer has improved the survival of patients with many types of cancer and is critical for future improvements in effectively treating the disease[1]. The detection of serum tumor markers is an effective and non-invasive diagnostic or prognostic tool for pancreatic cancer. The two major reasons that most tumor markers are not used for tumor screening are their low sensitivity and specificity, resulting in low detection rates and unacceptable false-positive diag-noses[2]. The examination of combined tumor markers might improve the sensitiv-ity or specificity[3].

The purpose of this study was to evaluate the diagnostic value of multi-tumor marker protein biochip detection for pancreatic cancer. This protein biochip system quantitatively measured 12 common tumor markers, including cancer an-tigen (CA)125, CA15-3, CA19-9, CA242, carcinoembryonic antigen (CEA), R-fetoprotein (AFP), prostate specific antigen (PSA), free-prostate specific antigen (f-PSA), humangrowth hormone (HGH), β-human chorionicgonadotropin (β-HCG), neuronspecific enolase (NSE) and ferritin (FER), in the serum and was tested in clinically confirmed cancer patients and apparently healthy individuals. The value of this biochip in cancer screening of apparently healthy populations and in cancer patients is discussed.

2. Methods

2.1. Patients and Serum Samples

From June 2012 to October 2013, 235 patients (150 men and 85 women, median age 61 years, range 20 to 78 years) with pancreatic cancer were included in the studygroup. One hundred and fifteen patients were treated with pancreaticoduodenectomy or distal pancreatectomy and 120 patients underwent a palliative operation. According to the TNM Classification, fifth edition[4], there were 22 stage I patients, 140 stage II patients and 73 stage III patients. The location of tumor was divided into head (48 cases), body/tail (146 cases) and the whole pancreas (59 cases). The tumor size was divided into equal to (12 cases) and smaller than 5cm (154 cases), or larger than 5cm (69 cases) in diameter. All diagnoses were confirmed by histology of postoperative or cytology of intraoperative biopsy examination. In addition, there were 230 benign pancreatic diseases (100 chronic pancreatitis and 130 benign adenomas, including 61 men and 39 women, age ranging from 20 to 82 years), and 240 blood donors and other volunteers known to be ingood health.

2.2. Sample Preparation

Horseradish peroxidase (HRP) and chemiluminescence sub strates (Super-Signal Femto maximum sensitivity) were purchased from Pierce (Rockford, IL, USA). Antigens and antibodies were produced in our laboratory. Antibody conjugation was done according to Nakane and Kawaio's article[5].

2.3. Sample Measurement

One point five microliters of each of the 12 capture antibodies, with an average concentration of 1mg/mL, were arrayed in duplicates on a 1×1cm nitrocellulose membrane. The array consisted of a 5×5 matrix with 12 pairs of antibody spots and 1 blank spot as control. After spotting, the membrane was mounted with a plastic mold and blocked with 10% BSA. Each protein chip was incubated with 100μL of serum, rinsed and washed with TBST (0.1 mol Tris-HCl, 8.5g NaCl, 1 mL Tween 20, pH 7.6). The chip was then incubated with 100μL of HRP-labeled antibodies for 30 minutes at 37°C and again rinsed and washed with TBST. Chemiluminescence substrates were added for 1 minute. Light signals were captured with the self-built chip reader based on a CCD camera and controlled with a computer system using self-developed software. The workflow of the chip detection system is shown in **Figure 1**.

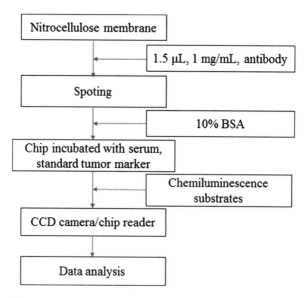

Figure 1. The workflow of the chip detection system.

2.4. Statistical Analysis

Due to non-normal distribution of the raw data, a logarithmic transformation was needed. Data collected were subjected to appropriate transformation (square root) before analysis of variance was performed and means were separated by SAS-SNK (P < 0.05) test (SAS Institute, Cary, NC, USA; 1989).

3. Results

Positive detection rates of tumor markers were: CA19-9 (49.3%), CA125 (45.1%), FER (44.2%), CA242 (42.5%), CEA (38.6%), CA15-3 (36.7%), β-HCG (29.6%), AFP (24.5%), NSE (18.2%), PSA (19.5%), f-PSA (9.4%) and HGH (8.7%) respectively (**Table 1**).

There was significant difference in CA19-9, NSE, CEA, CA242, CA125 by multi-tumor marker protein biochip detection among patients with cancer, benign disease and apparently healthy people (P < 0.05). We took the normal value of tumor marker serum level as cut-off value to determine the negative or positive likelihood of pancreatic cancer. The positive rate of 5 tumor markers was 94.9%,

Table 1. Twelve (C-12) protein biochip test results of healthy, benign pancreatic and pancreatic cancer subjects.

	Pancreatic cancer (n = 235)	Benign pancreatic disease (n = 230)
CA19-9 (U/ml)	49.3%	14.2%
CA125 (U/ml)	47.3%	13.6%
FER (ng/ml)	43.2%	49.2%
CA242 (U/ml)	42.7%	23.6%
CEA (ng/ml)	36.4%	14.8%
CA15-3 (U/ml)	28.7%	0
β-HCG (mIU/ml)	25.5%	0
AFP (ng/ml)	20.4%	0
NSE (ng/ml)	18.9%	0
PSA (ng/ml)	13.5%	0
f-PSA (ng/ml)	14.1%	0

Source of the curve: —— The combined five markers, − − - CEA, · · · CA125, · · · CA15-3, —— Reference line.

which was much higher than that of any single marker (**Table 2**). **Figure 2** shows the receiver operating characteristic (ROC) curves of the 5 markers. The diagnostic performance of markers was ranked according to the area under the curves.

It was noticed that the CA19-9 levels were significantly higher in patients with cancer of the pancreatic body and tail than of the pancreatic head ($P = 0.047$). There was no correlation of serum CEA and CA242 with tumor location ($P > 0.05$). The serum levels of CEA, CA19-9, and CA242 were obviously higher in stage III patients than in stages I and II ($P < 0.05$). However, the serum levels of CEA, CA19-9 and CA242 in patients with pancreatic cancer were not affected by the tumor size ($P > 0.05$) (**Table 3**).

4. Discussion

Due to their limited specificity, the measurement of a single tumor marker is

Table 2. Positive rate of pancreatic cancer versus benign pancreatic disease.

	Healthy (n = 240)	Benign pancreatic (n = 230)	Pancreatic cancer (n = 235)	P-value (SNK method)
CA19-9 (U/ml)	4.5 ± 2. 8	16.4 ± 19.2	203.8 ± 296.5	0. 0008
CA125 (U/ml)	2.9 ± 2. 6	18.9 ± 28.7	174.6 ± 266.2	0. 0016
FER (ng/ml)	118.9 ± 62.6	320.9 ± 285	373.8 ± 385.5	0. 5579
CA242 (U/ml)	2.3 ± 0.8	9.3 ± 14.7	130.5 ± 150.5	0. 0035
CEA (ng/ml)	1.1 ± 0.5	1.87 ± 2.3	13.5 ± 27.1	0. 0392
CA15-3 (U/ml)	5.1 ± 4.2	13.4 ± 6.8	79.4 ± 82.3	0. 0584
β-HCG (mIU/ml)	0.1 ± 0.1	0.5 ± 0.4	8.96 ± 12.8	0. 0694
AFP (ng/ml)	3.3 ± 2.4	1.6 ± 1.8	14.5 ± 36.8	0. 0568
NSE (ng/ml)	1.3 ± 0.8	2.1 ± 2.3	7.9 ± 12.8	0. 0179
PSA (ng/ml)	0.3 ± 0.2	0.6 ± 0.5	1.5 ± 2.38	0. 0575
f-PSA (ng/ml)	0.1 ± 0.1	0.2 ± 0.2	0.6 ± 0.6	0. 1046
HGH (ng/ml)	0.1 ± 0.2	0.8 ± 0.7	4.5 ± 4.8	0. 0564

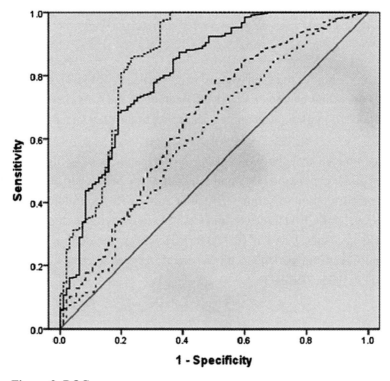

Figure 2. ROC curve.

Table 3. The relationship between the serum markers and the location, size, and TNM stage of pancreatic cancer.

Group	Number	CEA		CA19-9		CA242	
		Value (ng/ml)	P-value	Value (ng/ml)	P-value	Value (ng/ml)	P-value
Tumor location head	48	20.6 ± 42.6		756.6 ± 1,228.2		58.3 ± 55.3	
Body/tail	146	28.0 ± 33.1		2,902.5 ± 3,308.3		76.1 ± 72.1	
Whole	59	74.9 ± 232.1	$P > 0.5$	1,517.3 ± 2,928.6	$P < 0.5$	72.6 ± 60.3	$P > 0.5$
Tumor size							
≤5cm	166	23.7 ± 39.1		1,113.4 ± 2,660.4		45.2 ± 48.1	
>5cm	69	23.9 ± 36.3	$P > 0.5$	1,258.9 ± 5,002.3	$P > 0.5$	59.1 ± 60.3	$P > 0.5$
TNM stage							
I	22	14.1 ± 16.6		1,126.6 ± 1,425.9		57.6 ± 54.4	
II	140	12.7 ± 28.3		845.0 ± 2,000.7		53.9 ± 52.1	
III	73	90.3 ± 212.8	$P < 0.5$	2,976.6 ± 3,513.2	$P < 0.5$	97.6 ± 67.1	$P < 0.5$

usually not sufficient to diagnose cancer. Impressive integration efforts are demonstrated by the ability to perform on-chip trypsin digestion, separation and injection into a mass spectrometer with a single device[6]. Elevated levels of the proteins CEA, AFP, hCG-β, FER, CA15-3, CA19-9, and CA125 can be associated with lung, pancreatic, breast, colorectal, and other types of cancer[7]–[10]. Several studies have shown that the measurement of panels of tumor markers can improve their diagnostic value[5]–[8]. In previous reports, the levels of serum CEA, CA19- 9 and CA242 in patients with pancreatic cancer were higher than those of other malignant diseases and benign pancreatic diseases[7][11]. Here, we found that the combination of CEA and CA242 could increase the specificity to 94.9% in the diagnosis of pancreatic cancer. This is important in helping to differentiate pancreatic cancer from other malignancies and benign pancreatic diseases.

5. Conclusion

The biosensor system described here is suitable for the measurement of a wide range of biomarkers. We compared the serum levels of CA19-9, CA125, FER, CA242, CEA, CA15-3, β-HCG, AFP, NSE, PSA, f-PSA and HGH associated with pancreatic cancer, and found that simultaneous analysis of them was important for the diagnosis of pancreatic cancer. The detection of CA19-9, NSE, CEA, CA242 and CA125 in the multi-tumor markers protein biochip system is helpful in the diagnosis of pancreatic cancer.

6. Statement

The study was approved by the local ethical committee and all individuals provided written informed consent for study participation.

7. Abbreviations

CT: computed tomography; ROC: Receiver operating characteristic; CA15-3: carbohydrate antigen 15-3; β-HCG: β-human chorionic gonadotrophin; AFP: α-fetoprotein; NSE: 2-phospho-D-glycerate hydrolase; PSA: prostate specific antigen; f-PSA: free-prostate specific antigen; HGH: human growth Hormone.

Competing Interests

The authors declare that they have no competing interests.

Authors' Contribution

LF and DF conceived of and designed the experiments. LF performed the experiments and wrote the paper. DF analyzed the data. CX contributed reagents/materials/analysis tools. All authors read and approved the final manuscript.

Source: Liu F, Du F, Xiao C. Multiple tumor marker protein chip detection system in diagnosis of pancreatic cancer[J]. World Journal of Surgical Oncology, 2014, 12(12):1–4.

References

[1] Hollingsworth MA: Translational Implications of Molecular genetics for Early Diagnosis of Pancreatic Cancer. Springer New York: Molecular genetics of Pancreatic Cancer; 2013:75–82.

[2] Sun Z, Fu X, Zhang L, Yang X, Liu F, Hug: A protein chip system for parallel analysis of multi-tumor markers and its application in cancer detection. Anticancer Res 2004, 24(2C):1159–1166.

[3] Zhao XY, Yu SY, Da SP, Dai L,guo XZ, Dai XJ, Wang YM: A clinical evaluation of serological diagnosis for pancreatic cancer. World J gastroenterol 1998, 4:147–149.

[4] Sobin LH, Fleming ID: TNM classification of malignant tumors. Cancer1997, 80(9):1803–1804.

[5] Nakane PK, Kawaoi A: Peroxidase-labeled antibody a new method of conjugation. J Histochem Cytochem 1974, 22(12):1084–1091.

[6] Mouradian S: Lab-on-a-chip: applications in proteomics. Curr Opin Chem Biol 2002, 6(1):51–56.

[7] Carpelan-Holmstrom M, Louhimo J, Stenman UH, Alfthan H, Haglund C: CEA, CA 19-9 and CA 72-4 improve the diagnostic accuracy ingastrointestinal cancers. Anticancer Res 2001, 22(4):2311–2316.

[8] Louhimo J, Finne P, Alfthan H, Stenman UH, Haglund C: Serum HCGβ, CA 72-4 and CEA are independent prognostic factors in colorectal cancer. Int J Cancer 2002, 101(6):545–548.

[9] Hayakawa T, Naruse S, Kitagawa M, Ishiguro H, Kondo T, Kurimoto K, Fukushima M, Takayama T, Horiguchi Y, Kuno N, Noda A, Furukawa T: A prospective multicenter trial evaluating diagnostic validity of multivariate analysis and individual serum marker in differential diagnosis of pancreatic cancer from benign pancreatic diseases. Int J Pancreatol 1999, 25(1):23–29.

[10] Wilson MS, Nie W: Multiplex measurement of seven tumor markers using an electrochemical protein chip. Anal Chem 2006, 78(18):6476–6483.

[11] Haglund C: Tumour marker antigen CA125 in pancreatic cancer: a comparison with CA19-9 and CEA. Br J Cancer 1986, 54:897–901.

Chapter 16

Serum Irisin Levels Are Lower in Patients with Breast Cancer: Association with Disease Diagnosis and Tumor Characteristics

Xeni Provatopoulou[1], Georgia P. Georgiou[2], Eleni Kalogera[1], Vasileios Kalles[3], Maira A. Matiatou[2], Ioannis Papapanagiotou[2], Alexandros Sagkriotis[1], George C. Zografos[2], Antonia Gounaris[1]

[1]Research Center, Hellenic Anticancer Institute, Athens, Greece
[2]1st Department of Propaedeutic Surgery, Hippokratio Hospital, School of Medicine, University of Athens, Athens, Greece
[3]2nd Department of Surgery, Naval and Veterans Hospital of Athens, Athens, Greece.

Abstract: Background: Irisin is a recently discovered myokine, involved in the browning of white adipose tissue. To date, its function has been mainly associated with energy homeostasis and metabolism, and it has been proposed as a promising therapeutic target for obesity and metabolic diseases. This is the first study investigating the role of irisin in human breast cancer. Methods: Participants included one hundred and one (101) female patients with invasive ductal breast cancer and fifty one (51) healthy women. Serum levels of irisin, leptin, adiponectin and resistin were quantified in duplicates by ELISA. Serum levels of CEA, CA 15-3 and Her-2/neu were measured on an immunology analyzer. The association between irisin and breast cancer was examined by logistic regression analysis. The feasibility of serum irisin in discriminating breast cancer patients was assessed by ROC curve analysis. Potential correlations with demographic, anthropometric and clinical parameters, with markers of adiposity and with breast tumor characteristics were also investigated. Results: Serum levels of irisin were significantly lower in breast cancer patients compared to controls (2.47 ± 0.57 and $3.24 \pm 0.66 \mu g/ml$, respectively, $p < 0.001$). A significant independent association between irisin and breast cancer was observed by univariate and multivariate analysis ($p < 0.001$). It was estimated that a 1 unit increase in irisin levels leads to a reduction in the probability of breast cancer by almost 90%. Irisin could effectively discriminate breast cancer patients at a cut-off point of $3.21 \mu g/ml$, with 62.7% sensitivity and 91.1% specificity. A positive association with tumor stage and marginal associations with tumor size and lymph node metastasis were observed ($p < 0.05$, $p < 0.01$, $p < 0.01$, respectively). Conclusions: Our novel findings implicate irisin in breast cancer and suggest its potential application as a new diagnostic indicator of the presence of disease.

Keywords: Irisin, Serum Levels, Breast Cancer, Diagnostic Indicator

1. Background

Irisin is a newly discovered myokine, secreted from muscle tissue as a cleavage product of fibronectin type III domain containing 5 (FNDC5), after shedding of the extracellular portion of the transmembrane protein into extracellular space[1]. It has a molecular weight of approximately 12 KDa and its amino acid sequence is highly conserved among most mammalian species, suggesting a highly conserved function[1]. Even though the predominant source of irisin is skeletal muscle, it was recently reported that adipose tissue also expresses and secretes irisin, suggesting that it may function not only as a myokine, but also as an adipokine[2]. Interestingly, irisin has a different pattern of secretion depending on the anatomical location of adipose tissue, with subcutaneous adipose tissue secreting more protein than visceral adipose tissue[2]. A recent comprehensive immunohistochemical study of irisin expression in human tissues indicated that the protein is locally produced in several central and peripheral tissues, potentially acting as a gatekeeper of metabolic energy regulation[3].

Irisin appears to exert a variety of functions, which are not yet fully eluci-dated. One of its main roles appears to be associated with the browning of white adipose tissue (beige cell formation), known to be involved in thermo-genesis and energy expenditure[4][5]. According to the proposed mechanism, skeletal muscle releases several myokines to the circulation during physical activity, in-cluding peroxisome proliferator-activated receptor Y coactivator 1α (PGC1α). The activation of PGC1α induces FNDC5 secretion, which is proteolytically cleaved to irisin. Irisin subsequently acts on both brown and white adipose tissue (BAT and WAT, respectively)[6]. Its primary effect on BAT is the activation of uncoupling protein 1 (UCP1) in mitochondria, resulting in the dissipation of energy in the form of heat also known as energy expenditure[7][8]. The effect of irisin on WAT is the induction of BAT-like phenotypic changes. More specifical-ly, it increases the expression of PGC1α and UCP1 as well as oxygen consump-tion, while it downregulates genes that are characteristic of WAT, process known as browning[1]. Altogether, these effects are associated with higher energy ex-penditure, which can further lead to the reduction of body weight and the im-provement of metabolic parameters. As a result, irisin was originally proposed and investigated for its role as an exercise hormone and as a potential new agent for the treatment of obesity and metabolic diseases[9]-[18].

Obesity is a well-recognized risk factor for numerous diseases including metabolic, cardiovascular, and malignant diseases[19][20]. Obese women are at an increased risk of breast cancer and typically present more aggressive disease, poorer outcomes and higher mortality rates[21]-[25]. A number of mechanisms have been proposed to mediate the link between obesity and breast cancer development, including adipose tissue-induced increased secretion of estrogens, insulin and in-sulin-like growth factors and altered production of adipokines[26][27]. Adipokines have been recognized to participate in breast carcinogenesis providing a potential underlying molecular link between obesity and cancer development[28]. These fac-tors can act on breast tissue in an endocrine, paracrine and autocrine manner ex-erting direct and indirect effects on breast cancer risk and progression[29]-[31]. Con-sidering that alterations in adipokine secretion have been closely associated with breast cancer, it would be interesting to investigate the potential implication of irisin in disease development through its function as an adipokine.

The present study is the first attempt to explore the role of irisin in human breast cancer, by quantitatively determining serum levels of irisin in patients with invasive ductal breast cancer and healthy individuals. We aimed to examine the association between irisin and breast cancer and to evaluate the ability of serum irisin levels to discriminate between breast cancer patients and controls. We analyzed potential associations between irisin and various demographic, anthropometric and clinical parameters, as well as with established markers of obesity. Finally, potential correlations between irisin and breast tumor characteristics were assessed.

2. Methods

2.1. Participants

One hundred one (101) female patients with primary invasive ductal breast cancer were recruited from the 1st Department of Propaedeutic Surgery of Hippokratio Hospital of Athens upon disease diagnosis. In addition, fifty one (51) female healthy volunteers were recruited during their annual breast cancer screening, after exclusion of the presence of breast cancer or other suspicious breast lesions. Participants with other malignancies, impaired liver function, severe psychiatric conditions, cardiovascular diseases, metabolic diseases, diabetes, chronic kidney disease, diseases of the central nervous system, or under immunosuppressive agents were excluded from the study. Similarly, subjects under strenuous exercise within one month of the study were also excluded. Clinicopathological characteristics of patients and controls are presented in **Table 1**. The study protocol was approved by the Ethics Committee of the Hippokratio Hospital of Athens, Greece. All participants gave their written informed consent prior to entering the study.

2.2. Sample Analysis

Peripheral venous blood samples were collected from all patients preoperatively as well as from healthy controls. Serum samples were prepared by centrifugation according to standard protocols, aliquoted and stored at $-80°C$ until assayed. Irisin levels were quantitatively determined in duplicates using commercial enzyme-linked immunosorbent (ELISA) assays (AdipoGen International, Liestal, SW), according to the manufacturer's instructions. Serum levels of leptin, adiponectin

Table 1. Baseline participants' characteristics.

	Controls	Cases	p-value
Demographic characteristics			
N	51	101	
Age (years)	55.7 ± 18.2	60.2 ± 13.7	0.131
Female gender	51 (100%)	101 (100%)	-
Menopausal status			0.183
Pre-menopausal	17 (34.0%)	24 (23.8%)	
Post-menopausal	33 (66.0%)	77 (76.2%)	
Anthropometric characteristics			
BMI (Kgr/m^2)	25.7 ± 3.8	27.4 ± 5.1	0.021
BMI status			0.036
Normal weight	21 (42.0%)	36 (36.4%)	
Overweight	24 (48.0%)	35 (35.4%)	
Obese	5(10.0%)	28 (28.3%)	
Chronic Diseases			
Dyslipidemia	23 (46.0%)	13 (12.9%)	<0.001
Cancer History			
Personal history of breast benign disease	3(6.0%)	4 (4.0%)	0.685
Personal history of previous neoplasms	0(0%)	8 (7.9%)	0.053
Family history of breast and/or gynecological cancer	7(14.0%)	38 (38.0%)	0.002

and resistin were also quantified by corresponding ELISA assays (BioVendor, Brno, CZ). Serum levels of cancer markers CEA, CA 15-3 and Her-2/neu were measured on an Advia Centaur Immunology Analyzer (Siemens, Tarrytown, US).

2.3. Statistical Analysis

Normality of distribution was evaluated through the Shapiro-Wilk test. Continuous variables are presented as mean ± standard deviation (SD) when they are normally distributed and as median (25th–75th percentile) when they are skewed. Categorical variables are summarized as absolute (n) and relative frequencies (%).

Associations between categorical variables were tested by the use of contingency tables and the calculation of chi-square tests without the correction of continuity or Fisher's exact test as appropriate. Associations between continuous variables and categorical variables with two categories were evaluated through Student's t-test or Mann-Whitney when continuous variables were normally distributed or skewed, respectively. Associations between continuous variables and categorical variables with three or more categories were evaluated through one way ANOVA. However, due to multiple significance comparisons, we used the Bonferroni correction in order to account for the increase in Type I error.

Correlations between irisin levels and normally distributed continuous variables were evaluated by the Pearson's correlation coefficient, while Spearman correlation coefficient was used to assess the correlation between irisin levels and skewed continues variables.

Logistic regression analysis was performed in order to determine whether the irisin levels are independently associated with the probability of women having breast cancer. Patients' characteristics found to be significantly associated with the group were entered in the model as potential confounders. The results are presented as odds ratios (OR) and 95% confidence intervals (95% CI).

Cut-off point analysis was used to identify the optimal value of irisin levels that differentiates healthy women from women with breast cancer. The threshold was defined by the largest distance from the diagonal line of the receiver operating characteristic curve (ROC) [sensitivity x (1-specificity)]. Using the cut-off points obtained from the analysis mentioned above, the sensitivity and specificity of the index for the aforementioned health outcomes were calculated. As sensitivity was defined the probability of a Ca patient having irisin level equal to or lower than a specific value, and as specificity was defined the probability of a healthy woman having irisin level higher than a specific value. A probability value of 5% was considered statistically significant. All statistical calculations were performed on the SPSS version 21.0 software (SPSS Inc, Chicago, II, USA).

3. Results

3.1. Demographic Characteristics

Table 1 presents baseline demographic characteristics of breast cancer patients and healthy controls. The two groups had no significant differences regarding age, gender and menopausal status. Significant differences BMI was higher in cancer patients compared to controls (p = 0.021). A significant difference was observed regarding the presence of dyslipidemia, as a higher percentage of controls was dyslipidemic (p < 0.001) As far as cancer history is concerned, a significant difference was reported with a higher percentage of cancer patients having a family history of breast and/or gynecological cancer (p = 0.002), but not in personal history of benign breast diseases or previous neoplasms.

3.2. Comparison of Irisin Levels between Patients and Controls

Serum irisin levels were quantitatively determined in breast cancer patients and healthy controls. Cancer patients exhibited significantly lower serum levels of irisin compared to controls (2.47 ± 0.57 and 3.24 ± 0.66μg/ml, respectively, p < 0.001) (**Figure 1**). According to simple logistic regression analysis, there was a significant independent association between irisin levels and the presence of breast cancer (**Table 2**). It has been estimated that 1 unit increase in irisin levels results to almost 87% reduction in the probability of women having breast cancer. The finding remained significant after controlling for potential confounders, and more specifically for BMI, dyslipidemia and family history of breast/gynecologic malignancy. After adjustment, it was estimated that 1 unit increase in irisin levels leads to almost 90% reduction in the probability of women having breast cancer (**Table 2**).

Subsequently, ROC curve analysis was used to investigate the potential application of irisin for the discrimination between patients with breast cancer and healthy women. Our results indicate that irisin can effectively discriminate between patients and healthy individuals at an optimal value of 3.21μg/ml. At this cut-off point, the sensitivity and specificity of detection is 62.7% and 91.1%, respectively (**Figure 2**).

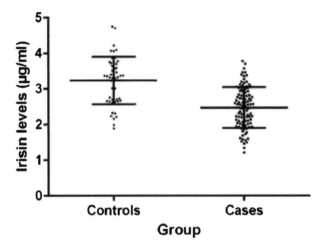

Figure 1. Scatter dot plots of serum irisin levels in patients with invasive breast cancer and controls. Mean values ± standard deviation are also denoted. Serum irisin levels were significantly lower in breast cancer patients compared to controls (2.47 ± 0.57 and 3.24 ± 0.66μg/ml, respectively, p < 0.001).

Table 2. Association of serum irisin levels with the probability of women having breast cancer (Logistic regression analysis).

	Un-adjusted model		Adjusted model	
Patients' characteristics	OR (95% CI)	p-value	OR (95% CI)	p-value
Irisin levels	0.131 (0.064 - 0.270)	<0.001	0.107 (0.045 - 0.255)	<0.001
BMI	-	-	1.117 (1.004 - 1.242)	0.041
Dyslipidemia	-	-	0.114 (0.039 - 0.330)	<0.001
Family history of breast/ gynecological neoplasms	-	-	3.774 (1.114 - 12.784)	0.033

3.3. Associations between Irisin Levels and Tumor/Patient Characteristics

Potential associations between serum irisin levels and tumor characteristics were investigated within the breast cancer group of patients (**Table 3**). Irisin levels were positively associated with tumor stage (p = 0.039), in particular stage I and stage III disease. A marginal association with tumor size and lymph node metastasis was observed (p = 0.084 and p = 0.098, respectively). There was no significant

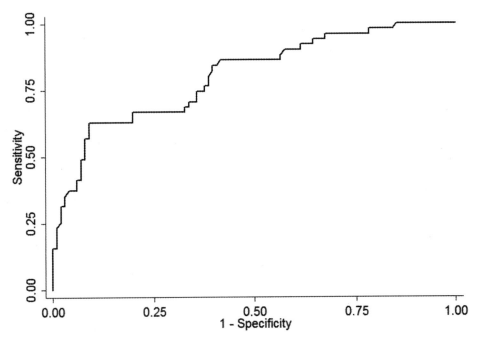

Figure 2. ROC curve analysis assessing the feasibility of serum irisin as a diagnostic indicator of breast cancer. Serum irisin can discriminate between breast cancer patients and healthy individuals at a cut-off point of 3.21μg/ml, with 62.7% sensitivity and 91.1% specificity.

Table 3. Association between irisin levels and breast tumor characteristics.

Characteristics	N(%)	Irisin levels (μg/ml)	p-value
Tumor size (cm)			0.084
≤2.0	43 (48.3%)	2.34 ± 0.52	
2.1 - 5.0	31 (34.8%)	2.58 ± 0.59	
>5.0	15 (16.9%)	2.65 ± 0.57	
Grade			0.450
I	14 (14.3%)	2.35 ± 0.59	
II	29 (29.6%)	2.42 ± 0.59	
III	55 (56.1%)	2.54 ± 0.56	
Stage			0.039
I	21 (30.4%)	2.31 ± 0.54	

II	28 (40.6%)	2.52 ± 0.58	
III	20 (29.0%)	2.75 ± 0.50a	
Lymph nodes			0.098
Negative	40 (56.3%)	2.44 ± 0.58	
Positive	31 (43.7%)	2.66 ± 0.53	
Concurrent DCIS			0.161
No	34 (34.0%)	2.37 ± 0.58	
Yes	66 (66.0%)	2.54 ± 0.56	
ER status			0.966
Negative	24 (25.3%)	2.46 ± 0.58	
Positive	71 (74.7%)	2.46 ± 0.56	
PR status			0.904
Negative	30 (29.7%)	2.47 ± 0.57	
Positive	65 (68.4%)	2.46 ± 0.57	
c-erb-B2 status			0.226
Negative	64 (68.1%)	2.41 ± 0.52	
Positive	30 (31.9%)	2.56 ± 0.66	
Ki67 Value			0.243
<10%	23 (24.5%)	2.27 ± 0.54	
10% - 15%	16 (17.0%)	2.53 ± 0.67	
16% - 30%	25 (26.6%)	2.58 ± 0.54	
>30%	30 (31.9%)	2.49 ± 0.53	
P53 status			0.759
<10%	52 (57.8%)	2.45 ± 0.55	
>10%	38 (42.2%)	2.49 ± 0.57	

Data are presented as mean ± standard deviation; [a]compared to stage I after Bonferroni correction for multiple comparisons.

association between irisin and tumor grade or the presence of concurrent DCIS. Irisin levels were not associated with ER, PR and c-erb-B2 status, or with Ki67 and p53 expression. No associations with serum levels of the established cancer markers CEA, CA15-3 and Her2/neu were observed (**Table 4**).

In breast cancer patients, irisin levels were not associated with BMI (p = 0.892). A positive association with leptin was observed, but not with adiponectin or resistin (**Table 4**). Finally, no associations between irisin and age, dyslipidemia or family history of breast and/or gynecological cancer were observed in the patients' group (p = 0.098, p = 0.712 and p = 0.236, respectively).

4. Discussion

Irisin is a muscle-derived factor, discovered and characterized three years ago[1]. Even though it is a relatively new molecule, a significant number of reports has already been published investigating its biology and function in several healthy and disease states. Originally, studies focused on the regulation of irisin by exercise with variable observations[1][9]–[15]. At the same time, extensive research is being carried out on the role of irisin in metabolic diseases, while new findings regarding its implication in other chronic conditions gradually accumulate[32]–[42]. As far as the role of irisin in cancer is concerned, current data are scarce and only include in vitro reports[43][44]. To our knowledge, the present study is

Table 4. Associations between serum irisin levels, and serum levels of cancer biomarkers and of markers of adiposity.

Biomarker	Median (25th - 75th percentile)	rho	p-value
CEA (ng/ml)	1.36 (0.86 - 2.04)	0.082	0.455
CA 15-3(U/ml)	15.90 (10.35 - 23.43)	−0.067	0.539
HER2/neu (ng/ml)	11.80 (10.05 - 14.90)	0.147	0.274
Adiponectin (μg/ml)[a]	12.30 ± 4.46	0.174	0.201
Resistin (ng/ml)	5.06 (4.35 - 5.94)	−0.203	0.134
Leptin (ng/ml)	18.99 (9.95 - 27.72)	0.399	0.003

[a]Data are presented as mean ± standard deviation.

the first aiming to investigate the potential role of the newly discovered irisin in human breast cancer. Our results demonstrate that serum irisin levels are significantly lower in breast cancer patients compared to healthy controls. Logistic regression analysis indicated that decreased irisin expression is closely associated with the presence of breast cancer. Most importantly, multivariate analysis showed that serum irisin is an independent predictor of breast cancer. It was estimated that 1 unit increase in irisin levels leads to almost 90% reduction in the probability of women having breast cancer. According to ROC curve analysis, irisin can effectively discriminate between patients and healthy individuals with 62.7% sensitivity and 91.1% specificity at a cut-off point of 3.21μg/ml, suggesting its potential value in breast cancer early detection.

Our observation of lower expression levels of irisin in breast cancer is supported by the findings of Gannon et al. evaluating the effect of various concentrations of irisin on the behavior of malignant and non-malignant breast epithelial cell lines[44]. The authors reported a significant suppressive effect of irisin on cell number, migration and viability in breast cancer cells, the induction of apoptotic cell death and the suppression of NFκB activity in malignant cell lines. Based on these data, they hypothesized that irisin may alter malignant characteristics similarly to other myokines and affect the development and aggressiveness of breast cancer[44]. It is thus reasonable to assume that reduced levels of irisin would favor breast cancer initiation, in agreement with our observations. The findings of Gannon et al. oppose previous data that reported lack of regulation of cell proliferation and malignant potential of other obesity-related cancer cell lines, including endometrial, colon, thyroid and esophageal, by irisin[43]. Nevertheless, these discrepancies have been attributed to different experimental techniques[44]. Since these are the only currently available data on the function of irisin in cancer, further studies are warranted to elucidate its molecular effects during disease development and to identify the implicated mechanisms.

Interestingly, a decreased expression of irisin has been associated with other chronic conditions, known to be associated with altered energy expenditure and metabolism. Most data arise from studies on patients with diabetes mellitus type 2 (DMT2), indicating a close relationship between the presence of disease and decreased circulating irisin levels[18][32]–[34]. These observations are further supported by reports of down-regulation of the FNDC5 gene in these patients[18][45]. Similarly,

426

circulating irisin levels have been found significantly decreased in patients with chronic kidney disease (CKD)[35]–[37]. Since the development of DMT2 and CKD is often associated with insulin resistance, it has been suggested that irisin may play an important role in the pathology of insulin-resistance related disorders while it may provide a novel therapeutic target for the treatment of metabolic diseases[18][32][35]. Two recent reports provide evidence for the implication of irisin in the development of polycystic ovary syndrome (PCOS) and also suggest that it may be a marker of insulin resistance in these individuals[41][42].

Adiponectin is another adipocyte-derived peptide hormone, able to stimulate the sensitivity of peripheral tissues to insulin, thus acting to enhance insulin sensitivity and protect against conditions of insulin-resistance[46]. Indeed, it has been documented that decreased levels of adiponectin are associated with increased insulin levels that accompany insulin resistance[47]. Low circulating levels of adiponectin have been observed in several diseases characterized by insulin resistance and hyperinsulinemia, including obesity, DMT2 and cancer[48]–[56]. Evidence from studies on breast cancer cell lines and animal models indicate that adiponectin can suppress cell proliferation, inhibit tumor growth, increase apoptosis and inhibit angiogenesis through multiple pathways[29]–[31]. Moreover, epidemiological data support that it exerts a protective role against breast cancer development, by displaying anti-proliferating, pro-apoptotic, anti-estrogen and anti-inflammatory properties[31]. More specifically, several studies on breast cancer patients have observed reduced adiponectin expression, particularly in post-menopausal women, suggesting a close association with breast cancer risk and providing a potential mechanistic link between obesity and breast cancer[53]–[55][57]–[60]. Among the many mechanisms proposed to mediate adiponectin function in breast cancer, the mitogenic effect of hyperinsulinemia appears to be of particular importance[57]. According to our results, serum levels of both irisin and adiponectin were lower in breast cancer patients compared to controls (data not presented) but there was no significant association between them. Current knowledge on the functions of irisin and the mechanisms involved inexerting its actions is exceptionally limited and only allows for hypotheses to be made. Nevertheless, the decreased expression levels of both molecules in ourcohort of patients support that irisin may play a rolesimilar to that of adiponectin. Moreover, irisin's downregulationin conditions characterized by insulin resistance suggest that this mechanism may be a majordeterminant of its function. Whether the effect of irisin on breast cancer can be attributed to obesity related hyperinsulinemia and insulin resistance extends beyond the scope of this work, but is a particularly interesting field of research that is worthy of thorough investigation in future studies.

Interestingly, we found that irisin levels were higher in stage III disease compared to stage I, resulting in a positive association with tumor stage. Based on our observation of reduced levels of irisin in breast cancer compared to controls, a further down regulation with the extent or progression of the disease would possibly be expected. This, however, may be a rather simplified hypothesis. Cancer is an exceptionally complex disease, accompanied by major dys regulation of a vast number of interacting molecular mechanisms and signaling pathways. At present, it is still impossible to know how irisin may behave and interact either in physiological conditions or in disease states. One assumption for our observation would be that, after the establishment of breast cancer, the secretion and metabolism of irisin may be affected by other, yet unidentified, cancer-related pathways and factors, resulting in alterations in its expression levels. Otherwise, irisin might exert a different function trying to counteract disease progression that is reflected in its expression levels. Nevertheless, it should be noted that even at stage III disease, irisin levels remained significantly lower than in healthy controls. Since this the first approach, our findings arise from a relatively restricted patient group and their verification in larger cohorts of patients is mandatory.

According to our findings, irisin levels were not associated with serum levels of the established cancer markers CEA, CA15-3 and Her2/neu. Despite their widespread use in routine clinical practice, it is well-recognized that the traditional tumor markers are only suitable for detection of recurrent or metastatic breast cancer as well as for management and surveillance of patients with advanced disease[61]–[63]. Their lack of specificity and sensitivity for in situ and primary breast cancer bears serious limitations and renders them rather inappropriate biomarkers for screening and diagnosis of low-volume disease[61][63]. Thus, our observation of no association between irisin and cancer markers is rather expected and may further support the potential diagnostic value of irisin.

Aiming to explore a potential link between irisin and obesity in human breast malignancy, we investigated potential correlations of irisin levels with body mass index (BMI) and with levels of the adipokines leptin, adiponectin and resistin in breast cancer patients. Our results indicate that irisin was positively associated with leptin, but not with adiponectin, resistin or BMI. Previously, several studies have investigated irisin expression in relation to obesity. BMI is the most traditional and widelyused measure of obesity. It has not yet been clarified if irisin levels are associated with BMI, as some studies have found positive correlations while others negative or no correlation[9][10][16]–[18]. It was recently proposed that irisin is positively correlated to BMI in healthy individuals but negatively correlated in subjects with metabolic diseases, suggesting a different function according to the metabolic state[64][65].

Leptin is the most prominent and best studied adipokine, and has been suggested to be implicated in the development of hormone-dependent malignancies including breast cancer[66]. Many studies have investigated leptin as a risk factor for breast cancer mainly in postmenopausal women, with conflicting and opposing findings[67]–[73]. At the same time, few reports have explored the role of leptin during disease progression and/or in relation to its clinical behavior. Although data are diverse, studies have provided evidence that increased expression of leptin in patients with breast cancer is associated with large tumor size, advanced tumor stage, high tumor grade and lymph node metastasis[59][60][67][74]–[76]. These observations have led to hypotheses that leptin is not only involved in breast cancer initiation but also in disease progression, and that it may be associated with more aggressive phenotypes[59][60][67][74][75]. In addition, leptin has been associated with distant metastasis and short survival, suggesting that it may have a negative prognostic value[76][77]. Considering the potential relationship of leptin expression with the characteristics and biological behavior of breast tumors, we consider the association between irisin and leptin levels in our patients is a reflection of the positive correlations of irisin with tumor stage and marginally with tumor size and lymph node involvement. The association of irisin levels with the presence of disease and tumor characteristics but not with BMI suggests that this factor is more likely to be related to systemic disease and tumor extent rather than to adiposity, as previously reported for leptin[76].

Altogether, our findings provide preliminary data for the implication of irisin in breast cancer development and suggest that it may serve as a potential novel biomarker of the presence of disease. Cancer serum markers may have a number of clinical applications including early diagnosis, differential diagnosis, prognosis, prediction of response and resistance to therapy, patient monitoring and surveillance. In breast cancer, established tumor markers are characterized by limited specificity and sensitivity precluding their use for screening and early diagnosis[60][63]. Mammography, in combination with clinical examination and breast self-examination, remains the primary modality for breast cancer screening and early detection of the disease, and has significant contribution to the decrease in mortality rates[78]. Nevertheless, mammography has important limitations particularly regarding the detection of suspicious lesions in women with very dense breasts and the early diagnosis of interval tumors[78]. As a result, improvements in the detection and early diagnosis of breast cancer are required and are expected to have a major impact on morbidity and mortality from the disease. In that aspect, intensive research is being carried out to exploit the use of novel serum biomarkers in screening, early diagnosis and differential diagnosis of breast cancer[79]. The identification of irisin, as well as other novel proteins, as candidate biomarkers that could assist in the early detection of the disease is an exciting perspective, and re- mains to be further investigated and verified by future prospective studies.

5. Conclusions

Significant evidence implicating irisin in various diseases, both metabolic and other chronic conditions, are gradually accumulating. Nevertheless, there is still lack of knowledge on its exact function and mode of action either in healthy or in disease states. To our knowledge, this is the first study attempting to investigate the role and clinical relevance of irisin in human breast cancer. Our findings provide significant preliminary evidence that serum irisin may serve as a novel indicator for breast cancer detection and early diagnosis. Forthcoming studies aimed to clarify these aspects are awaited with anticipation and are expected to add significant benefit for these patients.

6. Abbreviations

ANOVA: Analysis of variance; BAT: Brown adipose tissue; BMI: Body mass index; CA 15-3: Cancer antigen 15-3; CEA: Carcinoembryonic antigen; CI: Confidence interval; CKD: Chronic kidney disease; DMT2: Diabetes mellitus type 2; ELISA: Enzyme-linked immunosorbent assay; ER: Estrogen receptor; FNDC5:

Fibronectin type III domain containing 5; HER-2/neu: Human epidermal growth factor receptor 2; ml: Milligram; µg: Microgram; NFκB: Nuclear factor-kappaB; OR: Odds ratio; PCOS: Polycystic ovary syndrome; PGC1α: Peroxisome proliferator-activated receptor Y coactivator 1α; PR: Progesterone receptor; ROC: Receiver-operating characteristic; SD: Standard deviation; UCP1: Uncoupling protein 1; WAT: White adipose tissue.

Competing Interests

All authors declare they have no competing interests.

Authors' Contributions

XP: Experimental analysis, data assembly, data interpretation, manuscript writing. GPG: Patient recruitment, sample and clinical data collection. EK: Experimental analysis, assembly of data. VK, MAM, IP: Clinical data compilation. AS: Statistical analysis and data interpretation. GCZ: Patient selection, manuscript revision. AG: Conception and design, manuscript editing and study supervision. All authors read and approved the final manuscript.

Acknowledgements

This work was financially supported by the Hellenic Anticancer Institute. The authors thank the president of the Institute Mr. E. Fragkoulis and Ms V. Stasinopoulou for their contribution and continuous support.

Source: Provatopoulou X, Georgiou G P, Kalogera E, *et al*. Serum irisin levels are lower in patients with breast cancer: association with disease diagnosis and tumor characteristics[J]. Bmc Cancer, 2015, 15(1):1–9.

References

[1]   Boström P, Wu J, Jedrychowski MP, Korde A, Ye L, Lo JC, et al. A PGC1- al-

pha-dependent myokine that drives brown-fat-like development of white fat and thermogenesis. Nature. 2012; 481:463–8.

[2]   Roca-Rivada A, Castelao C, Senin LL, Landrove MO, Baltar J, Belén Crujeiras A, et al. FNDC5/irisin is not only a myokine but also an adipokine. PLoS One. 2013; 8, e60563.

[3]   Aydin S, Kuloglu T, Aydin S, Kalayci M, Yilmaz M, Cakmak T, et al. A comprehensive immunohistochemical examination of the distribution of the fat-burning protein irisin in biological tissues. Peptides. 2014; 61:130–6.

[4]   Nedergaard J, Bengtsson T, Cannon B. Unexpected evidence for active brown adipose tissue in adult humans. Am J Physiol Endocrinol Metab. 2007; 293:E444–52.

[5]   Wu J, Boström P, Sparks LM, Ye L, Choi JH, Giang AH, et al. Beige adipocytes are a distinct type of thermogenic fat cell in mouse and human. Cell. 2012; 150:366–76.

[6]   Novelle MG, Conteras C, Romero-Picó A, López M, Diéguez C. Irisin, two year later. Int J Endocrinol. 2013; 2013:746281.

[7]   Cannon B, Nedergaard J. Brown adipose tissue: function and physiological significance. Physiol Rev. 2004; 84:277–359.

[8]   Puigserver P, Wu Z, Park CW, Graves R, Wright M, Spiegelman BM. A cold-inducible coactivator of nuclear receptors linked to adaptive thermogenesis. Cell. 1998; 92:829–39.

[9]   Huh JY, Panagiotou G, Mougios V, Brinkoetter M, Vamvini MT, Schneider BE, et al. FNDC2 and irisin in humans: I. Predictors of circulating concentrations in serum and plasma and II. mRNA expression and circulating concentrations in response to weight loss and exercise. Metabolism. 2012; 61:1725–38.

[10] Timmons JA, Baar K, Davidsen PK, Atherton PJ. Is irisin a human exercise gene? Nature. 2012; 488:E9–10.

[11] Pekkala S, Wiklund PK, Hulmi JJ, Ahtiainen JP, Horttanainen M, Pöllänen E, et al. Are skeletal muscle FNDC5 gene expression and irisin release regulated by exercise and related to health? J Physiol. 2013; 591:5393–400.

[12] Anastasilakis AD, Polyzos SA, Saridakis ZG, Kynigopoulos G, Skouvaklidou EC, Molyvas D, et al. Circulating irisin in healthy, young individuals: Day-night rhythm, effects of food intake and exercise, and associations with gender, physical activity, diet and body composition. J Clin Endocrinol Metab. 2014; 99:3247–55.

[13] Huh JY, Siopi A, Mougios V, Park KH, Mantzoros CS. Irisin in response to exercise in humans with and without metabolic syndrome. J Clin Endocrinol Metab. 2015; 100:E453–7.

[14] Norheim F, Langleite TM, Hjorth M, Holen T, Kielland A, Stadheim HK, et al. The effects of acute and chronic exercise on PGC-1α, irisin and browning of subcutaneous adipose tissue in humans. FEBS J. 2014; 281:739–49.

[15] Löffler D, Müller U, Scheuermann K, Friebe D, Gesing J, Bielitz J, et al. Serum irisin levels are regulated by acute strenuous exercise. J Clin Endocrinol Metab. 2015; 100:1289–99.

[16] Park KH, Zaichenko L, Brinkoetter M, Thakkar B, Sahin-Efe A, Joung KE, et al. Circulating irisin in relation to insulin resistance and the metabolic syndrome. J Clin Endocrinol Metab. 2013; 98:4899–907.

[17] Stengel A, Hofmann T, Goebel-Stengel M, Elbert U, Kobelt P, Klapp BF. Circulating levels of irisin in patients with anorexia nervosa and different stages of obesity – correlation with body mass index. Peptides. 2013; 39:125–30.

[18] Moreno-Navarrete JM, Ortega F, Serrano M, Guerra E, Pardo G, Tinahones F, et al. Irisin is expressed and produced by human muscle and adipose tissue in association with obesity and insulin resistance. J Clin Endocrinol Metabol. 2013; 98:E769–78.

[19] Guh DP, Zhang W, Bansback N, Amarsi Z, Birmingham CL, Anis AH. The incidence of co-morbidities related to obesity and overweight: a systematic review and meta-analysis. BMC Public Health. 2009; 9:88.

[20] Renehan AG, Tyson M, Egger M, Heller RF, Zwahlen M. Body-mass index and incidence of cancer: a systematic review and meta-analysis of prospective observational studies. Lancet. 2008; 371:569–78.

[21] Lahmann PH, Hoffmann K, Allen N, van Gils CH, Khaw KT, Tehard B, et al. Body size and breast cancer risk: findings from the European Prospective Investigation into Cancer And Nutrition (EPIC). Int J Cancer. 2004; 111:762–71.

[22] Chan DS, Vieira AR, Aune D, Bandera EV, Greenwood DC, McTiernan A, et al. Body mass index and survival in women with breast cancer-systematic literature review and meta-analysis of 82 follow-up studies. Ann Oncol. 2014; 25:1901–14.

[23] Ewertz M, Jensen MB, Gunnarsdóttir KÁ, Højris I, Jakobsen EH, Nielsen D, et al. Effect of obesity on prognosis after early-stage breast cancer. J Clin Oncol. 2011; 29:25–31.

[24] Haakinson DJ, Leeds SG, Dueck AC, Gray RJ, Wasif N, Stucky CC, et al. The impact of obesity on breast cancer: a retrospective review. Ann Surg Oncol. 2012; 19:3012–8.

[25] Scholz C, Andergassen U, Hepp P, Schindlbeck C, Friedl TW, Harbeck N, et al. Obesity as an independent risk factor for decreased survival in node-positive high-risk breast cancer. Breast Cancer Res Treat. 2015; 151:569–76.

[26] McTiernan A. Obesity and cancer: the risks, science, and potential management strategies. Oncology (Williston Park). 2005; 19:871–81.

[27] Coughlin SS, Smith SA. The insulin-like growth factor axis, adipokines, physical activity, and obesity in relation to breast cancer incidence and recurrence. Cancer Clin Oncol. 2015; 4:24–31.

[28] Housa D, Housová J, Vernerová Z, Haluzík M. Adipocytokines and cancer. Physiol

Res. 2006; 55:233–44.

[29] Vona-Davis L, Rose DP. Adipokines as endocrine, paracrine and autocrine factors in breast cancer risk and progression. Endocr Relat Cancer. 2007; 14:189–206.

[30] Lorincz AM, Sukumar S. Molecular links between obesity and breast cancer. Endocr Relat Cancer. 2006; 13:279–92.

[31] Jardé T, Perrier S, Vasson MP, Caldefie-Chézet F. Molecular mechanisms of leptin and adiponectin in breast cancer. Eur J Cancer. 2011; 47:33–43.

[32] Choi YK, Kim MK, Bae KH, Seo HA, Jeong JY, Lee WK, et al. Serum irisin levels in new-onset type 2 diabetes. Diabetes Res Clin Pract. 2013; 100:96–101.

[33] Liu JJ, Wong MD, Toy WC, Tan CS, Liu S, Ng XW, et al. Lower circulating irisin is associated with type 2 diabetes mellitus. J Diabetes Complications. 2013; 27:365–9.

[34] Zhang C, Ding Z, Lv G, Li J, Zhou P, Zhang J. Lower Irisin Level in Patients with Type 2 Diabetes Mellitus: a Case–control Study and Meta-analysis. J Diabetes. 2015. doi:10.1111/1753-0407.12256

[35] Wen MS, Wang CY, Lin SL, Hung KC. Decrease in irisin in patients with chronic kidney disease. PLoS One. 2013; 8, e64025.

[36] Ebert T, Focke D, Petroff D, Wurst U, Richter J, Bachmann A, et al. Serum levels of the myokine irisin in relation to metabolic and renal function. Eur J Endocrinol. 2014; 170:501–6.

[37] Yang S, Xiao F, Pan L, Zhang H, Ma Z, Liu S, et al. Association of serum irisin and body composition with chronic kidney disease in obese Chinese adults: a cross-sectional study. BMC Nephrol. 2015; 16:16.

[38] Aronis KN, Moreno M, Polyzos SA, Mareno-Navarrete JM, Ricart W, Delgado E, et al. Circulating irisin levels and coronary heart disease association with future acute coronary syndrome and major adverse cardiovascular events. Int J Obes (Lond). 2015; 39:156–61.

[39] Kuloglu T, Aydin S, Eren MN, Yilmaz M, Sahin I, Kalayi M, et al. Irisin: a potential candidate marker for myocardial infarction. Peptides. 2014; 55:85–91.

[40] Lecker SH, Zavin A, Cao P, Arena R, Allsup K, Daniels KM, et al. Expression of the irisin precursor FNDC5 in skeletal muscle correlates with aerobic exercise performance in patients with heart failure. Circ Heart Fail. 2012; 5:812–8.

[41] Chang CL, Huang SY, Soong YK, Cheng PJ, Wang CJ, Liang IT. Circulating irisin and glucose-dependent insulinotropic peptide are associated with the development of polycystic ovary syndrome. J Clin Endocrinol Metab. 2014; 99: E2539–48.

[42] Li M, Yang M, Zhou X, Fang X, Hu W, Zhu W, et al. Elevated circulating levels of irisin and the effect of metformin treatment in women with polycystic ovary syndrome. J Clin Endocrinol Metab. 2015; 100:1485–93.

[43] Moon HS, Mantzoros CS. Regulation of cell proliferation and malignant potential by irisin in endometrial, colon, thyroid and esophageal cell lines. Metabolism. 2014; 63:188–93.

[44] Gannon NP, Vaughan RA, Garcia-Smith R, Bisoffi M, Trujillo KA. Effects of the exercise-inducible myokine irisin on malignant and non-malignant breast epithelial cell behavior in vitro. Int J Cancer. 2015; 136:E197–202.

[45] Kurdiova T, Balaz M, Vician M, Maderova D, Vlcek M, Valkovic L, et al. Effects of obesity, diabetes and exercise on Fndc5 gene expression and irisin release in human skeletal muscle and adipose tissue: in vivo and in vitro studies. J Physiol. 2014; 152:1091–107.

[46] Matsuzawa Y. Adiponectin: identification, physiology and clinical relevance in metabolic and vascular disease. Atheroscler Suppl. 2005; 6:7–14.

[47] Cnop M, Havel PJ, Utzschneider KM, Carr DB, Sinha MK, Boyko EJ, et al. Relationship of adiponectin to body fat distribution, insulin sensitivity and plasma lipoproteins: evidence for independent roles of age and sex. Diabetologia. 2003; 46:459–69.

[48] Arita Y, Kihara S, Ouchi N, Takahashi M, Maeda K, Miyagawa J, et al. Paradoxical decrease of an adipose-specific protein, adiponectin, in obesity. Biochem Biophys Res Commun. 1999; 257:79–83.

[49] Weyer C, Funahashi T, Tanaka S, Hotta K, Matsuzawa Y, Pratley RE, et al. Hypoadiponectinemia in obesity and type 2 diabetes: close association with insulin resistance and hyperinsulinemia. J Clin Endocrinol Metab. 2001; 86:1930–5.

[50] Petridou E, Mantzoros C, Dessypris N, Koukoulomatis P, Addy C, Voulgaris Z, et al. Plasma adiponectin concentrations in relation to endometrial cancer: a case–control study in Greece. J Clin Endocrinol Metab. 2003; 88:993–7.

[51] Dal Maso L, Augustin LS, Karalis A, Talamini R, Franceschi S, Trichopoulos D, et al. Circulating adiponectin and endometrial cancer risk. J Clin Endocrinol Metab. 2004; 89:1160–3.

[52] Soliman PT, Wu D, Tortolero-Luna G, Schmeler KM, Slomovitz BM, Bray MS, et al. Association between adiponectin, insulin resistance, and endometrial cancer. Cancer. 2006; 106:2376–81.

[53] Miyoshi Y, Funahashi T, Kihara S, Taquchi T, Tamaki Y, Matsuzawa Y, et al. Association of serum adiponectin levels with breast cancer risk. Clin Cancer Res. 2003; 9:5699–704.

[54] Mantzoros C, Petridou E, Dessypris N, Chavelas C, Dalamaga M, Alexe DM, et al. Adiponectin and breast cancer risk. J Clin Endocrinol Metab. 2004; 89:1102–7.

[55] Tworoger SS, Eliassen A, Kelesidis T, Colditz GA, Willett WC, Mantzoros CS, et al. Plasma adiponectin concentrations and risk of incident breast cancer. J Clin Endocrinol Metab. 2004; 92:1510–6.

[56] Wei EK, Giovannucci E, Fuchs CS, Willett WC, Mantzoros CS. Low plasma adiponectin levels and risk of colorectal cancer in men: a prospective study. J Natl Cancer Inst. 2005; 97:1688–4.

[57] Tian YF, Chu CH, Wu MS, Chang CL, Yang T, Chou YC, et al. Anthropometric measures, plasma adiponectin, and breast cancer risk. Endocr Related Cancer. 2007; 14:669–77.

[58] Kang JH, Yu BY, Youn DS. Relationship of serum adiponectin and resistin levels with breast cancer risk. J Korean Med Sci. 2007; 22:117–21.

[59] Hou WK, Xu YX, Yu T, Zhang L, Zhang WW, Fu CL, et al. Adipocytokines and breast cancer risk. Chin Med J (Engl). 2007; 120:1592–6.

[60] Chen DC, Chung YF, Yeh YT, Chaung HC, Kuo FC, Fu OY, et al. Serum adiponectin and leptin levels in Taiwanese breast cancer patients. Cancer Lett. 2006; 237:109–14.

[61] Duffy MJ. Serum tumor markers in breast cancer: are they of clinical value? Clin Chem. 2006; 52:345–51.

[62] Cheung KL, Graves CR, Robertson JF. Tumour marker measurements in the diagnosis and monitoring of breast cancer. Cancer Treat Rev. 2000; 26:91–102.

[63] Duffy MJ, Evoy D, McDermott EW. CA15-3 uses and limitation as a biomarker for breast cancer. Clin Chim Acta. 2010; 411:1869–74.

[64] Polyzos SA, Kountouras J, Anastasilakis AD, Geladari EV, Mantzoros CS. Irisin in patients with nonancoholic fatty liver disease. Metabolism. 2014; 63:207–17.

[65] Pardo M, Crujeiras AB, Amil M, Aguera Z, Jiménez-Murcia S, Baños R, et al. Association of irisin with fat mass, resting energy expenditure, and daily activity in conditions of extreme body mass index. Int J Endocrinol. 2014; 2014:857270.

[66] Garofalo C, Surmacz E. Leptin and cancer. J Cell Physiol. 2006; 207:12–22.

[67] Cust AE, Stocks T, Lukanova A, Lundin E, Hallmans G, Kaaks R, et al. The influence of overweight and insulin resistance on breast cancer risk and tumour stage at diagnosis: a prospective study. Breast Cancer Res Treat. 2009; 113:567–76.

[68] Tessitore L, Visio B, Pesola D, Cecchini F, Mussa A, Argiles JM, et al. Adipocyte expression and circulating levels of lepton increase in both gynecological and breast cancer patients. Int J Oncol. 2004; 24:1529–35.

[69] Wu MH, Chou YC, Chou XY, Hsu GC, Chu CH, Yu CP, et al. Circulating levels of leptin, adiposity and breast cancer risk. Br J Cancer. 2009; 100:578–82.

[70] Han C, Zhang HT, Du L, Liu X, Jing J, Zhao X, et al. Serum levels of leptin, insulin, and lipids in relation to breast cancer in China. Endocrine. 2005; 26:19–24.

[71] Petridou E, Papadiamantis Y, Markopoulos C, Spanos E, Dessypris N, Trichopoulos D. leptin and insulin growth factor I in relation to breast cancer (Greece). Cancer Causes Control. 2000; 11:383–8.

[72] Coskun U, Gűnel N, Toruner FB, Sancak B, Onuk E, Bayram O, et al. Serum leptin, prolactin and vascular endothelial growth factor (VEGF) levels in patients with breast cancer. Neoplasma. 2003; 50:41–6.

[73] Sauter ER, Garofalo C, Hewett J, Hewett JE, Morelli C, Surmasz E. Leptin expression in nipple aspirate fluid (NAF) and serum is influenced by body mass index (BMI) but not by the presence of breast cancer. Horm Metab Res. 2004; 36:336–40.

[74] Garofalo C, Koda M, Cascio S, Sulkowska M, Kanczuga-Koda L, Golasxewska J, et al. Increased expression of leptin and the leptin receptor as a marker of breast cancer progression: possible role of obesity-related stimuli. Clin Cancer Res. 2006; 15:1447–53.

[75] Liu CL, Chang YC, Cheng SP, Chern SR, Yang TL, Lee JJ, et al. The roles of serum leptin concentration and polymorphism in leptin receptor gene at codon 109 in breast cancer. Oncology. 2007; 72:75–81.

[76] Macciò A, Madeddu C, Gramignano G, Mulas C, Floris C, Massa D, et al. Correlation of body mass index and leptin with tumor size and stage of disease in hormone-dependent postmenopausal breast cancer: preliminary results and therapeutic implications. J Mol Med. 2010; 88:677–86.

[77] Ishikawa W, Kitayama J, Nagawa H. Enhanced expression of leptin and leptin receptor (OB-R) in human breast cancer. Clin Cancer Res. 2004; 10:4325–31.

[78] Euhus D, Di Carlo PA, Khouri NF. Breast cancer screening. Surg Clin N Am. 2015; 95:991–1011.

[79] Brooks M. Breast cancer screening and biomarkers. Methods Mol Biol. 2009; 472:307–21.

Chapter 17

A Mutation Screening of Oncogenes, Tumor Suppressor Gene TP53 and Nuclear Encoded Mitochondrial Complex I Genes in Oncocytic Thyroid Tumors

Cecilia Evangelisti[1,2], Dario de Biase[3], Ivana Kurelac[1], Claudio Ceccarelli[4], Holger Prokisch[5], Thomas Meitinger[5], Paola Caria[6], Roberta Vanni[6], Giovanni Romeo[1], Giovanni Tallini[3], Giuseppe Gasparre[1], Elena Bonora[1]

[1]Department of Medical and Surgical Sciences (DIMEC), Policlinico S. Orsola-Malpighi, Unit of Medical Genetics, University of Bologna, Bologna, Italy
[2]Department of Biomedical and Neuromotor Sciences (DIBINEM), Cell Signaling Laboratory, University of Bologna, Bologna, Italy
[3]Department of Diagnostic, Experimental and Specialty Medicine (DIMES), Unit of Anatomic Pathology, Bellaria Hospital, University of Bologna, Bologna, Italy
[4]Department of Diagnostic, Experimental and Specialty Medicine (DIMES), Unit of Anatomy, Policlinico S. Orsola-Malpighi, University of Bologna, Bologna, Italy
[5]Helmholtz Zentrum München Deutsches Forschungszentrum für Gesundheit und Umwelt, Neuherberg, Germany
[6]Department of Biomedical Sciences, University of Cagliari, Cagliari, Italy.

Abstract: Background: Thyroid neoplasias with oncocytic features represent a specific phenotype in non-medullary thyroid cancer, reflecting the unique biological phenomenon of mitochondrial hyperplasia in the cytoplasm. Oncocyticthyroid cells are characterized by a prominent eosinophilia (or oxyphilia) caused by mitochondrial abundance. Although disruptive mutations in the mitochondrial DNA (mtDNA) are the most significant hallmark of such tumors, oncocytomas may be envisioned as heterogeneous neoplasms, characterized by multiple nuclear and mitochondrial gene lesions. We investigated the nuclear mutational profile of oncocytic tumors to pinpoint the mutations that may trigger the early oncogenic hit. Methods: Total DNA was extracted from paraffin-embedded tissues from 45 biopsies of oncocytic tumors. High-resolution melting was used for mutation screening of mitochondrial complex I subunits genes. Specific nuclear rearrangements were investigated by RT-PCR (RET/PTC) or on isolated nuclei by interphase FISH (PAX8/PPARγ). Recurrent point mutations were analyzed by direct sequencing. Results: In our oncocytic tumor samples, we identified rare TP53 mutations. The series of analyzed cases did not include poorly or undifferentiated thyroid carcinomas, and none of the TP53 mutated cases had significant mitotic activity or high-grade features. Thus, the presence of disruptive TP53 mutations was completely unexpected. In addition, novel mutations in nuclear-encoded complex I genes were identified. Conclusions: These findings suggest that nuclear genetic lesions altering the bioenergetics competence of thyroid cells may give rise to an aberrant mitochondria-centered compensatory mechanism and ultimately to the oncocytic phenotype.

Keywords: Oncocytic Carcinoma, Nuclear Mitochondrial Complex I Subunits, Oncogene Mutation Analysis

1. Background

Non-medullary thyroid carcinoma (NMTC) is a well-differentiated thyroid cancer of follicular cell origin, either papillary thyroid carcinoma (PTC) or follicular thyroid carcinoma (FTC), which represents the most common endocrine malignancy. The annual incidence rate throughout the world ranges from 0.5 to 10 cases per 100,000 individuals with a two-fold to four-fold higher incidence of new thyroid cancer cases in women than in men[1]. The major known environmental risk factor for PTC, which represents about 80% of all thyroid cancers, is a prior exposure to radiation, with a dose-dependent effect on cancer risk. Other risk factors include iodine deficiency and excess, previous history of benign/autoimmune thyroid disease, as well as a positive family history[2].

A specific sub-phenotype in NMTC is represented by thyroid tumors with oncocytic features, which reflects the unique biological phenomenon of mitochondrial hyperplasia in the cytoplasm of oncocytic cells, characterized by their prominent eosinophilia (or oxyphilia) caused by mitochondrial abundance, from where the histopathological feature of swollen (oncòs) cells originate. For a thyroid cancer to be diagnosed as oncocytic, at least 75% of neoplastic cells ought to display the typical mitochondrial hyperplasia according to the 2004 World Health Organization classification[3].

Thyroid oncocytic tumors (with the exception of the rare oncocytic variant of medullary carcinoma) originate from follicular cells. They can be benign (oncocytic adenomas) or malignant (oncocytic carcinomas). It is generally accepted that oncocytic tumors in the thyroid and in other organs alike should be considered as distinct subtypes, since their features are peculiar enough to set them apart from corresponding neoplasms lacking accumulation of mitochondria (World Health Organization, 2004). Accordingly, oncocytic thyroid carcinomas are now classified as variants of follicular carcinoma (commonly) or of papillary carcinoma (less commonly). Interestingly, oncocytic carcinoma (OC) have long been considered a more aggressive subtype than PTC or FTC, particularly since they often appear to be refractory to radioactive iodine treatment and have poor chemo-sensitivity[4]. Overall, canonical histopathological criteria such as invasion of the tumor capsule or blood vessels are considered in order to distinguish benign versus malignant forms, regardless of the occurrence of an oncocytic phenotype. Among the molecular hallmarks of this phenotype, it has to be underlined that, in keeping with the observation that most of the time oncocytic cells mitochondria display a deranged morphology and function[5], disruptive mutations in the mitochondrial DNA (mtDNA) are nowadays univocally considered as the most prominent and frequent genetic signature for oncocytic tumors of the thyroid and other organs as well[6].

We and other groups have thereby demonstrated that pathogenic mutations in mtDNA encoded-genes impairing complex I are genetic markers of thyroid oncocytic tumors[7]–[9], albeit it has to be noted that in other organs, such as kidney and pituitary gland, the correlation between the occurrence of such mutations, the oncocytic phenotype and the functional disruption of complex I activity is far more stringent than in the thyroid[6][10]–[13]. Thyroid tumors may present as heterogeneous neoplasms, in which oncocytic cells are more or less a predominant component, and heterogeneity of nuclear and mitochondrial gene lesions may be envisioned[5][14]. Overall, since oncocytic features are present both in PTC and FTC and a number of oncocytic thyroid cancers are devoid of mtDNA disruptive mutations[7], the nuclear profile of oncocytic thyroid tumors is worth investigating, in order to pinpoint the mutations that may trigger the first hit in thyroid oncogenesis and may help in distinguishing, together with histological and cytological data, oncocytic tumors subtypes.

In forty-five oncocytic tumors of known mitochondrial DNA mutation status we therefore performed a screening survey of the nuclear encoded subunits of mitochondrial complex I, and of genes typically altered in thyroid-specific tumors such as B-Raf proto-oncogene (BRAF), Harvey rat sarcoma viral oncogene homolog (H-RAS), Neuroblastoma RAS viral oncogene homolog (N-RAS), and Kirsten rat sarcoma viral oncogene homolog (K-RAS), the fusion genes REarranged during Transfection (RET)/PTC1, RET/PTC3, Paired Box 8 (PAX8)/peroxisome proliferator-activated receptor gamma (PPARγ), and Tumor Protein p53 (TP53).

2. Methods

2.1. Tissue Samples Features

Forty-five tumor tissues samples were obtained from the Department of Experimental, Diagnostic and Specialty Medicine (DIMES), University of Bologna. Clinical and histological characterization was performed as previously described[7]. Briefly, 16 were hyperplastic oncocytic thyroid nodules, 7 were thyroid follicular adenomas (FA) and 22 were oncocytic thyroid carcinomas. Average patient age was 53 for patients with oncocytic lesions. All tumors were sporadic. The study was approved by the Ethical Committee of Azienda Ospedaliero-Universitaria of Bologna, protocol number 26/2009/U/Tess and handling of samples and clinical data proceeded accordingly. Patients' description is reported in Additional file 1: Table S1. Written informed consent was obtained for each patient included in the study and all data from the patients were handled in accordance with the local ethical committee approved protocols and in compliance with the Helsinki declaration.

2.2. Screening of TP53, BRAF, H-RAS, K-RAS and N-RAS Genes

All thyroid oncocytic samples were screened for TP53 mutations by polymerase chain reaction (PCR) and direct sequencing, as reported before[15]. PCR products were purified onto Millipore PCR clean-up plates, resuspended in bi-distilled water, and directly sequenced on both strands using BigDye v1.1 (Life Technologies) according to manufacturer's instructions. Samples were loaded on an ABI3730 automated sequencing machines (Life Technologies) and analyzed using Sequencer v2.1.

Detection of BRAF p.600 V > E and RAS codon 61 mutations was performed using PCR primers as reported in[16], sequenced using a CEQ2000 Genetic Analysis Systems (Beckman Coulter, Fullerton, CA, USA) and analyzed using CEQanalyzer software (Beckman Coulter, Fullerton, CA, USA) as previously described[16].

2.3. RET/PTC Analysis

Total RNA was extracted using the RecoverAll kit (Ambion Inc., Austin, Texas, USA) starting from four 20-μm-thick slides, in accordance to the manufacturer's instructions. RNA concentration was measured using Reverse-transcription PCR was performed using the Transcriptor High Fidelity cDNA Synthesis Sample Kit (Roche Diagnostic, Mannheim, Germany) and cDNA amplified using the FastStartTaq DNA polymerase reagents (Roche Applied Science, Mannheim, Germany), starting from about 100 ng of extracted RNA. RET rearrangement was analyzed by real time RT-PCR using primers specific for c-RET exons 10–11, c-RET exons 12–13, RET/PTC1 and RET/PTC3 as previously described[17]. Real time RT-PCR reactions were run in duplicate. The beta-Actin reference gene was used as RNA control. Real-time PCR was performed using an ABI SDS 7000™ instrument (Applied Biosystems, Foster City, CA, USA).

2.4. PAX8/PPARγ Analysis

To identify the PAX8/PPARγ rearrangement, a dual-color single-fusion home-brew probe containing BACs RP11–339 F22 (for PAX8) labeled with Spectrum Orange (Abbott Molecular/Vysis Downers Grove, IL) and RP11–167 M22 (for PPARγ) labeled with Spectrum Green (Abbott Molecular/Vysis) was designed. Cytogenetic and fluorescence in situ hybridization (FISH) studies were performed as described[18]. Evaluation of the results was done by counting 25–105 nuclei (mean 65) per case, depending on the quality of preparations, using a digital image analysis system based on an epifluorescence Olympus BX41 microscope and charge-coupled device camera (Cohu), interfaced with the CytoVysion system (software 2.81 Applied Imaging, Pittsburg, PA, USA). Normal nuclei were identified by two orange and two green FISH signals, nuclei with PAX8/PPARγ gene fusion were identified by one orange, one green and one fused orange/green signal. An example of the observed nuclear pattern is reported in **Figure 1**.

2.5. Mutation Screening of Nuclear Mitochondrial Complex I Subunits

Total DNA was extracted from tissues by the use of NucleoSpin Tissue extraction kit (Machery-Nagel) according to the manufacturer's instructions. All DNAs were pre-amplified using the GenomiPhi Illustra v2.0 amplification kit starting from 10 ng genomic DNA from tumor tissues according to the manufacturer's instructions (GE Healthcare, UK). A screening analysis for mutations in the nuclear subunits of mitochondrial complex I and assembly factors for complex I was carried out by high resolution melting point analysis (HRMA, Idaho Technology, USA) of PCR products of the coding and flanking intronic regions of these genes from preamplified DNA as described[19][20].

All PCR products presenting an aberrant melting pro-file were re-amplified from the corresponding original genomic DNA with the same PCR primers included in the screening. Sequence analysis (ABI3730, Life Technologies) was performed according to the manufacturer. PCR primer sequences and conditions were performed as reported[19][20].

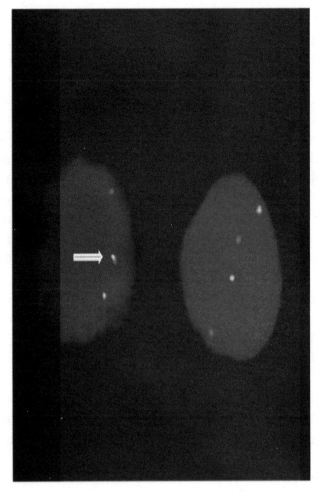

Figure 1. PAX8/PPARγ rearrangement observed in isolated nuclei from an oncocytic tumor biopsy. The white arrow indicates the gene fusion observed with the two differently labeled probes. See text for details.

3. Results

3.1. Nuclear Mitochondrial Complex I Mutation Screening

The DNA extracted from 45 sporadic thyroid oncocytic tumors was screened for mutations in the 38 nuclear genes encoding the subunits of mitochondrial complex I and two known complex I assembly factors (ECSIT; C6orf66). For all tumor samples the mtDNA mutation status has been previously determined[7]. We identified four heterozygous changes in four complex I genes. Two of these were variants already present in public databases: the missense change p. 81Arg > Gln in NDUFB1 (NM_004545.3, c.242G > A, rs72691104), with a very low frequency in control population (A = 1, G = 8599; m.a.f. = 0.0116, http://evs.gs. washington.edu/EVS/) and a common silent change in NDUFC2, corresponding to dbSNP ID rs534418 (m.a.f = 0.8546). Furthermore, an in-frame deletion of one amino acid residue was identified, c.398_400del3 p.(K133_I134delinsI) in NDUFA12, which despite having no dbSNP entry, was found in the control population at a low frequency (**Table 1**). Moreover, a novel variant was detected, namely the missense change p.8Glu > Val in NDUFB6, in an oncocytic carcinoma. The change was absent from 400 control chromosomes (blood-derived DNA) and from public databases (1000 Genomes and NIH-Exome Variant Server). In silico prediction of the putative functional effect was carried out with the programs PolyPhen-2, Provean and SIFT, all of which indicated as damaging the variant p.8 Glu > Val in NDUFB6, whereas conflicting results arose for the p. 81 Arg > Gln in NDUFB12 (**Table 1** and Additional file 1: Table S2). This sample also carried the mtDNA m.11403G > A, inserting a premature stopcodon in ND4 (p.W215Ter, Additional file 1: Table S1).

The NDUFB6 affecting p.8 Glu residue maps to the mitochondrial targeting sequence (MTS) of the protein, in a position highly conserved throughout species (Additional file 2: Figure S1A); therefore, it is reasonable to hypothesize that such

Table 1. Coding variants identified in nuclear mitochondrial complex I genes. Het = heterozygotes.

Gene	Position in cDNA	Number of het Oncocytic Thyroid	Number of het in EVSa	Type of change	PolyPhen-2 score (HumVar)
NDUFA12	c. 398 - 400 del_AGA (NM_018838.4)	1/45	21/6259	p.133del (Lys_Ile134insIle)	—
NDUFB1rs72691104	c. 242G > A (NM_004545.3)	1/45	1/4300	p.Arg81Gln	0.890
NDUFB6	c. 125A > T (NM_002493.4)	1/45	—	p.Glu8Val	0.852

aEVS (http://evs.gs.washington.edu/EVS/) accession as by June, 26th 2014.

a non-conservative change may be highly deleterious for the correct mitochondrial localization of the protein. In addition, this change resulted to be tumor-specific (Additional file 2: Figure S1B). The one-amino acid deletion in NDUFA12 was instead present also in the non-cancer tissue surrounding the lesion. This case also carried the PAX8/PPARγ rearrangement (see below).

3.2. Evaluation of Mutations in BRAF and RAS, and RET/PTC1-3 and PAX8-PPARγ Rearrangements

The BRAFV600E mutation was found in 2/45 samples (4.4%); RAS genes (H-RAS, K-RAS and N-RAS) were collectively mutated in 3/45 samples (6.7%). The RET/PTC1 rearrangement was analyzed in 26 cases and it was found in 1 out of 26 (3.8%). Results are presented in **Table 2**.

Considering the high frequency of mtDNA mutations in these samples and the role of PPARγ in mitochondrial biogenesis[21][22], we next hypothesized that PPARγ rearrangement might be preferentially associated with occurrence of mtDNA mutations. As a pilot study, PAX8-PPARγ rearrangements were analyzed in 10 samples, previously characterized for mtDNA mutations, in order to investigate whether this event is an alternative or concurrent mutational hit with mtDNA mutations in oncocytic thyroid lesions. The PAX8–PPARγ rearrangement was found in 5 out of 10 cases (mean fusion: 12.46%). Three samples carried concurrently the rearrangement and mtDNA mutations, and three samples negative for

Table 2. Oncogenes altered in oncocytic thyroid tumors.

Oncogene	Type of mutation	Type of change	Number of Oncogenic eventsa
RET/PTC	rearrangement	RET/PTC1	1/26
PAX8-PPARγ	rearrangement	—	5/10
RAS (H-RAS, K-RAS, and N-RAS)	point mutation	p.61 Gln > Arg (Q61R H-, N-, and K-RAS)	3/45
BRAF	point mutation	p.600Val > Glu (V600E)	2/45

aTotal numbers of tested samples are different, since the different analyses were not possible in all tissues.

the rearrangement carried mtDNA mutations (Additional file 1: Table S1). These findings suggest the lack of a stringent association between PAX8–PPARγ and mtDNA mutations.

3.3. TP53 Mutation Screening

All 45 tumor samples were screened for TP53 mutations: we identified two frameshift deletions and one missense change in 3 cases (6.7%; **Table 3**). All changes were detected as heterozygous variants. The missense change p.364 Ala > Thr was present in a sample from an oncocytic carcinoma, carrying also a frameshift mutation in mtDNA-encoded ND4 subunit (m.11038delA). The TP53 missense change was not present in databases of controls (*i.e.* ESP), but it has been reported in COSMIC as somatic mutation in ovarian cancer (accession n: COSM46361). Different prediction programs gave discrepant results on its pathogenicity (Additional file 1: Table S2).

One heterozygous deletion at c.728 was present in a sample from an oncocytic carcinoma, carrying the m.10885del, inserting a stop codon at amino acid 61 in mtDNA-encoded subunit ND4. The frameshift c.1248del was present in one sample, from an oncocytic adenoma, carrying also the N-RAS mutation. None of the TP53 mutated cases had poorly or undifferentiated histologic features.

The (co)occurrence of all genetic lesions identified is reported in Additional file 1: Table S1.

4. Discussion

Previous work carried out by our group has shed light on the tight correlation

Table 3. Mutations in TP53 tumor suppressor gene.

Base change (NM_000546)	Amino acid change	Number of het samples
c. 728delC	frameshift	1/45
c. 1248delC	frameshift	1/45
c. 1341G > A	missense change (p.364Ala > Thr)	1/45

between the co-occurrence of mtDNA alterations, the oncocytic phenotype, and a heavy dysfunction in the oxidative phosphorylation (OXPHOS) complexes activity, in particular in complex I[4][13]. The strength of a correlation between mtDNA mutations and functional impairment of complex I is even more striking in other oncocytomas, e.g. renal and pituitary oncocytic tumors[11]–[14].

Oncocytic thyroid tumors of follicular cell derivation are classified by the World Health Organization 2004 as distinctive histologic variants of FTC and PTC. This would suggest that they carry genetic abnormalities similar to those of their corresponding non-oncocytic counterparts (FTC and PTC)[23].

In comparison with other tumor types comprehensive molecular analyses of oncoytic thyroid tumors, including comparative genomic hybridization studies, have not been widely reported[24]. Recent work on oncocytic thyroid carcinomas found a series of recurrent deletion/ amplification in different chromosomes[25], confirming previously reported associations with chromosome instability[26]. This level of chromosome instability is remarkable when compared with that of other types of non-oncocytic differentiated thyroid cancer. BRAF mutations, RET/PTC or PAX8-PPARγ rearrangements were not identified[25]. RAS mutations were found in oncocytic FTCs with a much lower prevalence compared to the one of the corresponding non-oncocytic FTCs[25].

The finding of chromosome instability in oncocytic thyroid carcinoma may contribute to explain the peculiar phenotype of the tumors, i.e. the aberrant mitochondrial hyperplasia that, in a relatively high percentage of cases, is tightly associated to the occurrence of clearly pathogenic mitochondrial DNA mutations.

A complete analysis of the genomic landscape of oncocytic thyroid tumors, correlated with the co-occurrence of mtDNA mutations and in other complex I nuclear-encoded genes, has not been reported so far. Therefore, we performed an extensive mutation analysis of oncocytic tumor biopsies, previously characterized for the presence of mtDNA mutations. The presence of the best-known oncogenic events in thyroid cancer, including BRAF, RAS, TP53 mutations, RET/PTC and PAX8/PPARγ rearrangements, was assessed in addition to a high-throughput mutation screening for the nuclear-encoded complex I subunits[27], which may account for those cases lacking mtDNA mutations. The resulting data show that, in our samples, the BRAF, RAS, RET/PTC oncogenic events are relatively rare, similar to what observed by Ganly *et al.*[25]. On the other hand, the PAX8/PPARγ rearrangement did not show any significant correlation with the presence of mtDNA mutations, although the analysis was performed as a pilot study on a small number cases, which may also explain the relatively high frequency of PAX8/ PPARγ rearrangement with respect to previously published data.

Our study shows that heterozygous TP53 disruptive mutations are present in a small subset of oncocytic tumors. Two cases were oncocytic follicular carcinomas and one was diagnosed as oncocytic follicular adenoma. TP53 mutations are typically associated with poorly differentiated and anaplastic thyroid carcinoma[28]. The series of cases that we analyzed did not include poorly or undifferentiated thyroid carcinomas, and none of our TP53 mutated cases had significant mitotic activity or high-grade features. Thus, the presence of disruptive TP53 mutations, albeit in a subset of cases, was completely unexpected. Interestingly, TP53 mutations have been recently reported in 4 of 18 oncocytic carcinomas using Targeted Next-Generation Sequencing[29].

The occurrence of TP53 mutations in oncocytic tumors that do not carry the features of poorly-differentiated or anaplastic thyroid cancers is intriguing. Two of our TP53 mutated samples also harboured mtDNA mutations. Tumor suppressor p53 has been largely implicated in the metabolic remodeling that cancer cells develop during progression, particularly through the regulation of mitochondrial respiration via TIGAR and COXIV of the respiratory chain[30]. Nevertheless, several studies have shown that in thyroid oncocytic tumors a burden of mtDNA mutations all impinging on the bioenergetics competence of thyroid cells may give rise to an aberrant mitochondria-centered compensatory mechanisms and ultimately to the oncocytic phenotype[14].

In contrast to the findings that disruptive mtDNA mutations, in particular in genes encoding complex I subunits, are fairly common in oncocytic tumors, we did not identify a large number of nuclear-encoded complex I genetic abnormalities, suggesting that mutations in these genes do not play a major role in oncocytic thyroid cancer. This indicates that other genomic alterations may induce metabolic microenvironment changes drivers of tumorigenesis, coupled to mitochondrial abnormalities[13][31].

5. Conclusions

Characterizing the genomic landscape both at nuclear and mitochondrial levels in oncocytic thyroid tumors reveals a complex genetic interplay that may also confer prognostic differences. Available massive sequencing technologies, leading to the simultaneous analysis of hundreds of different genetic regions, are increasing the molecular characterization of solid tumors. Based on our data that show the co-occurrence of multiple genetic damages, a similar approach is indicated also for the characterization of oncocytic thyroid tumors, in order to identify the best therapeutic targets for a personalized treatment of thyroid cancer subtypes.

6. Additional Files

Additional file 1: Table S1. Clinical characteristics and molecular defects nuclear genes and mtDNA alterations. Table S2. PROVEAN and SIFT output for the rare variants identified in oncocytic tumors.

Additional file 2: Figure S1. (A) Protein sequence alignment showing the conservation across species of NDUFB6 p.8 Glu. (B) Electropherograms showing the novel missense change in NDFUB6 p.8 Glu > Val. Tumor tissue sample showing a somatic heterozygous profile, compared to perilesional tissue. The two different alleles were distinguished by cloning the PCR products into pcDNAII vector and sequencing the different clones.

7. Abbreviations

NMTC: Non-medullary thyroid carcinoma; PTC: Papillary thyroid carcinoma; FTC: Follicular thyroid carcinoma; OC: Oncocytic carcinoma; mtDNA: Mitochondrial DNA (mtDNA); FA: Follicular adenoma.

Competing Interests

The authors declare that they have no competing interests.

Authors' Contributions

EB, GG, GT conceived and designed the experiments. CE, IK, DdB, CC, PC, RV performed the experiments. TM and HP were in charge of high resolution melting analysis and interpretation. GT and GR recruited patients and provided data interpretation and manuscript organization. CE, EB, GG wrote the paper. All authors read and approved the final manuscript.

Authors' Information

Cecilia Evangelisti and Dario de Biase share first authorship.

Acknowledgements

We thank Ms. D. Rosano and Ms. D.V. Frau for technical help. This work was supported by the Associazione Italiana per la Ricerca sul Cancro (AIRC) grants "TRANSMIT" (IG8810) to G.R. and "JANEUTICS" (IG14242) to G.G., by grant GRERGENE "DIANE" from the Regione Emilia-Romagna-Italian Ministry of Health to E.B. and by an Italian Government MIUR grant (20074ZW8LA) to G. T.; I.K. is supported by a triennial "Borromeo" AIRC fellowship.

Source: Evangelisti C, Biase D D, Kurelac I, *et al*. A mutation screening of oncogenes, tumor suppressor gene TP53, and nuclear encoded mitochondrial complex I genes in oncocytic thyroid tumors[J]. Bmc Cancer, 2015, 15(1):1–7.

References

[1]   Bonora E, Tallini G, Romeo G. Genetic predisposition to familial nonmedullary thyroid cancer: an update of molecular findings and state-of-the-Art studies. J Oncol. 2010; 2010:385206.

[2]   Alsanea O, Clark OH. Familial thyroid cancer. Curr Opin Oncol. 2001; 13(1):44–51.

[3]   Tallini G. Oncocytic tumours. Virchows Arch. 1998; 433(1):5–12.

[4]   Gasparre G, Bonora E, Tallini G, Romeo G. Molecular features of thyroid oncocytic

tumors. Mol Cell Endocrinol. 2010; 321(1):67–76.

[5]   Maximo V, Rios E, Sobrinho-Simoes M. Oncocytic lesions of the thyroid, kidney, salivary glands, adrenal cortex, and parathyroid glands. Int J Surg Pathol. 2014; 22(1):33–6.

[6]   Gasparre G, Romeo G, Rugolo M, Porcelli AM. Learning from oncocytic tumors: why choose inefficient mitochondria? Biochim Biophys Acta. 2011; 1807(6):633–42.

[7]   Gasparre G, Porcelli AM, Bonora E, Pennisi LF, Toller M, Iommarini L, et al. Disruptive mitochondrial DNA mutations in complex I subunits are markers of oncocytic phenotype in thyroid tumors. Proc Natl Acad Sci U S A. 2007; 104(21):9001–6.

[8]   Maximo V, Soares P, Lima J, Cameselle-Teijeiro J, Sobrinho-Simoes M. Mitochondrial DNA somatic mutations (point mutations and large deletions) and mitochondrial DNA variants in human thyroid pathology: a study with emphasis on Hurthle cell tumors. Am J Pathol. 2002; 160(5):1857–65.

[9]   Pereira L, Soares P, Maximo V, Samuels DC. Somatic mitochondrial DNA mutations in cancer escape purifying selection and high pathogenicity mutations lead to the oncocytic phenotype: pathogenicity analysis of reported somatic mtDNA mutations in tumors. BMC Cancer. 2012; 12:53.

[10] Gasparre G, Porcelli AM, Lenaz G, Romeo G. Relevance of mitochondrial genetics and metabolism in cancer development. Cold Spring Harb Perspect Biol. 2013; 5:2. doi: 10.1101/cshperspect.a011411.

[11] Mayr JA, Meierhofer D, Zimmermann F, Feichtinger R, Kogler C, Ratschek M, et al. Loss of complex I due to mitochondrial DNA mutations in renal oncocytoma. Clin Cancer Res. 2008; 14(8):2270–5.

[12] Gasparre G, Hervouet E, de Laplanche E, Demont J, Pennisi LF, Colombel M, et al. Clonal expansion of mutated mitochondrial DNA is associated with tumor formation and complex I deficiency in the benign renal oncocytoma. Hum Mol Genet. 2008; 17(7):986–95.

[13] Kurelac I, MacKay A, Lambros MB, Di Cesare E, Cenacchi G, Ceccarelli C, et al. Somatic complex I disruptive mitochondrial DNA mutations are modifiers of tumorigenesis that correlate with low genomic instability in pituitary adenomas. Hum Mol Genet. 2013; 22(2):226–38.

[14] Porcelli AM, Ghelli A, Ceccarelli C, Lang M, Cenacchi G, Capristo M, et al. The genetic and metabolic signature of oncocytic transformation implicates HIF1alpha destabilization. Hum Mol Genet. 2010; 19(6):1019–32.

[15] Bartoletti-Stella A, Mariani E, Kurelac I, Maresca A, Caratozzolo MF, Iommarini L, et al. Gamma rays induce a p53-independent mitochondrial biogenesis that is counter-regulated by HIF1alpha. Cell Death Dis. 2013; 4:e663.

[16] Piana S, Ragazzi M, Tallini G, de Biase D, Ciarrocchi A, Frasoldati A, et al. Papillary thyroid microcarcinoma with fatal outcome: evidence of tumor progression in

lymph node metastases: report of 3 cases, with morphological and molecular analysis. Hum Pathol. 2013; 44(4):556–65.

[17] Rhoden KJ, Johnson C, Brandao G, Howe JG, Smith BR, Tallini G. Real-time quantitative RT-PCR identifies distinct c-RET, RET/PTC1 and RET/PTC3 expression patterns in papillary thyroid carcinoma. Lab Invest. 2004; 84(12):1557–70.

[18] Caria P, Dettori T, Frau DV, Di Oto E, Morandi L, Parmeggiani A, et al. Simultaneous occurrence of PAX8-PPARg and RET-PTC3 rearrangements ina follicular variant of papillary thyroid carcinoma. Am J Surg Pathol.2012; 36(9):1415–20.

[19] Haack TB, Madignier F, Herzer M, Lamantea E, Danhauser K, Invernizzi F,et al. Mutation screening of 75 candidate genes in 152 complex I deficiencycases identifies pathogenic variants in 16 genes including NDUFB9. J MedGenet. 2012; 49(2):83–9.

[20] Haack TB, Gorza M, Danhauser K, Mayr JA, Haberberger B, Wieland T, et al. Phenotypic spectrum of eleven patients and five novel MTFMT mutation sidentified by exome sequencing and candidate gene screening. Mol Genet Metab. 2014; 111(3):342–52.

[21] Skildum A, Dornfeld K, Wallace K. Mitochondrial amplification selectively increases doxorubicin sensitivity in breast cancer cells with acquired antiestrogen resistance. Breast Cancer Res Treat. 2011; 129(3):785–97.

[22] Corona JC, de Souza SC, Duchen MR. PPARgamma activation rescue smitochondrial function from inhibition of complex I and loss of PINK1.Exp Neurol. 2014; 253:16–27.

[23] Salvadori B, Greco M, Clemente C, De Lellis R, Delledonne V, Galluzzo D, et al.Prognostic factors in operable breast cancer. Tumori. 1983; 69(5):477–84.

[24] Stephens PJ, Tarpey PS, Davies H, Van Loo P, Greenman C, Wedge DC, et al.The landscape of cancer genes and mutational processes in breast cancer. Nature. 2012; 486(7403):400–4.

[25] Ganly I, Ricarte Filho J, Eng S, Ghossein R, Morris LG, Liang Y, et al. Genomicdissection of Hurthle cell carcinoma reveals a unique class of thyroid malignancy. J Clin Endocrinol Metab. 2013; 98(5):E962–72.

[26] Dettori T, Frau DV, Lai ML, Mariotti S, Uccheddu A, Daniele GM, et al.Aneuploidy in oncocytic lesions of the thyroid gland: diffuse accumulation of mitochondria within the cell is associated with trisomy 7 and progressive numerical chromosomal alterations. Genes Chromosomes Cancer.2003; 38(1):22–31.

[27] Ugalde C, Janssen RJ, van den Heuvel LP, Smeitink JA, Nijtmans LG.Differences in assembly or stability of complex I and other mitochondrial OXPHOS complexes in inherited complex I deficiency. Hum Mol Genet.2004; 13(6):659–67.

[28] Romitti M, Ceolin L, Siqueira DR, Ferreira CV, Wajner SM, Maia AL. Signalingpathways in follicular cell-derived thyroid carcinomas (review). Int J Oncol.2013;

42(1):19–28.

[29] Nikiforova MN, Wald AI, Roy S, Durso MB, Nikiforov YE. Targeted next generation sequencing panel (ThyroSeq) for detection of mutations in thyroid cancer.J Clin Endocrinol Metab. 2013; 98(11):E1852–60.

[30] Gerin I, Noel G, Bolsee J, Haumont O, Van Schaftingen E, Bommer GT.Identification of TP53-induced glycolysis and apoptosis regulator (TIGAR) asthe phosphoglycolate-independent 2,3-bisphosphoglycerate phosphatase. Biochem J. 2014;458(3):439–48.

[31] Iommarini L, Kurelac I, Capristo M, Calvaruso MA, Giorgio V, Bergamini C,*et al.* Different mtDNA mutations modify tumor progression in dependence of the degree of respiratory complex I impairment. Hum Mol Genet.2014; 23(6):1453–66.

Chapter 18

Tumor Phenotype and Breast Density in Distinct Categories of Interval Cancer: Results of Population-Based Mammography Screening in Spain

Laia Domingo[1,2]**, Dolores Salas**[3,4]**, Raquel Zubizarreta**[5]**, Marisa Baré**[2,6,7]**, Garbiñe Sarriugarte**[8]**, Teresa Barata**[9]**, Josefa Ibáñez**[3,4]**, Jordi Blanch**[1]**, Montserrat Puig-Vives**[10]**, Ana Belén Fernández**[5]**, Xavier Castells**[1,2,7]**, Maria Sala**[1,2,7] **and on behalf of the INCA Study Group**

[1]Department of Epidemiology and Evaluation, IMIM (Hospital del Mar Medical Research Institute), Barcelona, Spain

[2]Research network on health services in chronic diseases (REDISSEC), Barcelona, Spain

[3]General Directorate Public Health, Valencia, Spain

[4]Centre for Public Health Research (CSISP), FISABIO, Valencia, Spain

[5]Galician Breast Cancer Screening Program, Directorate for innovation and management of public health, Santiago de Compostela, Spain

[6]Epidemiology and Assessment Unit UDIAT-Diagnostic Centre, Corporació Sanitària Parc Taulí, Sabadell, Spain

[7]Department of Pediatrics, Obstetrics and Gynecology, Preventive Medicine and Public Health, Universitat Autònoma de Barcelona (UAB), Bellaterra, Spain

[8]Osakidetza Breast Cancer Screening Programme, Basque Country Health Service, Bilbao, Spain

[9]General Directorate of Health Care Programmes, Canary Islands Health Service, Las Palmas de Gran Canaria, Spain

[10]Epidemiology Unit and Girona Cancer Registry, University of Girona, Girona, Spain

Abstract: Introduction: Interval cancers are tumors arising after a negative screening episode and before the next screening invitation. They can be classified into true interval cancers, false-negatives, minimal-sign cancers, and occult tumors based on mammographic findings in screening and diagnostic mammograms. This study aimed to describe tumor-related characteristics and the association of breast density and tumor phenotype within four interval cancer categories. Methods: We included 2,245 invasive tumors (1,297 screening-detected and 948 interval cancers) diagnosed from 2000 to 2009 among 645,764 women aged 45 to 69 who underwent biennial screening in Spain. Interval cancers were classified by a semi-informed retrospective review into true interval cancers (n = 455), false-negatives (n = 224), minimal-sign (n = 166), and occult tumors (n = 103). Breast density was evaluated using Boyd's scale and was conflated into: <25%; 25% to 50%; 50% to 75%; >75%. Tumor-related information was obtained from cancer registries and clinical records. Tumor phenotype was defined as follows: luminal A: ER+/HER2− or PR+/HER2−; luminal B: ER+/HER2+ or PR+/HER2+; HER2: ER−/PR−/HER2+; triple-negative: ER−/PR−/HER2−. The association of tumor phenotype and breast density was assessed using a multinomial logistic regression model. Adjusted odds ratios (OR) and 95% confidence intervals (95% CI) were calculated. All statistical tests were two-sided. Results: Forty-eight percent of interval cancers were true interval cancers and 23.6% false-negatives. True interval cancers were associated with HER2 and triple-negative phenotypes (OR = 1.91 (95% CI: 1.22–2.96), OR = 2.07 (95% CI: 1.42–3.01), respectively) and extremely dense breasts (>75%) (OR = 1.67 (95% CI: 1.08–2.56)). However, among true interval cancers a higher proportion of triple-negative tumors was observed in predominantly fatty breasts (<25%) than in denser breasts (28.7%, 21.4%, 11.3% and 14.3%, respectively; <0.001). False-negatives and occult tumors had similar phenotypic characteristics to screening-detected cancers, extreme breast density being strongly associated with occult tumors (OR = 6.23 (95% CI: 2.65–14.66)). Minimal-sign cancers were biologically close to true interval cancers but showed no association with breast density. Conclusions: Our findings revealed that both the distribution of tumor phenotype and breast density play specific and independent roles in each category of interval cancer. Further research is needed to understand the biological basis of the overre-presentation of triple-negative phenotype among predominantly fatty breasts in true interval cancers.

1. Introduction

The main goal of mammographic screening is to reduce mortality and morbidity from breast cancer through early detection. However, women with interval cancer do not benefit from early detection, as their tumors are detected clinically after a negative screening episode and before the following screening invitation[1].

Interval cancers can be distinguished into four categories by the retrospective review of both screening and diagnostic mammograms: a) true interval cancers are those that showed normal or benign features in the previous screening mammogram; b) false-negative cancers are detected when signs suspicious for malignancy are retrospectively seen on a mammogram; c) minimal-signs are cancers showing detectable but non-specific signs at the latest screening; and d) occult tumors are those that present clinical signs of the disease despite a lack of mammographic abnormalities either at screening or at diagnosis. The European guidelines recommend first reviewing the screening films without histopathological information, and then using the screening and diagnostic films for the definitive classification. This practice involves substantial effort and is not normally routinely performed[1][2]. This explains why there are few large series with specific information on interval cancer categories, especially series providing biological information[3]. Studies evaluating interval cancers and following the recommendations of the European guidelines have found that about half are true interval cancers, over 20% are false negatives[3]–[5], and fewer than 20% are occult tumors and minimal-sign cancers[5][6].

There is evidence that interval cancers are more likely to have less favorable molecular features than screening-detected cancers, such as a high proportion of tumors not expressing estrogen receptor (ER negative, ER−) or progesterone receptor (PR negative, PR−)[4][7]–[9]. Some studies have reported a higher proportion of triple-negative cancers (ER−, PR−, human epidermal growth factor receptor 2 (HER2)−) among interval cancers[7][10] and this increase is even higher if only the subset of true interval cancers is considered in comparison to screening- detected cancers[4]. So far, this tumor phenotype lacks the benefit of specific adjuvant therapy and is associated with an aggressive behavior pattern and poor prognosis[11].

Breast density has also been related to interval cancer. There is increasing evidence that women with dense breasts are more likely to be diagnosed with interval cancer[12]−[14], but the role of breast density has not yet been elucidated[13][15]. A masking effect, which would contribute to hide the tumors[15], as well as a biological effect related to tumor growth[16], has been purposed. Because breast density influences both the risk and detection of breast cancer, as well as the likelihood of developing certain pathological subtypes[17][18], studying this factor in interval cancers would be of great interest.

We hypothesized that the roles of tumor phenotype and that of breast density differ in distinct categories of interval cancers. The aim of this study was to describe the tumor-related characteristics of true interval cancers, false negatives, minimal-sign cancers and occult tumors, and to assess the association of breast density and tumor phenotype in the four interval cancer categories. This study provides a comprehensive approach to the four categories of interval breast cancer identified from one of the largest cohorts of women participating in population-based breast cancer screening.

2. Methods

2.1. Setting

We performed a case-control study nested in a cohort of 645,764 women aged 45 to 69 years, screened in Spain between 1 January 2000 and 31 December 2006, and followed up until June 2009. These women underwent a total of 1,508,584 screening mammograms. During the study period, 5,309 cancers were detected in routine screening mammograms and 1,669 emerged as interval cancers, including both invasive and in situ carcinomas.

All women resident in Spain aged 50 to 69 years are actively invited to participate in the population-based screening program by a written letter every 2 years, following the European guidelines for Quality Assurance in Mammographic Screening Recommendations[1]. This nationwide program achieves the required standards[19].

We gathered data from five Spanish regions (Basque Country, Canary Islands, Catalonia, Galicia, and Valencia), covering a population of 752,487 women in 2005. Two mammographic projections (mediolateral-oblique and craniocaudal views) were made both in the initial and in successive rounds, except in one program. All mammograms were read by two radiologists, except in two programs, and the classification used for mammogram reading was BI-RADS[20]. Two regions switched to digital mammography during 2003 to 2005.

All screening programs keep mammography registers with data from participants and the final outcome of screening. Once a tumor is histologically confirmed, the woman is referred to a hospital for treatment and follow up. They are not further invited to screening, as they are controlled in the health care system.

Study data were collected using a protocol approved by the ethics committee of Parc de Salut Mar (CEIC-Parc de Salut MAR), Barcelona. Specific patient consent was not required because we used retrospective data from screening participants who had previously signed information release documents.

2.2. Study Population: Case and Control Definitions

Case subjects with interval cancer and control subjects with screening-detected cancer were drawn from women enrolled in any of the screening programs. We used the definition of interval cancers purposed in the European guidelines: "primary breast cancer arising after a negative screening episode, with or without further assessment, and before the next invitation to screening, or within 24 months for women who reached the upper age limit"[1]. The overall 1,669 interval cancers were matched by screening program and the year of the last screening mammogram to one screening-detected cancer, that is, a pathologically-confirmed malignant lesion identified during the screening process. We excluded those cases and controls with no available information on screening and diagnostic (only for interval cancers) mammograms. Finally, we analyzed 948 interval cancers, and 1,297 screening-detected cancers. Ductal in situ carcinomas were excluded from the analysis.

2.3. Assessment of Interval Cancers and Breast Density Classification

Interval cancers were identified by merging data from the registers of screening programs with population-based cancer registries, the regional Minimum Basic Data Set (MBDS) and hospital-based cancer registries. The use of different data sources ensured the quality and homogeneity of the process across the study period and regions. Population-based cancer registries covered four out of five regions. The MBDS (based on hospital discharges with information on the principal diagnosis) is updated yearly and is available in all regions. All data sources kept information on the time of diagnosis, which allowed us to ensure that all interval cancers fitted the case definition.

For interval cancer classification, three panels with three experienced radiologists performed a semi-informed retrospective review of both screening and diagnostic mammograms through independent double reading with arbitration. Screening mammograms were first reviewed alone, without the radiologists seeing the diagnostic mammogram and without histological information (blind review). Interval cancers were provisionally classified into positive (abnormality clearly visible and warrants assessment), negative (normal mammogram), and minimal-sign (subtle abnormality, not necessarily regarded as warranting assessment). Later, the diagnostic and screening mammograms were reviewed together and interval cancers were definitively classified into true interval cancers, false negatives, minimal-sign cancers, and occult tumors[1]. In the definitive classification, we ensured that the site where the minimal signs were identified correlated with the site of the interval cancer. When there was no correlation, the case was considered a true interval cancer.

One radiologist from each panel determined the breast density of the cancer-free breast, for both interval and screening-detected cancers. Breast density was evaluated using Boyd's scale, a semiquantitative score of six categories using percentages of density: A: 0%; B: 1% to 10%; C: 10% to 25%; D: 25% to 50%; E: 50% to 75%; F: 75% to 100%[21]. For purposes of assessing the impact of predominately fatty versus increasingly dense breasts, the first three categories were combined into the <25% group[22].

2.4. Study Variables

The woman's age at diagnosis was obtained from the date of birth and date of the screening mammogram. Tumor-related information (the tumor histology, grade, size, lymph node involvement, and ER, PR, HER2, p53 and Ki67 status) was obtained from the cancer registries, hospital-based registers, and from the clinical records. Biomarker assessment was performed as part of the diagnostic process in the hospitals. The positivity criteria used by each hospital followed international recommendations and their updates throughout the study period[23][24]. Tumors were considered positive when more than 20% and 10% of cells stained positive for Ki67 and p53, respectively. For the histological classification, we used ICD-O, 3rd edition. Histological grade was defined according to the Scarff-Bloom-Richardson criteria, modified by Elson[25].

Based on the expression of ER, PR and HER2, tumors were classified into four phenotypes: 1) luminal A: ER+/HER2− or PR+/HER2−; 2) luminal B: ER+/HER2+ or PR+/HER2+; 3) HER2: ER−/PR−/HER2+; and 4) triple-negative: ER−, PR−, HER2−[26].

2.5. Statistical Analysis

Comparisons were established between screening-detected cancers, true interval cancers, false negatives, minimal-sign cancers, and occult tumors. Statistical significance was assessed using the Chi-square or Fisher exact test for categorical variables, and one-way analysis of variance (ANOVA) for continuous variables. If a significant difference was found, we calculated standardized Pearson residuals as a measure of deviation between the observed and expected values to determine which cells contributed most to the Chi-square estimator[27]. Clinical features, age at diagnosis, breast density, bio-marker expression, and the phenotypic classification were compared between study groups. Then, we carried out a stratified analysis of tumor phenotype and breast density by study groups.

A multinomial regression analysis was computed to determine the effect of tumor phenotype and breast density on the odds of developing a true interval cancer, a false negative, a minimal-sign cancer, or an occult tumor versus screening-detected cancers. Our final multinomial regression model was adjusted for screening program (categorical), age (continuous), and tumor size (categorical, <11mm; 11 to 20mm; 21 to −50mm; >50mm). The outputs were plotted, showing the adjusted odds ratio (OR) and the 95% CI for each category of interval cancer, which served as the endpoints of the multinomial model.

We conducted sensitivity analyses by including or excluding screening-detected cancers diagnosed in prevalent screening. We tested different reference categories for breast density ($\leq 10\%$, $\leq 50\%$), and we checked the inclusion of covariates into the multivariate models (year of screening mammogram, histological grade, Ki67 and p53 status, the use of digital or analog mammography, and menopausal status). The sensitivity analyses showed no significant differences with respect to the definitive multinomial model. We examined the interaction between breast density and phenotype and found a non-significant effect within the multiple endpoints of the multinomial model.

All P-values were based on two-sided tests and were considered statistically significant if <0.05. Statistical analyses were performed using the SPSS (version 12.0) and R statistical software programs.

3. Results

A total of 1,297 screening-detected cancers and 948 interval cancers were included in the analyses. Most interval cancers were true interval cancers (n = 455, 48.0%), followed by false negatives (n = 224, 23.6%), minimal-sign cancers (n = 166, 17.5%) and occult tumors (n = 103, 10.9%).

Table 1 summarizes information on age at diagnosis and tumor-related characteristics of screening-detected cancers and interval cancer categories. Women

Table 1. Comparison of age at diagnosis and tumor characteristics at diagnosis between screening-detected cancers (n = 1,297) and interval cancers (n = 948).

	Screening-detected cancers n = 1,297	True interval cancers n = 455	False negatives n = 224	Minimal-sign cancers n = 166	Occult tumors n = 103	P-value[†]
Interval cancer entities, n (%)[‡]		455 (48.0)	224 (23.6)	166 (17.5)	103 (10.9)	
Time since last screening, n (%)						
<=12 months		89 (19.6)	73 (32.7)	53 (32.1)	44 (42.7)	
>12 months		364 (80.4)	150 (67.3)	112 (67.9)	59 (57.3)	<0.001
Age, y, mean (95% CI)	57.6 (57.3, 57.9)	56.4 (55.9, 57.0)	57.4 (56.6, 58.1)	56.8 (56.0, 57.6)	55.1 (54.0, 56.2)	<0.001
Tumor size,mm, mean (95% CI)	15.7 (15.1, 16.3)	25.3 (23.6, 26.9)	23.9 (22.1, 25.8)	22.7 (20.5, 24.8)	19.3 (17.0, 21.6)	<0.001
Focality, n (%)						
Unifocal	1030 (82.8)	341 (79.1)	171 (78.4)	118 (74.7)	83 (85.6)	
Multifocal and/or multicentric	214 (17.2)	90 (20.9)	47 (21.6)	40 (25.3)	14 (14.4)	0.041
Unknown	53	24	6	8	6	
Tumor size, n (%)						
<= 10mm	452 (34.8)[*]	36 (7.9)[*]	18 (8.0)[*]	22 (13.3)[*]	13 (12.6)[*]	
11 to 20mm	521 (40.2)	147 (32.3)	79 (35.3)	53 (31.9)	45 (43.7)	
21 to 50mm	233 (18.0)[*]	171 (37.6)[*]	78 (34.8)[*]	62 (37.3)[*]	23 (22.3)	
>50mm	91 (7.0)[*]	101 (22.2)[*]	49 (21.9)[*]	29 (17.5)	22 (21.4)[*]	<0.001
Unknown	0	0	0	0	0	
Lymph node involvement, n (%)						
Negative	872 (70.2)[*]	195 (50.4)[*]	102 (54.5)	76 (49.7)[*]	54 (62.1)	
Positive	371 (29.8)[*]	192 (49.6)[*]	85 (45.5)	77 (50.3)[*]	33 (37.9)	<0.001
Unknown	54	68	37	13	16	

Histological type, n (%)						
Ductal	1039 (80.5)	349 (77.6)	165 (74.0)	129 (77.7)	70 (68.6)	
Lobular	109 (8.4)[*]	54 (12.0)	36 (16.1)[*]	16 (9.6)	21 (20.6)[*]	
Other	143 (11.1)	47 (10.4)	22 (9.9)	21 (12.7)	11 (10.8)	<0.001
Unknown	6	5	1	0	1	
Histological grade, n (%)						
I	390 (34.9)[*]	57 (14.9)[*]	41 (21.4)	33 (22.9)	19 (22.6)	
II	474 (42.4)	149 (39.0)	88 (45.8)	62 (43.1)	42 (50.0)	
III	241 (21.6)[*]	171 (44.8)[*]	61 (31.8)	47 (32.6)	20 (23.8)	
NA	13 (1.2)	5 (1.3)	2 (1.0)	2 (1.4)	3 (3.6)	<0.001
Breast density, n (%)						
<25%	510 (39.3)[*]	139 (30.5)[*]	81 (36.2)	64 (38.6)	15 (14.6)[*]	
25% to 50%	359 (27.7)	127 (27.9)	60 (26.8)	47 (28.3)	20 (19.4)	
51% to 75%	277 (21.4)[*]	114 (25.1)	45 (20.1)	39 (23.5)	39 (37.9)[*]	
>75%	151 (11.6)	75 (16.5)	38 (17.0)	16 (9.6)	29 (28.2)[*]	<0.001
Unknown	0	0	0	0	0	

Missing values were excluded from the calculations of percentages. [*]Standardized Pearson residuals with statistically significant deviation between observed and expected values. [†]P-values for comparison of characteristics among the five study groups were obtained by one-way analysis of variance for continuous variables and the Chi-square test for categorical variables. All tests were two-sided. [‡]Row percentages.

with true interval cancers and occult tumors were younger (mean age 56.4 years and 55.1 years, respectively) than women in the remaining subsets (P < 0.001). Over 80% of true interval cancers were detected 12 months after the last screening or later, whereas 42.7% of occult tumors developed within the first 12 months. As expected, the highest percentage of tumors ≤10mm in size was found among screening-detected cancers (34.8%; P < 0.001). Among interval cancers, the percentage ranged from 7.9% to 13.3% in true interval cancers and occult tumors, respectively. Extremely dense breasts (>75%) were most frequently associated with occult tumors followed by false-negative cancers and true interval cancers

(28.2%, 17.0% and 16.5%, respectively, versus 11.6% in screening-detected cancers; P < 0.001).

The expression of biomarkers among study groups is detailed in **Table 2**. True interval cancers were less likely to express ER and PR than screening-detected cancers but were more likely to over express HER2, p53, and Ki67. In contrast, the molecular profile observed among occult tumors revealed a higher percentage of ER+ cancers (88.4 versus 82.5%) and a lower percentage of HER2+ cancers (14.1 versus 21.9%) compared with screening-detected cancers. Molecularly, false-negative tumors were similar to screening-detected cancers, although they showed a higher proportion of tumors over expressing Ki67 (50.3 versus 40.2%). Almost 35% of minimal-sign cancers over expressed p53.

Table 2. Biomarker expression among screening-detected cancers (n = 1,297) and distinct categories of interval cancers (n = 948).

	Screening-detected cancers	True interval cancers	False negatives	Minimal-sign cancers	Occult tumors	
	n = 1,297	n = 455	n = 224	n = 166	n = 103	P-value[†]
Estrogen receptor	1022 (82.5)[*]	283 (63.2)[*]	178 (81.7)	114 (71.3)	84 (88.4)	<0.001
Missing values	58	7	6	6	8	
Progesterone receptor	775 (63.7)[*]	214 (48.2)[*]	128 (59.0)	86 (54.4)	60 (64.5)	<0.001
Missing values	81	11	7	8	10	
HER2	203 (21.9)	113 (29.1)[*]	44 (24.0)	31 (23.1)	11 (14.1)	0.018
Missing values	371	67	41	32	25	
p53	149 (22.7)	86 (36.6)[*]	23 (21.5)	27 (34.6)	17 (28.8)	<0.001
Missing values	641	228	117	88	44	
Ki67	381 (40.2)	169 (52.5)[*]	83 (50.3)	50 (41.7)	26 (39.4)	0.001
Missing values	349	133	59	46	37	

Number of cases and percentage of tumors with positive biomarker expression. [*]Standardized Pearson residuals with statistically significant deviation between observed and expected values. [†]P-values for comparison of characteristics among the five study groups were obtained by two-sided Chi-square test. HER2, human epidermal growth factor receptor 2.

The distribution of tumor phenotypes among study groups is shown in **Table 3**. True interval cancers and minimal-sign tumors showed a higher proportion of triple-negative cancers (19.9% and 17.3%, respectively), whereas false-negative and occult tumors showed a similar tumor phenotype profile to screening-detected cancers.

In **Table 4** is shown the distribution of tumor phenotypes among study groups, stratified by breast density. According to breast density, differences in phenotype distribution were statistically significant among true interval cancers. The highest proportion of triple-negative cancers among true interval cancers was observed in breasts with 25% lower density than in denser breasts (28.7, 21.4, 11.3 and 14.3%, respectively; P < 0.001).

Adjusted OR and 95% CI estimated by multinomial regression analysis are plotted in **Figure 1**. True interval cancers were associated with HER2 and triple-negative phenotypes (OR 1.91, 95% CI 1.22, −2.96; OR 2.07, 95% CI 1.42, 3.01, respectively) and extremely dense breasts (OR 1.67, 95% CI 1.08, 2.56). Occult

Table 3. Distribution of tumor phenotypes among screening-detected cancers (n = 1,297) and categories of interval cancers (n = 948).

	Screening-detected cancers	True interval cancers	False negatives	Minimal-sign cancers	Occult tumors	
	n = 1,297	**n = 455**	**n = 224**	**n = 166**	**n = 103 (%)**	**P value†**
Tumor phenotype						
Luminal A	629 (68.3)	197 (50.9)*	124 (68.1)	79 (59.4)	62 (79.5)	
Luminal B	139 (15.1)	60 (15.5)	29 (15.9)	18 (13.5)	8 (10.3)	
HER2	62 (6.7)	53 (13.7)*	14 (7.7)	13 (9.8)	3 (3.8)	
Triple-negative	91 (9.9)*	77 (19.9)*	15 (8.2)	23 (17.3)	5 (6.4)	<0.001
Unknown	376	68	42	33	25	

Results are expressed as number (%). Tumor phenotype = Luminal A (ER+/HER2− or PR+/HER2−); Luminal B (ER+/HER2+ or PR+/HER2+); HER2 (ER−/PR−/HER2+); Triple-negative (ER−/PR−/HER2−). *Standardized Pearson residuals with statistically significant deviation between observed and expected values. †The distribution of tumor phenotype was compared among the study groups using the two-sided Chi-square test. ER, estrogen receptor; PR, progesterone receptor; HER2, human epidermal growth factor receptor 2.

Table 4. Distribution of tumor phenotypes among screening-detected cancers (n = 1,297) and categories of interval cancers (n = 948) stratified by breast density.

	Breast density				P-value[†]
	<25%	25% to 50%	50% to 75%	>75%	
Tumor phenotype					
Screening-detected cancers					
Luminal A	247 (68.6)	165 (65.5)	142 (70.3)	75 (71.4)	
Luminal B	51 (36.7)	49 (19.3)	24 (11.9)	15 (14.3)	
HER2	20 (5.6)	16 (6.3)	17 (8.4)	9 (8.6)	
Triple negative	42 (11.7)	24 (9.4)	19 (9.4)	6 (5.7)	
Unknown	150	105	25	46	0.306
True interval cancers					
Luminal A	60 (52.2)	51 (45.5)	49 (50.5)	37 (58.7)	
Luminal B	13 (11.3)	17 (15.2)	15 (15.5)	15 (23.8)	
HER2	9 (7.8)	20 (17.9)	22 (22.7)*	2 (3.2)*	
Triple negative	33 (28.7)*	24 (21.4)	11 (11.3)	9 (14.3)	
Unknown	24	15	17	12	<0.001
False negatives					
Luminal A	40 (62.5)	39 (75.0)	22 (64.7)	23 (71.9)	
Luminal B	10 (15.6)	4 (7.7)	9 (26.5)	6 (18.8)	
HER2	6 (9.4)	4 (7.7)	2 (5.9)	2 (6.3)	
Triple negative	8 (12.5)	5 (9.6)	1 (2.9)	1 (3.1)	
Unknown	17	8	11	6	0.375
Minimal-sign cancers					
Luminal A	30 (60.0)	26 (66.7)	16 (55.2)	7 (46.7)	
Luminal B	6 (12.0)	3 (7.7)	5 (17.2)	4 (26.7)	
HER2	2 (4.0)	5 (12.8)	2 (6.9)	4 (26.7)	
Triple negative	12 (24.0)	5 (12.8)	6 (20.7)	0 (0)	
Unknown	14	8	10	1	0.081
Occult tumors					
Luminal A	8 (80.0)	12 (80.0)	26 (78.8)	16 (80.0)	
Luminal B	0 (0)	2 (13.3)	4 (12.1)	2 (10.0)	
HER2	0 (0)	1 (6.7)	0 (0)	2 (10.0)	
Triple negative	2 (20.0)	0 (0)	3 (9.1)	0 (0)	
Unknown	5	5	6	9	0.296

Results are expressed as number (%). Tumor phenotypes = Luminal A (ER+/HER2− or PR+/HER2−); Luminal B (ER+/HER2+ or PR+/HER2+); HER2 (ER−/PR−/HER2+); Triple-negative (ER−/PR−/HER2−). *Standardized Pearson residuals with statistically significant deviation between observed and expected values. [†]P-value assesses the distribution of tumor phenotype distribution among breast density categories within study groups, using the two-sided Chi-square test, or Fisher exact test when appropriate. ER, estrogen receptor; PR, progesterone receptor; HER2, human epidermal growth factor receptor 2.

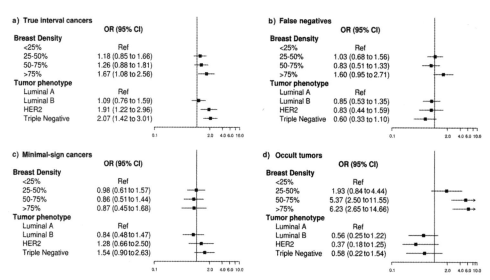

Figure 1. Multinomial logistic regression model of the association of breast density and tumor phenotypes with categories of interval cancer, adjusted for age at screening, screening program, and tumor size. The association of breast density with tumor phenotype, adjusted by screening program (categorical), age (continuous), and tumor size (categorical, <11mm; 11 to 20mm; 21 to 50mm; >50mm), is shown for the multiple endpoints of the multinomial logistic regression models, which are (a) true interval cancers; (b) false negatives; (c) minimal sign cancers and (d) occult tumors. The reference category (Ref) is screening-detected cancers. The black squares and the horizontal lines represent the odds ratios (OR) and corresponding 95% CI, respectively. ORs are presented on the log scale. Tumor phenotype = Luminal A: ER/HER2− or PR+/HER2−; Luminal B: ER+/HER2+ or PR+/HER2+; HER2: ER−/PR−/HER2−; Triple-negative: ER−/PR−/HER2−.

tumors were over six times more likely to develop in extremely dense breasts (OR 6.23, 95% CI 2.65, 14.66). False-negative cancers showed a non-significant tendency to occur in extremely dense breasts, whereas in the adjusted model, minimal-sign cancers showed no association with either breast density or tumor phenotype.

4. Discussion

This comprehensive study suggests that true interval and minimal-sign cancers showed similar tumor phenotype distribution, with almost 20% of these tumors being triple negative. In contrast, false-negative and occult tumors were phenotypically closer to screening-detected cancers. High breast density was mainly associated with occult tumors, and to a lesser extent, to true interval cancers and false negatives. However, among true interval cancers, those with the triple-negative phenotype were more likely to occur in predominately fatty breasts than in extremely dense breasts.

As expected by the lead time, all interval cancers were larger at diagnosis and were more likely to show lymph node involvement than screening-detected cancers. In agreement with previous work[4][8], true interval cancers were those with the longest waiting time to breast cancer diagnosis and were also the largest. However, some studies that analyzed occult tumors and true interval cancers together have reported that the clinical features of this subset differed less than those of screening-detected tumors[8]. As occult tumors were those detected earliest after screening, resulting in a higher proportion of small carcinomas and showing a molecular pattern similar to screening-detected cancers, grouping true interval and occult tumors together may lead to underestimation of the less prognostically favorable features of true interval cancers.

True interval and minimal-sign cancers showed similarities in their patterns of biomarker expression and tumor phenotype. Our results confirm that true interval cancers were less likely to express hormonal receptors[4][8][9][29] and support previous series reporting over expression of HER2, p53, and Ki67[4][9][30]. To our knowledge, this is the first study that provides complete molecular characterization of minimal-sign cancers. In line with previous evidence for the overrepresentation of triple-negative tumors among interval cancers[4][7][10], we found that most triple-negative tumors were concentrated among true interval and minimal-sign cancers. The biological similarities shared by both entities suggest that some minimal-sign tumors could be a more advanced form of true interval cancer, whereas false negatives seem to be a clearly distinct entity from minimal-sign cancers. These two entities should not be classified together, as has been done in some previous studies[31][32].

Breast density is a well-known risk factor for breast cancer and particularly interval cancer[13][14], but its association with tumor phenotypes remains controversial. Our findings revealed that luminal cancers were more likely to be detected in extremely dense breasts than in predominately fatty breasts, in agreement in with some previous studies[10][33][34], but contrasting with others[18]. Yanhjyan et al.[18] reported a higher proportion of triple-negative cancers among women with dense breasts. However, their study design was not comparable with ours, as these authors did not take into account whether the cancers were detected by screening. Unless the detection mode is considered, the association of triple- negative cancers and breast density may be overestimated, because tumors detected between two screenings are more likely to be detected in women with dense breasts and to be triple negative[15][17].

Our findings support the association of breast density and interval cancer independently of phenotype. The association of breast density and true interval cancers reinforces the hypothesis that some tumors are stimulated by growth factors found in dense breasts[35]. However, the overrepresentation of triple-negative tumors among predominantly fatty breasts in true interval cancers may reflect the aggressive behavior, rapid carcinogenesis and nonlinear progression of this tumor phenotype, regardless of breast density[11][36]. Further research is still needed to understand the biological basis of the association of breast density and tumor phenotypes, taking into account the mode of detection. The knowledge of epidemiological factors and radiological features predictive of an aggressive tumor subtype, such as the triple-negative phenotype, could add information for future personalized screening programs in women at risk of interval cancer.

The strong association of breast density and occult tumors pointed to a masking effect, confirming the assumptions noted years ago by Houssami[2]. Our findings also reinforce the idea that a masking effect mainly affects cancers that developed up to 12 months after screening[15]. Nevertheless, breast density appears to play a lesser role in false negatives, in line with previous series[13][37]. Breast density remains a major issue in breast cancer screening because it is one of the variables proposed to tailor screening[38]. Information on its role among interval cancer categories along with data on its relationship with tumor phenotypes may be useful to estimate the potential benefit of personalizing screening strategies on the basis of this factor.

The strengths of the current study are the large sample size and the completeness of the information. These factors have allowed us to study the role of breast density and tumor phenotype for each interval cancer category and to describe some features that may help to better understand their etiology.

There are, however, some limitations that should be considered. First, misclassification among interval cancers cannot be excluded. Some interval cancers could be classified as screening-detected if symptomatic women waited for the screening visit instead of making an immediate appointment with a physician. However, such misclassification would attenuate differences in tumor characteristics among study groups. Second, not all cases would have been phenotypically classified. Since this lack of information affects both screening-detected cancers and interval cancers, and was similar in all screening programs we do not believe that it affects the results. However, data on p53 and Ki67 were not always available because they were not routinely checked in all centers. Given that their lack of availability was not random, these data were not entered into the multinomial model. Third, grouping breast density into four categories reduced the sample size in the stratified analyses, but allowed the role of extremely dense breasts to be assessed. Collapsing breast density into two categories (≤ 50 and $>50\%$) diminished the magnitude of the association of breast density and distinct categories of interval cancer (data not shown). Fourth, some important variables associated with breast density, such as body mass index, age at menarche or childbirth, are not routinely collected by screening programs, and therefore we could not adjust for these potential confounders.

5. Conclusions

Our findings revealed that both the distribution of tumor phenotype and breast density play specific and independent roles in each category of interval cancer. Almost half of the interval cancers were true interval cancers, which encompassed a high percentage of tumors with a molecular profile associated with poor prognosis on the one hand and were more likely to be detected among women with extremely dense breasts on the other. False-negative and occult tumors had similar phenotypic characteristics to screening-detected cancers, high breast density being strongly associated with occult tumors. Minimal-sign cancers were biologically close to true interval cancers but showed no association with breast density. In view of the heterogeneity within interval cancers, further studies aiming to characterize interval cancers should avoid grouping true interval cancers and occult tumors, or false-negative and minimal-sign cancers. Knowledge of the clinical and biological particularities of interval cancers and of the role of breast density may be useful for the design of new risk-based screening strategies.

6. Abbreviations

ANOVA: analysis of variance; CI: confidence intervals; ER: estrogen receptor; HER2: human epidermal growth factor receptor 2; MBDS: Minimum Basic Data Set OR: odds ratio; PR: progesterone receptor.

Competing Interests

The authors declare that they have no competing interests.

Authors' Contributions

LD drafted the first version of the manuscript, performed the statistical analysis, and participated in the design of the study. MS, DS, RZ, and XC, conceived the study and participated in its design and coordination, and critically revised the manuscript for important intellectual content. MB, GS, TB, JI, JB, LD, MPV and ABF participated in the acquisition of data from screening programs and from clinical records, helped in the interpretation of the results, and helped to draft the manuscript. JB supported the statistical analysis, gathered data, and validated the whole database. ABF, JI, LD, DS and MS coordinated the review process for interval cancer classification and for the assessment of breast density. All authors critically reviewed the manuscript. All of them read and approved the final manuscript.

Acknowledgements

This work was supported by Instituto de Salud Carlos III-FEDER (PI 09/01153, PI09/02385, PI09/01340). The authors acknowledge the dedication and support of the entire Interval Cancer (INCA) Study Group (alphabetical order): IMIM (Hospital del Mar Medical Research Institute), Barcelona: Jordi Blanch, Xavier Castells, Mercè Comas, Laia Domingo, Francesc Macià, Juan Martínez, Ana Rodríguez-Arana, Marta Román, Anabel Romero, Maria Sala. General Directorate Public Health and Centre for Public Health Research (CSISP), FISABIO,

Valencia: Carmen Alberich, María Casals, Josefa Ibáñez, Amparo Lluch, Inmaculada Martínez, Josefa Miranda, Javier Morales, Dolores Salas, Ana Torrella. Galician Breast Cancer Screening Program, Xunta de Galicia: Raquel Almazán, Miguel Conde, Montserrat Corujo, Ana Belén Fernández, Joaquín Mosquera, Alicia Sarandeses, Manuel Vázquez, Raquel Zubizarreta. General Directorate of Health Care Programmes. Canary Islands Health Service: Teresa Barata, Isabel Díez de la Lastra, Juana María Reyes. Basque Country Breast Cancer Screening Program. Osakidetza: Arantza Otegi, Garbiñe Sarriugarte. Corporació Sanitària Parc Taulí, Sabadell: Marisa Baré, Núria Torà. Hospital Santa Caterina, Girona: Joana Ferrer, Francesc Castanyer, Gemma Renart. Epidemiology Unit and Girona Cancer Registry; and University of Girona: Rafael Marcos-Gragera, Montserrat Puig-Vives. Biomedical Research Institut of Lleida (IRBLLEIDA): Carles Forné, Montserrat Martínez-Alonso, Albert Roso, Montse Rué, Ester Vilaprinyó. Universitat Rovira i Virgili, Tarragona: Misericordia Carles, Aleix Gregori, María José Pérez, Roger Pla.

Source: Domingo L, Salas D, Zubizarreta R, *et al*. Tumor phenotype and breast density in distinct categories of interval cancer: results of population-based mammography screening in Spain[J]. Breast Cancer Research Bcr, 2013, 16(1):1–11.

References

[1] Perry N, Broeders M, de Wolf C, Törnberg C, Holland R, von Karsa L: European guidelines for quality assurance in breast cancer screening and diagnosis. 4th edition. Luxembourg: Office for Official Publications of the European Communities; 2006.

[2] Houssami N, Irwig L, Ciatto S: Radiological surveillance of interval breast cancers in screening programmes. Lancet Oncol 2006, 7:259–265.

[3] Hofvind S, Geller B, Skaane P: Mammographic features and histopathological findings of interval breast cancers. Acta Radiol 2008, 49:975–981.

[4] Domingo L, Sala M, Servitja S, Corominas JM, Ferrer F, Martinez J, Macia F, Quintana MJ, Albanell J, Castells X: Phenotypic characterization and risk factors for interval breast cancers in a population-based breast cancer screening program in Barcelona, Spain. Cancer Causes Control 2010, 21:1155–1164.

[5] Vitak B: Invasive interval cancers in the Ostergotland Mammographic Screening Programme: radiological analysis. Eur Radiol 1998, 8:639–646.

[6]   Bare M, Sentis M, Galceran J, Ameijide A, Andreu X, Ganau S, Tortajada L, Planas J:
        Interval breast cancers in a community screening programme: frequency, radiological
        classification and prognostic factors. Eur J Cancer Prev 2008, 17:414–421.

[7]   Collett K, Stefansson IM, Eide J, Braaten A, Wang H, Eide GE, Thoresen SO,
        Foulkes WD, Akslen LA: A basal epithelial phenotype is more frequent in interval
        breast cancers compared with screen detected tumors. Cancer Epidemiol Biomarkers
        Prev 2005, 14:1108–1112.

[8]   Kirsh VA, Chiarelli AM, Edwards SA, O'Malley FP, Shumak RS, Yaffe MJ, Boyd
        NF: Tumor characteristics associated with mammographic detection of breast cancer
        in the Ontario breast screening program. J Natl Cancer Inst 2011, 103:942–950.

[9]   Musolino A, Michiara M, Conti GM, Boggiani D, Zatelli M, Palleschi D, Bella MA,
        Sgargi P, Di Blasio B, Ardizzoni A: Human epidermal growth factor receptor 2 status
        and interval breast cancer in a population-based cancer registry study. J Clin Oncol
        2012, 30:2362–2368.

[10]   Caldarella A, Puliti D, Crocetti E, Bianchi S, Vezzosi V, Apicella P, Biancalani M,
        Giannini A, Urso C, Zolfanelli F, Paci E: Biological characteristics of interval can-
        cers: a role for biomarkers in the breast cancer screening. J Cancer Res Clin Oncol
        2013, 139:181–185.

[11]   Chacon RD, Costanzo MV: Triple-negative breast cancer. Breast Cancer Res 2010,
        12:S3.

[12]   Kerlikowske K, Grady D, Barclay J, Sickles EA, Ernster V: Effect of age, breast
        density, and family history on the sensitivity of first screening mammography. JAMA
        1996, 276:33–38.

[13]   Mandelson MT, Oestreicher N, Porter PL, White D, Finder CA, Taplin SH, White E:
        Breast density as a predictor of mammographic detection: comparison of interval-
        and screen-detected cancers. J Natl Cancer Inst 2000, 92:1081–1087.

[14]   Pollan M, Ascunce N, Ederra M, Murillo A, Erdozain N, Ales-Martinez JE, Pas-
        tor-Barriuso R: Mammographic density and risk of breast cancer according to tumor
        characteristics and mode of detection: a Spanish population-based case-control study.
        Breast Cancer Res 2013, 15:R9.

[15]   Boyd NF, Guo H, Martin LJ, Sun L, Stone J, Fishell E, Jong RA, Hislop G, Chiarelli
        A, Minkin S, Yaffe MJ: Mammographic density and the risk and detection of breast
        cancer. N Engl J Med 2007, 356:227–236.

[16]   Martin LJ, Boyd NF: Mammographic density. Potential mechanisms of breast cancer
        risk associated with mammographic density: hypotheses based on epidemiological
        evidence. Breast Cancer Res 2008, 10: 201.

[17]   Eriksson L, Czene K, Rosenberg L, Humphreys K, Hall P: The influence of mam-

mographic density on breast tumor characteristics. Breast Cancer Res Treat 2012, 134:859–866.

[18] Yaghjyan L, Colditz GA, Collins LC, Schnitt SJ, Rosner B, Vachon C, Tamimi RM: Mammographic breast density and subsequent risk of breast cancer in postmenopausal women according to tumor characteristics. J Natl Cancer Inst 2011, 103:1179–1189.

[19] Ascunce N, Salas D, Zubizarreta R, Almazan R, Ibanez J, Ederra M: Cancer screening in Spain. Ann Oncol 2010, 21:iii43–iii51.

[20] American College of Radiology (ACR): Breast Imaging Reporting and Data System Atlas (BI-RADS®Atlas). Reston, VA: American College of Radiology (ACR); 2003.

[21] Boyd NF, Byng JW, Jong RA, Fishell EK, Little LE, Miller AB, Lockwood GA, Tritchler DL, Yaffe MJ: Quantitative classification of mammographic densities and breast cancer risk: results from the Canadian National Breast Screening Study. J Natl Cancer Inst 1995, 87:670–675.

[22] Boyd NF, Lockwood GA, Byng JW, Tritchler DL, Yaffe MJ: Mammographic densities and breast cancer risk. Cancer Epidemiol Biomarkers Prev 1998, 7:1133–1144.

[23] Hammond ME, Hayes DF, Dowsett M, Allred DC, Hagerty KL, Badve S, Fitzgibbons PL, Francis G, Goldstein NS, Hayes M, Hicks DG, Lester S, Love R, Mangu PB, McShane L, Miller K, Osborne CK, Paik S, Perlmutter J, Rhodes A, Sasano H, Schwartz JN, Sweep FC, Taube S, Torlakovic EE, Valenstein P, Viale G, Visscher D, Wheeler T, Williams RB, *et al*: American Society of Clinical Oncology/College of American Pathologists guideline recommendations for immunohistochemical testing of estrogen and progesterone receptors in breast cancer (unabridged version). Arch Pathol Lab Med 2010, 134:e48–e72.

[24] Wheeler TM, Hayes DF, Van DV, Wolff AC, Hammond ME, Schwartz JN, Hagerty KL, Allred DC, Cote RJ, Dowsett M, Fitzgibbons PL, Hanna WM, Langer A, McShane LM, Paik S, Pegram MD, Perez EA, Press MF, Rhodes A, Sturgeon C, Taube SE, Tubbs R, Vance GH: American Society of Clinical Oncology/College of American Pathologists guideline recommendations for human epidermal growth factor receptor 2 testing in breast cancer. Arch Pathol Lab Med 2007, 131:18–43.

[25] Elston CW, Ellis IO: Pathological prognostic factors in breast cancer. I. The value of histological grade in breast cancer: experience from a large study with long-term follow-up. Histopathology 1991, 19:403–410.

[26] Goldhirsch A, Wood WC, Coates AS, Gelber RD, Thurlimann B, Senn HJ: Strategies for subtypes-dealing with the diversity of breast cancer: highlights of the St. Gallen International Expert Consensus on the Primary Therapy of Early Breast Cancer 2011. Ann Oncol 2011, 22:1736–1747.

[27] Agresti A: An Introduction to Categorical Data Analysis. 2nd edition. New York: Willey; 2007.

[28] Ciatto S, Catarzi S, Lamberini MP, Risso G, Saguatti G, Abbattista T, Martinelli F, Houssami N: Interval breast cancers in screening: the effect of mammography review method on classification. Breast 2007, 16:646–652.

[29] Rayson D, Payne JI, Abdolell M, Barnes PJ, MacIntosh RF, Foley T, Younis T, Burns A, Caines J: Comparison of clinical-pathologic characteristics and outcomes of true interval and screen-detected invasive breast cancer among participants of a Canadian breast screening program: a nested case-control study. Clin Breast Cancer 2011, 11:27–32.

[30] Crosier M, Scott D, Wilson RG, Griffiths CD, May FE, Westley BR: Differences in Ki67 and c-erbB2 expression between screen-detected and true interval breast cancers. Clin Cancer Res 1999, 5:2682–2688.

[31] Payne JI, Caines JS, Gallant J, Foley TJ: A review of interval breast cancers diagnosed among participants of the Nova Scotia Breast Screening Program. Radiology 2013, 266:96–103.

[32] Vitak B, Olsen KE, Manson JC, Arnesson LG, Stal O: Tumour characteristics and survival in patients with invasive interval breast cancer classified according to mammographic findings at the latest screening: a comparison of true interval and missed interval cancers. Eur Radiol 1999, 9:460–469.

[33] Conroy SM, Pagano I, Kolonel LN, Maskarinec G: Mammographic density and hormone receptor expression in breast cancer: the Multiethnic Cohort Study. Cancer Epidemiol 2011, 35:448–452.

[34] Ding J, Warren R, Girling A, Thompson D, Easton D: Mammographic density, estrogen receptor status and other breast cancer tumor characteristics. Breast J 2010, 16:279–289.

[35] Guo YP, Martin LJ, Hanna W, Banerjee D, Miller N, Fishell E, Khokha R, Boyd NF: Growth factors and stromal matrix proteins associated with mammographic densities. Cancer Epidemiol Biomarkers Prev 2001, 10:243–248.

[36] Yang XR, Chang-Claude J, Goode EL, Couch FJ, Nevanlinna H, Milne RL, Gaudet M, Schmidt MK, Broeks A, Cox A, Fasching PA, Hein R, Spurdle AB, Blows F, Driver K, Flesch-Janys D, Heinz J, Sinn P, Vrieling A, Heikkinen T, Aittomaki K, Heikkila P, Blomqvist C, Lissowska J, Peplonska B, Chanock S, Figueroa J, Brinton L, Hall P, Czene K, *et al*: Associations of breast cancer risk factors with tumor subtypes: a pooled analysis from the Breast Cancer Association Consortium studies. J Natl Cancer Inst 2011, 103:250–263.

[37] Ciatto S, Visioli C, Paci E, Zappa M: Breast density as a determinant of interval

cancer at mammographic screening. Br J Cancer 2004, 90:393–396.

[38] Schousboe JT, Kerlikowske K, Loh A, Cummings SR: Personalizing mammography by breast density and other risk factors for breast cancer: analysis of health benefits and cost-effectiveness. Ann Intern Med 2011, 155:10–20.

Chapter 19

The Clinical Trial Landscape in Oncology and Connectivity of Somatic Mutational Profiles to Targeted Therapies

Sara E. Patterson, Rangjiao Liu, Cara M. Statz, Daniel Durkin, Anuradha Lakshminarayana, Susan M. Mockus

The Jackson Laboratory for Genomic Medicine, 10 Discovery Dr., Farmington, CT 06032, USA

Abstract: Background: Precision medicine in oncology relies on rapid associations between patient-specific variations and targeted therapeutic efficacy. Due to the advancement of genomic analysis, a vast literature characterizing cancer-associated molecular aberrations and relative therapeutic relevance has been published. However, data are not uniformly reported or readily available, and accessing relevant information in a clinically acceptable time-frame is a daunting proposition, hampering connections between patients and appropriate therapeutic options. One important therapeutic avenue for oncology patients is through clinical trials. Accordingly, a global view into the availability of targeted clinical trials would provide insight into strengths and weaknesses and potentially enable research focus. However, data regarding the landscape of clinical trials in oncology is not readily available, and as a result, a comprehensive understanding of clinical trial availability is difficult. Results: To support clinical decision-making, we have developed a data loader and mapper that connects sequence information from oncology patients to data stored in an in-house database, the JAX Clinical Knowledgebase (JAX-CKB), which can be queried readily to access comprehensive data for clinical reporting via customized reporting queries. JAX-CKB functions as a repository to house expertly curated clinically relevant datasurrounding our 358-gene panel, the JAX Cancer Treatment Profile (JAX CTP), and supports annotation of functional significance of molecular variants. Through queries of data housed in JAX-CKB, we have analyzed the landscape of clinical trials relevant to our 358-gene targeted sequencing panel to evaluate strengths and weaknesses in current molecular targeting in oncology. Through this analysis, we have identified patient indications, molecular aberrations, and targeted therapy classes that have strong or weak representation in clinical trials. Conclusions: Here, we describe the development and disseminate system methods for associating patient genomic sequence data with clinically relevant information, facilitating interpretation and providing a mechanism for informing therapeutic decision-making. Additionally, through customized queries, we have the capability to rapidly analyze the landscape of targeted therapies in clinical trials, enabling a unique view into current therapeutic availability in oncology.

Keywords: Cancer, Precision Medicine, Actionability, Clinical Trials, Curation

1. Introduction

The advent of the genomic era has provided clinicians and researchers the ability to analyze molecular data from patients and identify genetic variants that may have an impact on their clinical outcome and treatment options. Cancer research has additionally identified a myriad of genetic variations that impact protein function, the pathology of tumor cells, and potential response to targeted therapies. Connecting this information to clinical patient data is critical for the implementation of precision medicine. However, this information is vast and disparate, which hampers the ability to access potentially crucial information in a clinically acceptable time frame. Access to this data requires several key components: a structured and well-organized database for deposition of clinically relevant data, accurate manual curation of data with limited variability, accessibility of connections between data elements via well-defined relationships, and a system for routinely and automatically mapping clinical sample data to the database. A number of publicly available databases exist that catalog cancer-related genomic variations or that connect variations to potentially relevant therapies, but none complement the need for connecting patient aberrations to targeted therapy—either through clinical trials or approved drugs, while incorporating supporting efficacy information. For instance, the COSMIC database provides an invaluable catalog of cancer-related somatic genetic aberrations but does not assess relationships between those variants and therapies[1]. The My Cancer Genome database from Vanderbilt incorporates efficacy data for well-studied molecular aberrations that could prove useful in clinical interpretation[2]. However, the content is confined to a small variant list and is not routinely updated and as a result, the depth and breadth of the coverage of molecular targets and targeted therapies, as well as patient indications and clinical trials curated is limited, effectively hindering its utility. In addition to the scarcity of databases populated with comprehensive targeted oncology clinical data, a system that can directly link patient sequence data to clinical information is lacking, and thus, the speed at which these data can be related to targetable mutations in tumor samples is greatly reduced.

To enable this process, we have developed a clinical bio-informatics and curation pipeline that operates within a Clinical Laboratory Improvements Amend- ment (CLIA) and College of American Pathologists (CAP)-accredited environment, the JAX Clinical Genome Analytics (CGA) system. This system enables systematic identification and annotation of clinically relevant cancer variants and facilitates connections to therapeutic interventions. JAX-CGA comprises several components, including an automated data loader and mapper, which loads called variants from clinical samples and transforms them to Human Genome Variation Society (HGVS) nomenclature using Human Genome Organisation (HUGO) gene symbols and subsequently maps the variants to the database. In addition, our in- house curation database, the JAX Clinical Knowledge-base (JAX-CKB) enables dynamic curation of data connecting genetic variant to phenotype and protein effect, as well as therapeutic relevance and potential treatment approaches, which can be queried readily for clinical reporting. To facilitate interoperability between databases, the JAX-CKB utilizes standardized variant nomenclature and incorporates specific ontologies. HUGO, through the HUGO Gene Nomenclature Committee (HGNC), maintains a catalog of unique approved gene names, which we have incorporated into the JAX-CKB, reducing ambiguity and enabling interoperability between databases[3]. Additionally, the Human Genome Variation Society (HGVS) provides guidelines for the standardization of variant nomenclature, which are actively maintained and updated, facilitating unambiguous variant naming[4].

A fundamental challenge to precision medicine is the ability to easily connect a patient's genetic variants with a therapeutic approach, which could include either FDA-approved targeted therapies or targeted therapies in recruiting clinical trials. Recent studies have demonstrated that linking patients to relevant targeted therapies based on genomic data has the potential to achieve higher clinical success relative to recruitment solely on histological subtype[5]. Leveraging the power of an integrated knowledgebase, we can identify opportunities for clinical intervention, including available clinical trials for targeted therapies. A comprehensive database can also provide a unique view into the landscape of molecular targets and therapies, uncovering potential opportunities for new research and development. In addition to supporting clinical reporting, the JAX-CKB allows visibility into deficiencies in the characterization of potentially actionable mutations and therapeutic interventions, exposing opportunities for research that have the potential to advance cancer treatment. Here, we detail and share the processes by which we map patient data to the knowledgebase and provide a detailed view of the clinical trial landscape in solid tumors.

2. Results and Discussion

The organization of the CGA system (**Figure 1**) incorporates several components, including the bioinformatics pipeline, the data loader and mapper, the JAX Clinical Knowledgebase, and reporting tools. The bioinformatics pipeline portion of the CGA system, including its validation, is discussed elsewhere[6].

The flow of data through the CGA-CKB system begins with the transformation and automated mapping of patient variants to JAX-CKB. Mapped variants are then filtered for actionability, which is defined as those with a related FDA-approved therapy or targeted therapy in clinical trials. Filtered actionable variants are then linked to treatment approaches and relevant recruiting clinical trials using unique clinical reporting tools through drug class or therapy, as well as by molecular criteria. This process is facilitated by the design of the JAX-CKB database,

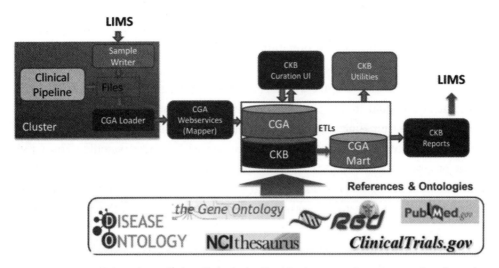

Figure 1. Flow of data through the clinical pipeline. Patient sample sequence data from the clinical genome analytics (CGA) pipeline is integrated with sample meta-data from the Laboratory Information Management System (LIMS), and called variants are mapped to the JAX-Clinical Knowledgebase (JAX-CKB) database. The JAX-CKB incorporates information populated from various incorporated ontologies and databases, and via the curation User Interface (UI), and is maintained using the CKB-Utilities tools. Using information from the JAX-CGA/CKB and the CKB reports, tools are used to generate datasets to enable clinical report generation.

which incorporates connectivity of various database attributes, through the use of standard language and ontologies. The user interface allows for annotation of the most current data surrounding genetic variants and targeted therapies, on top of a system that incorporates standard ontologies and controlled vocabularies. This data is then readily accessible via reporting and analysis queries for both patient clinical reporting applications and for comprehensive analysis of data, including data regarding clinical trials. To enable both clinical reporting and analysis of clinically relevant data surrounding the JAX-CTP-targeted gene panel, we have implemented a unique framework for managing and connecting patient molecular data to efficacy information and relevant treatment approaches in real-time.

2.1. Data Loader and Mapper

The data loader and mapper play a critical role in routine processing of large scale variation results from the CGA pipeline. The roles of the data loader and mapper are to upload genomic sequence data and integrate that sequence data with sample meta-data and to automatically map patient variants to JAX-CKB, enabling further queries for clinical interpretation.

The CGA loader (**Figure 2**) runs as a daemon program, which intermittently scans the file system in a cluster server searching for new runs from the clinical analytics (CGA) pipeline. New runs consist of either analysis results of a new sample or repeat analysis results from a previously mapped sample. The CGA loader program additionally extracts sample meta-data, such as patient diagnosis, from our Laboratory Information Management System (LIMS) and submits these data along with the variant call format (VCF) files to a Restful web service.

The web service, running in a Tomcat application server, saves all data files in the database with an initial "pending" file status and manages the workflow of all computational jobs in a queue. The format of each data file is defined as a template in the database allowing an integrated Java program, using Reflection, to

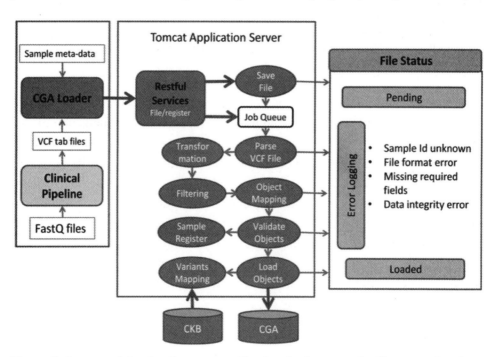

Figure 2. Automated data loading process. The data loader scans the file system hourly to find any new runs from the clinical pipeline and submits the variant call files (VCF) along with their sample meta-data to a web service. The web service manages the data loading jobs in a queue, to transform, filter, and upload the datasets to our CGA database and map the variants to the JAX-CKB.

dynamically parse, transform, and map file columns to database tables and columns. During this workflow, additional filtering or validation steps can be integrated for quality or biological reasons. If an error occurs in the loading process, the file status will be updated as "error" and a tracking message will be logged. Following successful completion of a job, the file status will be updated as "loaded."

The Mapper (**Figure 3**) is the nickname of the web service that manages the automated data loading and mapping jobs. During the data loading workflow, sequence variants, which include point mutations or small insertions or deletions (InDels), are transformed to standard Human Genome Variation Society (HGVS) nomenclature[4], which is consistent with the regular expression (regex) vocabulary of variants in the JAX-CKB. For example, the SnpEff and SnpSift programs annotate an amino acid from nucleotide sequence information using a three-letter

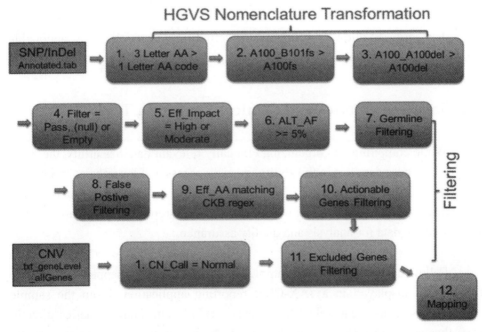

Figure 3. Automated variant mapping process. The genomic datasets are transformed to standard Human Genome Variation Society (HGVS) nomenclature, using a standardized Regular Expressions (regex) vocabulary incorporated into the JAX-CKB. This enables mapping and identification of clinically meaningful variants in a scalable and reproducible manner. The variant mapping program also includes several filtering steps, including removal of low-impact variants, those that did not pass metrics, and those that are likely germline or false-positive, to ensure reporting of only high-quality somatic variations.

amino acid code (e.g., "Gly" for Glycine). This three-letter code is then transformed to the single letter code for that amino acid, using the appropriate syntax (e.g., "G" for "Gly"). For example, p.Gly749Glu/c.2246G > A will be transformed to "G749E," and the frameshift Arg34_Val35fs/c.102_103insG will be transformed to "R34fs." Subsequent to transformation, several filtering steps have been implemented to ensure the use of only high-quality somatic variations and reduce false-positives. Filters include removal of variants with low coverage, variants with allele frequencies that do not meet minimum requirements for sensitivity, low impact variants including silent mutations, variants that are likely germline, and those that are likely false-positive or outside of coding regions. Simultaneously, Copy Number Variation (CNV) files are filtered to remove genes with fewer than six copies, based on the analytical validation of the assay[6]. Following filtering, CNV files are merged with the filtered VCFs. The analytics program will then automatically recognize and map the variants in the JAX-CKB, enabled by the transformation to the HGVS syntax used by JAX-CKB.

This process allows for direct connectivity between clinically actionable somatic variants present in patient tumor samples with applicable clinical data.

2.2. Database Queries and Clinical Reporting Tools

While compiling and organizing clinically relevant data has utility, the power to utilize these data lies in the ability to easily access and leverage complex data to inform clinical decision-making. To that end, we have designed and implemented several database queries, which both facilitate reporting and enable unique views into the data for analysis and quality assurance.

Following the mapping of samples to the JAX-CKB, mapped variants are filtered and displayed in a JAX-CKB reporting application. From the sample landing page, a user can select the relevant sample and launch queries directly from the sample results, allowing the user to tailor the queries to sample-specific molecular aberrations while providing traceability. Several queries have been built to generate result sets that support clinical reporting. The queries are designed to run based on all clinically relevant variants in a single sample simultaneously; however, the search page for each query incorporates a selection tool from which a user can deselect any variant in the sample to exclude as search parameters. This enables the user to run the queries on only variants that have clinical relevance, as well as limiting query results from samples with many actionable variants to produce multiple, more manageable, datasets. To retrieve the list of targeted therapies associated with sample-specific variants, we have designed a query that utilizes the associated drug class or individual therapy treatment approaches specific to variants to retrieve all drugs assigned to those treatment approaches. For example, the variant KIT D816V has the associated treatment approach "KIT Inhibitors." There are currently 31 drugs curated into JAX-CKB that have been assigned the drug class "KIT Inhibitors." If present in a mapped sample in CKB, launching the drug query retrieves the drug class treatment approach for KIT D816V and from this retrieves the list of drugs associated with this drug class. In addition, there are three separate queries that leverage different aspects of curated efficacy evidence. The approval status query retrieves data from the "approval status" attribute of curated efficacy evidence for all drugs related to treatment approaches for given variants. This enables identification of targeted therapies that are FDA-approved versus investigational therapies, related to a treatment approach for the patient variant(s). The drug resistance query retrieves efficacy evidence entries for all molecular profile responses with response type of "resistant" that contains the same parent gene of sample-specific variants. For example, for a sample containing a KRAS G12C variant, the resistance query would retrieve all resistance efficacy evidence associated with any molecular profile response containing a variant in KRAS. This would include the efficacy evidence related to KRAS G12C, as well as category variants "KRAS G12X" and closely related variants KRAS G12D and KRAS G13C. Relating to parent gene, rather than specific variant, enables visibility into all potential resistance mechanisms without requiring duplication of data in CKB. A third query pulls all evidence with sensitive response type related to the treatment approach for patient variants, to support rationale for therapies included on patient reports.

Clinical Trial Query

Clinical trials function as an avenue toward clinical intervention and constitute an important component of the therapeutic landscape for oncology patients. Thus, we have incorporated the identification of clinical trials relevant to patient variants into clinical reporting to provide multiple potential options for clinicians to direct patient treatment. Clinical trials can be relevant to patient variants via inclusion of drugs contained in variant treatment approaches, or through molecular inclusion criteria. To retrieve a list of open clinical trials related to sample variants, we have implemented a complex query that retrieves clinical trials both for drugs in treatment approaches and those that contain molecular criteria for the parent gene associated with sample variants, irrespective of therapy. Clinical trials are queried first by drugs contained in variant treatment approaches, and for resulting trials containing those drugs, data is retrieved and displayed including NCTID, sponsor, title, and therapy, as well as a column including the variant for which the trial was pulled. Clinical trials are also queried on parent gene, excluding all trials with a requirement for wild-type. Clinical trials can be further restricted through the selection of Disease Ontology terms, related to patient indication. The Disease Ontology (DO) is a robust, regularly maintained, ontology of standardized disease terms, each backed by individual unique identifiers (DOIDs), which facilitates precise mapping to patient diagnosis[7]. When selected, returned trials will include only those that are related to the selected DOID and all child terms. This process is enabled by the integration of the DO tree in clinical trial curation, which can be employed for retrieval of only those trials relevant to the patient's indication.

2.3. Clinical Trial Landscape

Outside of CKB, there are currently no publicly available comprehensive databases that curate information on molecular eligibility for clinical trials. Access of clinical trials recruiting on molecular criteria is not readily accessible through clinical trial registries, such as clinical-trials.gov, which is primarily the result of a lack of standardization of nomenclature and syntax for molecular eligibility criteria in clinical trial registries[8]. One significant potential outcome of this is an inadequate representation of potentially relevant clinical trials for clinicians performing a cursory keyword search. In addition, the lack of molecular criteria accessibility likely increases the time necessary for identifying potentially relevant trials, as a clinician must sort through the trial record to identify molecular inclusion criteria. To expedite retrieval of relevant clinical trials and streamline the path toward clinical intervention based on molecular variant, we have incorporated manual curation of molecular eligibility into the JAX-CKB database to easily connect patients with trials that are relevant to findings from next-generation sequencing.

In addition to providing a path to intervention in clinical reporting, the organization and design of the JAX-CKB (discussed below) allows us to readily analyze the current landscape of clinical trials. This analysis of the relative number of clinical trials for drug class or molecular criteria enables a view into the strengths and weaknesses in targeting actionable variants in clinical trials. Previous analysis of the landscape of cancer clinical trials in the USA, in the absence of a structured curated database, has required significant effort using data extracted manually via keyword search of clinicaltrials.gov[9]. The organization of data elements curated into the JAX-CKB database facilitates rapid analysis of data from clinical trials through customized queries of the database. Using these queries, we have analyzed the landscape of trials restricted to those currently open (defined as those with the recruitment status of "not yet recruiting," "recruiting," or "available") related to our 358-gene targeted panel.

When broken down by patient indication (**Figure 4**), 19.1% of open trials curated into the JAX-CKB are recruiting patients with advanced solid tumors with unspecified histology (398/2058; **Figure 4**). This comprises the largest proportion of curated clinical trials and likely represents early stage trials for therapeutics that have not demonstrated clinical utility in specific tumor types. Other well-studied indications are highly represented in clinical trials (**Figure 4**), particularly those for which a recurring molecular target has been identified. These include non-small cell lung cancer (13.23%; 274/2058), melanoma (8.0%; 167/2058), ERBB2 (Her2)-receptor negative breast cancer (4.8%; 100/2058), prostate adenocarcinoma (4.7%; 96/2058), glioblastoma multiforme (4.3%; 89/2058), and head and neck squamous cell carcinoma (4.0%; 83/2058) (**Figure 4**). There are 96 indications present as inclusion criteria in only a single open clinical trial for a targeted therapy, representing an unmet need for these patients. These indications include rare cancers, such as chordoma (NCT01407198) and hemangiopericytoma (NCT01396408), which have very little data surrounding targeted therapeutic efficacy, and accordingly very few promising treatment options[10][11].

Independent of histology, patients may enter clinical trials based on molecular eligibility, either through a molecular aberration that is targeted by an agent in the trial, or a trial that is directly recruiting on the presence of a specific molecular criterion, irrespective if the investigated therapy has demonstrated a connection to the molecular target. Drug classes are a proxy for treatment approach, and

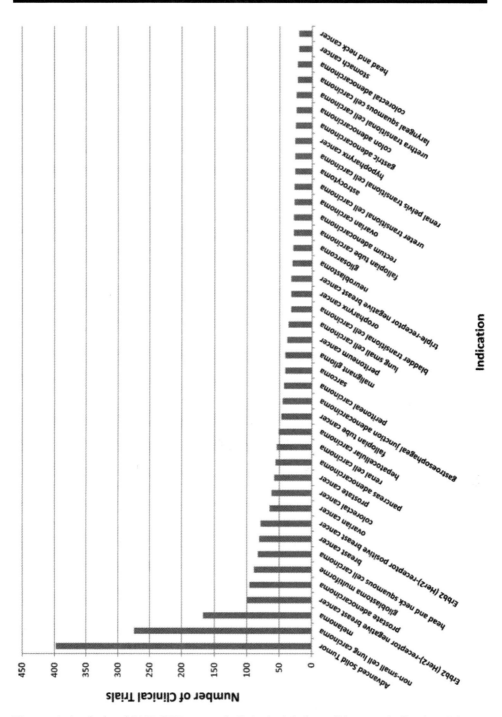

Figure 4. Analysis of JAX-CKB curated clinical trials by solid tumor indication. Disease Ontology terms selected as patient indication for greater than 20 clinical trials plotted relative to the number of open clinical trials recruiting on each indication.

identifying the number of clinical trials investigating drugs within specific drug classes provides insight into the availability of targeted therapies for molecular aberrations. In an analysis of the most frequent drug classes containing drugs currently under investigation in open clinical trials, we have determined that Pan-VEGFR Inhibitors (378/2168; 17.4%), KIT Inhibitors (312/2168; 14.4%), Pan-PDGFR Inhibitors (208/2168; 9.6%), and RET Inhibitors (205/2168; 9.5%) are most highly represented (**Figure 5**). This suggests that patients with activating mutations in KDR (VEGFR2), KIT, PDGFR, and RET, depending on indication, may have several options for potential therapeutic intervention through recruiting clinical trials. In contrast, the drug classes DNMT1 inhibitors, EZH2 inhibitors, and FGFR3 antibody are among those represented in a single open clinical trial, which suggests that patients harboring genetic aberrations targeted by these drug

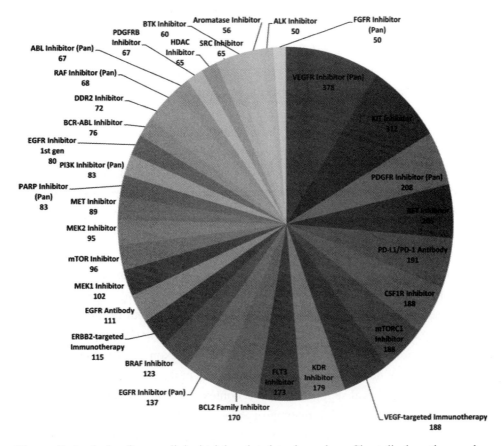

Figure 5. Analysis of open clinical trials related to drug class. Chart displays the number of clinical trials investigating targeted drugs within specified drug classes, for all drug classes represented in greater than 50 open clinical trials.

classes may have fewer options.

Clinical trials may also recruit patients based directly on molecular eligibility, which may be restricted to specific molecular aberrations, or a wider category of molecular aberrations. For instance, a patient with an exon 19 deletion in EGFR could potentially enroll in clinical trials recruiting patients with "EGFR mutations," "EGFR activating mutations," "EGFR exon 19 deletions," or the specific deletion harbored by this patient. Currently, the top 5 molecular criteria in open clinical trials are related to the expression of various hormone and growth factor receptors including ERBB2, PGR, and ESR1 (**Figure 6**), which is likely related to their long-standing clinical association with breast cancer subtyping and therapeutic relevance[12]. Mutations in BRAF V600 have demonstrated clinical utility as targetable aberrations[13] and are highly represented as molecular eligibility criteria in clinical trials, with 36 open trials recruiting on BRAF V600 mutations at the time of this manuscript [**Figure 6(b)**]. BRCA1 and BRCA2 mutations are also frequently included as molecular eligibility criteria, with 35 and 33 open trials recruiting on these variants, respectively [**Figure 6(b)**].

EGFR aberrations are a highly represented target for investigational therapies in clinical trials. EGFR is the fifth most common gene associated with molecular inclusion criteria for open clinical trials curated into CKB, with 86 clinical trials including EGFR-related molecular inclusion criteria [**Figure 6(a)**]. Most of these trials are related to the well-characterized EGFR L858R and exon 19 deletion mutations [**Figure 6(c)**], which have demonstrated sensitivity to EGFR tyrosine kinase inhibitors (TKIs)[14]. In contrast, EGFR exon 20 insertion mutations demonstrate de novo resistance to EGFR TKIs and have few options for clinical intervention[15][16]. At the time of this manuscript, EGFR exon 20 insertions are included as eligibility criteria for two open clinical trials. Both of these trials are investigating the HSP90 inhibitor AUY922 and are recruiting either specifically on exon 20 insertions or for EGFR mutations, including exon 20 insertions. HSP90 inhibitors have not demonstrated full clinical utility in the context of EGFR mutations but have preclinical support[17]. In this context, HSP90 inhibitors do not meet the stringency for a JAX-CKB treatment approach, and thus would not be an entry point for clinical trial association for patients with EGFR exon 20 insertion mutations. Therefore, the inclusion of molecular criteria in this instance represents a mechanism for therapeutic intervention that would not otherwise be available.

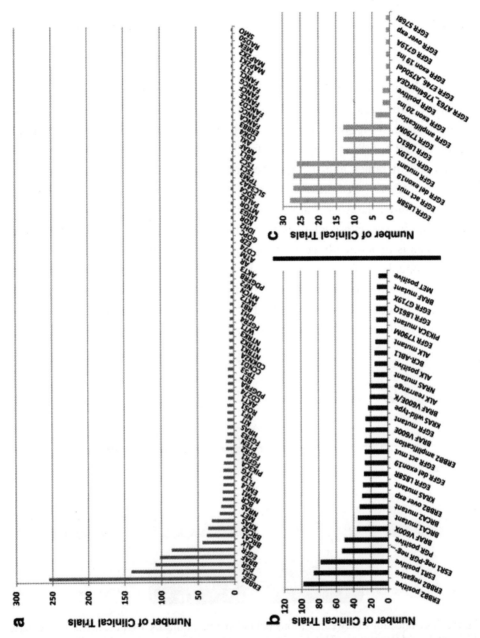

Figure 6. Analysis of number of open clinical trials relative to gene and gene variant as molecular criteria. a Combined total of clinical trials with eligibility criteria related to individual genes. Graph displays genes that are represented by molecular eligibility criteria in two or greater clinical trials. b Number of clinical trials for the top specific or category molecular criteria represented in clinical trials, limited to those in 10 or more clinical trials. c Number of clinical trials for each type of EGFR molecular criteria present in open clinical trials.

2.4. The JAX Clinical Knowledgebase and Curation User Interface

A critical component to accessing data for reporting or analysis is a comprehensive structured database. Thus, we have designed and implemented an in-house database to support clinical reporting and analysis of clinically relevant data. The JAX-CKB serves as a repository for data regarding oncology-relevant genetic variants and therapies and incorporates interconnectivity between protein effect, therapeutic efficacy, treatment approaches, and recruiting clinical trials. CKB features a structured database framework for managing clinical and biological data, into which clinical data content is entered through a curation user interface (**Figure 7**). Data is dynamically curated by experts to populate comprehensive content related to oncology, to support clinical reporting, and to maintain the most up-to-date information on therapies, response, and relevant clinical trials. While JAX-CKB content is currently tailored toward solid tumor clinical reporting, the framework of the JAX-CKB is versatile and can support additional applications.

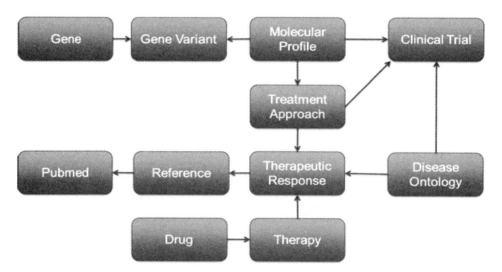

Figure 7. Connections between various data elements in the JAX Clinical Knowledgebase (JAX-CKB). Molecular profiles consist of one of more molecular entities, linked to gene variants and parent genes. Molecular profiles are assigned relevant treatment approaches based on available data from the literature on efficacy, as a therapeutic response. The therapeutic response additionally takes into account patient indication, which is represented by an integrated disease ontology. Treatment approaches contain therapies, which consist of a single drug or combination of drugs. These drugs can be either FDA-approved, or under investigation in clinical trials, which are additionally curated into the JAX-CKB.

The organization of the JAX-CKB is essential to its utility in supporting clinical reporting and includes several key elements (**Figure 3**), which are outlined below.

2.4.1. Data Elements

The JAX-CKB database incorporates several data elements, which are connected in various ways in curation of cancer-related data.

2.4.2. Genes and Gene Variants

To support standardization and mapping of genetic variants to JAX-CKB and facilitate interoperability with other databases, we have incorporated HUGO Gene No-menclature Committee (HGNC) nomenclature through the integration of approved symbols and gene names from the NCBI Gene database into the JAX-CKB[3][18]. By incorporating gene names from the Gene database, genes are assigned approved symbols, removing variability, and are additionally backed by unique numerical gene identifiers (NCBI GeneID). Although our current JAX Cancer Treatment Panel (JAX CTP) is limited to 358 cancer-related genes, the JAX-CKB incorporates all known annotated human genes. This supports the rapid pace of advancement in cancer research, as well as allowing for the flexibility to support additional assays, which would include sequencing assays for other disease types.

Naming of genetic variants in the JAX-CKB utilizes a Regular Expression (regex) system that conforms to Human Genome Variation Society (HGVS) nomenclature guidelines, restricting the entry of genetic variants to a predefined syntax and enabling mapping of variants to JAX-CKB. HGVS maintains standards for variant naming, which serves to eliminate ambiguity and ensure precision when reporting data related to genetic variants[4]. Conforming to these standards additionally provides a mechanism to promote interoperability between databases. Each variant type is assigned a specified syntax. For example, a mutation resulting in a single amino acid change, such as the gene variant KRAS G12C, would follow the syntax [ACDEFGHIKLMNPQRSTVWY] [0-9] + [ACDEF-GHIKLMN PQRSTVWY]. The regex syntax is periodically updated to maintain compliance with HGVS guidelines. The JAX-CKB additionally incorporates controlled vocabularies regarding protein effect, to annotate functional relevance of specific variants. This aids in the interpretation of actionability and provides a further mechanism for filtering gene variants. Gene variants are linked to a parent gene and can include any alteration to the gene, supporting multi-omic data curation. Examples of variants include mutations, changes to gene copy number, and expression changes. In addition, JAX-CKB supports annotation of category variants (e.g., activating mutation, inactivating mutation), which allows molecular profile responses and clinical trials to be curated to conditions where they are applicable to multiple or unknown/unspecified aberrations. For example, the category variant "EGFR activating mutation" represents any activating mutation in EGFR. There are also less broad category variants, such as "EGFR del exon 19," which represents a non-specified deletion within exon 19 of the EGFR gene. These variants are also subject to regex syntax and must meet predefined specifications. The inclusion of category variants enables capture of information that is relevant to bins of variants, rather than individual variants, or in conditions where the applicable variants are not specified.

Within the Gene Variant Curation User Interface (UI), there are multiple fields for data capture, each utilizing their own specific controlled vocabularies to minimize variability and allow for efficient analysis of curated information. The curation user interface allows users to capture information around genetic variants related to amino acid change, mutational impact to the protein (e.g., missense, deletion, and frameshift), and functional effect on the protein (e.g., gain-of function, and loss-of-function). In addition, gene variants can be linked to their impact on biological pathways, through the integration of a human pathway ontology from the Rat Genome Database[19]. The gene variant UI also incorporates a free-text annotation field for capture of specific information on the relationship of the variant to oncogenic transformation and protein function, which is supported by curated references from primary literature.

2.4.3. Molecular Profiles

A molecular profile in the JAX-CKB contains one or more genetic aberrations, which can include mutations, such as single nucleotide polymorphisms (SNPs), frame-shifts, insertions, and deletions, as well as gene fusions, copy number variations and/or changes in expression levels. The flexibility of the molecular profile and the ability to build complex molecular profiles allow for the curation of therapeutic efficacy to multiple aberrations simultaneously, rather than each variant in isolation. For example, a molecular profile may contain a mutation, such as the EGFR activating mutation EGFR L858R, as well as a copy number variation, such as amplification of the MET gene. MET amplification is a recognized mechanism for resistance to EGFR tyrosine kinase inhibitor therapy[20]–[22], and the ability to create a complex profile enables the curation of resistance data to the appropriate complex molecular conditions.

Current research supports the idea that targeted treatment of tumor driver mutations alone often leads to the up regulation of compensatory mechanisms and/or acquisition of secondary resistance mutations and that utilizing a multi-target approach may be beneficial in reducing the potential for resistance[23]. For example, the ability to assign treatment approaches and curate efficacy evidence to multiple aberrations simultaneously enables JAX-CKB and downstream clinical reporting to stay on-pace with clinical progress in the use of combination therapies in complex multi-omic conditions.

2.4.4. Drugs and Therapies

A key component to capture response data related to molecular targets is a comprehensive database of relevant drugs, which are incorporated as data elements into JAX-CKB. Attributes associated with drugs include drug name, trade name, and synonyms, in which each are required to be unique terms within a drug record, and among other records, to effectively eliminate redundancy. CKB currently contains 1108 unique targeted therapies relevant to treatment approaches or clinical trials for variants related to our 358-gene panel. When appropriate, drugs are assigned a "Drug Class," as a selectable field within the Therapy UI using an in-house controlled vocabulary. Drug class represents a rational group of drugs with a unified target, such as "PIK3CA Inhibitor" for drugs that target PIK3CA. These drug classes are then utilized as "Treatment Approaches" for a molecular profile, which provides a link between molecular aberrations and relevant targeted therapies.

Therapies, similar to molecular profiles, are comprised of one or more drugs. The ability to build complex therapies supports the therapeutic trend toward using targeted therapies in combination with other targeted therapies or chemotherapies and enables precision and accuracy in efficacy curation.

2.4.5. Treatment Approaches

The current utility of CKB is to support clinical reporting for our JAX CTP panel. To this end, we have incorporated the selection of potential treatment approaches for molecular profiles, which designates a relationship between a selected molecular profile and either a drug class or individual therapy. Treatment approaches are selected following extensive review of the literature supporting preclinical and/or clinical efficacy, which is additionally curated via molecular profile response. For example, the gene variant PIK3CA H1047R is a gain-of-function variant in PIK3CA[24]. Due to several lines of evidence, PIK3CA H1047R has been assigned the drug class treatment approaches "mTOR inhibitors", "PI3K inhibitors", and "AKT inhibitors". Each of these drug classes is linked to a milieu of drugs with the target mTOR, PI3K, and/or AKT, respectively. These treatment approaches are used in the reporting queries to identify relevant therapies and clinical trials.

2.4.6. Molecular Profile Response and Efficacy Evidence

An essential component of a clinical knowledgebase is the inclusion of evidence from primary literature sources supporting therapeutic efficacy in the context of specific molecular variants. The "Molecular Profile Response" element of the JAX-CKB represents the relationship between a molecular profile and indication, therapy, and related response type. The patient indication attribute integrates the cancer terms from the Disease Ontology[7], which are backed by unique identifiers (DOID) and represented in a navigable tree.

Associated with the molecular profile response is efficacy evidence, which is the point of entry for literature-based data supporting the molecular profile response. A molecular profile response can be associated with one or more lines of efficacy evidence. Efficacy evidence additionally includes information regarding the approval status of the associated therapy in relation to the curated evidence, using a controlled vocabulary to designate whether the study was preclinical, phase I, phase Ib/II, phase III, or FDA-approved, or if the therapy-molecular profile association is in National Comprehensive Cancer Network (NCCN), FDA, or European Society for Medical Oncology (ESMO) Guidelines. Curation of FDA-approval studies links tumor type to approval status, allowing for simultaneous identification of targeted therapies that have achieved FDA-approval in a patient indication. Efficacy evidence can be categorized, using controlled vocabulary, as actionable, which is characterized as data relating the efficacy of the selected therapy in the context of the selected profile response and is prioritized based on an in-house 25-tier ranking system. Additionally, the JAX-CKB supports the entry of prognostic and diagnostic evidence as well as emerging evidence, which supports potential emerging therapeutic targets.

2.4.7. Clinical Trials

To facilitate the inclusion of relevant clinical trials in patient reporting to provide an additional potential avenue for therapeutic intervention, we have incorporated clinical trial content into the JAX-CKB. This additionally provides a unique mechanism for the analysis of clinical trial data, which is cumbersome through direct extraction from clinical trial databases. For the import of clinical trials into CKB, we have built a utility that searches clinical trials from clinical-trials.gov using a predefined list of targeted therapies, restricted to trials in the USA or Canada in "cancer" that are "open," which are defined as those trials that have a recruitment status of "recruiting," "not yet recruiting," or "available." Returned trials are matched against those in the JAX-CKB to produce a unique list of new clinical trials. Information including NCTID, title, and recruitment status is imported, and remaining information from the trial record that cannot be automatically retrieved from clinicaltrials.gov is manually curated. The NCTID serves as a unique identifier for each clinical trial. The elements in the clinical trial user interface enable connectivity to molecular aberrations in two ways. First, an intervention attribute enables curation of therapies being tested in the clinical trial. These therapies are selected from a drop-down list of therapies that is populated from the therapy table. The drugs contained in those therapies can then be linked to a treatment approach via a drug class or individual therapy. Additionally, clinical trial curation integrates molecular eligibility criteria, so trials recruiting based on the presence or absence of specific molecular criteria can be easily identified. Therefore, a patient sample with an EGFR mutation would be linked to a trial testing erlotinib that is recruiting on EGFR activating mutations both by the targeted therapy and the required molecular criteria.

To ensure that we have the most up-to-date information in the JAX-CKB regarding clinical trial status, we have built a cron job that performs a nightly search of clinical-trials.gov for any change to recruitment status for trials in the JAX-CKB and automatically updates any changes to the database. Thus, only clinical trials that have open recruitment statuses are included on clinical reports.

The connectivity of data in JAX-CKB and the associated reporting tools enables a direct connection between molecular aberration and targeted therapy and connects patients to trials investigating a relevant targeted therapy, but which may not be specifically recruiting on a molecular aberration. This may have the unintentional, beneficial consequence of increasing success and development of targeted agents by prescreening patients outside of the clinical trial protocol for the presence of relevant genomic targets.

3. Conclusions

Progress in patient treatment in oncology is dependent on both a comprehensive understanding of the relationships between molecular variants in tumors and efficacy, and the power to access clinically relevant information in a timely manner. Here, we share methods and demonstrate the implementation of a data mapper and loader and queries for rapid retrieval of data related to clinical efficacy to inform clinical interpretation of molecular aberrations, supported by the structured and organized design of the JAX Clinical Knowledgebase. In addition, global analysis of the clinical trial landscape provides insight into the types of targeted agents and molecular targets that are focal points, as well as those that could be served by additional investigation.

4. Methods

4.1. JAX-CKB Mapper and JAX-CKB Schema

The following versions of the JAX-CKB mapper and database were used in analysis:

JAX-CKB mapper: Version 1.05.

JAX-CKB Schema: Version 1.4. JAX-CKB; 81 Tables.

4.2. Data Analysis

For data analysis, data was retrieved from the stage version of the JAX-CKB database using SQL queries. Due to the dynamic nature of the data in the production database due to continual curation, the stage database, which is not subject to continual update, was used to eliminate variability in the data. The stage database was last updated on September 18, 2015, from a snapshot of the production version of the JAX-CKB database.

4.3. Clinical Trial Recruitment Status Updating

A nightly cron job is implemented to query https://clinicaltrials.gov/ct2/results. It parses the HTML contents to obtain the trials that match the search criteria [cancer-related clinical trials in the United States and Canada] and check the recruitment status of all existing trials in the JAX-CKB database. Following comparison with the recruitment status of clinical trials in the JAX-CKB database, it updates the database and sends an email notification to data curators if any recruitment status is changed.

4.4. Abbreviations

CKB: Clinical Knowledgebase; CGA: Clinical Genome Analytics; CTP: Cancer Treatment Profile; DO: Disease Ontology; HGNC: HUGO Gene Nomenclature Committee; HGVS: Human Genome Variation Society; HUGO: Human Genome Organisation; regex: Regular Expression; VCF: variant call format.

Competing Interests

The authors declare that they have no competing interests.

Authors' Contributions

SEP prepared the manuscript and contributed to data analysis and interpretation and figure preparation. RL is the primary designer and developer of the JAX-CKB database and data loader and mapper and contributed to data analysis. SMM conceived of and participated in design of the database and contributed to data analysis. AL and DD designed queries and contributed to the database development. CMS participated in data analysis. All authors read and approved the final manuscript.

Acknowledgements

We would like to thank Taofei Yin, Sean Eddy, Guruprasad Ananda, and Danielle Ruby for their contributions to data curation and database support.

Source: Patterson S, RangjiaoLiu, Statz C, *et al*. The clinical trial landscape in oncology and connectivity of somatic mutational profiles to targeted therapies[J]. Human Genomics, 2016, 10(1).

References

[1]   Forbes SA, Beare D, Gunasekaran P, Leung K, Bindal N, Boutselakis H, *et al*. COSMIC: exploring the world's knowledge of somatic mutations in human cancer. Nucleic Acids Res. 2015; 43(Database issue): D805–811.

[2]   My Cancer Genome. Vanderbilt-Ingram Cancer Center. http://www. mycancerge-nome.org. Accessed 20 Oct 2015.

[3]   Gray KA, Yates B, Seal RL, Wright MW, Bruford EA. Genenames.org: the HGNC resources in. Nucleic Acids Res 2015. 2015; 43(Database issue):D1079–1085.

[4]   den Dunnen JT, Antonarakis SE. Mutation nomenclature extensions and suggestions to describe complex mutations: a discussion. Hum Mutat. 2000; 15:7–12.

[5]   Yuan Y, Van Allen EM, Omberg L, Wagle N, Amin-Mansour A, Sokolov A, *et al*. Assessing the clinical utility of cancer genomic and proteomic data across tumor types. Nat Biotechnol. 2014; 32:644–652.

[6]   Ananda G, Mockus S, Lundquist M, Spotlow V, Simons A, Mitchell T, *et al*. Devel-

opment and validation of the JAX Cancer Treatment Profile™ for detection of clinically actionable mutations in solid tumors. Exp Mol Pathol. 2015; 98:106–12.

[7]   Schriml LM, Mitraka E. The Disease Ontology: fostering interoperability between biological and clinical human disease-related data. Mamm Genome Off J Int Mamm Genome Soc. 2015; 26:584–9.

[8]   Mockus S, Patterson S, Statz C, Bult C, Tsongalis G. Clinical trials in precision oncology. Clin Chem. 2015.247437. [Epub ahead of print].

[9]   Roper N, Stensland KD, Hendricks R, Galsky MD. The landscape of precision cancer medicine clinical trials in the United States. Cancer Treat Rev. 2015; 41: 385–90.

[10] Di Maio S, Yip S, Al Zhrani GA, Alotaibi FE, Al Turki A, Kong E, et al. Novel targeted therapies in chordoma: an update. Ther Clin Risk Manag. 2015; 11:873–83.

[11] Ramakrishna R, Rostomily R, Sekhar L, Rockhill J, Ferreira M. Hemangiopericytoma: radical resection remains the cornerstone of therapy. J Clin Neurosci Off J Neurosurg Soc Australas. 2014; 21:612–5.

[12] Sana M, Malik HJ. Current and emerging breast cancer biomarkers. J Cancer Res Ther. 2015; 11:508–13.

[13] Spagnolo F, Ghiorzo P, Orgiano L, Pastorino L, Picasso V, Tornari E, et al. BRAF-mutant melanoma: treatment approaches, resistance mechanisms, and diagnostic strategies. OncoTargets Ther. 2015; 8:157–68.

[14] Kuan F-C, Kuo L-T, Chen M-C, Yang C-T, Shi C-S, Teng D, et al. Overall survival benefits of first-line EGFR tyrosine kinase inhibitors in EGFR-mutated non-small-cell lung cancers: a systematic review and meta-analysis. Br J Cancer. 2015; 113(10):1519–28.

[15] Naidoo J, Sima CS, Rodriguez K, Busby N, Nafa K, Ladanyi M, et al. Epidermal growth factor receptor exon 20 insertions in advanced lung adenocarcinomas: clinical outcomes and response to erlotinib. Cancer. 2015; 121(18):3212–20.

[16] Yasuda H, Park E, Yun C-H, Sng NJ, Lucena-Araujo AR, Yeo W-L, et al. Structural, biochemical, and clinical characterization of epidermal growth factor receptor (EGFR) exon 20 insertion mutations in lung cancer. Sci Transl Med. 2013; 5:216ra177.

[17] Choi YJ, Kim SY, So KS, Baek I-J, Kim WS, Choi SH, et al. AUY922 effectively overcomes MET- and AXL-mediated resistance to EGFR-TKI in lung cancer cells. PloS One. 2015; 10:e0119832.

[18] Brown GR, Hem V, Katz KS, Ovetsky M, Wallin C, Ermolaeva O, et al. Gene: a gene-centered information resource at NCBI. Nucleic Acids Res. 2015; 43(Database issue): D36–42.

[19] Petri V, Jayaraman P, Tutaj M, Hayman GT, Smith JR, De Pons J, et al. The pathway ontology—updates and applications. J Biomed Semant. 2014; 5:7.

[20] Costa DB, Nguyen K-SH, Cho BC, Sequist LV, Jackman DM, Riely GJ, *et al.* Effects of erlotinib in EGFR mutated non-small cell lung cancers with resistance to gefitinib. Clin Cancer Res Off J Am Assoc Cancer Res. 2008; 14:7060–7.

[21] Robinson KW, Sandler AB. The role of MET receptor tyrosine kinase in non-small cell lung cancer and clinical development of targeted anti-MET agents. The Oncologist. 2013; 18:115–22.

[22] Turke AB, Zejnullahu K, Wu Y-L, Song Y, Dias-Santagata D, Lifshits E, *et al.* Preexistence and clonal selection of MET amplification in EGFR mutant NSCLC. Cancer Cell. 2010; 17:77–88.

[23] Mancini M, Yarden Y. Mutational and network level mechanisms underlying resistance to anti-cancer kinase inhibitors. Semin Cell Dev Biol. 2015; pii: S1084-9521(15)00178-0. [Epub ahead of print].

[24] Gymnopoulos M, Elsliger M-A, Vogt PK. Rare cancer-specific mutations in PIK3CA show gain of function. Proc Natl Acad Sci U S A. 2007; 104:5569–74.

Chapter 20

Advancing Clinical Oncology Through Genome Biology and Technology

Anna M. Varghese[1], Michael F. Berger[2,3,4]

[1]Department of Medicine, Memorial Sloan Kettering Cancer Center, New York, NY 10065, USA

[2]Department of Pathology, Memorial Sloan Kettering Cancer Center, New York, NY 10065, USA

[3]Human Oncology and Pathogenesis Program, Memorial Sloan Kettering Cancer Center, New York, NY 10065, USA

[4]Center for Molecular Oncology, Memorial Sloan Kettering Cancer Center, New York, NY 10065, USA

Abstract: The use of genomic technologies for the molecular characterization of tumors has propelled our understanding of cancer biology and is transforming the way patients with cancer are diagnosed and treated.

1. Clinical Oncology - Facing up to the Next Steps

More than any other field of medicine, oncology has benefited from recent revolutionary advances in nucleic acid sequencing technology and genomic analysis. For increasingly lower costs and turnaround times, one can profile the full spectrum of genomic alterations in a tumor sample, including sequence mutations, copy number changes and structural rearrangements[1]. Research initiatives have capitalized on the availability of large numbers of tumors in order to delineate the most frequently mutated genes and pathways in a range of cancer types. Collectively these projects, including The Cancer Genome Atlas (TCGA) and the International Cancer Genome Consortium (ICGC), are characterizing the genomes and epigenomes of virtually all common tumor types and producing a more complete understanding of the biology of cancer[2]–[12]. Just as significantly, the introduction of genomic technologies is transforming clinical practice. Massively parallel "next-generation sequencing" (NGS) has proven to be a powerful molecular-diag- nostic tool, enabling the identification of prognostic and predictive biomarkers in individual clinical specimens. Challenges for the widespread implementation of clinical NGS platforms remain, including technical, operational, medical and societal considerations. However, by confronting these issues collectively, we can overcome these challenges and realize the maximum benefit to clinical oncology.

2. Opportunities for Applying Genomics to Oncology

Research initiatives such as TCGA and ICGC have led to an improved understanding of cancer biology through the genomic analysis of tumors procured from anonymized patients possessing many different types of cancer. A major goal of these and similar efforts is to identify genes and pathways important to cancer progression in order to design better therapies and interventions. As an early example, the identification of recurrent somatic mutations in the serine/threonine-protein kinase B-raf (BRAF) gene from systematic gene sequencing[13] prompted the development of multiple targeted inhibitors of BRAF (notably vemurafenib and dabrafenib), currently approved by the Food and Drug Administration (FDA) for melanoma and showing promise in a range of other cancer types[14][15]. Yet the most exciting and transformative applications of genomics in oncology involve the use of genomic techniques to analyze clinical tumor specimens. First, by sequencing tumors obtained from patients treated with approved and experimental targeted therapies, one can discover clinical biomarkers that predict outcomes and therapeutic response. Second, by prospectively sequencing patients' tumors as part of their care, one can select personalized therapies to employ based on the individual molecular profile of the tumors. We discuss both of these opportunities below.

2.1. Phenotype to Genotype: Retrospective Sequencing for Biomarker Discovery

Genomic alterations that predict the likelihood of response to therapeutic agents, especially novel targeted therapies, serve as powerful biomarkers and major determinants of treatment decisions. In many cases, the retrospective characterization of tumors procured from patients with documented clinical outcomes has revealed the molecular basis of drug response. For example, the discovery of epidermal growth factor receptor (EGFR) mutations in lung cancer was prompted by the clinical observation that a subset of patients exhibited a major response when administered tyrosine kinase inhibitors in clinical trials[16]–[18]. Today, a growing number of clinical trials in oncology are designed with correlative sequence analysis for biomarker discovery written into the study.

Recently, the analysis of "exceptional responders" cancer patients with an unexpected complete and/or durable response to therapy has proven to be particularly effective. Studying exceptional responders can reveal specific genomic alterations accounting for their exquisite sensitivity to certain drugs. One can hypothesize that other patients whose tumors bear similar alterations will benefit from the same drugs. Recent successful applications of whole-genome or exome sequencing in exceptional responders include the identification of tuberous sclerosis 1 protein/hamartin (TSC1) and serine/threonine-protein kinase mTOR/mammalian target of rapamycin (MTOR) mutations in bladder cancer patients responding to everolimus and a mutation in serine/threonine-protein kinase A-Raf (ARAF) in a lung cancer patient responding to sorafenib[19]–[21]. Owing to the promise of this approach, the US National Cancer Institute has launched a program to collect tissue samples and clinical data from up to 200 exceptional responders in an attempt to explain isolated responses to drugs that otherwise failed clinical trials[22].

Retrospective analysis of clinical tumor specimens can also reveal mechanisms of acquired resistance to targeted therapies. By collecting and comparing samples before treatment and at progression, one can discover genetic alterations that emerge during drug exposure and confer drug resistance. This approach has led to the identification of a broad spectrum of resistance mechanisms arising during inhibition of EGFR in lung cancer and during inhibition of BRAF in melanoma[23]–[27]. Other examples include single-nucleotide mutations conferring resistance to imatinib in leukemia[28], enzalutamide in prostate cancer[29] and anti-estrogen therapy in breast cancer[30][31]. Resistance mutations might be second hits to the drug target itself, could affect downstream genes that re- activate the targeted pathway or might activate alternative pathways that bypass or counteract the effects of the drug. The identification of such mutations in tumors can point to novel combination strategies and/or lead to the development of new, more potent drugs.

2.2. Genotype to Phenotype: Prospective Sequencing for Clinical Diagnosis

Based in part on the identification of predictive clinical biomarkers from retrospective analyses, there are several tumor types for which prospective mutation profiling as a diagnostic tool is now a standard of care. Patients with metastatic non-small cell lung cancer are routinely tested for EGFR mutations and rearrangements of the gene encoding the ALK tyrosine kinase receptor/anaplastic lymphoma kinase (ALK) to guide treatment. If a sensitizing mutation in EGFR or a rearrangement in ALK is identified, treatment with an inhibitor of EGFR or ALK is recommended. While drugs targeting these alterations are FDA approved, several targeted agents have demonstrated activity against lung cancers harboring other genetic alterations. For instance, cabozantinib has demonstrated activity in lung cancers harboring rearrangements in the gene encoding the tyrosine-protein kinase receptor Ret (RET), and crizotinib has demonstrated activity in lung cancers harboring amplifications in the gene encoding the hepatocyte growth factor receptor (MET) or rearrangements in the ROS1 gene encoding tyrosine-protein kinase ROS[32]–[34]. For patients with metastatic colorectal cancer, testing for the presence or absence of hotspot mutations in the genes encoding the GTPases KRAS and NRAS is recommended to assess whether patients might benefit from EGFR-directed monoclonal antibody therapies utilizing the drugs cetuximab or panitumumab. For patients with melanoma harboring V600 mutations in BRAF, treatment with vemurafenib or dabrafenib is recommended.

Molecular-diagnostics labs have traditionally relied on low-throughput, mutation-specific methods for DNA profiling in patients because there were so few actionable genetic alterations that altered treatment decisions in the clinical care of patients. However, given the growing number of biomarkers and clinical trials studying targeted agents, the approach of testing one mutation at a time is unsustainable. NGS-based assays are replacing these more-focused tests in both academic and commercial settings. The benefits of this are obvious. First, a single NGS test can encompass all "actionable" targets, eliminating the need for multiple parallel tests for different mutations and enabling more-efficient workflows and tissue utilization. Second, the entire coding sequence of target genes can be assayed (rather than only pre-specified sites), facilitating the detection of both common and rare mutations in oncogenes and tumor-suppressor genes. Third, NGS enables the detection of additional classes of genomic alterations, such as copy number changes and structural rearrangements. Finally, subclonal events in heterogeneous tumors can be detected more reliably owing to the high sensitivity afforded by NGS.

Some academic centers have implemented pilot programs for the comprehensive genomic characterization of tumors from selected patients by means of whole-genome or exome sequencing (DNA-Seq) and transcriptome sequencing (RNA-Seq)[35][36]. Through expert review and curation of these expansive data sets, clinically relevant alterations can often be identified that direct treatment with rationally chosen available therapies. "Genomic tumor boards" composed of clinicians and scientists trained in medical oncology, cell biology, genomics and bioinformatics, as pioneered by the University of Michigan and elsewhere, are forming at many leading cancer centers to review and interpret clinical genomic data in order to recommend and guide therapy[35]. These organizations also serve to educate members of the medical community as to the power and intricacies of genomic analysis and are catalyzing the development of communal frame- works for the clinical annotation and interpretation of somatic alterations.

Owing to practical barriers in the implementation of this comprehensive approach for all patients, namely its high cost and low throughput, large-volume molecular-diagnostics labs have focused instead on targeted sequencing of key cancer-associated genes as a feasible and economical alternative[37]-[42]. Furthermore, the deeper sequence coverage afforded by targeted sequencing enables low-allele-frequency mutations in heterogeneous or low-purity tumors to be detected with greater sensitivity. Multiplexing through the use of sample "bar-codes" permits many tumors to be profiled in a single NGS run[43]. This has enormous implications for the design and implementation of clinical trials in oncology. By systematically screening large numbers of patients with metastatic disease for common and rare "druggable" mutations, patients can be pre-identified for future trials involving the most promising targeted therapies, and new trials can rapidly accrue patients with the greatest likelihood of exhibiting a clinical response. Novel clinical trial designs have emerged as a direct result of advances in molecular profiling. One such trial, often called a "basket" study, involves a single targeted drug administered to patients across many different tumor types (baskets) that share a common genomic profile. Other clinical protocols utilize centralized NGS-based diagnostic testing to assign patients recruited through cooperative groups to multiple separate trials involving targeted agents, pioneered by the NCI-MATCH study and others[22].

3. Challenges in Applying Genomics to Oncology

In order for genomic insights and technologies to be truly transforming in oncology, we must develop and implement high-throughput molecular-diagnostic tests that exhibit both clinical validity and clinical utility. Assays must achieve rapid turnaround times at low cost, encompass all classes of sequence-based mutations and structural alterations, and operate on small biopsies, formalin-fixed paraffin embedded (FFPE) tissue and cytological specimens[44]. Furthermore, results must be annotated with associated genomic and clinical data pertaining to the specific set of mutations observed in each individual tumor in order for oncologists to make the most-informed treatment decisions. This endeavor, although very promising, is fraught with challenges.

3.1. Technical and Operational Considerations

The development of assays compatible with low-quality specimens and low input DNA amounts remains a technical challenge. For these suboptimal samples that are routinely encountered in clinical settings, comprehensive genomic analysis is not always possible. PCR-based capture technologies can produce deep-coverage sequence data with very little DNA, but targets are generally small, and the detection of copy-number alterations and structural rearrangements is compromised. With slightly more DNA, hybridization-based capture assays enable an expanded number of target genes and alteration types but still can exclude important regions of the genome. Even whole-exome sequencing, encompassing all protein-coding genes in the genome, will miss many structural alterations as well as nucleotide substitutions involving regulatory regions such as the promoter of the gene encoding telomerase reverse transcriptase (TERT), which rank among the most frequently observed mutations in all cancers[45]-[47]. Individual clinical labs are left to choose how many (and which particular) genes to sequence based largely on their anticipated volume and diversity of cases, desired turnaround time and cost, and bioinformatics capabilities.

Indeed, providing support for bioinformatics represents one of the most significant challenges for the widespread implementation of clinical NGS workflows. Historically, pathology departments at hospitals and academic cancer centers have not employed large numbers of bioinformaticians. As a result, the recruitment and training of capable computational staff is of utmost importance in order to develop, maintain and deploy pipelines for the analysis of clinical cancer genomic data. The bioinformatics algorithms and software that comprise these pipelines are continually evolving, with new tools emerging constantly, making it difficult to standardize analysis procedures. Additionally, issues pertaining to the management and storage of large data files and the establishment of high-performance computing infrastructures for data processing and analysis represent new challenges for clinical labs and departments. The complexity of most hospital information systems could further hinder efforts to deposit molecular-diagnostic results into a patient's electronic health record and to link genomic data to other clinical, phenotypic and demographic data. This integration of genomic and clinical data is crucial for the long-term goal of achieving better outcomes for patients with cancer.

In order for clinical NGS results to be used by oncologists to influence treatment decisions, tests must be performed in Clinical Laboratory Improvement Amendments (CLIA)-compliant laboratories, governed by the Centers for Medicare & Medicaid Services (CMS). Accordingly, extensive documentation and technical validation of sensitivity, accuracy and reproducibility are required before any genomic assay can be prospectively administered and/or billed to healthcare payers. While some institutions have initiated programs where large-scale genomic analysis is performed in research labs, followed by confirmatory testing in CLIA-compliant labs, this approach is unsustainable when NGS-related costs cannot be recovered through reimbursement.

3.2. Clinical Considerations

While use of comprehensive molecular profiling has produced success stories, such as the remarkable responses to erlotinib for patients with EGFR-mutant lung cancers or crizotinib for patients with ALK-positive lung cancers, these findings have also resulted in challenges and questions concerning how to proceed.

First, comprehensive molecular profiling using any of the assays or technologies described above will yield in- formation about both well-known molecular drivers in cancer and countless more alterations whose biological and clinical significance is unclear. It is often difficult for a clinician to make the crucially important distinction between key "driver alterations" that should impact treatment and less-relevant "passenger mutations". Some publicly available knowledge banks have been created to help doctors and patients interpret the significance of many commonly seen alterations, such as My Cancer Genome developed at the Vanderbilt-Ingram Cancer Center. While these sites are excellent resources to learn about clinically and pathologically annotated alterations, they are not comprehensive and cannot be expected to include information on all possible alterations that a clinician could encounter. Similarly, there is little guidance for the management of patients with multiple driver alterations in more than one gene. One might rationally assume to administer combinations of targeted therapies; however, without knowing the toxicity profiles or optimal dosing and scheduling of the combination, this strategy is problematic.

Also, the use of targeted therapies in the treatment of cancer is rarely straightforward, even in the presence of individual well-characterized driver alterations. NGS testing of heterogeneous tumors can reveal targetable mutations at subclonal allele frequencies, the clinical consequences of which are uncertain. Furthermore, the biological and clinical context can be extremely important. For instance, while patients with melanomas harboring BRAF V600E mutations almost always respond to inhibitors of BRAF, this direct treatment approach has not been replicated for patients with BRAF-mutant colon cancers. Colon cancers harboring BRAF V600E mutations do not respond to single-agent vemurafenib-this is thought to be related to feedback reactivation of alternative or upstream signaling

514

pathways[48][49]. Studies are ongoing to explore and exploit these mechanisms by using combination therapy in the treatment of BRAF-mutant colon cancer. In order for clinicians to make in- formed treatment decisions, molecular-diagnostic reports must display alongside each mutation disease-specific contextual annotations in a succinct and easily digestible form.

Which specimens to analyze and when to analyze them are also questions that arise in the clinical care of patients. Given emerging data about tumor hetero- geneity in metastatic disease, it is unclear that a single biopsy of a single site of metastatic disease will accurately capture driver alterations that would most im- pact a patient's clinical care. Additionally, it is unclear that biopsies obtained at the time of diagnosis remain relevant after patients have developed acquired resistance to targeted therapies or have developed recurrent disease after initial therapies for early-stage cancer. While biopsies taken at the time of acquired resistance are be- coming standard in many clinical trials of targeted agents, these biopsies are not routinely performed in the clinical care of patients.

Most importantly, targeted therapies are not curing patients of their cancer. While targeted therapies have yielded promising, dramatic and life-changing res- ponses for many patients with cancer, the reality is that these responses are gener- ally short lived. For instance, the average responses to erlotinib among patients with EGFR-mutant lung cancer and vemurafenib for patients with BRAF V600E mutant melanoma are 11 months and 5 months, respectively[14][50]. All of these pa- tients will ultimately acquire resistance and succumb to their disease. In fact, some have questioned the cost effectiveness of targeted therapies, given the rare fre- quency of some driver mutations and the high cost of these therapies[51].

3.3. Societal Considerations

The societal and ethical implications of comprehensive genetic testing must also be considered in this rapidly changing technological landscape. While focused diagnostic tests including targeted "hotspot" panels utilize only tumor-derived DNA, more-comprehensive NGS approaches typically require germline DNA to distinguish between novel somatic mutations and inherited variants. The use of germline DNA poses the risk that incidental findings could be revealed relating to inherited susceptibility to cancer or other diseases. This has led institutions to consider different strategies of informed consent and pre-test genetic counseling. However, given the time pressures of clinical care, the ability to perform thorough genetic counseling in a routine fashion is limited. For those patients in whom an inherited predisposition to cancer is discovered, care must be taken to ensure the patients' autonomy and privacy, protect them and their families from possible discrimination and also manage the unintended emotional and psychological consequences that such a diagnosis brings.

Additionally, it remains unclear whether NGS-based molecular profiling is cost-effective or even clinically effective in the care of patients outside of lung cancer, melanoma and colon cancer. As a result, insurance companies have demonstrated a reluctance to reimburse the cost of comprehensive testing in many tumor types. While large academic cancer centers might be able to offset costs temporarily through grants and philanthropic contributions, broad access to these tests for patients in the community has not been achieved. Demonstrating the general clinical utility of NGS-based molecular profiling is essential in this regard. A related hindrance is that, when actionable mutations are detected in unexpected tumor types, insurance companies are often unwilling to reimburse the off-label administration of therapies approved in other diseases.

4. Concluding Remarks

While genomic knowledge has been successfully applied to direct clinical decisions in several cases, the implementation of clinical genomic workflows for oncology has proven to be complex. Nevertheless, the introduction of NGS technology has the potential to transform clinical oncology, and it is incumbent upon clinicians, scientists, regulators, payers and patients to work collectively to overcome the obstacles that stand in its path.

5. Abbreviations

CLIA: Clinical Laboratory Improvement Amendments; CMS: Centers for Medicare & Medicaid Services; FDA: Food and Drug Administration; FFPE: Formalin-fixed paraffin embedded; ICGC: International Cancer Genome Consortium; NGS: Next-generation sequencing; TCGA: The Cancer Genome Atlas.

Competing Interests

The authors declare that they have no competing interests.

Acknowledgements

Writing of this paper was supported in part by the Farmer Family Foundation and a Melanoma Research Alliance Young Investigator Award (MFB).

Source: Varghese A M, Berger M F. Advancing clinical oncology through genome biology and technology[J]. Genome Biology, 2014, 15(8):1–7.

References

[1] Meyerson M, Gabriel S, Getz G: Advances in understanding cancer genomes through second-generation sequencing. Nat Rev Genet 2010, 11:685–696.

[2] The Cancer Genome Atlas Network: Comprehensive genomic characterization defines human glioblastoma genes and core pathways. Nature 2008, 455:1061–1068.

[3] The Cancer Genome Atlas Network: Integrated genomic analyses of ovarian carcinoma. Nature 2011, 474:609–615.

[4] The Cancer Genome Atlas Network: Comprehensive molecular characterization of human colon and rectal cancer. Nature 2012, 487:330–337.

[5] The Cancer Genome Atlas Network: Comprehensive genomic characterization of squamous cell lung cancers. Nature 2012, 489:519–525.

[6] The Cancer Genome Atlas Network: Comprehensive molecular portraits of human breast tumours. Nature 2012, 490:61–70.

[7] Kandoth C, Schultz N, Cherniack AD, Akbani R, Liu Y, Shen H, Robertson AG, Pashtan I, Shen R, Benz CC, Yau C, Laird PW, Ding L, Zhang W, Mills GB, Kucherlapati R, Mardis ER, Levine DA: Integrated genomic characterization of endometrial carcinoma. Nature 2013, 497:67–73.

[8] The Cancer Genome Atlas Network: Comprehensive molecular characterization of clear cell renal cell carcinoma. Nature 2013, 499:43–49.

[9] The Cancer Genome Atlas Network: Genomic and epigenomic landscapes of adult de novo acute myeloid leukemia. N Engl J Med 2013, 368:2059–2074.

[10] The Cancer Genome Atlas Network: Comprehensive molecular characterization of urothelial bladder carcinoma. Nature 2014, 507:315–322.

[11] Hudson TJ, Anderson W, Artez A, Barker AD, Bell C, Bernabe RR, Bhan MK, Calvo F, Eerola I, Gerhard DS, Guttmacher A, Guyer M, Hemsley FM, Jennings JL, Kerr D, Klatt P, Kolar P, Kusada J, Lane DP, Laplace F, Youyong L, Nettekoven G, Ozenberger B, Peterson J, Rao TS, Remacle J, Schafer AJ, Shibata T, Stratton MR, Vockley JG, et al: International network of cancer genome projects. Nature 2010, 464:993–998.

[12] Biankin AV, Waddell N, Kassahn KS, Gingras MC, Muthuswamy LB, Johns AL, Miller DK, Wilson PJ, Patch AM, Wu J, Chang DK, Cowley MJ, Gardiner BB, Song S, Harliwong I, Idrisoglu S, Nourse C, Nourbakhsh E, Manning S, Wani S, Gongora M, Pajic M, Scarlett CJ, Gill AJ, Pinho AV, Rooman I, Anderson M, Holmes O, Leonard C, Taylor D, et al: Pancreatic cancer genomes reveal aberrations in axon guidance pathway genes. Nature 2012, 491:399–405.

[13] Davies H, Bignell GR, Cox C, Stephens P, Edkins S, Clegg S, Teague J, Woffendin H, Garnett MJ, Bottomley W, Davis N, Dicks E, Ewing R, Floyd Y, Gray K, Hall S, Hawes R, Hughes J, Kosmidou V, Menzies A, Mould C, Parker A, Stevens C, Watt S, Hooper S, Wilson R, Jayatilake H, Gusterson BA, Cooper C, Shipley J, et al: Mutations of the BRAF gene in human cancer. Nature 2002, 417:949–954.

[14] Chapman PB, Hauschild A, Robert C, Haanen JB, Ascierto P, Larkin J, Dummer R, Garbe C, Testori A, Maio M, Hogg D, Lorigan P, Lebbe C, Jouary T, Schadendorf D, Ribas A, O'Day SJ, Sosman JA, Kirkwood JM, Eggermont AM, Dreno B, Nolop K, Li J, Nelson B, Hou J, Lee RJ, Flaherty KT, McArthur GA, BRIM-3 Study Group: Improved survival with vemurafenib in melanoma with BRAF V600E mutation. N Engl J Med 2011, 364:2507–2516.

[15] Hauschild A, Grob JJ, Demidov LV, Jouary T, Gutzmer R, Millward M, Rutkowski P, Blank CU, Miller WH Jr, Kaempgen E, Martín-Algarra S, Karaszewska B, Mauch C, Chiarion-Sileni V, Martin AM, Swann S, Haney P, Mirakhur B, Guckert ME, Goodman V, Chapman PB: Dabrafenib in BRAF-mutated metastatic melanoma: a multicentre, open-label, phase 3 randomised controlled trial. Lancet 2012, 380:358–365.

[16] Lynch TJ, Bell DW, Sordella R, Gurubhagavatula S, Okimoto RA, Brannigan BW, Harris PL, Haserlat SM, Supko JG, Haluska FG, Louis DN, Christiani DC, Settleman J, Haber DA: Activating mutations in the epidermal growth factor receptor underlying responsiveness of non-small-cell lung cancer to gefitinib. N Engl J Med 2004, 350:2129–2139.

[17] Paez JG, Janne PA, Lee JC, Tracy S, Greulich H, Gabriel S, Herman P, Kaye FJ, Lindeman N, Boggon TJ, Naoki K, Sasaki H, Fujii Y, Eck MJ, Sellers WR, Johnson BE, Meyerson M: EGFR mutations in lung cancer: correlation with clinical response to gefitinib therapy. Science 2004, 304:1497–1500.

[18] Pao W, Miller V, Zakowski M, Doherty J, Politi K, Sarkaria I, Singh B, Heelan R, Rusch V, Fulton L, Mardis E, Kupfer D, Wilson R, Kris M, Varmus H: EGF receptor gene mutations are common in lung cancers from "never smokers" and are asso-

ciated with sensitivity of tumors to gefitinib and erlotinib. Proc Natl Acad Sci U S A 2004, 36:13306–13311.

[19] Iyer G, Hanrahan AJ, Milowsky MI, Al-Ahmadie H, Scott SN, Janakiraman M, Pirun M, Sander C, Socci ND, Ostrovnaya I, Viale A, Heguy A, Peng L, Chan TA Bochner B, Bajorin DF, Berger MF, Taylor BS, Solit DB: Genome sequencing identifies a basis for everolimus sensitivity. Science 2012, 338:221.

[20] Wagle N, Grabiner BC, Van Allen EM, Hodis E, Jacobus S, Supko JG, Stewart M, Choueiri TK, Gandhi L, Cleary JM, Elfiky AA, Taplin ME, Stack EC, Signoretti S, Loda M, Shapiro GI, Sabatini DM, Lander ES, Gabriel SB, Kantoff PW, Garraway LA, Rosenberg JE: Activating mTOR mutations in a patient with an extraordinary response on a phase I trial of everolimus and pazopanib. Cancer Discov 2014, 4:546–553.

[21] Imielinski M, Greulich H, Kaplan B, Araujo L, Amann J, Horn L, Schiller J, Villalona-Calero MA, Meyerson M, Carbone DP: Oncogenic and sorafenib-sensitive ARAF mutations in lung adenocarcinoma. J Clin Invest 2014, 124:1582–1586.

[22] Abrams J, Conley B, Mooney M, Zwiebel J, Chen A, Welch JJ, Takebe N, Malik S, McShane L, Korn E, Williams M, Staudt L, Doroshow J: National Cancer Institute's precision medicine initiatives for the new national clinical trials network. Am Soc Clin Oncol Educ Book 2014, 34:71–76.

[23] Pao W, Miller VA, Politi KA, Riely GJ, Somwar R, Zakowski MF, Kris MG, Varmus H: Acquired resistance of lung adenocarcinomas to gefitinib or erlotinib is associated with a second mutation in the EGFR kinase domain. PLoS Med 2005, 2:e73.

[24] Sequist LV, Waltman BA, Dias-Santagata D, Digumarthy S, Turke AB, Fidias P, Bergethon K, Shaw AT, Gettinger S, Cosper AK, Akhavanfard S, Heist RS, Temel J, Christensen JG, Wain JC, Lynch TJ, Vernovsky K, Mark EJ, Lanuti M, Iafrate AJ, Mino-Kenudson M, Engelman JA: Genotypic and histological evolution of lung cancers acquiring resistance to EGFR inhibitors. Sci Transl Med 2011, 3:75ra26.

[25] Wagle N, Emery C, Berger MF, Davis MJ, Sawyer A, Pochanard P, Kehoe SM, Johannessen CM, Macconaill LE, Hahn WC, Meyerson M, Garraway LA: Dissecting therapeutic resistance to RAF inhibition in melanoma by tumor genomic profiling. J Clin Oncol 2011, 29:3085–3096.

[26] Van Allen EM, Wagle N, Sucker A, Treacy DJ, Johannessen CM, Goetz EM, Place CS, Taylor-Weiner A, Whittaker S, Kryukov GV, Hodis E, Rosenberg M, McKenna A, Cibulskis K, Farlow D, Zimmer L, Hillen U, Gutzmer R, Goldinger SM, Ugurel S, Gogas HJ, Egberts F, Berking C, Trefzer U, Loquai C, Weide B, Hassel JC, Gabriel SB, Carter SL, Getz G, et al: The genetic landscape of clinical resistance to RAF inhibition in metastatic melanoma. Cancer Discov 2014, 4:94–109.

[27] Shi H, Hugo W, Kong X, Hong A, Koya RC, Moriceau G, Chodon T, Guo R, Johnson DB, Dahlman KB, Kelley MC, Kefford RF, Chmielowski B, Glaspy JA, Sosman JA, van Baren N, Long GV, Ribas A, Lo RS: Acquired resistance and clonal evolution in melanoma during BRAF inhibitor therapy. Cancer Discov 2014, 4:80–93.

[28] Shah NP, Tran C, Lee FY, Chen P, Norris D, Sawyers CL: Overriding imatinib resistance with a novel ABL kinase inhibitor. Science 2004, 305:399–401.

[29] Balbas MD, Evans MJ, Hosfield DJ, Wongvipat J, Arora VK, Watson PA, Chen Y, Greene GL, Shen Y, Sawyers CL: Overcoming mutation-based resistance to antiandrogens with rational drug design. Elife 2013, 2:e00499.

[30] Toy W, Shen Y, Won H, Green B, Sakr RA, Will M, Li Z, Gala K, Fanning S, King TA, Hudis C, Chen D, Taran T, Hortobagyi G, Greene G, Berger M, Baselga J, Chandarlapaty S: ESR1 ligand-binding domain mutations in hormone-resistant breast cancer. Nat Genet 2013, 45:1439–1445.

[31] Robinson DR, Wu YM, Vats P, Su F, Lonigro RJ, Cao X, Kalyana-Sundaram S, Wang R, Ning Y, Hodges L, Gursky A, Siddiqui J, Tomlins SA, Roychowdhury S, Pienta KJ, Kim SY, Roberts JS, Rae JM, Van Poznak CH, Hayes DF, Chugh R, Kunju LP, Talpaz M, Schott AF, Chinnaiyan AM: Activating ESR1 mutations in hormone-resistant metastatic breast cancer. Nat Genet 2013, 45:1446–1451.

[32] Drilon A, Wang L, Hasanovic A, Suehara Y, Lipson D, Stephens P, Ross J, Miller V, Ginsberg M, Zakowski MF, Kris MG, Ladanyi M, Rizvi N: Response to cabozantinib in patients with RET fusion-positive lung adenocarcinomas. Cancer Discov 2013, 3:630–635.

[33] Bergethon K, Shaw AT, Ou SH, Katayama R, Lovly CM, McDonald NT, Massion PP, Siwak-Tapp C, Gonzalez A, Fang R, Mark EJ, Batten JM, Chen H, Wilner KD, Kwak EL, Clark JW, Carbone DP, Ji H, Engelman JA, Mino-Kenudson M, Pao W, Iafrate AJ: ROS1 rearrangements define a unique molecular class of lung cancers. J Clin Oncol 2012, 30:863–870.

[34] Ou SH, Kwak EL, Siwak-Tapp C, Dy J, Bergethon K, Clark JW, Camidge DR, Solomon BJ, Maki RG, Bang YJ, Kim DW, Christensen J, Tan W, Wilner KD, Salgia R, Iafrate AJ: Activity of crizotinib (PF02341066), a dual mesenchymal-epithelial transition (MET) and anaplastic lymphoma kinase (ALK) inhibitor, in a non-small cell lung cancer patient with de novo MET amplification. J Thorac Oncol 2011, 6:942–946.

[35] Roychowdhury S, Iyer MK, Robinson DR, Lonigro RJ, Wu YM, Cao X, Kalyana-Sundaram S, Sam L, Balbin OA, Quist MJ, Barrette T, Everett J, Siddiqui J, Kunju LP, Navone N, Araujo JC, Troncoso P, Logothetis CJ, Innis JW, Smith DC, Lao CD, Kim SY, Roberts JS, Gruber SB, Pienta KJ, Talpaz M, Chinnaiyan AM: Personalized oncology through integrative high-throughput sequencing: a pilot study. Sci Transl Med 2011, 3:111ra121.

[36] Van Allen EM, Wagle N, Stojanov P, Perrin DL, Cibulskis K, Marlow S, Jane-Valbuena J, Friedrich DC, Kryukov G, Carter SL, McKenna A, Sivachenko A, Rosenberg M, Kiezun A, Voet D, Lawrence M, Lichtenstein LT, Gentry JG, Huang FW, Fostel J, Farlow D, Barbie D, Gandhi L, Lander ES, Gray SW, Joffe S, Janne P, Garber J, MacConaill L, Lindeman N, et al: Whole-exome sequencing and clinical interpretation of formalin-fixed, paraffin-embedded tumor samples to guide precision cancer medicine. Nat Med 2014, 20:682–688.

[37] Wagle N, Berger MF, Davis MJ, Blumenstiel B, Defelice M, Pochanard P, Ducar M, Van Hummelen P, Macconaill LE, Hahn WC, Meyerson M, Gabriel SB, Garraway LA: High-throughput detection of actionable genomic alterations in clinical tumor samples by targeted, massively parallel sequencing. Cancer Discov 2012, 2:82–93.

[38] Frampton GM, Fichtenholtz A, Otto GA, Wang K, Downing SR, He J, Schnall-Levin M, White J, Sanford EM, An P, Sun J, Juhn F, Brennan K, Iwanik K, Maillet A, Buell J, White E, Zhao M, Balasubramanian S, Terzic S, Richards T, Banning V, Garcia L, Mahoney K, Zwirko Z, Donahue A, Beltran H, Mosquera JM, Rubin MA, Dogan S, et al: Development and validation of a clinical cancer genomic profiling test based on massively parallel DNA sequencing. Nat Biotechnol 2013, 31:1023–1031.

[39] Won HH, Scott SN, Brannon AR, Shah RH, Berger MF: Detecting somatic genetic alterations in tumor specimens by exon capture and massively parallel sequencing. J Vis Exp 2013,:e50710.

[40] Beadling C, Neff TL, Heinrich MC, Rhodes K, Thornton M, Leamon J, Andersen M, Corless CL: Combining highly multiplexed PCR with semiconductor-based sequencing for rapid cancer genotyping. J Mol Diagn 2013, 15:171–176.

[41] Cottrell CE, Al-Kateb H, Bredemeyer AJ, Duncavage EJ, Spencer DH, Abel HJ, Lockwood CM, Hagemann IS, O'Guin SM, Burcea LC, Sawyer CS, Oschwald DM, Stratman JL, Sher DA, Johnson MR, Brown JT, Cliften PF, George B, McIntosh LD, Shrivastava S, Nguyen TT, Payton JE, Watson MA, Crosby SD, Head RD, Mitra RD, Nagarajan R, Kulkarni S, Seibert K, Virgin HW 4th, et al: Validation of a next-generation sequencing assay for clinical molecular oncology. J Mol Diagn 2014, 16:89–105.

[42] Singh RR, Patel KP, Routbort MJ, Reddy NG, Barkoh BA, Handal B, Kanagal-Shamanna R, Greaves WO, Medeiros LJ, Aldape KD, Luthra R: Clinical validation of a next-generation sequencing screen for mutational hotspots in 46 cancer-related genes. J Mol Diagn 2013, 15:607–622.

[43] Craig DW, Pearson JV, Szelinger S, Sekar A, Redman M, Corneveaux JJ, Pawlowski TL, Laub T, Nunn G, Stephan DA, Homer N, Huentelman MJ: Identification of genetic variants using bar-coded multiplexed sequencing. Nat Methods 2008, 5:887–893.

[44] MacConaill LE, Van Hummelen P, Meyerson M, Hahn WC: Clinical implementation of comprehensive strategies to characterize cancer genomes: opportunities and challenges. Cancer Discov 2011, 1:297–311.

[45] Huang FW, Hodis E, Xu MJ, Kryukov GV, Chin L, Garraway LA: Highly recurrent TERT promoter mutations in human melanoma. Science 2013, 339:957–959.

[46] Horn S, Figl A, Rachakonda PS, Fischer C, Sucker A, Gast A, Kadel S, Moll I, Nagore E, Hemminki K, Schadendorf D, Kumar R: TERT promoter mutations in familial and sporadic melanoma. Science 2013, 339:959–961.

[47] Killela PJ, Reitman ZJ, Jiao Y, Bettegowda C, Agrawal N, Diaz LA Jr, Friedman AH, Friedman H, Gallia GL, Giovanella BC, Grollman AP, He TC, He Y, Hruban RH,

Jallo GI, Mandahl N, Meeker AK, Mertens F, Netto GJ, Rasheed BA, Riggins GJ, Rosenquist TA, Schiffman M, Shih IM, Theodorescu D, Torbenson MS, Velculescu VE, Wang TL, Wentzensen N, Wood LD, et al: TERT promoter mutations occur frequently in gliomas and a subset of tumors derived from cells with low rates of self-renewal. Proc Natl Acad Sci USA 2013, 110:6021–6026.

[48] Prahallad A, Sun C, Huang S, Di Nicolantonio F, Salazar R, Zecchin D, Beijersbergen RL, Bardelli A, Bernards R: Unresponsiveness of colon cancer to BRAF(V600E) inhibition through feedback activation of EGFR. Nature 2012, 483:100–103.

[49] Kopetz S, Desai J, Chan E, Hecht JR, O'Dwyer PJ, Lee RJ, Nolop KB, Saltz L: PLX4032 in metastatic colorectal cancer patients with mutant BRAF tumors. J Clin Oncol 2010, 28:15s.

[50] Maemondo M, Inoue A, Kobayashi K, Sugawara S, Oizumi S, Isobe H, Gemma A, Harada M, Yoshizawa H, Kinoshita I, Fujita Y, Okinaga S, Hirano H, Yoshimori K, Harada T, Ogura T, Ando M, Miyazawa H, Tanaka T, Saijo Y, Hagiwara K, Morita S, Nukiwa T, North-East Japan Study Group: Gefitinib or chemotherapy for non-small-cell lung cancer with mutated EGFR. N Engl J Med 2010, 362: 2380–2388.

[51] Djalalov S, Beca J, Hoch JS, Krahn M, Tsao MS, Cutz JC, Leighl NB: Cost effectiveness of EML4-ALK fusion testing and first-line crizotinib treatment for patients with advanced ALK-positive non-small-cell lung cancer. J Clin Oncol 2014, 32:1012–1019.

Chapter 21

Evidence-Based Medicine and Clinical Fluorodeoxyglucose PET/MRI in Oncology

Kenneth Miles[1,2], Liam McQueen[3], Stanley Ngai[1], Phillip Law[1]

[1]Department of Diagnostic Imaging, Princess Alexandra Hospital, Woolloongabba, Brisbane, Australia
[2]Institute of Nuclear Medicine, University College London, London, UK
[3]Department of Health, Health Technology Assessment & Evaluation, Queensland Government, Herston, Brisbane, Australia

Abstract: Positron Emission Tomography/Magnetic Resonance Imaging (PET/ MRI) is a hybrid of two technologies each with its own evidence for clinical effectiveness. This article amalgamates evidence for clinical effectiveness of fluoro-deoxyglucose (FDG) PET/CT and MRI as separate modalities with current evidence for hybrid PET/MRI and considers whether such an approach might provide a stronger case for the clinical use of PET/MRI at an earlier stage. Because links between diagnostic accuracy and health outcomes have already been established for FDG-PET/CT in the investigation of suspected residual or recurrent malignancies, evidence showing improved diagnostic performance and therapeutic impact from the use of PET/MRI as an alternative would imply clinical effectiveness of this modality for this application. A meta-analysis of studies comparing FDG-PET/ CT to MRI in patients with suspected residual disease or recurrence of tumours indicates complementary roles for these modalities. PET demonstrates greater sensitivity for recurrence within lymph nodes whereas MRI is more effective that PET/CT in the detection of skeletal and hepatic recurrence. A review of studies assessing therapeutic impact of PET/MRI suggests a greater likelihood for change in clinical management when PET/MRI is used for assessment of suspected residual or recurrent disease rather than tumour staging. Supplementing the evidence-base for FDG-PET/MRI with studies that compare the components of this hybrid-technology deployed separately indicates that FDG-PET/MRI is likely to be clinical effective for the investigation of patients with a range of suspected residual or recurrent cancers. This indication should therefore be prioritised for further health technology assessment.

1. Background

William Osler's description of medicine as "a science of uncertainty and an art of probability" is as pertinent now as it was in his time[1]. A frequent area of uncertainty in medicine today relates to the introduction of emerging health technologies, where early adoption is often associated with lack of clarity regarding the clinical applications that add value for patients and society. This situation reflects the current status of Positron Emission Tomography/Magnetic Resonance Imaging (PET/MRI) in oncology. The ability to simultaneously acquire PET images of tissue function and MRI images of soft tissue morphology represents a technological advance on PET/Computed Tomography (CT) which is currently used widely for staging and assessment of suspected residual or recurrent disease in patients with a range of tumour types.

Whilst recognising the potential for PET/MRI to impact on priority health areas, recent technology briefs in Australia and the UK have both highlighted the need for better evidence of clinical effectiveness for this technology[2][3]. Emerging technologies typically have a limited evidence-base from which to identify clinical applications and accumulation of sufficient evidence to justify clinical use may take a significant amount of time. However, hybrid devices such as PET/MRI do not represent a completely new technology, but integrate two pre-existing technologies each with its own evidence for clinical effectiveness. A different approach to evidence synthesis that assimilates data for PET/CT and MRI as separate modalities could therefore potentially supplement the currently limited evidence derived using hybrid PET/MRI systems. This article considers whether such an approach might provide a stronger case for the clinical use of PET/MRI at an earlier stage.

1.1. Technical Advantages of PET/MRI

An important technical advantage for PET/MRI is a reduction radiation exposure for patients. With PET/CT, the CT component is used for attenuation correction, and for the localisation and characterisation of lesions identified by PET. Although attenuation correction is achieved using a low-dose protocol, additional diagnostic quality CT acquisitions may be required for accurate lesion localisation and characterisation. If these CT acquisitions are replaced by MRI, it can be estimated that dose reductions of 1.5 to 19.4 mSv per examination could be achieved[4]. There are also opportunities to reduce the amount of radiotracer administered.

Secondly, the high tissue contrast afforded by MRI offers the potential to compensate for some diagnostic limitations of PET/CT, such as the constraints created by background physiological tracer uptake in certain organs. For the most commonly used clinical PET tracer, Fluorodeoxyglucose (FDG), the reduced sensitivity of PET for cerebral metastases due to high physiological radiotracer uptake is sufficiently well recognised for brain MRI to be frequently included in current care pathways. However, there is also significant physiological FDG uptake in liver and bone marrow and addition of appropriate MRI sequences to FDG-PET could similarly improve detection of metastatic disease in these organs. Appropriate whole-body MRI acquisitions for detection of skeletal metastases can be acquired concurrently with the whole-body PET images. For maximal detection of liver lesions, an additional dedicated series of acquisitions in a single bed-position can be readily appended to the whole-body acquisitions, including images with liver-specific contrast material[5]. The multiple MR sequences acquired in this way can also potentially improve tissue characterisation in comparison to CT, for example aiding the distinction between malignant and inflammatory causes of FDG uptake.

1.2. Advantages of PET/MRI over Separately Acquired PET/CT and MRI

An important consideration for clinical PET/MR is the extent to which simultaneous PET/MR benefits over sequential PET/CT and MRI acquisitions with either side-by-side interpretation or software fusion. Acquiring PET and MRI data sets on a single device avoids duplication of booking procedures, saves time and number of departmental visits for the patient, and avoids the radiation dose associated with the low-dose CT component of PET-CT. Simultaneous acquisition of PET and MR images results in highly accurate anatomical registration that is more readily integration into clinical workflow than software co-registration of separately acquired PET/MRI data sets. Furthermore, software fusion approaches cannot reliably compensate for the differences in respiration, peristalsis, and filling of bowel and bladder that frequently occur between images of thorax, abdomen and pelvis acquired at different times[6]. Image co-registration afforded by PET/MRI is also superior to that achievable with PET/CT devices which acquire the image datasets sequentially, albeit in close temporal proximity on the same imaging table, resulting in greater confidence in assignment of areas of radiotracer uptake to anatomical findings[7]. Studies comparing side-by-side interpretation with integrated image acquisition for other hybrid imaging modalities such as SPECT/CT and PET/CT have confirmed that more accurate co-registration of functional and anatomical datasets is associated with greater diagnostic specificity and fewer indeterminate reports and such benefits can be also be anticipated for PET/MRI[8][9]. There are also opportunities for PET/MR to improve quantification of radiotracer uptake by more accurate compensation for body composition and/or intra-lesional fat, analogous to methods proposed for brain PET/MRI[10].

1.3. Patient Groups Who May Benefit from PET/MRI

Reductions in radiation exposure due diagnostic imaging would be a particular advantage for paediatric patients. However, as the incidence of cancer in this population is relatively low, the burden of disease is unlikely to justify installation of PET/MR outside highly specialised centres. A second group of patients for whom radiation exposure from diagnostic tests is emerging is a significant issue comprises cancer survivors. A recent study has estimated the risk of second cancer induction by the use of CT in this group of patients to be between 0.1% and 10%[11]. With the growing success of first-line cancer therapy leading to an increasing population of cancer survivors, survivorship is emerging as a significant challenge for health care. For example, it has been estimated that 13.7 million cancer survivors were living in the US as of January 2012 as compared to 1.6 million new cancer cases diagnosed in the US that year, a ratio greater than 8:1[12]. Diagnostic imaging, including PET/CT, is frequently used in cancer survivors when residual or recurrent disease is suspected on the basis of symptoms or rising tumour markers. If tumour is excluded, patients can continue routine surveillance. If residual or recurrent tumour is confirmed, patients with localised disease may benefit from surgery or other local therapy such as stereotactic ablative radiotherapy, whereas second-line chemotherapy or best-supportive care would be appropriate for patients with extensive disease. Alternatively, imaging instigated for suspected recurrence may also reveal a second malignancy. In this clinical context, residual disease needs to be distinguished from post-treatment inflammatory change whilst the brain, liver and bone marrow are common sites for disease recurrence. Thus, this group of patients could also benefit from the potential for PET/MRI to overcome current limitations of PET/CT in this clinical context.

1.4. Evaluating Evidence for Clinical Effectiveness of Hybrid Imaging Technologies

Clinical effectiveness of a diagnostic test is defined by the extent to which incorporating the test into clinical practice improves health outcomes[13]. Direct evidence of the impact of a diagnostic test on health outcomes is rarely available due to a range of methodological difficulties. Clinical effectiveness can therefore also be demonstrated by using evidence that links test accuracy with evidence that the test result changes treatment practice, and with evidence that the alternative treatments have different effectiveness and safety profiles[13]. Links between diagnostic accuracy and health outcomes have already been established for a range of clinical applications for PET and MRI as separate modalities. For investigation of suspected residual or recurrent malignancies, strong links have been established between FDG-PET and clinical outcome for patients with lymphoma, sarcoma, malignant melanoma and cancers of the colon or rectum, ovary, uterine cervix, and head & neck. The key issues for the clinical effectiveness of hybrid PET/MRI devices in the assessment of suspected residual or recurrent malignancy are therefore a) the extent to which combining these modalities can improve diagnostic performance compared to either modality alone, and b) whether any improvements diagnostic performance lead to changes in treatment practice.

1.5. Comparative Studies of Diagnostic Accuracy of FDG-PET and MRI for Residual/Recurrent Malignancy

The Cochrane Collaboration has stipulated standards for the analysis of comparative studies of diagnostic accuracy[14]. To minimise bias, such studies employ a direct comparison of the tests in question by either applying both tests to each individual, or randomising each individual to receive one of the tests. A common reference standard should be consistently applied to both tests. Nine studies that meet these standards whilst reporting the accuracy of MRI and FDG-PET in patients with suspected residual or recurrent disease for the tumour types listed above are available[15]–[23].

1.5.1. Detection of Tumour Recurrence within Lymph Nodes, Bone and Liver

Seven publications have reported the diagnostic performances of PET/CT and MRI in the detection of nodal, skeletal or hepatic metastases in patients clinically suspected to have recurrent tumours[15]–[21]. Three of these reports considered patients with recurrent melanoma (total number of patients = 136), one study comprised patients with recurrent colorectal (24 patients), one study considered patients with head and cancer (179 patients) and 2 studies included patients with various non-central nervous system tumours (total number of patients = 72). For each study the reference standard consisted of histology or clinical follow-up for at least 6 months.

These studies indicate complementary roles for PET and MRI in identification of tumour recurrence. FDG-PET/CT demonstrates superior diagnostic performance for recurrence in lymph nodes whilst recurrences in the skeleton and liver are more reliably depicted by MRI (**Figure 1**). The weighted averages from the 5 studies reporting diagnostic performance for detection of nodal recurrence (**Table 1**) show superior sensitivity for PET/CT with no significant change in positive predictive value (PPV) whereas the weighted averages of the 5 studies reporting diagnostic performance for detection of skeletal recurrence (**Table 2**) and the 5 studies comparing PET/CT and MRI in the detection of tumour recurrence within the liver (**Table 3**) both confirm superior sensitivity for MRI with no significant difference in PPV.

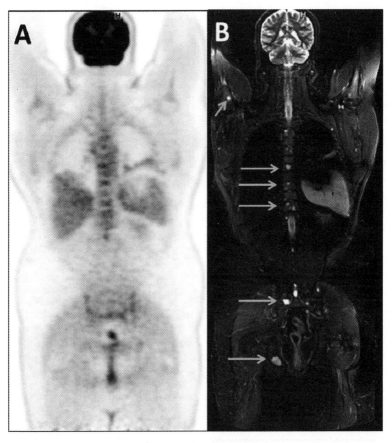

Figure 1. PET/MRI study comprising whole-body FDG-PET (A) and Short Tau Inversion Recovery (STIR) MRI (B) from a patient with recurrent myxoid liposarcoma. The skeletal metastases are more readily appreciated on the MRI than on FDG-PET.

1.5.2. Identification of Patients with Tumour Recurrence

Three studies compared the performance of FDG-PET/CT to combined reading of PET/CT and MRI in patients with suspected tumour recurrence (**Table 4**). The first comprised a meta-analysis which identified 4 studies that comparing the diagnostic performance on a per-patient basis of PET/CT alone to PET combined with WB-MRI in the detection of residual or recurrent tumour of the head and neck[22]. Combined reading improved the sensitivity for the identification of patients with residual or recurrent disease from 82% (95% CI: 69%–90%) to 89% (95% CI: 86%–96%) with no loss of specificity (PET-CT: 97 [94–98]%; combined reading: 98 [97–99]%). Additional to the above meta-analysis, in a study of

Table 1. Summary of the results of test accuracy in studies comparing whole-body MRI with FDG-PET/CT in the detection of sites of tumour recurrence within lymph nodes.

Study	Population & setting	Reference standard	Outcome [95%CI]			
			PET-CT		WB-MRI	
			Sensitivity	PPV	Sensitivity	PPV
Pfannenberg *et al.* (2007)[15]	Recurrent melanoma Self-controlled study (n = 64)	Histology or 8 months follow-up	85 [77–91]%	94% [87–97]%	66 [56–74]%	84% [74–90]%
Schmidt *et al.* (2009)[16]	Recurrent Colorectal Cancer Self-controlled study (n = 24)	Follow-up (mean 11 months)	93 [78–98]%	100 [86–100]%	62 [44–77]%	82 [61–93]%
Ng *et al.* (2010)[18]	Recurrent Head & Neck Cancer Self-controlled study (n = 179)	Histology or 12 months follow-up	80 [61–91]%	77 [58–89]%	88 [70–96]%	81 [63–92]%
Laurent *et al.* (2010)[19]	Recurrent melanoma Self-controlled study (n = 35)	Histology or 6 months follow-up	83 [65–92]%	100 [86–100]%	90 [74–96]%	96 [82–99]%
Jouvet *et al.* (2014)[20]	Recurrent melanoma Self-controlled study (n = 37)	Histology or ≥6 months follow-up	96 [79–99]%	96 [79–99]%	87 [68–95]%	100 [84–100]%
Weighted averages	(n = 339)		87 [81–91]%	93 [89–96]%	74 [67–79]%	87 [81–91]%

Table 2. Summary of the results of test accuracy in studies comparing whole-body MRI with FDG-PET/CT in the detection of sites of skeletal metastases.

Study	Population & setting	Reference standard	Outcome [95%CI]			
			PET-CT		WB-MRI	
			Sensitivity	PPV	Sensitivity	PPV
Pfannenberg et al. (2007) [15]	Recurrent melanoma Self-controlled study (n = 64)	Histology or 8 months follow-up	91 [78–97]%	91% [78–97]%	100 [90–100]%	90% [76–96]%
Schmidt et al. (2007)[16]	Non-CNS tumours and suspicion of bone metastases Self-controlled study (n = 35)	≥6 months imaging follow-up	77 [68–84]%	94 [67–97]%	94 [88–97]%	94 [88–97]%
Schmidt et al. (2009)[17]	Recurrent Colorectal Cancer Self-controlled study (n = 24)	Follow-up (mean 11 months)	50 [15–85]%	100 [51–100]%	100 [51–100]%	100 [51–100]%
Laurent et al. (2010)[19]	Recurrent melanoma Self-controlled study (n = 35)	Histology or 6 months follow-up	71 [45–88]%	100 [72–100]%	93 [69–99]%	100 [77–100]%
Jouvet et al. (2014)[20]	Recurrent melanoma Self-controlled study (n = 37)	Histology or ≥6 months follow-up	88 [64–97]%	93 [70–99]%	100 [81–100]%	76 [55–89]%
Weighted averages	(n = 195)		80 [74–85]%	94 [89–97]%	96 [92–98]%	92 [87–95]%

Table 3. Summary of the results of test accuracy in studies comparing whole-body MRI with FDG-PET/CT in the detection of sites of tumour recurrence within the liver.

Study	Population & setting	Reference standard	Outcome [95%CI]			
			PET-CT		WB-MRI	
			Sensitivity	PPV	Sensitivity	PPV
Donati et al. (2010)[21]	Various (n = 37, Colorectal Cancer: n = 20)	Histology or follow-up	76 [64–86]%	93 [82–98]%	91 [80–96]%	100 [93–100]%
Schmidt et al. (2009)[16]	Recurrent Colorectal Cancer Self-controlled study (n = 24)	Follow-up (mean 11 months)	86 [65–95]%	100 [82–100]%	100 [85–100]%	100 [85–100]%
Pfannenberg et al. (2007) [15]	Recurrent melanoma Self-controlled study (n = 64)	Histology or 8 months follow-up	94 [81–98]%	100 [90-100]%	100 [90–100]%	100 [90–100]%
Laurent et al. (2010)[19]	Recurrent melanoma Self-controlled study (n = 35)	Histology or 6 months follow-up	50 [15–85]%	100 [51–100]%	100 [51–100]%	100 [51–100]%
Jouvet et al. (2014)[20]	Recurrent melanoma Self-controlled study (n = 37)	Histology or ≥6 months follow-up	100 [76–100]%	100 k [76–100]%	100 [76–100]%	92 [67–99]%
Weighted averages	(n = 90)		84 [77–90]%	97 [92–99]%	96 [91–98]%	99 [96–100]%

67 patients undergoing both dedicated PET/MRI and PET/CT, Biederwellen et al.[23] reported a trend for improved sensitivity when using PET/MRI (100%, [95% CI: 72%–100%] versus 90% [68%–98%] for PET/CT) with no change in specificity (each 100%; [94–100]%). On the other hand, a study of 37 patients by Donati et al. found no significance difference in the ability of retrospectively fused PET and MRI data sets compared to PET-CT to identify patients with liver metastases[21].

Table 4. Summary of the results of test accuracy in studies comparing combined MRI and FDG-PET/CT to PET/CT alone for the classification of patients with or without tumour recurrence.

Study	Population & setting	Reference standard and comparator	Outcome [95%CI]			
			PET/CT		PET/MR	
			Sensitivity	Specificity	Sensitivity	Specificity
Xu *et al.* (2013)[22]	Meta-analysis of 4 studies comparing PET/CT and WB-MRI in the detection metastatic head & neck cancer (n = 511)	Reference standard variable. Combined reading of PET and WB-MRI	82 [69–90]%	97 [94–98]%	89 [86–96]%	98 [97–99]%
Donati *et al.* (2010)[21]	Hepatic metastases (n = 37, CRC: n = 20)	Histology or follow-up Fused PET/MR	100 [77–100]%	92 [67–99]%	100 [77–100]%	100 [77–100]%
Beiderwellen *et al.* (2014)[23]	Skeletal metastases (n = 67)	Histology or follow-up Dedicated PET/MR	90 [68–98]%	100 [72–100]%	100 [94–100]%	100 [94–100]%

1.6. Changes in Treatment Practice from FDG-PET/MRI for Patients Suspected Residual or Recurrent Malignancy

Three studies have reported therapeutic impact from the use of PET/MRI in place of PET/CT[7][24][25] (**Table 5**). Two of these studies[24][25] included patients with suspected residual disease or recurrence whereas the study by Al- Nabhani *et al.*[7] comprised only patients for staging. The likelihood of PET/MRI detecting additional findings not identified on PET/CT with impact on clinical management is much greater in the studies including patients with suspected recurrence (Odds ratio 14.4 or infinity versus 2.1). The largest of these studies (Catalano *et al.*) also reported the incidence of change in management for different categories of additional finding. Change in clinical management was significantly more likely when additional findings related to recurrent or residual disease (Odds ratio calculated from reported data = 10.4, 95% CI 2.9–37, p < 0.0001).

Table 5. Summary table for studies reporting therapeutic impact.

Study	Population	Outcome	New Technology n with event/N (%)	Comparator n with event/N (%)	Effect size (95% CI/p value)
Catalano et al. (2013)[24]	Cohort observational study. Staging or follow-up of non-CNS tumours (n = 134)	Patients additional findings not identified on alternate modality	6/134 (4.5%)	55/134 (41%)	OR: 14.9 (6.1–36.1 p < 0.0001)
		Patients with additional findings not identified on alternate modality affecting clinical management	24/134 (17.9%)	2/134 (1.5%)	OR: 14.4 (3.3–62.3 p < 0.0001)
Reine et al. (2014)[25]	Cohort observational study. Hepatic metastases (n = 55, CRC: n = 41)	Patients additional findings not identified on alternate modality	8/55 (9.1%)	0/55 (0%)	OR: Infinity OR: Infinity
		Patients with additional findings not identified on alternate modality affecting clinical management	5/55 (9.1%)	0/55 (0%)	
Al-Nabhani et al. (2014)[7]	Cohort observational study. Staging of non-CNS tumours (n = 50)	Patients with additional findings not identified on alternate modality affecting clinical management	4/50 (8%)	1/50 (2%)	OR: 2.1 (0.36–11.9 NS)

1.7. The Need for Further Clinical Evaluation of PET/MRI in Residual/Recurrent Malignancy

There are areas in which the evidence-based for PET/MRI in the assessment of suspected residual or recurrent malignancy is deficient. Current management of residual/recurrent tumour requires stratification of patients beyond the presence or absence of tumour. Local treatments such as surgery or radiotherapy may be appropriate for patients with localised recurrence whereas systemic treatment such as chemotherapy or palliative treatment would be most appropriate for disseminated

disease. Using the available literature, it has not been possible to assess the potential impact of PET/MRI over PET/CT in stratifying patients as described above and we highlight the need for such studies in future. Furthermore, even after the evidence-synthesis described in our study, current literature is not sufficiently mature to enable an assessment of whether the implied effectiveness of PET/MRI in recurrent/residual malignancy is likely to be cost-effective. The capital cost of PET/MRI devices are comparable to PET/CT and MRI systems purchased separately and therefore, to ensure cost-effectiveness, PET/MRI workflows need to minimise the amount of time when either component is idle. Where PET/MRI replaces PET/CT and MRI performed separately, streamlining of clerical, radiographer and nursing work related to imaging investigation of patients with residual or recurrent cancer into a single imaging episode may defray some of these costs. On the other hand, potential improvements in cost-effectiveness can be anticipated. The therapeutic impact study of Catalano et al. found the commonest change in management when PET/MRI was used for patient with residual or recurrent disease was avoidance of biopsy[24]. Further management changes of potential health economic importance include avoiding the cost and morbidity of futile local treatments that would have been inappropriately selected due to under-estimation of disease extent by current technology, earlier identification of limited or disseminated disease allowing timely instigation of local therapy or salvage therapy respectively, and avoidance of futile chemotherapy in the presence of advanced disease of an extent under-estimated by current technology. Future studies are also needed to address these aspects of PET/MRI deployment.

Other potential benefits of PET/MRI are less tangible than those that can be inferred from improved diagnostic performance and therapeutic impact over PET/CT. Combining into a single procedure, examinations that in some instances may have been performed on separate devices and/or separate occasions using current technology, will result in increased convenience for patients such as reduced travel costs and fewer attendance days, with more rapid availability of the results of imaging assessment allowing earlier clinical decision making. Deployment of PET/MRI could also usefully increase capacity for MRI at a time when utilisation of MRI for oncological applications is increasing[26]. The impact of the reduced radiation exposure for patients from the use of MRI in place of CT can also be anticipated to improve health outcomes by reducing the risks of second cancer induction which have been shown to be significant for cancer survivors[11]. However, such benefits are harder to quantify in health economic terms and are not typically included in economic analyses of diagnostic imaging technologies. The impact of reduced risk of adverse reaction to contrast material for those situations where PET/MRI has replaced PET/CT with contrast enhancement is similarly hard to quantify.

The approach to evidence-based synthesis outlined above for FDG-PET is currently not applicable for other PET tracers with emerging roles in oncology such as 68Ga-dotatate and 68Ga-Prostate Specific MembraneAntigen because the evidence-based for these tracers is underdeveloped in comparison to FDG. In particular, there is a paucity of data linking the use of these tracers with improvements in health outcomes and few studies comparing their use with PET/CT against whole-body MRI. Therefore, the clinical effectiveness of these emerging tracers will need to be evaluated using conventional approaches to health technology assessment approaches.

1.8. Considerations for PET/MRI Service Delivery

There are a range of further issues that would need to be addressed before implementing clinical PET/MRI for evaluation of suspected residual or recurrent disease. Firstly, there would need to be sufficient patients with relevant clinical need. Secondly, PET/MRI would need to co-located with PET/CT to ensure available of PET for patients with contraindications to MRI (e.g., MR incompatible implantable medical devices, previous ocular metallic foreign body) and to meet the circumstances when PET/CT may be superior to PET/MRI, for example the visualisation of small pulmonary nodules. Overall imaging demand would therefore need to justify 2 PET systems (one PET/MRI and one PET/CT) and thus a regional oncology centre would likely be the most appropriate location for such a service. Even under these circumstances, PET/MRI research and/or additional standalone MR examinations would likely be needed to completely fill the capacity of the PET/MRI installation. Although the clinical component of such a combined program may be based on a remote supply of FDG, colocation with a cyclotron would facilitate a parallel PET/MR research program by making other PET tracers available for oncological research. Furthermore, the clinical and research components of such a programme would each require availability and co-ordination of technical and radiological expertise in both nuclear medicine and oncologic MRI. Funding of a clinical FDG-PET/MRI service may also be problematic as, depending on the relevant health-care system, if accessible at all, re-imbursement may only be available at the same level as PET/CT. Studies demonstrating the cost-effectiveness of PET/MR in comparison to PET/CT may be required before a level of reimbursement reflecting the additional cost associated with PET/MRI becomes available.

2. Conclusion

This review has illustrated two issues related to evidence-based assessments of hybrid imaging technologies such as PET/MRI. Firstly, the requirement to demonstrate a link between diagnostic performance and health outcomes may have already been met by the existing evidence-base for either component of the hybrid technology deployed alone. In the case of FDG-PET/MRI for patients with suspected recurrent or residual malignancy, such links have already been demonstrated for the PET component for a range of tumour types. Secondly, rather than rely solely on technology assessments of the new device, the evidence-base for hybrid technologies such as PET/MRI can be supplemented by studies comparing the components of the hybrid technology deployed separately. In the current study, this approach to evidence-synthesis has identified additional support for the application of PET/MRI in the assessment of suspected recurrent of residual malignancy by providing supplementary evidence of improved detection of malignant lesions in bone and liver whilst preserving the effectiveness of PET for lymph node recurrence. Furthermore, a review of studies assessing therapeutic impact of FDG-PET/MRI suggests a greater likelihood for change in clinical management when FDG-PET/MRI is used for assessment of suspected residual or recurrent disease rather than tumour staging. Thus, supplementing the evidence-base for FDG-PET/MRI with studies that compare the components of this hybrid technology deployed separately suggests that FDG-PET/MRI is likely to be clinical effective for the investigation of patients with a range of suspected residual or recurrent cancers. This indication should therefore be prioritised for further health technology assessment.

Competing Interests

The authors declare that they have no competing interests.

Authors' Contributions

KM conceived the methodology used in this work. KM and LM undertook the literature review. KM, SN and PL developed the context of the work. All authors read and approved the manuscript.

Source: Miles K, Mcqueen L, Ngai S, *et al*. Evidence-based medicine and clinical fluoro deoxy glucose PET/MRI in oncology [J]. Cancer Imaging, 2014, 15(1):1–8.

References

[1]   Osler W. The Quotable Osler Eds Silverman ME, Murray TJ, Bryan CS. (ACP Press, Philadelphia) 2008.

[2]   Technology Brief: PET-MRI integrated hybrid scanners. Health Policy Advisory Committee on Technology [State of Queensland (Queensland Health), Brisbane] 2012.

[3]   Hybrid PET/MR systems for whole-body diagnostic imaging. (NIHR Horizon Scanning Centre, University of Birmingham) 2012.

[4]   Brix G, Lechel U, Glatting G, Ziegler SI, Münzing W, Müller SP, *et al*. Radiation exposure of patients undergoing whole-body dual-modality 18 F-FDG PET/CT examinations. J Nucl Med. 2005; 46:608–613.

[5]   Gaertner FC, Furst S, Schwaiger M. PET/MR: A paradigm shift. Cancer Imaging. 2013; 13:36–52.

[6]   Wehrl HF, Sauter AW, Divine MR, Pichler BJ. Combined PET/MR: a technology becomes mature. J Nucl Med. 2015; 56:165–168.

[7]   Al-Nabhani KZ, Syed R, Michopoulou S, Alkalbani J, Afaq A, Panagiotidis E, *et al*. Qualitative and quantitative comparison of PET/CT and PET/MR imaging in clinical practice. J Nucl Med. 2014; 55:88–94.

[8]   Blodgett TM, Meltzer CC, Townsend DW. PET/CT: form and function. Radiology.

2007; 242:360–385.

[9] Utsunomiya D, Shiraishi S, Imuta M, Tomiguchi S, Kawanaka K, Morishita S, *et al*. Added value of SPECT/CT fusion in assessing suspected bone metastasis: comparison with scintigraphy alone and nonfused scintigraphy and CT. Radiology. 2006; 238:264–271.

[10] Jochimsen TH, Schulz J, Busse H, Werner P, Schaudinn A, Zeisig V, *et al*. Lean body mass correction of standardized uptake value in simultaneous whole-body positron emission tomography and magnetic resonance imaging. Phys Med Biol. 2015; 60:4651–4664.

[11] Calandrino R, Ardu V, Corletto D, del Vecchio A, Origgi D, Signorotto P, *et al*. Evaluation of second cancer induction risk by follow-up in oncological long-surviving patients. Health Phys. 2012; 104:1–8.

[12] de Moor JS, Mariotto AB, Parry C, Alfano CM, Padgett L, Kent EE, *et al*. Cancer Survivors in the United States: Prevalence across the Survivorship Trajectory and Implications for Care. Cancer Epidemiol Biomarkers Prev. 2013; 22:561–570.

[13] Guidelines for the assessment of diagnostic technologies. Medical Services Advisory Committee (Commonwealth of Australia, Canberra) 2005.

[14] Macaskill P, Gatsonis C, Deeks JJ, Harboard RM, Takwoingi Y. Chapter 10: Analysing and Presenting Results. In: Deeks JJ, Bossuyt PM, Gatsonis C (editiors), Cochrane Handbook for Systematic Reviews of Diagnostic Test Accuracy Version 1.0. The Cochrane Collaboration, 2010. Available from: http://srdta.cochrane.org/. Accessed 11/11/2015.

[15] Pfannenberg C, Aschoff P, Schanza S, Eschmann SM, Plathow C, Eigentler TK, *et al*. Prospective comparison of 18 F-fluorodeoxyglucose positron emission tomography/computed tomography and whole-body magnetic resonance imaging in staging of advanced malignant melanoma. Europ J Cancer. 2007; 43:555–564.

[16] Schmidt GP, Schoenberg SO, Schmid R, Stahl R, Tiling R, Becker CR, *et al*. Screening for bone metastases: whole-body MRI using a 32-channel system versus dual-modality PET-CT. Eur Radiol. 2007; 17:939–949.

[17] Schmidt GP, Baur-Melnyk A, Haug A, Utzschneider S, Becker CR, Tiling R, *et al*. Whole-body MRI at 1.5 T and 3 T compared with FDG-PET-CT for the detection of tumour recurrence in patients with colorectal cancer. Eur Radiol. 2009; 19: 1366 –1378.

[18] Ng SH, Chan SC, Yen TC, Liao CT, Chang JT, Ko SF, *et al*. (2010) Comprehensive imaging of residual/ recurrent nasopharyngeal carcinoma using whole-body MRI at 3 T compared with FDG-PET-CT. Eur Radiol. 2010; 20:2229–2240.

[19] Laurent V, Trausch G, Bruot O, Olivier P, Felblingerd J, Régenta D. Comparative study of two whole-body imaging techniques in the case of melanoma metastases: Advantages of multi-contrast MRI examination including a diffusion-weighted sequence in comparison with PET-CT. Europ J Radiol. 2010; 75:376–383.

[20] Jouvet JC, Thomas L, Thomson V, Yanes M, Journe C, Morelec I, *et al*. Whole-body MRI with diffusion-weighted sequences compared with 18 FDG PET-CT, CT and superficial lymph node ultrasonography in the staging of advanced cutaneous melanoma: a prospective study. J Eur Acad Dermatol Venereol. 2014; 28:176–185.

[21] Donati OF, Hany TF, Reiner CS, von Schulthess GK, Marincek B, Seifert B, *et al*. Value of retrospective fusion of PET and MR images in detection of hepatic metastases: comparison with 18 F-FDG PET/CT and Gd-EOB-DTPA-enhanced MRI. J Nucl Med. 2010; 51:692–699.

[22] Xu GZ, Li CY, Zhao L, He ZY. Comparison of FDG whole-body PET/CT and gadolinium-enhanced whole-body MRI for distant malignancies in patients with malignant tumors: a meta-analysis. Ann Oncol. 2013; 24:96–101.

[23] Beiderwellen K, Huebner M, Heusch P, Grueneisen J, Ruhlmann V, Nensa F, *et al*. Whole-body[18 F]FDG PET/MRI vs. PET/CT in the assessment of bone lesions in oncological patients: initial results. Eur Radiol. 2014; 24:2023–2030.

[24] Catalano OA, Rosen BR, Sahani DV, Hahn PF, Guimaraes AR, Vangel MG, *et al*. Clinical impact of PET/MR imaging in patients with cancer undergoing same-day PET/CT: initial experience in 134 patients-a hypothesis-generating exploratory study. Radiology. 2013; 269:857–8569.

[25] Reiner CS, Stolzmann P, Husmann L, Burger IA, Hüllner MW, Schaefer NG, *et al*. Protocol requirements and diagnostic value of PET/MR imaging for liver metastasis detection. Eur J Nucl Med Mol Imaging. 2014; 41:649–658.

[26] Dinan MA, Curtis LH, Hammill BG, Patz EF Jr, Abernethy AP, Shea AM, *et al*. Changes in the use and costs of diagnostic imaging among medicare beneficiaries with cancer, 1999-2006. JAMA. 2010; 303(16):1625–1631.

Chapter 22

Current Concepts in Clinical Radiation Oncology

Michael Orth, Kirsten Lauber, Maximilian Niyazi, Anna A. Friedl,
Minglun Li, Cornelius Maihöfer, Lars Schüttrumpf, Anne Ernst,
Olivier M. Niemöller, Claus Belka

Department of Radiotherapy and Radiation Oncology,
Ludwig-Maximilians-University of Munich, Munich, Germany

Abstract: Based on its potent capacity to induce tumor cell death and to abrogate clonogenic survival, radiotherapy is a key part of multimodal cancer treatment approaches. Numerous clinical trials have documented the clear correlation between improved local control and increased overall survival. However, despite all progress, the efficacy of radiation-based treatment approaches is still limited by different technological, biological, and clinical constraints. In principle, the following major issues can be distinguished: (1) The intrinsic radiation resistance of several tumors is higher than that of the surrounding normal tissue, (2) the true patho-anatomical borders of tumors or areas at risk are not perfectly identifiable, (3) the treatment volume cannot be adjusted properly during a given treatment series, and (4) the individual heterogeneity in terms of tumor and normal tissue responses toward irradiation is immense. At present, research efforts in radiation oncology follow three major tracks, in order to address these limitations: (1) implementation of molecularly targeted agents and 'omics'-based screening and stratification procedures, (2) improvement of treatment planning, imaging, and accuracy of dose application, and (3) clinical implementation of other types of radiation, including protons and heavy ions. Several of these strategies have already revealed promising improvements with regard to clinical outcome. Nevertheless, many open questions remain with individualization of treatment approaches being a key problem. In the present review, the current status of radiation-based cancer treatment with particular focus on novel aspects and developments that will influence the field of radiation oncology in the near future is summarized and discussed.

Keywords: Radiotherapy, IMRT/IGRT, Particle Therapy, Targeted Therapy, Biomarkers, Personalized Medicine

1. Introduction

Cancer is the second most frequent cause of death within developed countries being responsible for 200–400 deaths per 100,000 people each year. The incidence of cancer is closely related to age, indicating that the probability of malignant transformation increases with life span. Additionally, cancer can evolve due to risk factors, such as cancer-causing lifestyle habits (e.g., cigarette smoking), genetic predisposition, and viral infections.

Radiotherapy, the clinical application of ionizing radiation, is one crucial treatment option in modern cancer therapy apart from surgery and systemic therapy as being corroborated by the fact that more than 60% of all cancer patients receive radiotherapy today. Radiotherapy can be used in various treatment settings ranging from definitive strategies to multimodal settings, e.g., in adjuvant and in neoadjuvant settings, with or without concomitant chemotherapy. The efficacy of radiotherapy has been proven in multiple randomized trials and has been described in metaanalyses that included multiple cancer types. Radiotherapy can significantly prolong patient survival and improve the local control rates of tumors. Furthermore, radiotherapy can help to avoid surgical amputation and to yield better cosmesis, and it can be used in palliative settings (Ringborg et al. 2003; Delaney et al. 2005).

For the treatment of head and neck cancer, radiotherapy may be used postoperatively, e.g., for patients with specific risk factors (Bernier et al. 2004; Cooper et al. 2004), but it has also been proven to be effective as primary definitive treatment strategy—particularly when being combined with concomitant chemotherapy (Pignon et al. 2009). In case of lung cancer, radiotherapy can be applied stereo-tactically for the treatment of early forms of bronchial carcinoma achieving high rates in local control (Guckenberger et al. 2009; Timmerman et al. 2010), and for advanced stages, it can be used in a neoadjuvant, adjuvant, or definitive manner as well as for palliation, respectively (Auperin et al. 2010; Albain et al. 2009; Douillard et al. 2006). For breast cancer, it was shown that breast-conserving surgery in combination with adjuvant radiotherapy results in survival rates that are equal to mastectomy (Fisher et al. 2002) and that omitting adjuvant radiotherapy causes a decrease by 4% in patient survival (Darby et al. 2011). Finally, in case of prostate cancer, radiotherapy with or without combined hormone therapy reveals comparable cure rates as surgical treatment efforts (Bolla et al. 2002), albeit randomized trials are missing. Taken together, all these findings demonstrate the importance of radiotherapy as one of today's crucial cancer treatment strategies, and the evidence for its effectiveness is still expanding.

2. Technical Improvements in Precision of Radiotherapy

Since ionizing radiation is extremely effective in killing any kind of euka-ryotic cell, a relevant therapeutic gain is only obtained when several prerequisites are met: adequate fractionation, optimal target delineation, radiation planning, image guidance, and toxicity diversification (radio- chemotherapy). In recent years, intensity-modulated radiotherapy (IMRT) and image-guided radiotherapy (IGRT) comprise the most important technological advances (**Figure 1**).

2.1. Intensity-Modulated Radiotherapy (IMRT) and Image-Guided Radiotherapy (IGRT)

In principle, all radiation techniques that employ a non- homogenous photon fluence over a given radiation field can be considered as "intensity modulated." In a more narrow sense, IMRT describes the sequential accumulation of multiple radiation fields resulting in a non-homogenous photon fluence from different gantry angles (Glatstein 2002). Currently, several variations in the IMRT principle are being used to achieve highly conformal radiation distributions: Classical IMRT, volumetric-modulated arc therapy (VMAT), Rapid Arc®, Tomotherapy, and

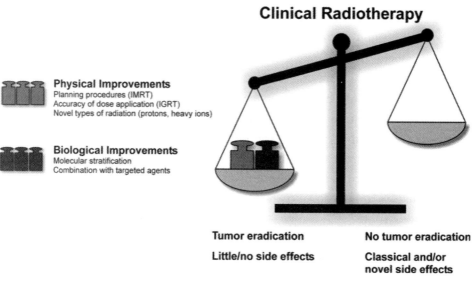

Figure 1. Improvements in clinical radiotherapy with decisive impact in recent years.

Cyber-knife are different technological/vendor-specific solutions that are used to achieve optimal dose distributions while sparing normal tissues in an optimal fashion. To date, it has been proven that the use of IMRT achieves better conformity of the high-dose region to the target volume when compared to 3D conformal approaches, especially for complex treatment situations (Bortfeld 1999), in which adjacent organs at risk might compromise full coverage of the target volume (Mok et al. 2011).

Up to now, many trials have been performed documenting the feasibility of increased target doses with reduced toxicity using IMRT. Probably, the best examples are sparing of the parotid gland in head and neck cancer (Hey et al. 2011) and sparing of the rectum and the bladder while concomitantly increasing the target dose in prostate cancer (Takeda et al. 2012). However, randomized data that compare IMRT with classical 3D conformal radio-therapy are rare (Gupta et al. 2012). This is clearly related to the fact that it is difficult to set up a randomized trial whenever obvious differences in high-dose distributions are visible already after radiation plan comparison. In the meantime, more advanced rotational IMRT techniques such as VMAT and RapidArc® have entered clinical practice and allow for even faster application of prescribed doses. However, the clinical benefits of these techniques need to be further investigated (Jiang et al. 2011; Wiezorek et al. 2011; Foroudi et al. 2012; Fogarty et al. 2011). At present, the development strategies in the field of IMRT and related techniques basically aim at further improving the underlying planning and optimization algorithms as well as the technology of the LINACs in use. However, several open issues are not yet fully solved: (1) dose optimization in case of non-homogenous dose distributions, (2) toxicity prediction in case of non-homogenous doses to organs at risk, (3) reproducibility and verification of treatments with strongly increasing degrees of freedom (rotation, rotation speed, dose rate, field shape, etc.), and (4) mechanical stability and reliability of all components in use. Therefore, one focus of research is the development of planning algorithms, including tools for biological optimization and improved dose calculation (Monte Carlo calculations or similar). In addition, the technology providers aim at developing LINACs that are more and more "ab initio" designed for the implementation of the technologies mentioned above. In parallel, with increasing precision of radiation planning and dose application, the need for better target acquisition raises strongly. The term "target acquisition" covers merely all aspects of patient positioning, patient movement, internal organ movement between fractions, and internal organ motion within a fraction. In this regard, many different visualization tools are in use or in clinical testing. IGRT tools range from classical electronic portal imaging devices (EPIDs) (Njeh et al. 2012) and MV and kV cone-beam CTs (Foster et al. 2012) to complex 3D ultrasound (Chadha et al. 2011) and surface scanners (Pallotta et al. 2012). The wide use of these imaging devices will change the classical target volume approaches considerably. To date, the gross target volume (GTV)-[clinical target volume (CTV)-[planning target volume (PTV) concept is rather static using predefined safety margins in order to compensate for any kind of movement. Replacing this paradigm by daily "online" controls allows for smaller margins, which only reflect biological uncertainties.

In a wider sense, the term "IGRT" describes the use of advanced imaging technology, in order to optimally define target volume sites and organs at risk. At present, several imaging modalities have entered clinical practice in radiation oncology. 18F-Fluorodeoxyglucose (FDG)-based positron emission tomography (PET)-CT is frequently helpful during target volume definition. Highly specific PET markers such as tetraazacyclo-dodecane-tetraacetic acid (DOTA)-octreotide (DOTATOC) and DOTA-octreotate (DOTATATE) strongly improve the definition of the target volume for meningioma (Gehler et al. 2009). Even less specific markers (e.g., 18F-fluoroethyltyrosine (FET)-PET) may strongly influence radiation treatment planning for glioma patients. In this regard, several groups have shown that FET-PET alters treatment volumes in roughly 50% of the cases (Niyazi et al. 2012b). Nevertheless, many issues are currently unsolved: Specificity and sensitivity of merely all tracers are not high enough to allow for automated segmentation of the target volumes. Besides PET-CT, other means of advanced imaging also influence target volume delineation in radiation oncology. At present, the definition of the adjuvant lymphatic drainage region follows empiric and pragmatic rules (Vorwerk and Hess 2011) rather than individual patient-oriented considerations. For the prostate, several groups have analyzed the feasibility of SPECT-based sentinel analysis to define individual lymphatic regions at risk (Vees et al. 2012; Ganswindt et al. 2007). Similarly, more specific MRI tracers would be of key importance for improved target volume definition in various disease sites (Weidner et al. 2011). Thus, it is clear that the combination of improved imaging, both for delineation of the target volume and during treatment, will play a key role in future radiation oncology (Xing et al. 2006). In this regard, the use of IGRT results already today in less acute toxicity during radio-therapy, e.g. in case of prostate cancer (Gill et al. 2011; Crehange et al. 2012).

2.2. Protons and Heavy Ions

Several recent developments like IMRT allow for the reduction in the dose exposed to normal tissue while keeping the prescribed dose on the tumor volume. However, these methods come at the cost of increasing the volume of normal tissues receiving low or moderate doses, and it has been assumed that this may increase the risk of radiation-induced secondary cancers (Hall 2009) although clinical or epidemiological data are not available yet. Charged particles such as protons or heavy ions deliver the highest dose near the end of their range, in the so-called Bragg peak. This allows for extremely steep dose gradients distal to the Bragg peak and thus for superior sparing of organs at risk in the vicinity of the target. Because there is, apart from a dose that is due to secondary particles or fragments, no exit dose and because entrance doses are lower than in the case of photons, this allows for an overall reduction in the integral dose outside the planned target area, which is expected to significantly reduce the risk of radiogenic secondary malignancies in long-term cancer survivors (Fontenot et al. 2010; Newhauser and Durante 2011). So far, no long-term epidemiological studies on the incidence of secondary cancer cases following a proton or a heavy ion-based cancer treatment are available, and given the latency period associated with radiation-induced tumors, these studies will also not be available in nearer future. The knowledge of radia-tion-induced tumorigenesis and the many parameters involved (e.g., radiation dose and quality, fractionation, age at exposure, genetic susceptibility) is limited, and therefore, risk estimations are difficult to perform. For example, passive beam scattering, which has been the predominant method for increasing the size of the proton pencil beam generated by the accelerator up to now, produces secondary neutrons with a broad range of energies for some of which the relative biological effectiveness (RBE) is poorly characterized (Hall 2009), and therefore, the impact of these neutrons on secondary tumor risk is difficult to estimate. It should be noted that part of secondary neutron production is reduced in particle therapy se-tups using active beam scanning (Clasie et al. 2010).

So far, only a few clinical studies have been performed on the efficacy and acute side effects of proton and ion therapy, and only very few of them have di-rectly compared the outcome of particle therapy and conventional radio- therapy. Brada et al. (2009) gave a detailed overview on the clinical impact of proton ther-apy based on a search within published, peer-reviewed literature. They identified 52 studies of proton therapy fulfilling their quality criteria (at least 20 patients with a follow-up period of at least 2 years), encompassing data of in total 13,736 pa-tients (Brada et al. 2009). Of these patients, 10,328 received treatments for ocular tumors and 1,642 were treated for prostate tumors and 880 for tumors of the cen-tral nervous system (CNS). Other tumor entities such as head and neck tumors, gastrointestinal tumors, lung cancer, and sarcomas were subjects of two to five studies each, encompassing between 97 and 375 patients per tumor site. This number must be compared to more than 60,000 patients who had undergone a proton-based cancer therapy by the end of 2008 (http://ptcog.web.psi.ch/Archive/Patientstatistics- update02Mar2009.pdf). Brada and coauthors concluded that the evaluated literature lacks any evidence demonstrating a clear benefit of proton-based therapy if compared to the best available conventional therapies with respect to tumor control, patient survival, and side effects. Others studies came to similar conclusions, even with respect to pediatric tumors (Bouyon-Monteau et al. 2010), prostate cancer (Kagan and Schulz 2010), lung cancer (Liao et al. 2011), head and neck cancers (Ramaekers et al. 2011), and tumors of the skull base treated by ra-diosurgery (Amichetti et al. 2012). A recent study even showed higher rates of ga-strointestinal side effects after a proton-based therapy if compared to conventional IMRT of prostate cancer (Sheets et al. 2012), but the methodology applied in this study is under debate (Deville et al. 2012; Mendenhall et al. 2012; Jacobs et al. 2012). Clearly, the absence of evidence is not evidence of absence of a superior efficacy or tolerance of proton therapy, but nevertheless, these analyses clearly stress the requirement of more clinical studies assessing the clinical impact of proton-based cancer therapy.

The better the conformity, the higher are the requirements for setup reproducibility, accuracy in patient immobilization, and consideration of changes in the patient's anatomy, such as the motion of organs (e.g., due to filling of the bladder or the rectum), or treatment- induced alterations, e.g., tumor shrinkage. This holds for a highly conformal therapy with both photons and protons. The impact of intrafraction mobility, which is affected by the duration of the treatment, may be of special importance in case of an active proton beam scanning, because this method takes considerably more time than passive scattering or photon irradiation. Importantly, in the case of protons, an additional level of complexity comes into play since absorption and scattering of protons largely depend on the material traversed so that the range and the lateral penumbra are affected by the inhomogeneity of the tissue. Uncertainty in estimating the particle range will automatically translate into dose uncertainties. In spite of demands for state-of-the-art imaging, image guidance, and dose verification, several authors raised concerns about the lack of optimal technologies at proton therapy facilities (Merchant 2009; Schippers and Lomax 2011). As already pointed out by Goitein in 2008, the possibility for treatment errors is much greater in case of protons than with photons and therefore, proton therapy has to be used exclusively in a highly controlled fashion (Goitein 2008).

Carbon ions are less affected by energy straggling and scattering as compared to protons, and therefore, the precision of the dose deposition achievable is even greater than in the case of protons. However, due to fragmentation processes, a dose tail is always present distally from the Bragg peak, which must be considered in treatment planning. These fragmentation processes come, however, also with an advantage, namely the generation of positron emitters that allow for in situ beam monitoring (Weber and Kraft 2009). One major potential of carbon ions lies in the fact that they can confer a significant higher RBE than photons within their Bragg peak region, and this not only means that the physical dose there is highest, but also the biological effect achievable per dose unit. The expenses for carbon-ion-based radiotherapy units are, however, even greater than for proton facilities, and only few facilities have been available in the past. Since 2009, the carbon ion radiotherapy unit at the Heidelberg Ion Therapy (HIT) center which uses active beam scanning is operating, and initial data on clinical experiences become available now (Combs et al. 2010b). At HIT, all patients are treated within clinical trials (Combs et al. 2010a, c; Jensen et al. 2011a, b), and recently, randomized phase III trials have been initiated to compare proton- and carbonion-based therapies for the treatment of chondrosarcomas and chordomas (Nikoghosyan et al. 2010a, b). Due to their higher RBE, the treatment with carbon ions might be more effective for the cure of radioresistant tumors. A recent meta-analysis performed in different head and neck cancers compared the efficacies of photons, protons, and carbon ions (Ramaekers et al. 2011) but, so far, only revealed a survival benefit for mucosal malignant melanomas after a carbon-ion-based therapy, which might reflect a high grade of resistance of this particular tumor entity toward irradiation in general. Other work suggests that due to the reduced volume of normal tissue that is exposed to modest doses, particle therapy may confer advantages in treatments using concurrent drug administration (Nystrom 2010). In a modeling study, Vogelius et al. (2011) estimated the pneumonitis risk after a treatment with photons or protons either in combination with or in the absence of chemotherapy and came to the conclusion that proton therapy could potentially minimize the risk by reducing the volume that is exposed to lower doses (Vogelius et al. 2011). Given the increasing role of multimodality treatment approaches, further investigations into the relative merit of particle therapy in these settings are clearly needed.

The controversial discussion on the necessity of clinical studies of particle therapy is, in part, fuelled by the high costs of this treatment if compared to established photon therapy. One part of such elevated costs is due to the size of the synchrotrons or cyclotrons used, and there are several developments that aim for provision of smaller accelerators (Schippers and Lomax 2011). One putative solution could be the acceleration of protons and also of heavier ions by laser acceleration (Tajima 2010). Although current technologies are far from clinical application, some research groups already started to address the question of whether the RBE of laser-driven particles may differ from that of conventionally accelerated particles, thereby focusing on the ultrashort pulsing process by which these particles are generated as well as on the ultra-high dose rates associated with it (Rigaud et al. 2010; Yogo et al. 2009; Kraft et al. 2010; Bin et al. 2012). By simulating the pulsed radiation conditions expected in therapy settings using laser-accelerated protons of a pulsed proton beam at the Munich ion microbeam SNAKE (Dollinger et al. 2009), an extensive series of experiments with various endpoints in cell monolayers, 3D tissue culture models, and tumor xenografts were conducted. However, no significant differences between a dose of a few Gy that was given in about 1 ns (the dose rate expected after laser acceleration) and the same dose given in about 100 ms (the dose rate at conventional irradiation settings) could be observed in these experiments (Schmid et al. 2009, 2010; Auer et al. 2011; Greubel et al. 2011; Zlobinskaya et al. 2012).

3. Biological Improvements of Radiotherapy

During the last decades, significant improvements have been made: A special focus has been placed on the development of advanced planning procedures (van Herk 2004), the physical accuracy of dose application (Bucci et al. 2005) and combined modality treatment approaches in terms of radiochemotherapy (Al-Sarraf et al. 1998) (**Figure 1**). However, dose escalation studies revealed that the combination of radiotherapy with classical chemotherapy has reached some kind of dead end (Budach et al. 2006). At this point, the combination of radiotherapy with molecularly designed agents specifically targeting the hallmarks of cancer has revealed significant improvements in clinical outcomes when compared to each treatment strategy alone (Begg et al. 2011). However, the effective integration of molecularly targeted drugs requires a detailed patient stratification, since only those patients with relevant signal aberrations will benefit. Furthermore, it has to be noted that stratification is urgently needed in order to avoid side effects induced by the addition of such targeted drugs (Niyazi et al. 2011b). In the following paragraphs, the key biological targets for specifically improved radiotherapy will be introduced.

3.1. The Hallmarks of Cancer

The emergence of cancer, in general, is due to failures within mechanisms or pathways that control the growth, the proliferation, and/or the death of cells in response to extracellular or intracellular signals. Deregulations within these mechanisms can commit cells to sustained proliferation, replicative immortality, evasion of growth suppression, and resistance to cell death—attributes commonly shared by malignantly transformed cells (Hanahan and Weinberg 2000). However, the transition from a single transformed cell toward the formation of a solid tumor requires additional features, such as the capacity to instigate the formation of blood vessels (angiogenesis and/or neovascularization), mechanisms to evade immune responses, as well as an increased potential to invade other tissues (metastasis) (Hanahan and Weinberg 2011).

3.1.1. Sustained Proliferation and Replicative Immortality

The growth as well as the proliferation of cells is orchestrated by a class of signaling molecules called mitogens. While in non-transformed cells, the synthesis and the release of mitogens are tightly controlled, these processes are often deregulated in cancer cells. Such deregulation can be due to the acquisition of genetic mutations (for instance due to exposure to tumor-initiating chemicals and/or ionizing radiation) or to the experience of growth-supporting signals, such as tumor-promoting chemicals and chronic inflammation. Two of the best-characterized mitogens are the platelet-derived growth factor (PDGF) and the epidermal growth factor (EGF). The binding of these ligands to their respective receptors, PDGFR and epidermal growth factor receptor (EGFR), activates sophisticated signaling pathways, including the mitogen-activated kinase (MAP kinase) pathway, thereby stimulating both the growth and the proliferation of cells (Seger and Krebs 1995). Mutations within the genes that encode for such mitogens/receptors can render the corresponding gene products in a state of constitutive activation culminating in uncontrolled growth and/or proliferation of cells. In this regard, the gene encoding the small GTPase K-Ras provides a prototypical example as activating mutations of K-Ras are found in diverse cancer entities, e.g., in more than 40% of all colorectal cancers (Karapetis et al. 2008). Similar examples can be found in other mitogenic signaling pathways, including the phospho-inositide-3-kinase (PI3K)/AKT kinase and the insulin-like growth factor (IGF) pathway (Chang et al. 2003; Fresno Vara et al. 2004; Samani et al. 2007; Frasca et al. 2008).

With regard to their impact on the outcome of radio- therapy, both overexpression and mutation of EGFR were shown to correlate with increased resistance of tumors to irradiation and poor clinical prognosis (Lammering et al. 2003, 2004; Giralt et al. 2005; Milas et al. 2004). Furthermore, ligand-independent activation of EGFR in response to irradiation and the subsequent activation of its downstream signaling cascades apparently contribute to radioresistance (Iyer et al. 2004;

Gupta et al. 2001; Toulany et al. 2005). Therefore, multiple strategies have been developed in order to interfere with EGFR function as being discussed in more detail later on.

A key step in malignant transformation is the acquirement of basically limitless replicative potential. After a certain number of division cycles, a normal cell exits the cell cycle and transits into senescence, a stage of metabolic activity devoid of further proliferation (Campisi and d'Adda di Fagagna 2007). The induction of senescence requires a group of proteins encoded by genes that are known as tumor-suppressor genes (e.g., p53, pRB). These genes negatively regulate the growth and/or the proliferation of cells, and hence, mutations that render their products inactive can support both immortalization and unrestrained proliferation. Another prerequisite for replicative immortality is the cell's capacity to protect its telomeres (Blasco 2005). Since expression of telomerase is almost absent in non-immortalized cells, their replicative potential is greatly limited by successive telomere shortening. In immortalized cells (including cancer cells), to the contrary, expression of telomerase is reinitiated, thereby counteracting the erosion of telomeres and, in consequence, the induction of senescence or apoptosis. Additionally, expression of telomerase and telomere length have been reported to contribute to radioresistance of tumor cells (Genesca et al. 2006).

3.1.2. Evasion of Growth Suppression and Resistance to Cell Death

Aside from extensive proliferation, the formation of solid tumors necessitates the cellular capacity for evading growth-suppressive signals, which mostly depend on tumor-suppressor proteins, such as p53 or the members of the retinoblastoma protein family. These proteins interfere with cell proliferation in response to growth-inhibiting signals and/or intracellular disorders including DNA damage either by blocking the expression of genes required for cell cycle progression or by initiating the expression of cell cycle-inhibiting genes such as p16^{INK4a} and p21^{WAF1} (Sherr and Roberts 1999). Alternatively, tumor-suppressor proteins (in particular p53) can also stimulate the induction of a programmed form of cell death called apoptosis, e.g., in response to DNA damage, explaining p53's pivotal role in determination of tumor radiosensitivity (Gudkov and Komarova 2003). In this context, p53 induces the expression of several pro-apoptotic proteins (e.g., PUMA) and thereby facilitates the induction of apoptosis. However, many cancer cells circumvent apoptosis, e.g., by inactivating p53, by down-regulating pro- apoptotic genes, or by up-regulating antiapoptotic genes.

3.1.3. Angiogenesis and Neovascularization

Since the formation of solid tumors demands for a continuous nutrient and oxygen supply, tumor cells must acquire the capacity to stimulate vascularization involving de novo formation of blood vessels (vasculogenesis) as well as sprouting of newly formed vessels from preexisting ones (angiogenesis). In adults, angiogenesis and vasculogenesis are tightly limited to certain physiological processes, such as wound healing. However, during tumor progression, angiogenesis is reinitiated (Bergers and Benjamin 2003). To this end, tumor cells secrete pro- angiogenic factors, such as the vascular endothelial growth factor (VEGF) that, upon binding to their respective receptors (VEGFR), stimulate the proliferation of endothelial cells resulting in increased vessel formation and tumor infiltration. VEGF expression in tumor cells is facilitated by certain oncogene products, including c-Myc or H-Ras, whereas non-transformed cells express VEGF almost exclusively under hypoxic conditions (Baudino et al. 2002; Chin et al. 1999). The degree of vascularization plays an important role in regard to the tumor's responsiveness to ionizing radiation. As the induction of DNA damage is supported by the presence of oxygen, increased hypoxia limits the efficacy of radiotherapy. Consequently, intense efforts are spent in order to increase tumor oxygenation and to improve the therapeutic effect of exposure to ionizing radiation (Wachsberger et al. 2003).

3.1.4. Evasion of Immune Responses

Another barrier limiting the formation and the progression of tumors is the immune system. This becomes clear by the fact that immunocompromised mice, e.g., mice that are deficient in $CD8^+$ T lymphocytes or natural killer (NK) cells, show a significant higher susceptibility to cancer than those that are immunocompetent (Schreiber et al. 2011). Consequently, it is no wonder that tumor cells acquire multiple mechanisms to evade immune responses, such as elimination and/or aberration of tumor antigens/MHC class I molecules, secretion of immunosuppressive cytokines such as transforming growth factor β (TGF-β) and interleukins, recruitment of immunosuppressive immune cells (e.g., $CD4^+$ $CD25^+$ regulatory T cells and myeloid-derived suppressor cells), or expression of indolamine-2, 3-dioxygenase (IDO) (Kaufman and Disis 2004; Munn and Mellor 2007; Garcia-Lora et al. 2003). Several lines of evidence support the notion that the immune system plays a pivotal role in tumor regression in response to radiotherapy (Lauber et al. 2012). This is of particular interest, since the induction of an antitumor immune response might not only be helpful for the elimination of the primary tumor within the irradiation field, but also for out-of-field metastases (Frey et al. 2012).

3.1.5. Tissue Invasion and Metastasis

Aside from their capacity to form primary tumors, some malignantly transformed cells also acquire the capacity to infiltrate neighboring tissues or even penetrate lymphatic and/or blood vessels, giving rise to several kinds of secondary tumors or metastases. Usually, metastasis starts with the detachment of tumor cells from the primary tumor site facilitated by the repression of factors that mediate cellular adhesion, such as E-cadherin, and by secretion of enzymes that degrade extracellular matrices (ECMs), thus liberating tumor cells from their surroundings (Valastyan and Weinberg 2011). These processes depend on the activation of a conserved cellular program termed the epithelial-mesenchymal transition (EMT), which regulates the formation of the mesoderm and the neural tube during embryonic development (Thiery et al. 2009). For several tumor entities, glioblastomas in particular, it was shown that irradiation increases their invasive potential and thus might even accelerate local dissemination and development of distant metastasis (Qian et al. 2002; Cordes et al. 2003; Wild-Bode et al. 2001; Camphausen et al. 2001).

3.2. Mechanisms of Cell Death

Radiotherapy is an important treatment modality in clinical cancer therapy because of its great potential to kill malignant cells and to abrogate clonogenic survival. Directly or indirectly, ionizing radiation induces different types of genome damage, including DNA double-strand breaks (DSBs), bulky lesions, and others, thereby activating a highly sophisticated signaling network termed the DNA damage response (DDR) culminating in transient or permanent cell cycle arrest and/or cell death, respectively (**Figure 2**).

3.2.1. DNA Damage Response (DDR)

The DDR mediates cellular responses to various kinds of DNA damage, a cell has to cope with. The DDR is regulated by two conserved protein kinases called Ataxia telangiectasia mutated (ATM) and Ataxia telangiectasia and Rad3 related (ATR) (Smith et al. 2010). ATM is recruited to DSBs by the Mre11-Rad50-Nbs1 (MRN) complex where it phosphorylates the histone H2 variant H2AX, thereby creating a recruitment platform for other DDR factors (Shiloh 2006). In parallel, ATM mediates resection of the broken DNA strand(s), and the resulting ssDNA repair intermediates specifically activate ATR kinase (Hurley and Bunz

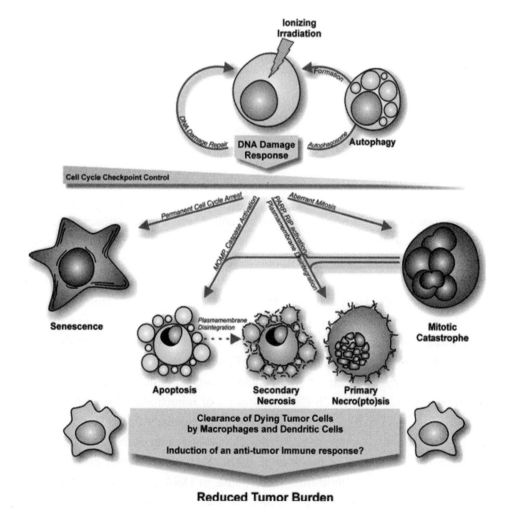

Figure 2. Mechanisms of cell death triggered by ionizing radiation.

2007). By phosphorylation of two respective downstream kinases termed CHK1 and CHK2, ATR and ATM trigger a multitude of signaling pathways, thereby initiating both a transient arrest within cell cycle progression and DNA damage repair. However, in case of excessive DNA damage, ATM/ATR can also induce cellular senescence and/or cell death (Jackson and Bartek 2009).

The major target of the ATM/ATR cascade in terms of arresting the cell cycle or committing the cell to cell death is the tumor-suppressor protein p53. In the absence of DNA damage, the overall levels of p53 within the cell are maintained rather low because of the association of p53 with the ubiquitin ligase MDM2 (HDM2 in human). MDM2 continuously ubiquitylates p53, thereby targeting p53 for proteasomal degradation. Yet, in the context of the DDR, p53 is phosphorylated by kinases of the ATM/ATR cascade leading to its dissociation from MDM2 and thus to stabilization of p53 (Meek 2009). Once being stabilized, the transcription factor p53 crucially regulates cell cycle arrest, DNA damage repair, and the induction of cell death or senescence by inducing or repressing the expression of several target genes that encode for factors involved in these processes (Sengupta and Harris 2005).

3.2.2. Apoptosis

Apoptosis is a form of programmed cell death, which is characterized by chromatin condensation/fragmentation, cell shrinkage, and blebbing of cell membranes. In response to irradiation, apoptosis is predominantly observed in cells of the hematopoietic system. Radiation-dependent induction of apoptosis mainly relies on the intrinsic death pathway (Rudner 2001), in which cytochrome c is released into the cytosol by permeabilization of the outer mitochondrial membrane. This, in turn, stimulates the formation of the apoptosome and subsequent activation of the caspase cascade. The cleavage of multiple caspase substrates within the cell finally results in chromatin fragmentation, organelle destruction, and cellular disintegration (Taylor et al. 2008). The process of mitochondrial permeabilization is essentially controlled by pro- and antiapoptotic members of the B-cell lymphoma-2 (Bcl-2) family, which regulate the channel-forming activity of the family members BAX and BAK (Chipuk et al. 2010; Youle and Strasser 2008). Protein p53 can modulate this equilibrium in response to DNA damage by inducing the expression of pro-apoptotic Bcl-2 family members, such as PUMA, NOXA, and BAX itself (Sengupta and Harris 2005).

Stimulation of apoptosis via the extrinsic death pathway, on the contrary, depends on the binding of death ligands (e.g., CD95L, TRAIL) to their respective cell surface receptors (Debatin and Krammer 2004). Subsequent death receptor clustering triggers the activation of the caspase cascade in this pathway. Although the expression levels of several key regulators of the extrinsic pathway have been described to increase upon exposure to ionizing radiation (Belka et al. 1998; Haupt et al. 2003), the intrinsic pathway appears to be the dominant pathway of apoptosis induction in response to DNA damage (Rudner 2001). Additionally, it should be noted that cells deficient in p53 function can undergo radiation-induced apoptosis as well, indicating that alternative mechanisms such as p63-/p73-dependent expression of pro-apoptotic factors can compensate for the lack of p53 in these cases (Afshar et al. 2006; Wakatsuki et al. 2008).

3.2.3. Necroptosis/Necrosis

When activation of caspases is prevented, DNA damage can induce an alternate form of cell death termed necroptosis. Necroptosis depends on hyperactivation of the poly-ADP-ribose-polymerase (PARP), a protein involved in DNA excision repair, and subsequent activation of receptor-interacting protein (RIP)—kinases as a response to depletion of intracellular ATP. Necroptosis, once being triggered by a structure called the necrosome, is characterized by the appearance of reactive oxygen species (ROS), lipid peroxidation, failure in calcium homeostasis, organelle swelling, and plasma membrane rupture (Van- denabeele et al. 2010). It appears to be of special importance in cancer cells of epithelial origin which reveal a limited apoptosis induction capacity in response to ionizing radiation, and also when irradiation is applied in high doses or in combination with hyperthermia (Mantel et al. 2010; Schildkopf et al. 2010). Additionally, high doses of ionizing radiation can stimulate necrosis, an accidental, uncontrolled type of cell death, which is predominantly characterized by rupture of the plasma membrane and a resulting release of intracellular contents, including danger signals, which can potently alert the immune system.

3.2.4. Mitotic Catastrophe

The term "mitotic catastrophe" describes a cellular condition, which results from aberrant cell cycle progression prior to mitotic entry or during cell division itself. Mitotic catastrophe is characterized by the formation of huge cells with multiple nuclei as well as hyperamplified centrosomes. It might constitute the pre-dominant mechanism of radiation-dependent cell death in cells with defective cell cycle checkpoints (Eriksson and Stigbrand 2010). However, cells, which have un-dergone mitotic catastrophe, might survive for several days, transit into senescence, or die by apoptosis and/or necro (pto)sis due to their high degrees of aneuploidy.

3.2.5. Cellular Senescence

Cellular senescence is a state of permanent cell cycle arrest, which can be instigated by DNA damage. Senescence induction requires function of certain cell cycle checkpoint components, such as p53 and the retinoblastoma protein pRB, but it has also been observed in the absence of functional p53 (Nardella et al. 2011). Senescent cells are active in terms of metabolism, but do not show further cell cycle progression. Central features of senescent cells comprise a flattened mor-phology, an increase in granularity, the up-regulation of cyclin-dependent kinase inhibitors, and a positive staining for β-galactosidase (SA-β-Gal). Furthermore, senescent cells have been reported to release factors that can support as well as inhibit malignant progression by influencing both the proliferation of neighboring cells and antitumor immune responses (Krtolica et al. 2001; Eriksson and Stig-brand 2010; Coppe et al. 2010).

3.2.6. Autophagy

Autophagy represents a cellular state that is currently being discussed as both a mechanism of cell death and cell survival (Apel et al. 2009). It is characte-rized by the sequestration of proteins and/or organelles within huge autophagic vesicles called autophagosomes. As fusion of these vesicles with lysosomes leads to the formation of autophagolysosomes and degradation of their content provid-ing material for de novo synthesis and regeneration, it is rather unclear whether autophagy represents a mechanism of survival or cell death, respectively. Auto-phagy involves the activation of multiple protein kinases, including the class I phosphatidylinositol-3-kinases (PI3 K-I), stress kinases, and the mammalian target of rapamycin (mTOR) kinase, and it has been observed in response to exposure to ionizing radiation (Apel et al. 2008).

3.2.7. Immunological Consequences

The induction of tumor cell death and the inhibition of clonogenic survival by the application of ionizing radiation are central elements of its therapeutic success. Yet, it is well accepted that mechanisms involving both the innate and the adaptive immune system contribute to tumor regression—particularly in the context of ablative radio-therapy, where irradiation is applied in high single doses of 10 Gy or more (Lauber et al. 2012). In this regard, local high-dose radiotherapy of transplanted mouse B16 melanoma has been reported to stimulate the generation of tumor antigen-specific, interferon-γ (IFN-γ)-producing T cells (Lugade et al. 2005). Moreover, ablative, but not fractionated, radiotherapy drastically enhanced T cell priming in tumor-draining lymph nodes, which was paralleled by a regression of the primary tumor as well as distant, out-of-field metastases in a CD8$^+$ T cell-dependent manner (Lee et al. 2009). Mechanistically, these T cells apparently have been primed by dendritic cells (DCs), which carry ingested tumor material and cross-present it in the tumor-draining lymph nodes. A recent study showed that the intratumoral production of type I interferons (IFN-α/β) in response to ablative radiotherapy is key in this scenario, since it enhances the cross-presenting capacity of tumor-infiltrating DCs (Burnette et al. 2011). This cascade of interferons, where IFN-α/β produced by CD11c$^+$ cells (presumably DCs and macrophages) enhances the crosspriming activity of CD8α^+ DCs thereby stimulating the generation of IFN-γ-producing CD8$^+$ T cells and, finally, tumor rejection, is well known from the field of tumor immunoediting (Diamond et al. 2011; Fuertes et al. 2013). Here, IFN-α/β and IFN-γ contribute on different levels to the reduction in tumor burden. Whereas IFN-α/β primarily exerts its effects on macrophages, DCs, and NK cells by facilitating their activation and maturation and by enhancing their capacity to induce adaptive immune responses (Dunn et al. 2006), IFN-γ directly affects the tumor via inhibition of tumor cell proliferation, apoptosis induction, inhibition of angiogenesis, and an overall enhancement of tumor immunogenicity (Dunn et al. 2006; Lugade et al. 2008; Reits et al. 2006). Additionally, IFN-c contributes to the stimulation of an antitumor immune response since it is essentially involved in T_H1/T_C1 cell responses and exerts similar effects as IFN-α/β in terms of innate immune cell activation and DC-mediated antigen cross-presentation (Dunn et al. 2006). This interferon cascade of innate and adaptive immune responses has only been described in case of ablative but not conventional, fractionated radiotherapy (Lee et al. 2009), and the question that needs to be addressed is why. One feasible explanation could be that ablative and fractionated radio- therapy trigger different tumor cell responses in terms of cell death and/or senescence induction with only high single-dose irradiation stimulating primary or secondary, postapoptotic secondary necro(pto)sis or senescence, respectively. The corresponding cellular releasates, a complex mixture of danger signals, and the senescence-associated secretome are well known to be potent inducers of IFN-α/β and other pro-inflammatory cytokines and hence could initiate the IFN-cascade described above and the DC-mediated instigation of antitumor T cell responses (Coppe et al. 2010; Apetoh et al. 2007; Peter et al. 2010; Kuilman and Peeper 2009).

3.3. Combination of Radiotherapy (RTX) with Targeted Agents

Despite the technical improvements in cancer radiotherapy in recent years, the combination of radiotherapy with classical chemotherapy has reached a dead end (Budach et al. 2006). Therefore, novel strategies encompassing the combination of conventional radiotherapy with agents that are specifically raised against key factors of malignant transformation have been designed and are currently being tested (**Figure 3**). In the following paragraphs, current efforts made in order to specifically target cellular compounds to improve the efficacy of clinical radiation oncology in the future are discussed.

3.3.1. Combination of RTX with Agents Targeting the DDR

As the cell-death-inducing potential of ionizing radiation is largely determined by the cells' capacity to cope with DNA damage, it is no wonder that both the expression and the functionality of DDR components have great impact on the efficacy of radiotherapy. This can be appreciated by the fact that the expression of DDR components within different tissues often correlates with the resistance or sensitivity of the respective tissue toward irradiation (Peters et al. 1982; Deacon et al. 1984). Therefore, targeted pharmaceutical agents, which interfere with proper function of the DDR, should be suitable to enhance the efficacy of conventional radiotherapy (Basu et al. 2012; Begg et al. 2011). Indeed, several studies revealed that interfering with ATM function (e.g., by using small-molecule inhibitors such as KU-55933) efficiently sensitizes human cancer cells to irradiation (Hickson et

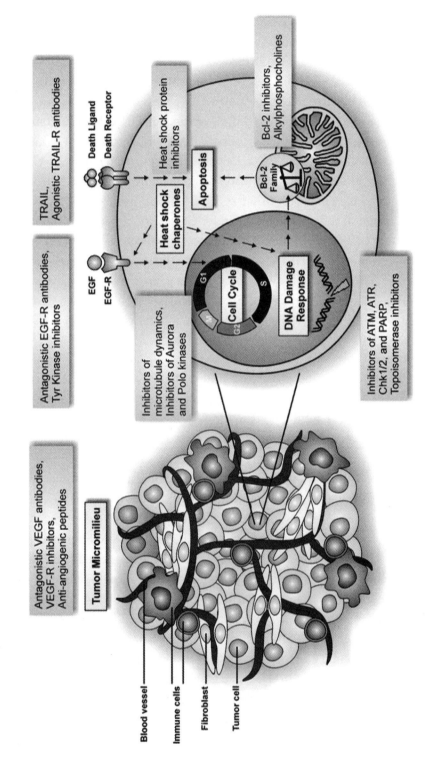

Figure 3. Survey of valuable targets for combined modality approaches.

561

al. 2004; Cowell et al. 2005; Golding et al. 2009). Similar results have been reported for inhibitors of other DDR kinases, e.g., the ATR inhibitors VE-821 and VE-822 (Prevo et al. 2012; Pires et al. 2012; Fokas et al. 2012) or the CHK1/2 inhibitor AZD7762 (Zabludoff et al. 2008; Mitchell et al. 2010; Morgan et al. 2010). Other targets within the DDR network are the PARPs as this class of enzymes is involved in repair of DNA single-strand breaks (SSBs)—a kind of DNA damage commonly induced by ionizing radiation. Indeed, several PARP inhibitors, such as olaparib (AZD-2281) and veliparib (ABT-888), have revealed great potentials in terms of sensitizing tumor cells to irradiation in combined modality approaches (Donawho et al. 2007; Barazzuol et al. 2013; Miura et al. 2012; Chalmers et al. 2004; Senra et al. 2011; Shelton et al. 2013) and are, therefore, tested in clinical trials (Audeh et al. 2010; Tutt et al. 2010; Kaye et al. 2012). Recently, a specific inhibitor of the non-homologous end joining (NHEJ)-associated DNA ligase IV has been published (Srivastava et al. 2012) and showed great potency in terms of radiosensitizing cancer cells both in vitro and in vivo (Srivastava et al. 2012). Further studies are needed in order to see whether this inhibitor is feasible for clinical purposes.

Meanwhile, the small-molecule-inhibitor-based interference with DDR function might also offer the possibility to specifically target cancer stem cells (CSCs)—a small subset of the tumor cell population that shares several features with normal stem cells, e.g., the potential to selfrenew, to proliferate excessively, to differentiate into multiple cellular lineages, and to induce de novo formation of blood vessels (Reya et al. 2001; Jordan et al. 2006). CSCs have moved into the focus of targeted therapies in recent years since complete eradication of a tumor inevitably demands for elimination of this particular kind of tumor cells that have the potential to self-renew and, in consequence, exhibit clonogenicity. Notably, CSCs exhibit an enormously high level of radioresistance (Bao et al. 2006; Firat et al. 2011), but the underlying mechanisms are unknown. It has been suggested that lower levels of ROS generated within the CSCs contribute to their high degree of radio-resistance as well as to their enormous capacity to cope with DNA damages (Bao et al. 2006; Diehn et al. 2009). Very recently, it has been reported that CSCs exhibit a great enhancement in ATM kinase activity, suggesting that ATM might be a valuable target for combined modality approaches aiming at overcoming CSC radiore-sistance (Yin and Glass 2011). Indeed, Yin and Glass show that the inhibition of ATM by a small-molecule inhibitor reduces the radioresistance of CSCs (Yin and Glass 2011), thereby offering novel therapeutic perspectives. Aside, multiple signal transduction pathways that are important for the development of non-transformed stem cells, including the notch-, the hedgehog-, and the Wnt-/β-catenin pathway, have been reported to contribute to radiore-sistance in CSCs (Chen et al. 2007; Phillips et al. 2006; Woodward et al. 2007; Wesbuer et al. 2010; Cerdan and Bhatia 2010). This might offer additional prospects for combinatorial approaches in future.

3.3.2. Combination of RTX with Agents Targeting Topoisomerases

Topoisomerases represent a class of enzymes that regulate the topology of DNA, e.g., during processes such as replication, transcription, recombination, and DNA repair. While topoisomerase I (Topo I) coordinates relaxation of super- helical DNA by introducing single-strand breaks (nicks) within the DNA duplex, topoisomerase II (Topo II) introduces transient double-strand breaks, thereby disentangling coiled DNA (Champoux 2001). As these functions are crucial both for the integrity and for the propagation of genomes, topoisomerases became one of the first classes of enzymes targeted in cancer therapy. Primarily, inhibitors that were derived from camptothecin (inhibits topoisomerase I) and etoposide/VP-16 (inhibits topoisomerase II) were deployed to target the function of topoisomerases. Aside from their immense chemotherapeutic potential per se, these drugs also turned out to possess an excellent potential in terms of sensitizing tumor cells toward ionizing radiation (Chen et al. 1999). In parallel, several synthetic analogues, such as topotecan and irinotecan, were raised and investigated for clinical purposes (Pommier 2013). The results obtained confirmed the notion that pharmaceutical inhibition of topoisomerases provides a good opportunity for combined modality treatment of multiple kinds of neoplasms (Mattern et al. 1991; Kim et al. 1992; Choy and MacRae 2001). This explains why respective combinations have been and still are enduringly tested within clinical trials (O'Leary and Muggia 1998; Hande 1998; Tao et al. 2013). In addition, multiple other classes of topoisomerase inhibitors, such as quinolines (inhibitors of topoisomerase I), quinolones, and anthracy- clines (inhibitors of topoisomerase II), have been deployed for clinical purpose (Pommier 2013).

3.3.3. Combination of RTX with Agents Targeting the Apoptosis Network

As the induction of cell death—at least in part—depends on the functionality of the apoptotic machinery, drugs that can directly stimulate apoptosis (for instance, by facilitating caspase activation) also moved into the view of clinically oriented research, especially as it can be assumed that targeting of apoptotic network components should efficiently sensitize tumor cells toward ionizing radiation. Moreover, many kinds of tumor cells circumvent efficient induction of apoptosis by down-regulation of pro-apoptotic genes or up-regulation of antiapoptotic ones (Kasibhatla and Tseng 2003). One prominent target among these components is the TNF-α-related apoptosis-inducing ligand (TRAIL/Apo2L). For several tumor cell lines, it could be shown that both recombinant TRAIL itself and TRAIL- receptor agonistic antibodies, e.g., mapatumumab and lexatumumab, efficiently sensitize tumor cells to ionizing radiation (Belka et al. 2001; Chinnaiyan et al. 2000; Gong and Almasan 2000; Marini et al. 2009a, b; Niyazi et al. 2009a, b). In particular, cells that displayed only weak responses to either treatment alone often showed strong sensitization effects while no effect could be detected for non- transformed cells, which is—at least in part—due to the high level of selectivity of TRAIL and TRAIL-receptor agonizing antibodies for malignant cells. Another class of proteins involved in the regulation of apoptosis and therefore representing a promising target for combined modality approaches are the members of the B-cell lymphoma 2 (Bcl-2) family (Vogler et al. 2009). This protein family regulates the permeabilization of the outer mito- chondrial membrane—a prerequisite for apoptosis induction via the intrinsic pathway. Therefore, inhibition of antia- poptotic Bcl-2 proteins should enhance the induction of apoptosis, especially when being combined with irradiation. In fact, several studies showed that inhibition of Bcl-2 sensitizes tumor cells toward ionizing radiation (Zerp et al. 2009; Moretti et al. 2010), revealing that Bcl-2 and, possibly, other members of this protein family may serve as candidates for targeted approaches in the future. Currently, navitoclax (ABT-263), a highly selective Bcl-2 inhibitor, is tested in clinical trials, and initial results strengthen the hope for its future implementation in the clinic (Gandhi et al. 2011; Rudin et al. 2012). A third class of compounds known to promote both intrinsic activation of apoptosis and radiosensitization are phospholipid analogues, such as the membrane-targeted alkylphosphocholines miltefosine and perifosine (Hilgard et al. 1997; Unger et al. 1989). The radiosensitizing capacity of this kind of drugs has already been proven in multiple tumor entities (Gao et al. 2011; Henke et al. 2012; Vink et al. 2006, 2007; Berkovic et al. 1997; Ruiter et al. 1999; Rubel et al. 2006).

3.3.4. Combination of RTX with Agents Targeting Cell Division

The cell cycle phase in which cell division takes place (M-phase) is considered to be the most vulnerable state in terms of radiotherapeutic intervention as it is well acknowledged that the sensitivity of cells to ionizing radiation peaks at this cell cycle stage (Sinclair and Morton 1966; Terasima and Tolmach 1963). Therefore and because of the fact that tumor cells, in contrast to most other non- transformed cell types, divide extensively, ancient approaches already aimed at arresting tumor cells within M-phase in order to achieve a maximum in radiosensitivity. For this purpose, drugs mainly derived from natural origin, such as taxol/paclitaxel, colchicine, and colcemid, were initially used. These compounds interfere with microtubule dynamics, thereby preventing accurate execution of cell division which results in a permanent arrest of the cells within M-phase. As to be expected, several of these drugs exhibited synergistic effects when being combined with exposure to ionizing radiation (Griem and Malkinson 1966; Brues et al. 1940; Tishler et al. 1992; Milas et al. 1994, 1996; Milross et al. 1997). This is why some of them (e.g., taxol) not only are adopted in radiochemotherapy but even still are in the focus of current clinical research (Pergolizzi et al. 2011; Combs et al. 2012). However, these drugs not only lack the level of specificity current therapies demand for, but they also exhibit side effects, which, in worst case, even limit the therapeutic effort. Progression through M-phase and the process of cell division itself both depend on the function of a multitude of cellular proteins including many protein kinases, which offers great opportunities for pharmaceutical intervention. In recent years, small-molecule inhibitors targeting protein kinases, which function more or less exclusively during cell division (e.g., Aurora kinases and Polo-like kinases), were designed and tested for their utility in combinatorial approaches. In these studies, several compounds, e.g., the Aurora kinase inhibitors AZD1152 (Barasertib), VX-680 (Tozasertib), and MLN8054, as well as the Polo-like kinase-1 inhibitor BI2536, have proven radiosensitizing potential (Moretti et al. 2011; Tao et al. 2008, 2009; Guan et al. 2007; Harris et al. 2012), nourishing the hope for their future implementation in the clinic.

3.3.5. Combination of RTX with Agents Targeting the Heat Shock Response

Heat shock proteins (HSPs) are molecular chaperones that catalyze the proper folding of other proteins and thereby avoid protein aggregations within cells. HSPs are often overexpressed in tumor cells as these cells are characterized by an overall increased level of protein synthesis, thus necessitating effective chaperone function in order to prevent misfolding and/or aggregation of proteins in these cells. In addition, HSP expression can be induced in response to multiple physiological or environmental insults, including irradiation, hypoxia, and/or chemical stress (Young et al. 2004). In this context, HSPs frequently function in an antiapoptotic fashion by associating with key components of the apoptotic machinery, thereby interfering with efficient apoptosis induction. For example, HSP70 and HSP90 can interfere with caspase-dependent and caspase- independent apoptosis induction as well as by binding to the pro-apoptotic proteins Apaf-1 and apoptosis-inducing factor (AIF) (Garrido et al. 2006).

These findings explain why compounds that obstruct HSP function came into the focus of clinical research in recent years. Initially, naturally derived inhibitors targeting HSPs, such as geldanamycin and radicicol, were tested for clinical purposes but turned out to exhibit fatal side effects such as liver toxicity, thus precluding their implementation in the clinic. Therefore, novel compounds have been designed molecularly in order to minimize these kinds of side effects concomitant with a maximum in HSP-inhibiting capacity (Chiosis et al. 2006). Among those, inhibitors of HSP90 such as 17-N-allylamino-17-demethox- ygeldanamycin (17-AAG), 17-dimethylaminoethylamino-17-demethoxygeldanamycin (17-DMAG), or NVP-AUY922, in particular, exhibited convincing potential in promoting tumor cell death as well as in sensitizing tumor cells to ionizing radiation (Bisht et al. 2003; Bull et al. 2004; Russell et al. 2003; Machida et al. 2005; Matsumoto et al. 2005; Kabakov et al. 2008; Stingl et al. 2010; Mil- anovi et al. 2013).

3.3.6. Combination of RTX with Agents Targeting the EGFR Pathway

Another promising target for combined modality approaches is the EGFR, one member of the epithelial tyrosine kinase-associated membrane receptor family, and its downstream signaling pathways (Davies et al. 1980). Activation of EGFR leads to cell proliferation, inhibition of apoptosis, and angiogenesis. EGFR expression is commonly increased in human cancers (Wernicke et al. 2010), and preclinical evidence suggests a direct impact of EGFR on the sensitivity of tumor cells toward ionizing radiation (Milas et al. 2000; Akimoto et al. 1999). In accordance, the expression of EGFR was reported to be up-regulated in response to irradiation, which might attenuate the effectiveness of fractionated radiotherapy (Fedrigo et al. 2011). Indeed, overexpression as well as mutations in the EGFR gene was shown to directly correlate with tumor radioresistance and poor clinical prognosis (Lammering et al. 2004; Giralt et al. 2005). Therefore, the EGFR pathway exhibits great influence on the overall effect that can be achieved by clinical irradiation, which in turn offers great opportunities for pharmaceutical intervention. Various kinds of EGFR-inhibiting molecules, such as the mono- clonal antibodies cetuximab and panitumumab as well as the tyrosine kinase inhibitors erlotinib and gefitinib, have been developed and demonstrated great therapeutic benefit both in preclinical reports and in randomized clinical trials when combined with ionizing radiation. Therefore, EGFR inhibition meanwhile has become an established part of the clinical routine in radiation oncology (Nieder et al. 2012).

3.3.7. Combination of RTX with Agents Targeting the Tumor Micromilieu

Solid tumors are usually composed of tumor cells and several other cell types that form the tumor micromilieu. Both the formation and the progression of a solid tumor depend on the tight interaction between transformed tumor cells and the cells in the tumor microenvironment. By secreting growth factors and cytokines that target endothelial cells, fibroblasts, and other cell types within the microenvironment, tumor cells actively shape their surrounding milieu, for instance by inducing de novo formation of blood vessels and extracellular matrices (Carmeliet and Jain 2011). Moreover, tumor cells can also acquire the capacity to skew or evade antitumor immune responses and even to induce a milieu of immune tolerance (Dunn et al. 2004).

The complex interplay between tumor cells and the tumor stroma has strong impact on the tumor's sensitivity to exposure to ionizing radiation and, therefore, on longterm tumor control following radiotherapeutic attendance. In this respect, understanding the effects of ionizing radiation on the tumor microenvironment rather than on isolated tumor cells is one of the greatest interests in current radiobiological science. One promising candidate for radiotherapeutic approaches is the tumor microvasculature (Garcia-Barros et al. 2003). Recent reports suggest that directly targeting angiogenesis might increase the therapeutic ratio when being combined with irradiation (Beal et al. 2011). In accordance, the monoclonal antibody bevacizumab, which blocks angiogenesis by preventing the binding of VEGF to its respective receptor (Willett et al. 2004), significantly improves clinical outcome when combined with radiotherapy (Velenik et al. 2011; Shin et al. 2011; Niyazi et al. 2012a), and similar results were obtained for the VEGF-R inhibitor vandetanib and, primarily, for the antiangiogenetic peptide cilengitide (Albert et al. 2006; Williams et al. 2004; Brazelle et al. 2006; Drappatz et al. 2010; Yang et al. 2010). However, a recent phase III trial on cilengitide in combination with radiochemotherapy failed to show a significant increase in overall survival in glioblastoma patients.

Another mediator of the microenvironment's response to irradiation is transforming growth factor-b (TGF-β), which is activated in response to ROS (Barcellos-Hoff and Dix 1996). TGF-β regulates the proliferation, the differentiation, and the migration of cells (Massague' et al. 2000) and also contributes to metastasis and cell invasion (Heldin et al. 2009; Pardali and Moustakas 2007). This explains why interfering with TGF-β signaling may decrease tumor cell growth, as well as their motility and their metastasizing capacity (Ikushima and Miyazono 2010). Thus, inhibition of TGF-β can actively modulate the tumors' response to ionizing radiation, thereby providing an interesting tool for combinatorial approaches (Flanders and Burmester 2003; Rabbani et al. 2003; Xavier et al. 2004).

4. Side Effects

As exposure to ionizing radiation induces cell death, radiotherapy inevitably coincides with side effects, including degeneration of normal tissues, acute inflammation, and even fibrotic tissue remodeling. The implementation of modern techniques such as IMRT has greatly facilitated the reduction in these classical kinds of side effects. On the other hand, novel, combined modality approaches that employ novel, molecularly designed compounds have led to rise of new, so far unknown side effects.

4.1. Classical Side Effects

Both acute inflammation and chronic fibrosis are classical side effects that coincide with the radiotherapeutic treatment of neoplasms and may limit radiation doses and thus the efficacy of the treatment (Abratt et al. 2004; Plathow et al. 2004; Abdollahi et al. 2005). In some cases, e.g., lung cancer, dose limitations due to the restricted tolerance of normal tissues even preclude successful radiotherapy in many patients with advanced disease progression (McDonald et al. 1995; Rosenzweig et al. 2000). In general, the severity of irradiation-induced pneumonitis depends on treatment factors, such as totality of the dose, the volume of irradiated lung, the schedule of fractionation, and the chemotherapy administered (Taghian et al. 2001; Rosen et al. 2001; Shi et al. 2010; Blom Goldman et al. 2010), but also on patient- and/or disease-related factors, such as preexisting lung diseases, poor pulmonary function, or genetic predispositions (Movsas et al. 1997; Mertens et al. 2002; Abratt et al. 2004). However, the mechanisms underlying these side effects are still poorly understood.

Although irradiation-induced primary damages in target cells such as apoptosis and necrosis have been sufficiently documented (Eriksson and Stigbrand 2010; McBride 1995), subsequent biological reactions in irradiated organs are quite sophisticated and not well defined (Lindroos et al. 1995; Zhang and Phan 1996). Recent studies suggest that cytokine cascades that govern the signaling pathways involved in irradiation response may play a pivotal role within these processes (Pohlers et al. 2009; Li et al. 2007; Lee et al. 2010), and a growing body of evidence demonstrates an increased expression of cytokines in radiation- induced pulmonary lesions (Johnston et al. 1996; Abdollahi et al. 2005). Among these, some pro-inflammatory cytokines such as the TNF- and the CD95 ligands are of importance for acute inflammation (Johnston et al. 1996; Heinzelmann et al. 2006), while others, such as TGF-β and PDGF, are more involved in the regulation of chronic fibrotic response (Abdollahi et al. 2005; Dancea et al. 2009).

Recently described strategies that directly interfere with intracellular signaling pathways have revealed encouraging results in terms of attenuating radiation-caused side effects (Abdollahi et al. 2005; Anscher et al. 2008; Puthawala et al. 2008). However, as the cytokine signaling pathways that are activated in response to irradiation are broadly overlapping, rather than being independent of each other, it is unlikely that a complete blockage of these reactions can be achieved by blocking only one of them (Li et al. 2009; Wynn 2008). Thus, multi-targeted agents should exhibit higher effectiveness in attenuation of radiation-induced inflammation and fibrogenesis.

4.2. Novel Side Effects Due to Employment of Targeted Agents

With the increase in clinical relevance of novel, molecularly targeted agents, novel kinds of side effects are emerging (Niyazi et al. 2011b). Unfortunately, clinical data that would allow the assessment of these side effects are scarce. Additionally, the heterogeneity of both targeted agents and study designs does not allow abstraction these side effects. The examples presented here are meant to give an insight into the wide variety of side effects that may arise due to employment of targeted agents.

On the one hand, huge clinical trials exist for targeted agents such as trastuzumab, a humanized monoclonal antiher-2/neu antibody approved for the treatment of her-2/neu-positive breast cancers, showing no significant additional effects if being combined with radiation in a shorttime follow-up (Halyard et al. 2009). On the other hand, there are agents such as sorafenib or erlotinib belonging to the group of kinase inhibitors for which toxicity data upon combined usage are extremely rare. However, case reports exist, in which combinational or sequential application of radiotherapy and kinase inhibitors were shown to lead to severe or even fatal toxicities such as diarrhea (Silvano et al. 2008), bowel perforation (Peters et al. 2008), and bronchial fistula (Basille et al. 2010).

The most prominent and rather well-documented example of a non-classical side effect can be observed for the EGFR-antagonizing antibody cetuximab which, for example, has been successfully used in combination with radio- therapy for the treatment of head and neck cancers (Bonner et al. 2006). In the trial conducted by Bonner and colleagues, a significant improvement in overall survival of patients that were treated with radioimmunotherapy was observed when compared to patients treated with radiotherapy alone. During this trial, the combinational treatment was reported to be rather well tolerated; however, during the years of clinical use, multiple reports pointing out an increase in skin toxicity and cases of even severe skin toxicity have been published (Walsh et al. 2011; Koutcher et al. 2009; Giro et al. 2009; Berger and Belka 2008).

Another targeted agent that exemplifies the heterogeneity of putative toxicities is the VEGF-antagonizing antibody bevacizumab that is used in combination with radiotherapy in different anatomical regions. Promising attempts were made in the combination of radiotherapy with bevacizumab for the treatment of (recurrent) glioblastomas (Beal et al. 2011; Vredenburgh et al. 2012). While no increased infield bleeding was reported for the application of ionizing radiation to the CNS, some cases of wound dehiscence of the previously operated site as well as increased levels of toxicity at late stages with some cases of optic neuropathy and one single case of Brown-Se'quard syndrome have been documented (Gutin et al. 2009; Niyazi et al. 2012a; Lai et al. 2008; Kelly et al. 2011). Concerning the combination of bevacizumab and radiotherapy in case of the gastrointestinal tract, some studies pointed out an increased toxicity level, such as ischemic bowel complications (Lordick et al. 2006), mucosal tumor-associated bleeding (Crane et al. 2010), GI-bleeding, ulceration (Crane et al. 2010), and wound complications (Dipetrillo et al. 2012). Finally, in case of the mediastinal region, an increased rate of tracheoesophageal fistula has been reported (Spigel et al. 2010).

5. Prognosis and Prediction

To date, therapeutic decisions are taken on increasing individualized and personalized bases. Important criteria in this regard are markers that help to predict the overall prognosis of the patient, the potential success of a particular kind of therapy, and the occurrence of unwanted side effects. In particular, the combination of ionizing radiation with molecularly targeted agents requires an a priori identification of patients that will benefit most (or at all) from a respective therapy. Here, classical parameters such as age, tumor node metastasis (TNM) stage, and histology of the tumor might not be sufficient, and additional information concerning the molecular tumor characteristics is needed in order to find the best therapeutic approach for the individual patient. "Prognostic" markers, in general, provide information concerning the natural course of the respective disease independently of the treatment applied. In contrast, the term "predictive" refers to markers for which it is likely that a specific subgroup among the patient collective will benefit from a certain intervention. For example, the EGFR1 mutation has a predictive value in adeno-NSCLC patients, but not a prognostic one (Oldenhuis et al. 2008).

5.1. Biomarkers for Tumors

In patients with malignant gliomas, it should be of standard to test for the mutational status of the genes encoding for isocitrate dehydrogenases 1 and 2 (IDH-1/-2) as well as for codeletion of the 1p/19q loci. While mutations within the IDH-1/-2 genes can be found in more than 70% of all primary astrocytomas (WHO grades II/III), oligodendrogliomas, and secondary glioblastomas, the respective mutation rate is only about 5% in primary glioblastomas and mutations within IDH-1/-2 are associated with positive clinical prognosis in astrocytoma and glioblastoma (Yan et al. 2009; Combs et al. 2011). In parallel, the codeletion of 1p/19q was shown to correlate with reduced tumor aggressiveness and better response in anaplastic oligodendroglioma (Cairncross et al. 2006; Quon and Abdul-karim 2008; van den Bent et al. 2006). In addition, also the methylation status of the O-(6)-methylguanine-DNA methyltransferase (MGMT) gene promoter should be investigated. MGMT is a DNA-repairing enzyme that decreases the effects achievable by alkylating agent (e.g., temozolomide)-based chemotherapy (Esteller et al. 2000). Temozolomide is routinely used for concomitant radio- chemotherapy in malignant gliomas as it was shown that combining temozolomide with radio-therapy results in significant prolongation of patient survival (Hegi et al. 2005; Stupp et al. 2009). As methylation of the MGMT promoter represses the expression of MGMT, this leads to a better response and thus, the methylation status of the MGMT promoter should be tested in routine before starting a temozolomide-based therapy.

Carcinogenesis in squamous cell carcinomas of the head and neck (HNSCC) can be linked either to the frequent use of tobacco and alcohol or to human papillomavirus (HPV) infection. In HPV-positive tumors, p53 and pRB tumor- suppressor function is blocked by viral proteins called E6 and E7, respectively, culminating in high levels of genome instability and increased expression of the se-nescence- associated Cdk1-inhibitor p16[Ink4a]. Detection of the HPV status can be accomplished by real-time PCR, and p16[Ink4a] can be detected by immunohistoche-mistry (Snow and Laudadio 2010). Approximately one-quarter of all HNSCC patients are positive for HPV (Deacon et al. 1984), and in oropharyngeal carcinomas, the prevalence of a positive HPV status is even around 40%. Moreover, HPV- positive tumors not only genetically differ from negative ones (Martinez et al. 2007), but they also differ in terms of capacity to cope with DNA damage which is reduced in the HPV-positive tumors (Rieckmann et al. 2013). This can also explain, at least in part, why the HPV status is such an important prognostic factor in HNSCC patients, as it is often associated with superior outcome in case of patients treated with surgery followed by adjuvant radiotherapy or definitive radiochemotherapy (Ihloff et al. 2010; Fischer et al. 2010; Prestwich et al. 2010).

5.2. Biomarkers for Side Effects

One limitation in the radiotherapeutic treatment for malignant tumors is given by the need to minimize toxic effects that may harm normal tissues. In this context, late complications are of special importance because of frequently showing progression and thus association with long-life risk (Jung et al. 2001). Meanwhile, the extent of tissue toxicity introduced by irradiation greatly varies among different patients. Even though inherited hyper-sensitivity syndromes such as ataxia telangiectasia and the Nijmegen breakage syndrome that are characterized by severe side effects are rare, a wide range of reactions within normal tissues can be detected among the standard population. It was suggested that such individual variations in radiosensitivity are caused by genetic differences, such as single nucleotide polymorphisms (SNPs) (Turesson et al. 1996; Safwat et al. 2002). As these may serve as markers that would allow for estimating the individual risk of radiation-induced toxicity to non-transformed tissues, extensive efforts were made to identify such markers. Indeed, several SNPs could be identified that show tight relation with the degree of radiotoxicity as exemplified by SNPs that reside in the IL12RB2 and the ABCA1 genes (Isomura et al. 2008) as well as within the ATM gene (Edvardsen et al. 2007; Xiong et al. 2012). However, the studies performed so far often give rise to heterogeneous and/or even conflicting results. This can be seen for instance by the C-509 T polymorphism, an extensively studied SNP of the TGFβ1-encoding gene, for which conflicting results have been reported regarding its role in promoting inflammatory and fibrotic effects (Quarmby et al. 2003; Andreassen et al. 2005; De Ruyck et al. 2006; Barnett et al. 2010; Martin et al. 2010). Moreover, it was shown that significant coincidence of SNP occurrence and tissue toxicity is only found when several SNPs and/or other risk alleles are combined (Alsner et al. 2008; Andreassen et al. 2006; Zschenker et al. 2010). However, these data also have been contradicted by other studies (Raabe et al. 2012; Barnett et al. 2012). Therefore, analyzing the presence of SNPs as biomarkers that allow for individual prediction of side effects is still far from routine.

5.3. Personalized Medicine: Imaging for Prognosis and Prediction

[^{18}F]FDG-PET imaging has become the standard in oncologic treatment over the recent years especially for staging purposes due to its higher sensitivity and specificity if being compared to conventional imaging modalities such as CT and MRI. PET tracers may serve as prognostic and predictive markers for estimating responsiveness to radio-therapy or combined radiochemotherapy (Bussink et al. 2011). The outcome of head and neck cancer patients has been related to standardized uptake value (SUV) changes in PET imaging (Allal et al. 2004). Several tumor entities have been described in which PET gives early information as a marker for pathological response, especially in the cases of rectal cancer (de Geus-Oei et al. 2009), NSCLC (Pottgen et al. 2006), and esophageal cancer (Song et al. 2005). PET-CT was even described to be complimentary to conventional CT scan and able to predict early recurrences in breast cancer (Evangelista et al. 2011). Ongoing Hodgkin trials are in part based on PET imaging, and the stratification in these trials is done according to PET positivity after several chemotherapy cycles; however, this has still to be regarded as an experimental concept. Involved- node radiotherapy has been proposed as a means to further improve the therapeutic ratio by reduction of radiation-induced toxicity (Kobe et al. 2010) substantially based on proper PET/CT staging. Altogether, PET seems to be a substantial part of personalized medicine providing prognostic information and enabling the clinician to base treatment strategies on this information.

Meanwhile, PET-CT has gained an important place in radiotherapy planning (Yaromina and Zips 2010) as it provides detailed information about the tumor microenvironment in addition to anatomical imaging. In first instance, PET imaging data can be used for better delineation of the target volume. A second strategy, dose painting by contours (DPBC), consists in the creation of an additional PET-based target volume that is then treated with higher dose levels. In contrast, dose painting by numbers (DPBN) aims for a local variation in dose prescription according to the variation in the PET signal (Thorwarth et al. 2010). For instance, in case of lung cancer, several approaches already are available that directly depend on PET imaging (De Ruysscher et al. 2012). Currently, ^{11}C-choline and occasionally ^{18}F- or ^{11}C- acetate are used as tracers for prostate cancer, reflecting the phospholipid metabolism (Pinkawa et al. 2011). ^{11}C-choline-PET/CT might be considered as the imaging modality in radiation oncology to select and to delineate target volumes extending the prostate gland or fossa. In conjunction with IMRT and IGRT, it therefore might offer the opportunity for a dose escalation to selected sites while avoiding the irradiation of healthy tissues (Wurschmidt et al. 2011), and although the underlying assumption that PET correlates positively with more resistant subvolumes is still not proven for the broad variety of cancer types, data are coming forward that this is the case, e.g., in lung cancer. One open question is whether selective boosting with limited sensitivity of choline-PET indeed leads to higher tumor control rates (Niyazi et al. 2010).

Several trials are on their way to test PET imaging prospectively, e.g., in lung cancer [PET-PLAN trial (Fleckenstein et al. 2011)]. For malignant gliomas, FET-PET has been shown to significantly alter the target volumes (Niyazi et al. 2011a; Walter et al. 2012) and amino acid-PET in general, including 11C-methionine (MET)-PET, which was shown to be effective in target volume delineation (Grosu et al. 2005). The observation that meningioma cells overexpress the somatostatin receptor 2 (SSTR2) was the rationale to retrospectively analyze how far DOTATOC-PET/CT is helpful to improve target volume delineation for IMRT (Gehler et al. 2009). Many other tumor types are currently under investigation as PET provides additional information on tumor extent, involvement of lymph nodes, and putative distant metastases. Nevertheless, several problems have to be solved in the future, such as the inclusion of dynamic analyses and the correct procedures for thresholds.

6. Conclusions

Radiotherapy represents a crucial treatment option in the treatment for malignant diseases. In the recent years, the efficacy of radiotherapy has been improved by new techniques, among which IMRT and IGRT may constitute the most important ones. In parallel, novel approaches that combine radiotherapy with molecularly designed agents specifically targeting the hallmarks of cancer have been deployed and revealed promising results both in preclinical models and in clinical trials. However, employment of such targeted agents often coincides with new kinds of side effects demanding for biomarkers, which allow for detailed patient stratification. As the current availability of such markers is far from satisfying, efforts to identify novel candidates must be increased. In parallel, research focusing on multimodality approaches must be intensified as conventional radiochemo-therapy has reached its limits.

Source: Orth M, Lauber K, Niyazi M, et al. Current concepts in clinical radiation oncology [J]. Radiation & Environmental Biophysics, 2014, 53(1):1–29.

References

[1] Abdollahi A, Li M, Ping G, Plathow C, Domhan S, Kiessling F, Lee LB, McMahon G, Grone HJ, Lipson KE, Huber PE (2005) Inhibition of platelet-derived growth factor signaling attenuates pulmonary fibrosis. J Exp Med 201(6):925–935.

[2] Abratt RP, Morgan GW, Silvestri G, Willcox P (2004) Pulmonary complications of radiation therapy. Clin Chest Med 25(1):167–177. doi:10.1016/S0272-5231(03)00126-6.

[3] Afshar G, Jelluma N, Yang X, Basila D, Arvold ND, Karlsson A, Yount GL, Dansen TB, Koller E, Haas-Kogan DA (2006) Radiation-induced caspase-8 mediates p53-independent apoptosis in glioma cells. Cancer Res 66(8):4223–4232. doi:10.1158/ 0008-5472-05-1283.

[4] Akimoto T, Hunter NR, Buchmiller L, Mason K, Ang KK, Milas L (1999) Inverse relationship between epidermal growth factor receptor expression and radiocurability of murine carcinomas. Clin Cancer Res 5(10):2884–2890.

[5] Albain KS, Swann RS, Rusch VW, Turrisi AT 3rd, Shepherd FA, Smith C, Chen Y, Livingston RB, Feins RH, Gandara DR, Fry WA, Darling G, Johnson DH, Green MR, Miller RC, Ley J, Sause WT, Cox JD (2009) Radiotherapy plus chemotherapy with or without surgical resection for stage III non-small-cell lung cancer: a phase III randomised controlled trial. Lancet 374(9687):379–386. doi:10.1016/S0140-6736(09)60737-6.

[6] Albert JM, Cao C, Geng L, Leavitt L, Hallahan DE, Lu B (2006) Integrin avb3 antagonist Cilengitide enhances efficacy of radiotherapy in endothelial cell and non-small-cell lung cancer models. Int J Radiat Oncol Biol Phys 65(5):1536-1543. doi:10.1016/j.ijrobp. 2006.04.036.

[7] Allal AS, Slosman DO, Kebdani T, Allaoua M, Lehmann W, Dulguerov P (2004) Prediction of outcome in head-and-neck cancer patients using the standardized uptake value of 2-[18F]fluoro-2-deoxy-D-glucose. Int J Radiat Oncol Biol Phys 59(5): 1295–1300. doi:10.1016/j.ijrobp.2003.12.039.

[8] Al-Sarraf M, LeBlanc M, Giri PG, Fu KK, Cooper J, Vuong T, Forastiere AA, Adams G, Sakr WA, Schuller DE, Ensley JF (1998) Chemoradiotherapy versus radiotherapy in patients with advanced nasopharyngeal cancer: phase III randomized Intergroup study 0099. J Clin Oncol 16(4):1310–1317.

[9] Alsner J, Andreassen CN, Overgaard J (2008) Genetic markers for prediction of normal tissue toxicity after radiotherapy. Semin Radiat Oncol 18(2):126–135. doi:S1053-4296 (07)00095-1.

[10] Amichetti M, Amelio D, Minniti G (2012) Radiosurgery with photons or protons for benign and malignant tumours of the skull base: a review. Radiat Oncol 7(1):210. doi:10.1186/1748-717X-7-210.

[11] Andreassen CN, Alsner J, Overgaard J, Herskind C, Haviland J, Owen R, Homewood J, Bliss J, Yarnold J (2005) TGFB1 polymor- phisms are associated with risk of late normal tissue complications in the breast after radiotherapy for early breast cancer. Radiother Oncol 75(1):18–21.

[12] Andreassen CN, Alsner J, Overgaard M, Sorensen FB, Overgaard J (2006) Risk of radiation-induced subcutaneous fibrosis in relation to single nucleotide polymorphisms in TGFB1, SOD2, XRCC1, XRCC3, APEX and ATM-a study based on DNA from formalin fixed paraffin embedded tissue samples. Int J Radiat Biol 82(8): 577–586.

[13] Anscher MS, Thrasher B, Zgonjanin L, Rabbani ZN, Corbley MJ, Fu K, Sun L, Lee WC, Ling LE, Vujaskovic Z (2008) Small molecular inhibitor of transforming growth factor-beta protects against development of radiation-induced lung injury. Int J Radiat Oncol Biol Phys 71(3):829–837.

[14] Apel A, Herr I, Schwarz H, Rodemann HP, Mayer A (2008) Blocked autophagy sensitizes resistant carcinoma cells to radiation therapy. Cancer Res 68(5):1485–1494. doi:10.1158 /0008-5472. CAN-07-0562.

[15] Apel A, Zentgraf H, Buchler MW, Herr I (2009) Autophagy-A double-edged sword in oncology. Int J Cancer 125(5):991–995. doi:10.1002/ijc.24500.

[16] Apetoh L, Ghiringhelli F, Tesniere A, Criollo A, Ortiz C, Lidereau R, Mariette C, Chaput N, Mira JP, Delaloge S, Andre F, Tursz T, Kroemer G, Zitvogel L (2007) The interaction between HMGB1 and TLR4 dictates the outcome of anticancer chemotherapy and radiotherapy. Immunol Rev 220:47–59.

[17] Audeh MW, Carmichael J, Penson RT, Friedlander M, Powell B, Bell-McGuinn KM, Scott C, Weitzel JN, Oaknin A, Loman N, Lu K, Schmutzler RK, Matulonis U, Wickens M, Tutt A (2010) Oral poly(ADP-ribose) polymerase inhibitor olaparib in patients with BRCA1 or BRCA2 mutations and recurrent ovarian cancer: a proof-of-concept trial. Lancet 376(9737): 245–251. doi:10. 1016/S0140-6736(10)60893-8.

[18] Auer S, Hable V, Greubel C, Drexler GA, Schmid TE, Belka C, Dollinger G, Friedl AA (2011) Survival of tumor cells after proton irradiation with ultra-high dose rates. Radiat Oncol 6:139. doi:10.1186/1748-717X-6-139.

[19] Auperin A, Le Pechoux C, Rolland E, Curran WJ, Furuse K, Fournel P, Belderbos J, Clamon G, Ulutin HC, Paulus R, Yamanaka T, Bozonnat MC, Uitterhoeve A, Wang X, Stewart L, Arriagada R, Burdett S, Pignon JP (2010) Meta-analysis of concomitant versus sequential radiochemotherapy in locally advanced non-small-cell lung

cancer. J Clin Oncol 28(13):2181–2190. doi:10.1200/JCO. 2009.26.2543.

[20] Bao S, Wu Q, McLendon RE, Hao Y, Shi Q, Hjelmeland AB, Dewhirst MW, Bigner DD, Rich JN (2006) Glioma stem cells promote radioresistance by preferential activation of the DNA damage response. Nature 444(7120):756–760.

[21] Barazzuol L, Jena R, Burnet NG, Meira LB, Jeynes JC, Kirkby KJ, Kirkby NF (2013) Evaluation of poly (ADP-ribose) polymerase inhibitor ABT-888 combined with radiotherapy and temozolomide in glioblastoma. Radiat Oncol 8(1):65. doi:10.116/1748-717X-8-65.

[22] Barcellos-Hoff MH, Dix TA (1996) Redox-mediated activation of latent transforming growth factor-beta 1. Mol Endocrinol 10(9):1077–1083. doi:10.1210/me.10.9.1077.

[23] Barnett GC, Coles CE, Burnet NG, Pharoah PD, Wilkinson J, West CM, Elliott RM, Baynes C, Dunning AM (2010) No association between SNPs regulating TGF-beta1 secretion and late radiotherapy toxicity to the breast: results from the RAPPER study. Radiother Oncol 97(1):9–14. doi:S0167- 8140(09)00664-1.

[24] Barnett GC, Coles CE, Elliott RM, Baynes C, Luccarini C, Conroy D, Wilkinson JS, Tyrer J, Misra V, Platte R, Gulliford SL, Sydes MR, Hall E, Bentzen SM, Dearnaley DP, Burnet NG, Pharoah PD, Dunning AM, West CM (2012) Independent validation of genes and polymorphisms reported to be associated with radiation toxicity: a prospective analysis study. Lancet Oncol 13(1):65–77. doi:S1470-2045(11)70302-3.

[25] Basille D, Andrejak M, Bentayeb H, Kanaan M, Fournier C, Lecuyer E, Boutemy M, Garidi R, Douadi Y, Dayen C (2010) Bronchial fistula associated with sunitinib in a patient previously treated with radiation therapy. Ann Pharmacother 44(2):383–386. doi:10.1345/aph.1M469.

[26] Basu B, Yap TA, Molife LR, de Bono JS (2012) Targeting the DNA damage response in oncology: past, present and future perspectives. Curr Opin Oncol 24(3):316–324. doi:10.1097/CCO. 0b013e32835280c6.

[27] Baudino TA, McKay C, Pendeville-Samain H, Nilsson JA, Maclean KH, White EL, Davis AC, Ihle JN, Cleveland JL (2002) c-Myc is essential for vasculogenesis and angiogenesis during development and tumor progression. Genes Dev 16(19):2530–2543. doi:10. 1101/gad.1024602.

[28] Beal K, Abrey L, Gutin P (2011) Antiangiogenic agents in the treatment of recurrent or newly diagnosed glioblastoma: analysis of single-agent and combined modality approaches. Radiat Oncol 6(1):2.

[29] Begg AC, Stewart FA, Vens C (2011) Strategies to improve radiotherapy with targeted drugs. Nat Rev Cancer 11(4):239-253 Belka C, Marini P, Budach W, Schulze-Osthoff K, Lang F, Gulbins E, Bamberg M (1998) Radiation-induced apoptosis in human lymphocytes and lymphoma cells critically relies on the upregulation of CD95/Fas/APO-1 ligand. Radiat Res 149(6): 588–595.

[30] Belka C, Schmid B, Marini P, Durand E, Rudner J, Faltin H, Bamberg M, Schulze-Osthoff K, Budach W (2001) Sensitization of resistant lymphoma cells to irradiation-induced apoptosis by the death ligand TRAIL. Oncogene 20(17):

2190–2196. doi:10. 1038/sj.onc.1204318.

[31] Berger B, Belka C (2008) Severe skin reaction secondary to concomitant radiotherapy plus cetuximab. Radiat Oncol 3:5. doi:10.1186/1748-717X-3-5.

[32] Bergers G, Benjamin LE (2003) Tumorigenesis and the angiogenic switch. Nat Rev Cancer 3(6):401-410. doi:10.1038/nrc1093 Berkovic D, Grundel O, Berkovic K, Wildfang I, Hess CF, Schmoll HJ (1997) Synergistic cytotoxic effects of ether phospholipid analogues and ionizing radiation in human carcinoma cells. Radiother Oncol 43(3):293–301.

[33] Bernier J, Domenge C, Ozsahin M, Matuszewska K, Lefebvre JL, Greiner RH, Giralt J, Maingon P, Rolland F, Bolla M, Cognetti F, Bourhis J, Kirkpatrick A, van Glabbeke M (2004) Postoperative irradiation with or without concomitant chemotherapy for locally advanced head and neck cancer. N Engl J Med 350(19): 1945–1952. doi:10.1056/N EJMoa032641.

[34] Bin J, Allinger K, Assmann W, Dollinger G, Drexler GA, Friedl AA, Habs D, Hilz P, Hoerlein R, Humble N, Karsch S, Khrennikov K, Kiefer D, Krausz F, Ma W, Michalski D, Molls M, Raith S, Reinhardt S, Roper B, Schmid TE, Tajima T, Wenz J, Zlobinskaya O, Schreiber J, Wilkens JJ (2012) A laser-driven nanosecond proton source for radiobiological studies. Appl Phys Lett 101(24):243701–243704.

[35] Bisht KS, Bradbury CM, Mattson D, Kaushal A, Sowers A, Markovina S, Ortiz KL, Sieck LK, Isaacs JS, Brechbiel MW, Mitchell JB, Neckers LM, Gius D (2003) Geldanamycin and 17-allylamino-17-demethoxy geldanamycin potentiate the in vitro and in vivo radiation response of cervical tumor cells via the heat shock protein 90-mediated intracellular signaling and cytotoxicity. Cancer Res 63(24):8984–8995.

[36] Blasco MA (2005) Telomeres and human disease: ageing, cancer and beyond. Nat Rev Genet 6(8):611–622. doi:10.1038/nrg1656.

[37] Blom Goldman U, Wennberg B, Svane G, Bylund H, Lind P (2010) Reduction of radiation pneumonitis by V20-constraints in breast cancer. Radiat Oncol 5:99. doi:10.1186/ 1748- 717X-5-99.

[38] Bolla M, Collette L, Blank L, Warde P, Dubois JB, Mirimanoff RO, Storme G, Bernier J, Kuten A, Sternberg C, Mattelaer J, Lopez Torecilla J, Pfeffer JR, Lino Cutajar C, Zurlo A, Pierart M (2002) Long-term results with immediate androgen suppression and external irradiation in patients with locally advanced prostate cancer (an EORTC study): a phase III randomised trial. Lancet 360(9327):103–106.

[39] Bonner JA, Harari PM, Giralt J, Azarnia N, Shin DM, Cohen RB, Jones CU, Sur R, Raben D, Jassem J, Ove R, Kies MS, Baselga J, Youssoufian H, Amellal N, Rowinsky EK, Ang KK (2006) Radiotherapy plus cetuximab for squamous-cell carcinoma of the head and neck. N Engl J Med 354(6):567–578.

[40] Bortfeld T (1999) Optimized planning using physical objectives and constraints. Semin Radiat Oncol 9(1):20–34.

[41] Bouyon-Monteau A, Habrand JL, Datchary J, Alapetite C, Bolle S, Dendale R, Feuvret L, Helfre S, Calugaru V, Cosset JM, Bey P (2010) Is proton beam therapy

the future of radiotherapy? Part I: clinical aspects. Cancer Radiother 14(8):727–738.

[42] Brada M, Pijls-Johannesma M, De Ruysscher D (2009) Current clinical evidence for proton therapy. Cancer J 15(4):319–324. doi:10.1097/PPO.0b013e3181b6127c.

[43] Brazelle WD, Shi W, Siemann DW (2006) VEGF-associated tyrosine kinase inhibition increases the tumor response to single and fractionated dose radiotherapy. Int J Radiat Oncol Biol Phys 65(3):836–841.

[44] Brues AM, Marble BB, Jackson EB (1940) Effects of colchicine and radiation on growth of normal tissues and tumors. Am J Cancer 38(2):159–168. doi:10.1158/ajc.1940.159.

[45] Bucci MK, Bevan A, Roach M 3rd (2005) Advances in radiation therapy: conventional to 3D, to IMRT, to 4D, and beyond. CA Cancer J Clin 55(2):117–134.

[46] Budach W, Hehr T, Budach V, Belka C, Dietz K (2006) A meta- analysis of hyperfractionated and accelerated radiotherapy and combined chemotherapy and radiotherapy regimens in unresected locally advanced squamous cell carcinoma of the head and neck. BMC Cancer 6:28.

[47] Bull EE, Dote H, Brady KJ, Burgan WE, Carter DJ, Cerra MA, Oswald KA, Hollingshead MG, Camphausen K, Tofilon PJ (2004) Enhanced tumor cell radiosensitivity and abrogation of G2 and S phase arrest by the Hsp90 inhibitor 17-(dimethyl laminoethylamino)-17-demethoxygeldanamycin. Clin Cancer Res 10(23):8077–8084.

[48] Burnette BC, Liang H, Lee Y, Chlewicki L, Khodarev NN, Weichselbaum RR, Fu YX, Auh SL (2011) The efficacy of radiotherapy relies upon induction of type i interferon-dependent innate and adaptive immunity. Cancer Res 71(7):2488–2496. doi:10.1158/0008-5472.CAN-10-2820.

[49] Bussink J, Kaanders JH, van der Graaf WT, Oyen WJ (2011) PET-CT for radiotherapy treatment planning and response monitoring in solid tumors. Nat Rev Clin Oncol 8(4):233–242.

[50] Cairncross G, Berkey B, Shaw E, Jenkins R, Scheithauer B, Brachman D, Buckner J, Fink K, Souhami L, Laperierre N, Mehta M, Curran W (2006) Phase III trial of chemotherapy plus radiotherapy compared with radiotherapy alone for pure and mixed anaplastic oligodendroglioma: Intergroup Radiation Therapy Oncology Group Trial 9402. J Clin Oncol 24(18): 2707–2714.

[51] Camphausen K, Moses MA, Beecken WD, Khan MK, Folkman J, O'Reilly MS (2001) Radiation therapy to a primary tumor accelerates metastatic growth in mice. Cancer Res 61(5): 2207–2211.

[52] Campisi J, d'Adda di Fagagna F (2007) Cellular senescence: when bad things happen to good cells. Nat Rev Mol Cell Biol 8(9):729–740.

[53] Carmeliet P, Jain RK (2011) Principles and mechanisms of vessel normalization for cancer and other angiogenic diseases. Nat Rev Drug Discov 10(6):417–427.

[54] Cerdan C, Bhatia M (2010) Novel roles for Notch, Wnt and Hedgehog in hematopoesis derived from human pluripotent stem cells. Int J Dev Biol 54(6-7): 955–963.

[55] Chadha M, Young A, Geraghty C, Masino R, Harrison L (2011) Image guidance using 3D-ultrasound (3D-US) for daily positioning of lumpectomy cavity for boost irradiation. Radiat Oncol 6:45. doi:10.1186/1748-717X-6-45.

[56] Chalmers A, Johnston P, Woodcock M, Joiner M, Marples B (2004) PARP-1, PARP-2, and the cellular response to low doses of ionizing radiation. Int J Radiat Oncol Biol Phys 58(2):410-419 Champoux JJ (2001) DNA topoisomerases: structure, function, and mechanism. Annu Rev Biochem 70:369–413.

[57] Chang F, Lee JT, Navolanic PM, Steelman LS, Shelton JG, Blalock WL, Franklin RA, McCubrey JA (2003) Involvement of PI3 K/Akt pathway in cell cycle progression, apoptosis, and neoplastic transformation: a target for cancer chemotherapy. Leukemia 17(3):590–603. doi:10.1038/sj.leu.2402824.

[58] Chen AY, Choy H, Rothenberg ML (1999) DNA topoisomerase I-targeting drugs as radiation sensitizers. Oncology (Williston Park) 13(10 Suppl 5):39–46.

[59] Chen MS, Woodward WA, Behbod F, Peddibhotla S, Alfaro MP, Buchholz TA, Rosen JM (2007) Wnt/b-catenin mediates radiation resistance of Sca1? progenitors in an immortalized mammary gland cell line. J Cell Sci 120(3):468–477. doi:10. 1242/jcs.03348.

[60] Chin L, Tam A, Pomerantz J, Wong M, Holash J, Bardeesy N, Shen Q, O'Hagan R, Pantginis J, Zhou H, Horner JW 2nd, Cordon- Cardo C, Yancopoulos GD, DePinho RA (1999) Essential role for oncogenic Ras in tumour maintenance. Nature 400(6743):468– 472. doi:10.1038/22788.

[61] Chinnaiyan AM, Prasad U, Shankar S, Hamstra DA, Shanaiah M, Chenevert TL, Ross BD, Rehemtulla A (2000) Combined effect of tumor necrosis factor-related apoptosis-inducing ligand and ionizing radiation in breast cancer therapy. Proc Natl Acad Sci USA 97(4):1754–1759. doi:10.1073/pnas.030545097.

[62] Chiosis G, Caldas Lopes E, Solit D (2006) Heat shock protein-90 inhibitors: a chronicle from geldanamycin to today's agents. Curr Opin Investig Drugs 7(6): 534–541.

[63] Chipuk JE, Moldoveanu T, Llambi F, Parsons MJ, Green DR (2010) The BCL-2 family reunion. Mol Cell 37(3):299–310. doi:10. 1016/j.molcel.2010.01.025.

[64] Choy H, MacRae R (2001) Irinotecan and radiation in combined-modality therapy for solid tumors. Oncology (Williston Park) 15(7 Suppl 8):22–28.

[65] Clasie B, Wroe A, Kooy H, Depauw N, Flanz J, Paganetti H, Rosenfeld A (2010) Assessment of out-of-field absorbed dose and equivalent dose in proton fields. Med Phys 37(1):311–321.

[66] Combs SE, Burkholder I, Edler L, Rieken S, Habermehl D, Jakel O, Haberer T, Haselmann R, Unterberg A, Wick W, Debus J (2010a) Randomised phase I/II study to evaluate carbon ion radiotherapy versus fractionated stereotactic radiotherapy in patients with recurrent or progressive gliomas: the CINDERELLA trial. BMC Cancer 10:533. doi: 10.1186/1471-2407-10-533.

[67] Combs SE, Ellerbrock M, Haberer T, Habermehl D, Hoess A, Jakel O, Jensen A, Klemm S, Munter M, Naumann J, Nikoghosyan A, Oertel S, Parodi K, Rieken S, Debus J (2010b) Heidelberg Ion Therapy Center (HIT): initial clinical experience in the first 80 patients. Acta Oncol 49(7):1132-1140. doi:10.3109/0284186X. 2010.498432.

[68] Combs SE, Jakel O, Haberer T, Debus J (2010c) Particle therapy at the Heidelberg Ion Therapy Center (HIT)—Integrated research- driven university-hospital-based radiation oncology service in Heidelberg, Germany. Radiother Oncol 95(1):41–44.

[69] Combs SE, Rieken S, Wick W, Abdollahi A, von Deimling A, Debus J, Hartmann C (2011) Prognostic significance of IDH-1 and MGMT in patients with glioblastoma: one step forward, and one step back? Radiat Oncol 6:115. doi:10.1186/1748-717X-6-115.

[70] Combs SE, Zipp L, Rieken S, Habermehl D, Brons S, Winter M, Haberer T, Debus J, Weber KJ (2012) In vitro evaluation of photon and carbon ion radiotherapy in combination with chemotherapy in glioblastoma cells. Radiat Oncol 7:9.doi:10. 1186/1748-717X-7-9.

[71] Cooper JS, Pajak TF, Forastiere AA, Jacobs J, Campbell BH, Saxman SB, Kish JA, Kim HE, Cmelak AJ, Rotman M, Machtay M, Ensley JF, Chao KS, Schultz CJ, Lee N, Fu KK (2004) Postoperative concurrent radiotherapy and chemotherapy for high-risk squamous-cell carcinoma of the head and neck. N Engl J Med 350(19):1937–1944. doi:10.1056/NEJMoa032646.

[72] Coppe JP, Desprez PY, Krtolica A, Campisi J (2010) The senescence- associated secretory phenotype: the dark side of tumor suppression. Annu Rev Pathol 5:99–118. doi:10. 1146/annurev-pathol-121808-102144.

[73] Cordes N, Hansmeier B, Beinke C, Meineke V, van Beuningen D (2003) Irradiation differentially affects substratum-dependent survival, adhesion, and invasion of glioblastoma cell lines. Br J Cancer 89(11):2122-2132. doi:10.1038/sj.bjc.6601429

[74] Cowell IG, Durkacz BW, Tilby MJ (2005) Sensitization of breast carcinoma cells to ionizing radiation by small molecule inhibitors of DNA-dependent protein kinase and ataxia telangiectsia mutated. Biochem Pharmacol 71(1-2):13–20.

[75] Crane CH, Eng C, Feig BW, Das P, Skibber JM, Chang GJ, Wolff RA, Krishnan S, Hamilton S, Janjan NA, Maru DM, Ellis LM, Rodriguez-Bigas MA (2010) Phase II trial of neoadjuvant bevacizumab, capecitabine, and radiotherapy for locally advanced rectal cancer. Int J Radiat Oncol Biol Phys 76(3):824–830. doi:10.1016/j.ijrobp.2009.02.037.

[76] Crehange G, Mirjolet C, Gauthier M, Martin E, Truc G, Peignaux- Casasnovas K, Azelie C, Bonnetain F, Naudy S, Maingon P (2012) Clinical impact of margin reduction on late toxicity and short-term biochemical control for patients treated with daily online image guided IMRT for prostate cancer. Radiother Oncol 103(2):244–246. doi:10.1016/ j.radonc.2011.10.025.

[77] Dancea HC, Shareef MM, Ahmed MM (2009) Role of radiation- induced TGF-beta

signaling in cancer therapy. Mol Cell Pharmacol 1(1):44–56.

[78] Darby S, McGale P, Correa C, Taylor C, Arriagada R, Clarke M, Cutter D, Davies C, Ewertz M, Godwin J, Gray R, Pierce L, Whelan T, Wang Y, Peto R (2011) Effect of radiotherapy after breast-conserving surgery on 10-year recurrence and 15-year breast cancer death: meta-analysis of individual patient data for 10,801 women in 17 randomised trials. Lancet 378(9804):1707–1716. doi:10.1016/S0140-6736(11) 61629-2.

[79] Davies RL, Grosse VA, Kucherlapati R, Bothwell M (1980) Genetic analysis of epidermal growth factor action: assignment of human epidermal growth factor receptor gene to chromosome 7. Proc Natl Acad Sci USA 77(7):4188–4192.

[80] de Geus-Oei LF, Vriens D, van Laarhoven HW, van der Graaf WT, Oyen WJ (2009) Monitoring and predicting response to therapy with 18F-FDG PET in colorectal cancer: a systematic review. J Nucl Med 50(Suppl 1):43S–54S.

[81] De Ruyck K, Van Eijkeren M, Claes K, Bacher K, Vral A, De Neve W, Thierens H (2006) TGFbeta1 polymorphisms and late clinical radiosensitivity in patients treated for gynecologic tumors. Int J Radiat Oncol Biol Phys 65(4):1240–1248.

[82] De Ruysscher D, Nestle U, Jeraj R, Macmanus M (2012) PET scans in radiotherapy planning of lung cancer. Lung Cancer 75(2):141–145. doi:10.1016/j.lungcan.2011.07.018.

[83] Deacon J, Peckham MJ, Steel GG (1984) The radioresponsiveness of human tumours and the initial slope of the cell survival curve. Radiother Oncol 2(4):317–323.

[84] Debatin K-M, Krammer PH (2004) Death receptors in chemotherapy and cancer. Oncogene 23(16):2950–2966.

[85] Delaney G, Jacob S, Featherstone C, Barton M (2005) The role of radiotherapy in cancer treatment: estimating optimal utilization from a review of evidence-based clinical guidelines. Cancer 104(6):1129–1137. doi:10.1002/cncr.21324.

[86] Deville C, Ben-Josef E, Vapiwala N (2012) Radiation therapy modalities for prostate cancer. JAMA 308 (5):451; author reply 451–452.

[87] Diamond MS, Kinder M, Matsushita H, Mashayekhi M, Dunn GP, Archambault JM, Lee H, Arthur CD, White JM, Kalinke U, Murphy KM, Schreiber RD (2011) Type I interferon is selectively required by dendritic cells for immune rejection of tumors. J Exp Med 208(10):1989–2003. doi:10.1084/jem. 20101158.

[88] Diehn M, Cho RW, Lobo NA, Kalisky T, Dorie MJ, Kulp AN, Qian D, Lam JS, Ailles LE, Wong M, Joshua B, Kaplan MJ, Wapnir I, Dirbas FM, Somlo G, Garberoglio C, Paz B, Shen J, Lau SK, Quake SR, Brown JM, Weissman IL, Clarke MF (2009) Association of reactive oxygen species levels and radioresistance in cancer stem cells. Nature 458(7239): 780–783. doi:10.1038/nature07733.

[89] Dipetrillo T, Pricolo V, Lagares-Garcia J, Vrees M, Klipfel A, Cataldo T, Sikov W, McNulty B, Shipley J, Anderson E, Khurshid H, Oconnor B, Oldenburg NB, Radie-Keane K, Husain S, Safran H (2012) Neoadjuvant bevacizumab, oxaliplatin, 5-fluorouracil, and radiation for rectal cancer. Int J Radiat Oncol Biol Phys

82(1):124–129. doi:10.1016/j.ijrobp.2010.08.005.

[90] Dollinger G, Bergmaier A, Hable V, Hertenberger R, Greubel C, Hauptner A, Reichart P (2009) Nanosecond pulsed proton microbeam. Nucl Instrum Methods Phys Res Sect B 267(12–13):2008–2012. doi:10.1016/j.nimb.2009.03.006.

[91] Donawho CK, Luo Y, Penning TD, Bauch JL, Bouska JJ, Bontcheva- Diaz VD, Cox BF, DeWeese TL, Dillehay LE, Ferguson DC, Ghoreishi-Haack NS, Grimm DR, Guan R, Han EK, Holley- Shanks RR, Hristov B, Idler KB, Jarvis K, Johnson EF, Kleinberg LR, Klinghofer V, Lasko LM, Liu X, Marsh KC, McGonigal TP, Meulbroek JA, Olson AM, Palma JP, Rodriguez LE, Shi Y, Stavropoulos JA, Tsurutani AC, Zhu GD, Rosenberg SH, Giranda VL, Frost DJ (2007) ABT-888, an orally active poly(ADP-ribose) polymerase inhibitor that potentiates DNA- damaging agents in preclinical tumor models. Clin Cancer Res 13(9):2728–2737.

[92] Douillard JY, Rosell R, De Lena M, Carpagnano F, Ramlau R, Gonzales-Larriba JL, Grodzki T, Pereira JR, Le Groumellec A, Lorusso V, Clary C, Torres AJ, Dahabreh J, Souquet PJ, Astudillo J, Fournel P, Artal-Cortes A, Jassem J, Koubkova L, His P, Riggi M, Hurteloup P (2006) Adjuvant vinorelbine plus cisplatin versus observation in patients with completely resected stage IB-IIIA non-small-cell lung cancer (Adjuvant Navelbine International Trialist Association [ANITA]): a randomised controlled trial. Lancet Oncol 7(9):719–727.

[93] Drappatz J, Norden AD, Wong ET, Doherty LM, Lafrankie DC, Ciampa A, Kesari S, Sceppa C, Gerard M, Phan P, Schiff D, Batchelor TT, Ligon KL, Young G, Muzikansky A, Weiss SE, Wen PY (2010) Phase I study of vandetanib with radiotherapy and temozolomide for newly diagnosed glioblastoma. Int J Radiat Oncol Biol Phys 78(1):85–90. doi:10.1016/j.ijrobp.2009. 07.1741.

[94] Dunn GP, Old LJ, Schreiber RD (2004) The immunobiology of cancer immunosurveillance and immunoediting. Immunity 21(2):137–148. doi:10.1016/j.immuni.2004.07.017.

[95] Dunn GP, Koebel CM, Schreiber RD (2006) Interferons, immunity and cancer immunoediting. Nat Rev Immunol 6(11):836–848.

[96] Edvardsen H, Tefre T, Jansen L, Vu P, Haffty BG, Fossa SD, Kristensen VN, Borresen-Dale AL (2007) Linkage disequilibrium pattern of the ATM gene in breast cancer patients and controls; association of SNPs and haplotypes to radio- sensitivity and post-lumpectomy local recurrence. Radiat Oncol 2:25.

[97] Eriksson D, Stigbrand T (2010) Radiation-induced cell death mechanisms. Tumor Biol 31(4):363–372. doi:10.1007/s13277-010-0042-8.

[98] Esteller M, Garcia-Foncillas J, Andion E, Goodman SN, Hidalgo OF, Vanaclocha V, Baylin SB, Herman JG (2000) Inactivation of the DNA-repair gene MGMT and the clinical response of gliomas to alkylating agents. N Engl J Med 343(19):1350–1354. doi:10. 1056/NEJM200011093431901.

[99] Evangelista L, Baretta Z, Vinante L, Cervino AR, Gregianin M, Ghiotto C, Saladini G, Sotti G (2011) Tumour markers and FDG PET/CT for prediction of disease re-

lapse in patients with breast cancer. Eur J Nucl Med Mol Imaging 38(2):293–301. doi:10. 1007/s00259-010-1626-7.

[100] Fedrigo CA, Grivicich I, Schunemann DP, Chemale IM, dos Santos D, Jacovas T, Boschetti PS, Jotz GP, Braga Filho A, da Rocha AB (2011) Radioresistance of human glioma spheroids and expression of HSP70, p53 and EGFr. Radiat Oncol 6:156. doi:10.1186/1748-717X-6-156.

[101] Firat E, Gaedicke S, Tsurumi C, Esser N, Weyerbrock A, Niedermann G (2011) Delayed cell death associated with mitotic catastrophe in gamma-irradiated stem-like glioma cells. Radiat Oncol 6(1):71.

[102] Fischer CA, Zlobec I, Green E, Probst S, Storck C, Lugli A, Tornillo L, Wolfensberger M, Terracciano LM (2010) Is the improved prognosis of p16 positive oropharyngeal squamous cell carci-noma dependent of the treatment modality? Int J Cancer 126(5):1256–1262. doi:10.1002/ijc.24842.

[103] Fisher B, Anderson S, Bryant J, Margolese RG, Deutsch M, Fisher ER, Jeong JH, Wolmark N (2002) Twenty-year follow-up of a randomized trial comparing total mastectomy, lumpectomy, and lumpectomy plus irradiation for the treatment of invasive breast cancer. N Engl J Med 347(16):1233–1241. doi:10.1056/NEJMoa022152.

[104] Flanders KC, Burmester JK (2003) Medical applications of transforming growth factor-b. Clin Med Res 1(1):13-20. doi:10.3121/cmr.1.1.13.

[105] Fleckenstein J, Hellwig D, Kremp S, Grgic A, Groschel A, Kirsch CM, Nestle U, Rube C (2011) F-18-FDG-PET confined radio- therapy of locally advanced NSCLC with concomitant chemo-therapy: results of the PET-PLAN pilot trial. Int J Radiat Oncol Biol Phys 81(4):e283–e289.

[106] Fogarty GB, Ng D, Liu G, Haydu LE, Bhandari N (2011) Volumetric modulated arc therapy is superior to conventional intensity modulated radiotherapy-a comparison among prostate cancer patients treated in an Australian centre. Radiat Oncol 6:108. doi:10.1186/ 1748-717X-6-108.

[107] Fokas E, Prevo R, Pollard JR, Reaper PM, Charlton PA, Cornelissen B, Vallis KA, Hammond EM, Olcina MM, Gillies McKenna W, Muschel RJ, Brunner TB (2012) Targeting ATR in vivo using the novel inhibitor VE-822 results in selective sensitization of pancreatic tumors to radiation. Cell Death Dis 3:e441. doi:10. 1038/cddis.2012.181.

[108] Fontenot JD, Bloch C, Followill D, Titt U, Newhauser WD (2010) Estimate of the uncertainties in the relative risk of secondary malignant neoplasms following proton therapy and intensity- modulated photon therapy. Phys Med Biol 55(23):6987–6998.

[109] Foroudi F, Wilson L, Bressel M, Haworth A, Hornby C, Pham D, Cramb J, Gill S, Tai KH, Kron T (2012) A dosimetric comparison of 3D conformal vs intensity modulated vs volumetric arc radiation therapy for muscle invasive bladder cancer. Radiat Oncol 7:111. doi:10.1186/1748-717X-7-111.

[110] Foster RD, Pistenmaa DA, Solberg TD (2012) A comparison of radiographic techniques and electromagnetic transponders for localization of the prostate. Radiat On-

col 7:101. doi:10.1186/1748-717X-7-101.

[111] Frasca F, Pandini G, Sciacca L, Pezzino V, Squatrito S, Belfiore A, Vigneri R (2008) The role of insulin receptors and IGF-I receptors in cancer and other diseases. Arch Physiol Biochem 114(1):23-37. doi:10.1080/13813450801969715.

[112] Fresno Vara JA, Casado E, de Castro J, Cejas P, Belda-Iniesta C, Gonzalez-Baron M (2004) PI3 K/Akt signalling pathway and cancer. Cancer Treat Rev 30(2):193–204. doi: 10. 1016/j.ctrv. 2003.07.007.

[113] Frey B, Rubner Y, Wunderlich R, Weiss EM, Pockley AG, Fietkau R, Gaipl US (2012) Induction of abscopal anti-tumor immunity and immunogenic tumor cell death by ionizing irradiation—implications for cancer therapies. Curr Med Chem 19(12):1751– 1764 Fuertes MB, Woo SR, Burnett B, Fu YX, Gajewski TF (2013) Type I interferon response and innate immune sensing of cancer. Trends Immunol 34(2):67–73. doi:10.1016/ j.it.2012.10.004.

[114] Gandhi L, Camidge DR, de Oliveira MR, Bonomi P, Gandara D, Khaira D, Hann CL, McKeegan EM, Litvinovich E, Hemken PM, Dive C, Enschede SH, Nolan C, Chiu YL, Busman T, Xiong H, Krivoshik AP, Humerickhouse R, Shapiro GI, Rudin CM (2011) Phase I study of Navitoclax (ABT-263), a novel Bcl-2 family inhibitor, in patients with small-cell lung cancer and other solid tumors. J Clin Oncol 29(7):909–916.

[115] Ganswindt U, Paulsen F, Corvin S, Hundt I, Alber M, Frey B, Stenzl A, Bares R, Bamberg M, Belka C (2007) Optimized coverage of high-risk adjuvant lymph node areas in prostate cancer using a sentinel node-based, intensity-modulated radiation therapy technique. Int J Radiat Oncol Biol Phys 67(2):347–355.

[116] Gao Y, Ishiyama H, Sun M, Brinkman KL, Wang X, Zhu J, Mai W, Huang Y, Floryk D, Ittmann M, Thompson TC, Butler EB, Xu B, Teh BS (2011) The alkylphospholipid, perifosine, radiosensitizes prostate cancer cells both in vitro and in vivo. Radiat Oncol 6:39. doi:10.1186/1748-717X-6-39.

[117] Garcia-Barros M, Paris F, Cordon-Cardo C, Lyden D, Rafii S, Haimovitz-Friedman A, Fuks Z, Kolesnick R (2003) Tumor response to radiotherapy regulated by endothelial cell apoptosis. Science 300(5622):1155–1159. doi:10.1126/science.1082504.

[118] Garcia-Lora A, Algarra I, Garrido F (2003) MHC class I antigens, immune surveillance, and tumor immune escape. J Cell Physiol 195(3):346–355. doi:10.1002/jcp.10290.

[119] Garrido C, Galluzzi L, Brunet M, Puig PE, Didelot C, Kroemer G (2006) Mechanisms of cytochrome c release from mitochondria. Cell Death Differ 13(9): 1423–1433.

[120] Gehler B, Paulsen F, Oksuz MO, Hauser TK, Eschmann SM, Bares R, Pfannenberg C, Bamberg M, Bartenstein P, Belka C, Ganswindt U (2009) [68 Ga]-DOTATOC-PET/CT for meningioma IMRT treatment planning. Radiat Oncol 4:56. doi:10.1186/1748-717X- 4-56.

[121] Genesca A, Martin M, Latre L, Soler D, Pampalona J, Tusell L (2006) Telomere

dysfunction: a new player in radiation sensitivity. BioEssays 28(12):1172–1180. doi:10.1002/ bies.20501.

[122] Gill S, Thomas J, Fox C, Kron T, Rolfo A, Leahy M, Chander S, Williams S, Tai KH, Duchesne GM, Foroudi F (2011) Acute toxicity in prostate cancer patients treated with and without image-guided radiotherapy. Radiat Oncol 6:145. doi:10.116/1748-717X-6-145.

[123] Giralt J, de las Heras M, Cerezo L, Eraso A, Hermosilla E, Velez D, Lujan J, Espin E, Rosello J, Majo J, Benavente S, Armengol M, de Torres I (2005) The expression of epidermal growth factor receptor results in a worse prognosis for patients with rectal cancer treated with preoperative radiotherapy: a multicenter, retrospective analysis. Radiother Oncol 74(2):101–108.

[124] Giro C, Berger B, Bolke E, Ciernik IF, Duprez F, Locati L, Maillard S, Ozsahin M, Pfeffer R, Robertson AG, Langendijk JA, Budach W (2009) High rate of severe radiation dermatitis during radiation therapy with concurrent cetuximab in head and neck cancer: results of a survey in EORTC institutes. Radiother Oncol 90(2):166–171. doi:10.1016/ j.radonc.2008.09.007.

[125] Glatstein E (2002) Intensity-modulated radiation therapy: the inverse, the converse, and the perverse. Semin Radiat Oncol 12(3): 272–281.

[126] Goitein M (2008) Magical protons? Int J Radiat Oncol Biol Phys 70(3):654–656.

[127] Golding SE, Rosenberg E, Valerie N, Hussaini I, Frigerio M, Cockcroft XF, Chong WY, Hummersone M, Rigoreau L, Menear KA, O'Connor MJ, Povirk LF, van Meter T, Valerie K (2009) Improved ATM kinase inhibitor KU-60019 radiosensitizes glioma cells, compromises insulin, AKT and ERK prosurvival signaling, and inhibits migration and invasion. Mol Cancer Ther 8(10):2894–2902. doi:10.1158/1535-7163.MCT-09-0519.

[128] Gong B, Almasan A (2000) Apo2 ligand/TNF-related apoptosis- inducing ligand and death receptor 5 mediate the apoptotic signaling induced by ionizing radiation in leukemic cells. Cancer Res 60(20):5754–5760.

[129] Greubel C, Assmann W, Burgdorf C, Dollinger G, Du G, Hable V, Hapfelmeier A, Hertenberger R, Kneschaurek P, Michalski D, Molls M, Reinhardt S, Roper B, Schell S, Schmid TE, Siebenwirth C, Wenzl T, Zlobinskaya O, Wilkens JJ (2011) Scanning irradiation device for mice in vivo with pulsed and continuous proton beams. Radiat Environ Biophys 50(3):339–344. doi:10.1007/s00411-011-0365-x.

[130] Griem ML, Malkinson FD (1966) Modification of radiation response of tissue by colchicine. A clinical evaluation. Am J Roentgenol Radium Ther Nucl Med 97(4): 1003–1006.

[131] Grosu AL, Weber WA, Riedel E, Jeremic B, Nieder C, Franz M, Gumprecht H, Jaeger R, Schwaiger M, Molls M (2005) L-(methyl-11C) methionine positron emission tomography for target delineation in resected high-grade gliomas before radio- therapy. Int J Radiat Oncol Biol Phys 63(1):64–74.

[132] Guan Z, Wang XR, Zhu XF, Huang XF, Xu J, Wang LH, Wan XB, Long ZJ, Liu JN,

Feng GK, Huang W, Zeng YX, Chen FJ, Liu Q (2007) Aurora-A, a negative prognostic marker, increases migration and decreases radiosensitivity in cancer cells. Cancer Res 67(21):10436–10444.

[133] Guckenberger M, Wulf J, Mueller G, Krieger T, Baier K, Gabor M, Richter A, Wilbert J, Flentje M (2009) Dose-response relationship for image-guided stereotactic body radiotherapy of pulmonary tumors: relevance of 4D dose calculation. Int J Radiat Oncol Biol Phys 74(1):47–54. doi:10.1016/j.ijrobp.2008. 06.1939.

[134] Gudkov AV, Komarova EA (2003) The role of p53 in determining sensitivity to radiotherapy. Nat Rev Cancer 3(2):117–129. doi:10.1038/nrc992.

[135] Gupta AK, Bakanauskas VJ, Cerniglia GJ, Cheng Y, Bernhard EJ, Muschel RJ, McKenna WG (2001) The Ras radiation resistance pathway. Cancer Res 61(10): 4278–4282.

[136] Gupta T, Agarwal J, Jain S, Phurailatpam R, Kannan S, Ghosh-Laskar S, Murthy V, Budrukkar A, Dinshaw K, Prabhash K, Chaturvedi P, D'Cruz A (2012) Three-dimensional conformal radiotherapy (3D-CRT) versus intensity modulated radiation therapy (IMRT) in squamous cell carcinoma of the head and neck: a randomized controlled trial. Radiother Oncol 104(3):343–348. doi:10.1016/j. radonc.2012.07.001.

[137] Gutin PH, Iwamoto FM, Beal K, Mohile NA, Karimi S, Hou BL, Lymberis S, Yamada Y, Chang J, Abrey LE (2009) Safety and efficacy of bevacizumab with hypofractionated stereotactic irradiation for recurrent malignant gliomas. Int J Radiat Oncol Biol Phys 75(1):156–163. doi:10.1016/j.ijrobp.2008.10.043.

[138] Hall EJ (2009) Is there a place for quantitative risk assessment? J Radiol Prot 29(2A): A171–A184.

[139] Halyard MY, Pisansky TM, Dueck AC, Suman V, Pierce L, Solin L, Marks L, Davidson N, Martino S, Kaufman P, Kutteh L, Dakhil SR, Perez EA (2009) Radiotherapy and adjuvant trastuzumab in operable breast cancer: tolerability and adverse event data from the NCCTG Phase III Trial N9831. J Clin Oncol 27(16): 2638–2644. doi:10.1200/ JCO. 2008.17.9549.

[140] Hanahan D, Weinberg RA (2000) The hallmarks of cancer. Cell 100(1):57–70. doi: 10.1016/s0092-8674(00)81683-9.

[141] Hanahan D, Weinberg RA (2011) Hallmarks of cancer: the next generation. Cell 144(5):646-674. doi:10.1016/j.cell.2011.02.013 Hande KR (1998) Etoposide: four decades of development of a topoisomerase II inhibitor. Eur J Cancer 34(10): 1514–1521 Harris PS, Venkataraman S, Alimova I, Birks DK, Donson AM, Knipstein J, Dubuc A, Taylor MD, Handler MH, Foreman NK, Vibhakar R (2012) Polo-like kinase 1 (PLK1) inhibition suppresses cell growth and enhances radiation sensitivity in medulloblastoma cells. BMC Cancer 12:80. doi:10.1186/1471-2407-12-80.

[142] Haupt S, Berger M, Goldberg Z, Haupt Y (2003) Apoptosis-the p53 network. J Cell Sci 116(Pt 20):4077–4085. doi:10.1242/jcs. 00739.

[143] Hegi ME, Diserens AC, Gorlia T, Hamou MF, de Tribolet N, Weller M, Kros JM,

Hainfellner JA, Mason W, Mariani L, Bromberg JE, Hau P, Mirimanoff RO, Cairncross JG, Janzer RC, Stupp R (2005) MGMT gene silencing and benefit from temozolomide in glioblastoma. N Engl J Med 352(10):997–1003.

[144] Heinzelmann F, Jendrossek V, Lauber K, Nowak K, Eldh T, Boras R, Handrick R, Henkel M, Martin C, Uhlig S, Kohler D, Eltzschig HK, Wehrmann M, Budach W, Belka C (2006) Irradiation- induced pneumonitis mediated by the CD95/CD95-ligand system. J Natl Cancer Inst 98(17):1248–1251.

[145] Heldin C-H, Landstro¨ m M, Moustakas A (2009) Mechanism of TGF- b signaling to growth arrest, apoptosis, and epithelial-mesen-chymal transition. Curr Opin Cell Biol 21(2):166–176. doi:10. 1016/j.ceb.2009.01.021.

[146] Henke G, Meier V, Lindner LH, Eibl H, Bamberg M, Belka C, Budach W, Jendrossek V (2012) Effects of ionizing radiation in combination with Erufosine on T98G glioblastoma xenograft tumours: a study in NMRI nu/nu mice. Radiat Oncol 7(1): 172. doi: 10.11 86/1748-717X-7-172.

[147] Hey J, Setz J, Gerlach R, Janich M, Hildebrandt G, Vordermark D, Gernhardt CR, Kuhnt T (2011) Parotid gland-recovery after radiotherapy in the head and neck region-36 months follow-up of a prospective clinical study. Radiat Oncol 6:125. doi:10.1186/1748- 717X-6-125.

[148] Hickson I, Zhao Y, Richardson CJ, Green SJ, Martin NM, Orr AI, Reaper PM, Jackson SP, Curtin NJ, Smith GC (2004) Identification and characterization of a novel and specific inhibitor of the ataxia-telangiectasia mutated kinase ATM. Cancer Res 64(24): 9152– 9159.

[149] Hilgard P, Klenner T, Stekar J, Nossner G, Kutscher B, Engel J (1997) D-21266, a new heterocyclic alkylphospholipid with antitumour activity. Eur J Cancer 33(3):442–446.

[150] Hurley PJ, Bunz F (2007) ATM and ATR: components of an Integrated Circuit. Cell Cycle 6(4):414–417.

[151] Ihloff AS, Petersen C, Hoffmann M, Knecht R, Tribius S (2010) Human papilloma virus in locally advanced stage III/IV squamous cell cancer of the oropharynx and impact on choice of therapy. Oral Oncol 46(10):705–711. doi:10.1016/j. oraloncology.2010.07.006.

[152] Ikushima H, Miyazono K (2010) TGFb signalling: a complex web in cancer progression. Nat Rev Cancer 10(6):415–424.

[153] Isomura M, Oya N, Tachiiri S, Kaneyasu Y, Nishimura Y, Akimoto T, Hareyama M, Sugita T, Mitsuhashi N, Yamashita T, Aoki M, Sai H, Hirokawa Y, Sakata K, Karasawa K, Tomida A, Tsuruo T, Miki Y, Noda T, Hiraoka M (2008) IL12RB2 and ABCA1 genes are associated with susceptibility to radiation dermatitis. Clin Cancer Res 14(20): 6683–6689.

[154] Iyer R, Thames HD, Tealer JR, Mason KA, Evans SC (2004) Effect of reduced EGFR function on the radiosensitivity and proliferative capacity of mouse jejunal crypt clonogens. Radiother Oncol 72(3):283–289. doi:10.1016/j.radonc.2004.07.012.

[155] Jackson SP, Bartek J (2009) The DNA-damage response in human biology and disease. Nature 461(7267):1071–1078.

[156] Jacobs BL, Zhang Y, Hollenbeck BK (2012) Radiation therapy modalities for prostate cancer. JAMA 308 (5):450; author reply 451–452.

[157] Jensen AD, Nikoghosyan AV, Ecker S, Ellerbrock M, Debus J, Herfarth KK, Munter MW (2011a) Raster-scanned carbon ion therapy for malignant salivary gland tumors: acute toxicity and initial treatment response. Radiat Oncol 6:149. doi:10.1186/1748-717X-6-149.

[158] Jensen AD, Nikoghosyan AV, Windemuth-Kieselbach C, Debus J, Munter MW (2011b) Treatment of malignant sinonasal tumours with intensity-modulated radiotherapy (IMRT) and carbon ion boost (C12). BMC Cancer 11:190. doi:1471-2407-11-190.

[159] Jiang X, Li T, Liu Y, Zhou L, Xu Y, Zhou X, Gong Y (2011) Planning analysis for locally advanced lung cancer: dosimetric and efficiency comparisons between intensity-modulated radio- therapy (IMRT), single-arc/partial-arc volumetric modulated arc therapy (SA/PA-VMAT). Radiat Oncol 6:140. doi:10.1186/1748-717X-6-140.

[160] Johnston CJ, Piedboeuf B, Rubin P, Williams JP, Baggs R, Finkelstein JN (1996) Early and persistent alterations in the expression of interleukin-1 alpha, interleukin-1 beta and tumor necrosis factor alpha mRNA levels in fibrosis-resistant and sensitive mice after thoracic irradiation. Radiat Res 145(6):762–767.

[161] Jordan CT, Guzman ML, Noble M (2006) Cancer stem cells. N Engl J Med 355(12):1253– 1261. doi:10.1056/NEJMra061808.

[162] Jung H, Beck-Bornholdt HP, Svoboda V, Alberti W, Herrmann T (2001) Quantification of late complications after radiation therapy. Radiother Oncol 61(3):233–246.

[163] Kabakov AE, Makarova YM, Malyutina YV (2008) Radiosensitization of human vascular endothelial cells through Hsp90 inhibition with 17-N-allilamino-17- demethoxygel danamycin. Int J Radiat Oncol Biol Phys 71(3):858–865.

[164] Kagan AR, Schulz RJ (2010) Proton-beam therapy for prostate cancer. Cancer J 16(5):405–409. doi:10.1097/PPO.0b013e 3181f8c25d.

[165] Karapetis CS, Khambata-Ford S, Jonker DJ, O'Callaghan CJ, Tu D, Tebbutt NC, Simes RJ, Chalchal H, Shapiro JD, Robitaille S, Price TJ, Shepherd L, Au HJ, Langer C, Moore MJ, Zalcberg JR (2008) K-ras mutations and benefit from cetuximab in advanced colorectal cancer. N Engl J Med 359(17):1757–1765. doi:10. 1056/NEJMoa0804385.

[166] Kasibhatla S, Tseng B (2003) Why target apoptosis in cancer treatment? Mol Cancer Ther 2(6):573–580.

[167] Kaufman HL, Disis ML (2004) Immune system versus tumor: shifting the balance in favor of DCs and effective immunity. J Clin Invest 113(5):664–667. doi:10.1172/JCI21148.

[168] Kaye SB, Lubinski J, Matulonis U, Ang JE, Gourley C, Karlan BY, Amnon A,

Bell-McGuinn KM, Chen LM, Friedlander M, Safra T, Vergote I, Wickens M, Lowe ES, Carmichael J, Kaufman B (2012) Phase II, open-label, randomized, multicenter study comparing the efficacy and safety of olaparib, a poly (ADP- ribose) polymerase inhibitor, and pegylated liposomal doxorubicin in patients with BRCA1 or BRCA2 mutations and recurrent ovarian cancer. J Clin Oncol 30(4):372–379. doi:10.1200/JCO. 2011.36.9215.

[169] Kelly PJ, Dinkin MJ, Drappatz J, O'Regan KN, Weiss SE (2011) Unexpected late radiation neurotoxicity following bevacizumab use: a case series. J Neurooncol 102(3):485–490. doi:10.1007/s11060-010-0336-0.

[170] Kim JH, Kim SH, Kolozsvary A, Khil MS (1992) Potentiation of radiation response in human carcinoma cells in vitro and murine fibrosarcoma in vivo by topotecan, an inhibitor of DNA topoisomerase I. Int J Radiat Oncol Biol Phys 22(3):515–518.

[171] Kobe C, Dietlein M, Fuchs M (2010) Interpretation and validation of interim positron emission tomography in Hodgkin lymphoma. Leuk Lymphoma 51(3):552–553. doi: 10.3109/104281909 03585468.

[172] Koutcher LD, Wolden S, Lee N (2009) Severe radiation dermatitis in patients with locally advanced head and neck cancer treated with concurrent radiation and cetuximab. Am J Clin Oncol 32(5):472–476. doi:10.1097/COC.0b013e318193125c.

[173] Kraft SD, Richter C, Zeil K, Baumann M, Beyreuther E, Bock S, Bussmann M, Cowan TE, Dammene Y, Enghardt W, Helbig U, Karsch L, Kluge T, Laschinsky L, Lessmann E, Metzkes J, Naumburger D, Sauerbrey R, Schu"rer M, Sobiella M, Woithe J, Schramm U, Pawelke J (2010) Dose-dependent biological damage of tumour cells by laser- accelerated proton beams. New J Phys 12(8):085003.

[174] Krtolica A, Parrinello S, Lockett S, Desprez PY, Campisi J (2001) Senescent fibroblasts promote epithelial cell growth and tumorigenesis: a link between cancer and aging. Proc Natl Acad Sci USA 98(21):12072–12077. doi:10.1073/pnas.211053698.

[175] Kuilman T, Peeper DS (2009) Senescence-messaging secretome: SMS-ing cellular stress. Nat Rev Cancer 9(2):81–94. doi:10. 1038/nrc2560.

[176] Lai A, Filka E, McGibbon B, Nghiemphu PL, Graham C, Yong WH, Mischel P, Liau LM, Bergsneider M, Pope W, Selch M, Cloughesy T (2008) Phase II pilot study of bevacizumab in combination with temozolomide and regional radiation therapy for up-front treatment of patients with newly diagnosed glioblastoma multiforme: interim analysis of safety and tolerability. Int J Radiat Oncol Biol Phys 71(5):1372–1380. doi:10. 1016/ j.ijrobp.2007.11.068.

[177] Lammering G, Hewit TH, Valerie K, Contessa JN, Amorino GP, Dent P, Schmidt-Ullrich RK (2003) EGFRvIII-mediated radioresistance through a strong cytoprotective response. Oncogene 22(36):5545–5553. doi:10.1038/sj.onc.1206788.

[178] Lammering G, Valerie K, Lin PS, Hewit TH, Schmidt-Ullrich RK (2004) Radiation-induced activation of a common variant of EGFR confers enhanced radioresistance. Radiother Oncol 72(3):267–273. doi:10.1016/j.radonc.2004.07.004.

[179] Lauber K, Ernst A, Orth M, Herrmann M, Belka C (2012) Dying cell clearance and

its impact on the outcome of tumor radiotherapy. Front Oncol 2:116. doi:10.3389/fonc. 2012.00116.

[180] Lee Y, Auh SL, Wang Y, Burnette B, Meng Y, Beckett M, Sharma R, Chin R, Tu T, Weichselbaum RR, Fu YX (2009) Therapeutic effects of ablative radiation on local tumor require CD8? T cells: changing strategies for cancer treatment. Blood 114(3):589–595. doi:10.1182/blood-2009-02-206870.

[181] Lee JW, Zoumalan RA, Valenzuela CD, Nguyen PD, Tutela JP, Roman BR, Warren SM, Saadeh PB (2010) Regulators and mediators of radiation-induced fibrosis: gene expression profiles and a rationale for Smad3 inhibition. Otolaryngol Head Neck Surg 143(4):525–530. doi:10.1016/j.otohns.2010.06.912.

[182] Li M, Jendrossek V, Belka C (2007) The role of PDGF in radiation oncology. Radiat Oncol 2:5.

[183] Li M, Abdollahi A, Grone HJ, Lipson KE, Belka C, Huber PE (2009) Late treatment with imatinib mesylate ameliorates radiation- induced lung fibrosis in a mouse model. Radiat Oncol 4:66. doi:10.1186/1748-717X-4-66.

[184] Liao Z, Lin SH, Cox JD (2011) Status of particle therapy for lung cancer. Acta Oncol 50(6):745–756. doi:10.3109/0284186X. 2011.590148.

[185] Lindroos PM, Coin PG, Osornio-Vargas AR, Bonner JC (1995) Interleukin 1 beta (IL-1 beta) and the IL-1 beta-alpha 2-macro- globulin complex upregulate the plate-let-derived growth factor alpha-receptor on rat pulmonary fibroblasts. Am J Respir Cell Mol Biol 13(4):455–465.

[186] Lordick F, Geinitz H, Theisen J, Sendler A, Sarbia M (2006) Increased risk of ischemic bowel complications during treatment with bevacizumab after pelvic irradiation: report of three cases. Int J Radiat Oncol Biol Phys 64(5):1295–1298.

[187] Lugade AA, Moran JP, Gerber SA, Rose RC, Frelinger JG, Lord EM (2005) Local radiation therapy of B16 melanoma tumors increases the generation of tumor antigen-specific effector cells that traffic to the tumor. J Immunol 174(12):7516–7523.

[188] Lugade AA, Sorensen EW, Gerber SA, Moran JP, Frelinger JG, Lord EM (2008) Radiation-induced IFN-gamma production within the tumor microenvironment influences antitumor immunity. J Immunol 180(5):3132–3139.

[189] Machida H, Nakajima S, Shikano N, Nishio J, Okada S, Asayama M, Shirai M, Kubota N (2005) Heat shock protein 90 inhibitor 17-allylamino-17-demethoxy geldanamycin potentiates the radiation response of tumor cells grown as monolayer cultures and spheroids by inducing apoptosis. Cancer Sci 96(12):911–917.

[190] Mantel F, Frey B, Haslinger S, Schildkopf P, Sieber R, Ott O, Lo¨ dermann B, Ro¨del F, Sauer R, Fietkau R, Gaipl U (2010) Combination of ionising irradiation and hyperthermia activates programmed apoptotic and necrotic cell death pathways in human colorectal carcinoma cells. Strahlenther Onkol 186(11):587–599. doi:10.1007/s00066-010- 2154-x.

[191] Marini P, Budach W, Niyazi M, Junginger D, Stickl S, Jendrossek V, Belka C (2009a)

Combination of the pro-apoptotic TRAIL-receptor antibody mapatumumab with io-nizing radiation strongly increases long-term tumor control under ambient and hy-poxic conditions. Int J Radiat Oncol Biol Phys 75(1):198–202.

[192] Marini P, Junginger D, Stickl S, Budach W, Niyazi M, Belka C (2009b) Combined treatment with lexatumumab and irradiation leads to strongly increased long term tumour control under normoxic and hypoxic conditions. Radiat Oncol 4:49. doi:10.1186/1748- 717X-4-49.

[193] Martin S, Sydenham M, Haviland J, A'Hern R, Owen R, Bliss J, Yarnold J (2010) Test of association between variant tgbeta1 alleles and late adverse effects of breast radiotherapy. Radiother Oncol 97(1):15–18.

[194] Martinez I, Wang J, Hobson KF, Ferris RL, Khan SA (2007) Identification of diffe-rentially expressed genes in HPV-positive and HPV-negative oropharyngeal squam-ous cell carcinomas. Eur J Cancer 43(2):415–432.

[195] Massague' J, Blain SW, Lo RS (2000) TGFb Signaling in Growth control, cancer, and heritable disorders. Cell 103(2):295–309. doi:10.1016/s0092-8674(00)00121-5.

[196] Matsumoto Y, Machida H, Kubota N (2005) Preferential sensitization of tumor cells to radiation by heat shock protein 90 inhibitor geldanamycin. J Radiat Res 46(2):215–221.

[197] Mattern MR, Hofmann GA, McCabe FL, Johnson RK (1991) Synergistic cell killing by ionizing radiation and topoisomerase I inhibitor topotecan (SK&F 104864). Can-cer Res 51(21):5813–5816.

[198] McBride WH (1995) Cytokine cascades in late normal tissue radiation responses. Int J Radiat Oncol Biol Phys 33(1):233-234 McDonald S, Rubin P, Phillips TL, Marks LB (1995) Injury to the lung from cancer therapy: clinical syndromes, measurable endpoints, and potential scoring systems. Int J Radiat Oncol Biol Phys 31(5):1187–1203.

[199] Meek DW (2009) Tumour suppression by p53: a role for the DNA damage response? Nat Rev Cancer 9(10):714–723.

[200] Mendenhall WM, Henderson RH, Hoppe BS, Nichols RC, Menden- hall NP (2012) Salvage of locally recurrent prostate cancer after definitive radiotherapy. Am J Clin Oncol. doi:10.1097/COC. 0b013e31824be3b4.

[201] Merchant TE (2009) Proton beam therapy in pediatric oncology. Cancer J 15(4):298–305. doi:10.1097/PPO.0b013e3181b6d4b7.

[202] Mertens AC, Yasui Y, Liu Y, Stovall M, Hutchinson R, Ginsberg J, Sklar C, Robison LL (2002) Pulmonary complications in survivors of childhood and adolescent cancer. A report from the Childhood Cancer Survivor Study. Cancer 95(11): 2431–2441. doi:10. 1002/cncr.10978.

[203] Milanovi DA, Firat E, Grosu AL, Niedermann G (2013) Increased radiosensitivity and radiothermo sensitivity of human pancreatic MIA PaCa-2 and U251 glioblasto-ma cell lines treated with the novel Hsp90 inhibitor NVP-HSP990. Radiat Oncol

8(1):42. doi:10.1186/1748-717X-8-42.

[204] Milas L, Hunter NR, Mason KA, Kurdoglu B, Peters LJ (1994) Enhancement of tumor radioresponse of a murine mammary carcinoma by paclitaxel. Cancer Res 54(13):3506–3510.

[205] Milas L, Saito Y, Hunter N, Milross CG, Mason KA (1996) Therapeutic potential of paclitaxel-radiation treatment of a murine ovarian carcinoma. Radiother Oncol 40(2):163– 170. doi:0167814096017781.

[206] Milas L, Mason K, Hunter N, Petersen S, Yamakawa M, Ang K, Mendelsohn J, Fan Z (2000) In vivo enhancement of tumor radioresponse by C225 antiepidermal growth factor receptor antibody. Clin Cancer Res 6(2):701–708.

[207] Milas L, Fan Z, Andratschke NH, Ang KK (2004) Epidermal growth factor receptor and tumor response to radiation: in vivo preclinical studies. Int J Radiat Oncol Biol Phys 58(3):966–971. doi:10. 1016/j.ijrobp.2003.08.035.

[208] Milross CG, Mason KA, Hunter NR, Terry NH, Patel N, Harada S, Jibu T, Seong J, Milas L (1997) Enhanced radioresponse of paclitaxel-sensitive and -resistant tumours in vivo. Eur J Cancer 33(8):1299–1308.

[209] Mitchell JB, Choudhuri R, Fabre K, Sowers AL, Citrin D, Zabludoff SD, Cook JA (2010) In vitro and in vivo radiation sensitization of human tumor cells by a novel checkpoint kinase inhibitor, AZD7762. Clin Cancer Res 16(7):2076–2084. doi:10.1158/1078- 0432.CCR-09-3277.

[210] Miura K, K-i Sakata, Someya M, Matsumoto Y, Matsumoto H, Takahashi A, Hareyama M (2012) The combination of olaparib and camptothecin for effective radiosensitization. Radiat Oncol 7(1):62.

[211] Mok H, Crane CH, Palmer MB, Briere TM, Beddar S, Delclos ME, Krishnan S, Das P (2011) Intensity modulated radiation therapy (IMRT): differences in target volumes and improvement in clinically relevant doses to small bowel in rectal carcinoma. Radiat Oncol 6:63. doi:10.1186/1748-717X-6-63.

[212] Moretti L, Li B, Kim KW, Chen H, Lu B (2010) AT-101, a pan-Bcl-2 inhibitor, leads to radiosensitization of non-small cell lung cancer. J Thorac Oncol 5(5):680–687. doi: 10. 1097/JTO.0b013e 3181d6e08e.

[213] Moretti L, Niermann K, Schleicher S, Giacalone NJ, Varki V, Kim KW, Kopsombut P, Jung DK, Lu B (2011) MLN8054, a small molecule inhibitor of aurora kinase a, sensitizes androgen- resistant prostate cancer to radiation. Int J Radiat Oncol Biol Phys 80(4):1189–1197. doi:10.1016/j.ijrobp.2011.01.060.

[214] Morgan MA, Parsels LA, Zhao L, Parsels JD, Davis MA, Hassan MC, Arumugarajah S, Hylander-Gans L, Morosini D, Simeone DM, Canman CE, Normolle DP, Zabludoff SD, Maybaum J, Lawrence TS (2010) Mechanism of radiosensitization by the Chk1/2 inhibitor AZD7762 involves abrogation of the G2 checkpoint and inhibition of homologous recombinational DNA repair. Cancer Res 70(12):4972–4981. doi:10.1158/0008-5472. CAN-09-3573.

[215] Movsas B, Raffin TA, Epstein AH, Link CJ Jr (1997) Pulmonary radiation injury. Chest 111(4):1061–1076.

[216] Munn DH, Mellor AL (2007) Indoleamine 2, 3-dioxygenase and tumor-induced tolerance. J Clin Invest 117(5):1147–1154. doi:10.1172/JCI31178.

[217] Nardella C, Clohessy JG, Alimonti A, Pandolfi PP (2011) Pro-senescence therapy for cancer treatment. Nat Rev Cancer 11(7):503-511 Newhauser WD, Durante M (2011) Assessing the risk of second malignancies after modern radiotherapy. Nat Rev Cancer 11(6):438–448.

[218] Nieder C, Pawinski A, Dalhaug A, Andratschke N (2012) A review of clinical trials of cetuximab combined with radiotherapy for non- small cell lung cancer. Radiat Oncol 7:3. doi:10.1186/1748- 717X-7-3.

[219] Nikoghosyan AV, Karapanagiotou-Schenkel I, Munter MW, Jensen AD, Combs SE, Debus J (2010a) Randomised trial of proton vs. carbon ion radiation therapy in patients with chordoma of the skull base, clinical phase III study HIT-1-Study. BMC Cancer 10:607. doi:10.1186/1471-2407-10-607.

[220] Nikoghosyan AV, Rauch G, Munter MW, Jensen AD, Combs SE, Kieser M, Debus J (2010b) Randomised trial of proton vs. carbon ion radiation therapy in patients with low and intermediate grade chondrosarcoma of the skull base, clinical phase III study. BMC Cancer 10:606. doi:10.1186/1471-2407-10-606.

[221] Niyazi M, Marini P, Daniel PT, Humphreys R, Jendrossek V, Belka C (2009a) Efficacy of a triple treatment with irradiation, agonistic TRAIL receptor antibodies and EGFR blockade. Strahlenther Onkol 185(1):8–18. doi:10.1007/s00066-009-1856-4.

[222] Niyazi M, Marini P, Daniel PT, Humphreys R, Jendrossek V, Belka C (2009b) Efficacy of triple therapies including ionising radiation, agonistic TRAIL antibodies and cisplatin. Oncol Rep 21(6): 1455–1460.

[223] Niyazi M, Bartenstein P, Belka C, Ganswindt U (2010) Choline PET based dose-painting in prostate cancer-modelling of dose effects. Radiat Oncol 5:23.doi:10.1186/1748- 717X-5-23.

[224] Niyazi M, Geisler J, Siefert A, Schwarz SB, Ganswindt U, Garny S, Schnell O, Suchorska B, Kreth FW, Tonn JC, Bartenstein P, la Fougere C, Belka C (2011a) FET-PET for malignant glioma treatment planning. Radiother Oncol 99(1):44–48.

[225] Niyazi M, Maihoefer C, Krause M, Rodel C, Budach W, Belka C (2011b) Radiotherapy and "new" drugs-new side effects? Radiat Oncol 6:177. doi:10.1186/1748-717X-6-177.

[226] Niyazi M, Ganswindt U, Schwarz SB, Kreth FW, Tonn JC, Geisler J, la Fougere C, Ertl L, Linn J, Siefert A, Belka C (2012a) Irradiation and bevacizumab in high-grade glioma retreatment settings. Int J Radiat Oncol Biol Phys 82(1):67–76. doi:10.1016/j.ijrobp. 2010.09.002.

[227] Niyazi M, Schnell O, Suchorska B, Schwarz SB, Ganswindt U, Geisler J, Bartenstein P, Kreth FW, Tonn JC, Eigenbrod S, Belka C, la Fougere C (2012b) FET-PET as-

sessed recurrence pattern after radio-chemotherapy in newly diagnosed patients with glioblastoma is influenced by MGMT methylation status. Radiother Oncol 104(1):78–82. doi: 10.1016/j.radonc.2012.04.022.

[228] Njeh CF, Caroprese B, Desai P (2012) A simple quality assurance test tool for the visual verification of light and radiation field congruent using electronic portal images device and computed radiography. Radiat Oncol 7:49. doi:10.1186/1748-717X-7-49.

[229] Nystrom H (2010) The role of protons in modern and biologically guided radiotherapy. Acta Oncol 49(7):1124–1131. doi:10.3109/0284186X.2010.498436.

[230] Oldenhuis CN, Oosting SF, Gietema JA, de Vries EG (2008) Prognostic versus predictive value of biomarkers in oncology. Eur J Cancer 44(7):946–953. doi:10.1016/ j.ejca. 2008. 03.006.

[231] O'Leary J, Muggia FM (1998) Camptothecins: a review of their development and schedules of administration. Eur J Cancer 34(10):1500–1508.

[232] Pallotta S, Marrazzo L, Ceroti M, Silli P, Bucciolini M (2012) A phantom evaluation of Sentinel(TM), a commercial laser/camera surface imaging system for patient setup verification in radio- therapy. Med Phys 39(2):706–712. doi:10.1118/1.3675973.

[233] Pardali K, Moustakas A (2007) Actions of TGF-b as tumor suppressor and pro-metastatic factor in human cancer. Biochimica et Biophysica Acta (BBA) 1775(1):21–62. doi:10. 1016/j.bbcan. 2006.06.004.

[234] Pergolizzi S, Santacaterina A, Adamo B, Franchina T, Denaro N, Ferraro P, Ricciardi GR, Settineri N, Adamo V (2011) Induction chemotherapy with paclitaxel and cisplatin to concurrent radio- therapy and weekly paclitaxel in the treatment of loco-regionally advanced, stage IV (M0), head and neck squamous cell carcinoma. Mature results of a prospective study. Radiat Oncol 6:162. doi:10.1186/1748-717X-6-162.

[235] Peter C, Wesselborg S, Herrmann M, Lauber K (2010) Dangerous attraction: phagocyte recruitment and danger signals of apoptotic and necrotic cells. Apoptosis 15(9):1007– 1028. doi:10.1007/s10495-010-0472-1.

[236] Peters LJ, Withers HR, Thames HD Jr, Fletcher GH (1982) Tumor radioresistance in clinical radiotherapy. Int J Radiat Oncol Biol Phys 8(1):101–108.

[237] Peters NA, Richel DJ, Verhoeff JJ, Stalpers LJ (2008) Bowel perforation after radiotherapy in a patient receiving sorafenib. J Clin Oncol 26(14):2405–2406. doi:10.1200/ JCO. 2007.15. 8451.

[238] Phillips TM, McBride WH, Pajonk F (2006) The response of CD24-/low/CD44? breast cancer-initiating cells to radiation. J Natl Cancer Inst 98(24):1777–1785. doi:10.1093/ jnci/djj495.

[239] Pignon JP, le Maitre A, Maillard E, Bourhis J (2009) Meta-analysis of chemotherapy in head and neck cancer (MACH-NC): an update on 93 randomised trials and 17,346 patients. Radiother Oncol 92(1):4–14. doi:10.1016/j.radonc.2009.04.014.

[240] Pinkawa M, Eble MJ, Mottaghy FM (2011) PET and PET/CT in radiation treatment planning for prostate cancer. Expert Rev Anticancer Ther 11(7):1033–1039. doi:10.1586/ era.11.51.

[241] Pires IM, Olcina MM, Anbalagan S, Pollard JR, Reaper PM, Charlton PA, McKenna WG, Hammond EM (2012) Targeting radiation- resistant hypoxic tumour cells through ATR inhibition. Br J Cancer 107(2):291–299. doi:10.1038/bjc.2012.265.

[242] Plathow C, Li M, Gong P, Zieher H, Kiessling F, Peschke P, Kauczor HU, Abdollahi A, Huber PE (2004) Computed tomography monitoring of radiation-induced lung fibrosis in mice. Invest Radiol 39(10):600–609.

[243] Pohlers D, Brenmoehl J, Loffler I, Muller CK, Leipner C, Schultze- Mosgau S, Stallmach A, Kinne RW, Wolf G (2009) TGF-beta and fibrosis in different organs—molecular pathway imprints. Biochim Biophys Acta 1792(8):746–756.

[244] Pommier Y (2013) Drugging topoisomerases: lessons and challenges. ACS Chem Biol 8(1):82–95. doi:10.1021/cb300648v.

[245] Pottgen C, Levegrun S, Theegarten D, Marnitz S, Grehl S, Pink R, Eberhardt W, Stamatis G, Gauler T, Antoch G, Bockisch A, Stuschke M (2006) Value of 18F-fluoro-2- deoxy-D-glucose-positron emission tomography/computed tomography in non- small-cell lung cancer for prediction of pathologic response and times to relapse after neoadjuvant chemoradiotherapy. Clin Cancer Res 12(1):97–106. doi:12/1/97.

[246] Prestwich RJ, Kancherla K, Oksuz DC, Williamson D, Dyker KE, Coyle C, Sen M (2010) A single centre experience with sequential and concomitant chemoradiotherapy in locally advanced stage IV tonsillar cancer. Radiat Oncol 5:121. doi:10.1186/1748- 717X-5-121.

[247] Prevo R, Fokas E, Reaper PM, Charlton PA, Pollard JR, McKenna WG, Muschel RJ, Brunner TB (2012) The novel ATR inhibitor VE-821 increases sensitivity of pancreatic cancer cells to radiation and chemotherapy. Cancer Biol Ther 13(11): 1072–1081. doi:10.4161/cbt.21093.

[248] Puthawala K, Hadjiangelis N, Jacoby SC, Bayongan E, Zhao Z, Yang Z, Devitt ML, Horan GS, Weinreb PH, Lukashev ME, Violette SM, Grant KS, Colarossi C, Formenti SC, Munger JS (2008) Inhibition of integrin alpha(v)beta6, an activator of latent transforming growth factor-beta, prevents radiation-induced lung fibrosis. Am J Respir Crit Care Med 177(1):82–90.

[249] Qian LW, Mizumoto K, Urashima T, Nagai E, Maehara N, Sato N, Nakajima M, Tanaka M (2002) Radiation-induced increase in invasive potential of human pancreatic cancer cells and its blockade by a matrix metalloproteinase inhibitor, CGS27023. Clin Cancer Res 8(4):1223–1227.

[250] Quarmby S, Fakhoury H, Levine E, Barber J, Wylie J, Hajeer AH, West C, Stewart A, Magee B, Kumar S (2003) Association of transforming growth factor beta-1 single nucleotide polymor- phisms with radiation-induced damage to normal tissues in breast cancer patients. Int J Radiat Biol 79(2):137–143.

[251] Quon H, Abdulkarim B (2008) Adjuvant treatment of anaplastic oligodendrogliomas and oligoastrocytomas. Cochrane Database Syst Rev 16(2):CD007104. doi:10.1002/14 651858.CD007104.

[252] Raabe A, Derda K, Reuther S, Szymczak S, Borgmann K, Hoeller U, Ziegler A, Petersen C, Dikomey E (2012) Association of single nucleotide polymorphisms in the genes ATM, GSTP1, SOD2, TGFB1, XPD and XRCC1 with risk of severe erythema after breast conserving radiotherapy. Radiat Oncol 7:65. doi:10.1186/1748-717X-7-65.

[253] Rabbani ZN, Anscher MS, Zhang X, Chen L, Samulski TV, Li C-Y, Vujaskovic Z (2003) Soluble TGFb TYPE II receptor gene therapy ameliorates acute radiation-induced pulmonary injury in rats. Int J Radiat Oncol Biol Phys 57(2):563–572. doi:10.1016/ s0360-3016(03)00639-4.

[254] Ramaekers BLT, Pijls-Johannesma M, Joore MA, van den Ende P, Langendijk JA, Lambin P, Kessels AGH, Grutters JPC (2011) Systematic review and meta-analysis of radiotherapy in various head and neck cancers: comparing photons, carbon-ions and protons. Cancer Treat Rev 37(3):185–201. doi:10.1016/j.ctrv.2010.08.004.

[255] Reits EA, Hodge JW, Herberts CA, Groothuis TA, Chakraborty M, Wansley EK, Camphausen K, Luiten RM, de Ru AH, Neijssen J, Griekspoor A, Mesman E, Verreck FA, Spits H, Schlom J, van Veelen P, Neefjes JJ (2006) Radiation modulates the peptide repertoire, enhances MHC class I expression, and induces successful antitumor immunotherapy. J Exp Med 203(5): 1259–1271.

[256] Reya T, Morrison SJ, Clarke MF, Weissman IL (2001) Stem cells, cancer, and cancer stem cells. Nature 414(6859):105-111 Rieckmann T, Tribius S, Grob TJ, Meyer F, Busch CJ, Petersen C, Dikomey E, Kriegs M (2013) HNSCC cell lines positive for HPV and p16 possess higher cellular radiosensitivity due to an impaired DSB repair capacity. Radiother Oncol 107(2):242–246. doi:10.1016/j.radonc.2013.03.013.

[257] Rigaud O, Fortunel NO, Vaigot P, Cadio E, Martin MT, Lundh O, Faure J, Rechatin C, Malka V, Gauduel YA (2010) Exploring ultrashort high-energy electron-induced damage in human car-cinoma cells. Cell Death Dis 1:e73.

[258] Ringborg U, Bergqvist D, Brorsson B, Cavallin-Stahl E, Ceberg J, Einhorn N, Frodin JE, Jarhult J, Lamnevik G, Lindholm C, Littbrand B, Norlund A, Nylen U, Rosen M, Svensson H, Moller TR (2003) The Swedish Council on Technology Assessment in Health Care (SBU) systematic overview of radiotherapy for cancer including a prospective survey of radiotherapy practice in Sweden 2001-summary and conclusions. Acta Oncol 42(5-6):357–365.

[259] Rosen II, Fischer TA, Antolak JA, Starkschall G, Travis EL, Tucker SL, Hogstrom KR, Cox JD, Komaki R (2001) Correlation between lung fibrosis and radiation therapy dose after concurrent radiation therapy and chemotherapy for limited small cell lung cancer. Radiology 221(3):614–622.

[260] Rosenzweig KE, Mychalczak B, Fuks Z, Hanley J, Burman C, Ling CC, Armstrong J, Ginsberg R, Kris MG, Raben A, Leibel S (2000) Final report of the 70.2-Gy and 75.6-Gy dose levels of a phase I dose escalation study using three-dimensional con-

formal radiotherapy in the treatment of inoperable non-small cell lung cancer. Cancer J 6(2):82–87.

[261] Rubel A, Handrick R, Lindner LH, Steiger M, Eibl H, Budach W, Belka C, Jendrossek V (2006) The membrane targeted apoptosis modulators erucylphosphocholine and erucylphosphohomocho- line increase the radiation response of human glioblastoma cell lines in vitro. Radiat Oncol 1:6. doi:10.1186/1748-717X-1-6.

[262] Rudin CM, Hann CL, Garon EB, Ribeiro de Oliveira M, Bonomi PD, Camidge DR, Chu Q, Giaccone G, Khaira D, Ramalingam SS, Ranson MR, Dive C, McKeegan EM, Chyla BJ, Dowell BL, Chakravartty A, Nolan CE, Rudersdorf N, Busman TA, Mabry MH, Krivoshik AP, Humerickhouse RA, Shapiro GI, Gandhi L (2012) Phase II study of single-agent navitoclax (ABT-263) and biomarker correlates in patients with relapsed small cell lung cancer. Clin Cancer Res 18(11):3163–3169. doi:1078-0432. CCR-11-3090.

[263] Rudner CBPMRJWHFAL-WMBWBJ (2001) Radiation sensitivity and apoptosis in human lymphoma cells. Int J Radiat Biol 77(1):1–11. doi:10.1080/095530001453069.

[264] Ruiter GA, Zerp SF, Bartelink H, van Blitterswijk WJ, Verheij M (1999) Alkyl- lysophospholipids activate the SAPK/JNK pathway and enhance radiation-induced apoptosis. Cancer Res 59(10):2457–2463.

[265] Russell JS, Burgan W, Oswald KA, Camphausen K, Tofilon PJ (2003) Enhanced cell killing induced by the combination of radiation and the heat shock protein 90 inhibitor 17-allylamino-17- demethoxygeldanamycin: a multitarget approach to radiosensitization. Clin Cancer Res 9(10 Pt 1):3749–3755.

[266] Safwat A, Bentzen SM, Turesson I, Hendry JH (2002) Deterministic rather than stochastic factors explain most of the variation in the expression of skin telangiectasia after radiotherapy. Int J Radiat Oncol Biol Phys 52(1):198–204.

[267] Samani AA, Yakar S, LeRoith D, Brodt P (2007) The role of the IGF system in cancer growth and metastasis: overview and recent insights. Endocr Rev 28(1):20–47.

[268] Schildkopf P, Frey B, Mantel F, Ott OJ, Weiss EM, Sieber R, Janko C, Sauer R, Fietkau R, Gaipl US (2010) Application of hyperthermia in addition to ionizing irradiation fosters necrotic cell death and HMGB1 release of colorectal tumor cells. Biochem Biophys Res Commun 391(1):1014–1020. doi:10. 1016/j.bbrc.2009.12.008.

[269] Schippers JM, Lomax AJ (2011) Emerging technologies in proton therapy. Acta Oncol 50(6):838–850. doi:10.3109/0284186X. 2011.582513.

[270] Schmid TE, Dollinger G, Hauptner A, Hable V, Greubel C, Auer S, Friedl AA, Molls M, Roper B (2009) No evidence for a different RBE between pulsed and continuous 20 MeV protons. Radiat Res 172(5):567–574. doi:10.1667/RR1539.1.

[271] Schmid TE, Dollinger G, Hable V, Greubel C, Zlobinskaya O, Michalski D, Molls M, Roper B (2010) Relative biological effectiveness of pulsed and continuous 20 MeV protons for micronucleus induction in 3D human reconstructed skin tissue. Radiother

Oncol 95(1):66–72.

[272] Schreiber RD, Old LJ, Smyth MJ (2011) Cancer immunoediting: integrating immunity's roles in cancer suppression and promotion. Science 331(6024):1565–1570. doi:10.1126/ science. 1203486.

[273] Seger R, Krebs EG (1995) The MAPK signaling cascade. FASEB J 9(9):726–735.

[274] Sengupta S, Harris CC (2005) p53: traffic cop at the crossroads of DNA repair and recombination. Nat Rev Mol Cell Biol 6(1):44–55.

[275] Senra JM, Telfer BA, Cherry KE, McCrudden CM, Hirst DG, O'Connor MJ, Wedge SR, Stratford IJ (2011) Inhibition of PARP-1 by olaparib (AZD2281) increases the radiosensitivity of a lung tumor xenograft. Mol Cancer Ther 10(10):1949–1958. doi:10.1158/ 1535-7163.MCT-11-0278.

[276] Sheets NC, Goldin GH, Meyer AM, Wu Y, Chang Y, Sturmer T, Holmes JA, Reeve BB, Godley PA, Carpenter WR, Chen RC (2012) Intensity-modulated radiation therapy, proton therapy, or conformal radiation therapy and morbidity and disease control in localized prostate cancer. JAMA 307(15):1611–1620.

[277] Shelton JW, Waxweiler TV, Landry J, Gao H, Xu Y, Wang L, El- Rayes B, Shu HK (2013) In Vitro and In Vivo Enhancement of Chemoradiation Using the Oral PARP Inhibitor ABT-888 in Colorectal Cancer Cells. Int J Radiat Oncol Biol Phys 86(3):469–476. doi:10.1016/j.ijrobp.2013.02.015.

[278] Sherr CJ, Roberts JM (1999) CDK inhibitors: positive and negative regulators of G1-phase progression. Genes Dev 13(12): 1501–1512.

[279] Shi A, Zhu G, Wu H, Yu R, Li F, Xu B (2010) Analysis of clinical and dosimetric factors associated with severe acute radiation pneumonitis in patients with locally advanced non-small cell lung cancer treated with concurrent chemotherapy and intensity- modulated radiotherapy. Radiat Oncol 5:35. doi:10.1186/1748-717X-5-35.

[280] Shiloh Y (2006) The ATM-mediated DNA-damage response: taking shape. Trends Biochem Sci 31(7):402–410. doi:10.1016/j.tibs. 2006.05.004.

[281] Shin S, Yoon H, Kim N, Lee K, Min B, Ahn J, Keum K, Koom W (2011) Upfront systemic chemotherapy and preoperative short- course radiotherapy with delayed surgery for locally advanced rectal cancer with distant metastases. Radiat Oncol 6(1):99.

[282] Silvano G, Lazzari G, Lovecchio M, Palazzo C (2008) Acute and fatal diarrhoea after erlotinib plus abdominal palliative hypofractionated radiotherapy in a metastatic non-small cell lung cancer patient: a case report. Lung Cancer 61(2):270–273. doi:10.1016/ j.lungcan.2008.03.004.

[283] Sinclair WK, Morton RA (1966) X-ray sensitivity during the cell generation cycle of cultured Chinese hamster cells. Radiat Res 29(3):450–474.

[284] Smith J, Mun Tho L, Xu N, A. Gillespie D (2010) Chapter 3: The ATM-Chk2 and ATR-Chk1 Pathways in DNA Damage Signaling and Cancer. In: George FVW, George K (eds) Advances in Cancer Research, vol Volume 108. Academic Press, pp

73–112. doi:10.1016/b978-0-12-380888-2.00003-0.

[285] Snow AN, Laudadio J (2010) Human papillomavirus detection in head and neck squamous cell carcinomas. Adv Anat Pathol 17(6):394–403. doi:10.1097/PAP.0b013e3181f895c1.

[286] Song SY, Kim JH, Ryu JS, Lee GH, Kim SB, Park SI, Song HY, Cho KJ, Ahn SD, Lee SW, Shin SS, Choi EK (2005) FDG-PET in the prediction of pathologic response after neoadjuvant chemora- diotherapy in locally advanced, resectable esophageal cancer. Int J Radiat Oncol Biol Phys 63(4):1053–1059.

[287] Spigel DR, Hainsworth JD, Yardley DA, Raefsky E, Patton J, Peacock N, Farley C, Burris HA 3rd, Greco FA (2010) Tracheoesophageal fistula formation in patients with lung cancer treated with chemoradiation and bevacizumab. J Clin Oncol 28(1):43–48. doi:10.1200/JCO.2009.24.7353.

[288] Srivastava M, Nambiar M, Sharma S, Karki SS, Goldsmith G, Hegde M, Kumar S, Pandey M, Singh RK, Ray P, Natarajan R, Kelkar M, De A, Choudhary B, Raghavan SC (2012) An inhibitor of nonhomologous end-joining abrogates double-strand break repair and impedes cancer progression. Cell 151(7):1474–1487. doi:10.1016/j.cell.2012.11.054.

[289] Stingl L, Stuhmer T, Chatterjee M, Jensen MR, Flentje M, Djuzenova CS (2010) Novel HSP90 inhibitors, NVP-AUY922 and NVP- BEP800, radiosensitise tumour cells through cell-cycle impairment, increased DNA damage and repair protraction. Br J Cancer 102(11):1578–1591.

[290] Stupp R, Hegi ME, Mason WP, van den Bent MJ, Taphoorn MJ, Janzer RC, Ludwin SK, Allgeier A, Fisher B, Belanger K, Hau P, Brandes AA, Gijtenbeek J, Marosi C, Vecht CJ, Mokhtari K, Wesseling P, Villa S, Eisenhauer E, Gorlia T, Weller M, Lacombe D, Cairncross JG, Mirimanoff RO (2009) Effects of radiotherapy with concomitant and adjuvant temozolomide versus radiotherapy alone on survival in glioblastoma in a randomised phase III study: 5-year analysis of the EORTC-NCIC trial. Lancet Oncol 10(5): 459–466. doi:10.1016/S1470- 2045(09)70025-7.

[291] Taghian AG, Assaad SI, Niemierko A, Kuter I, Younger J, Schoenthaler R, Roche M, Powell SN (2001) Risk of pneumonitis in breast cancer patients treated with radiation therapy and combination chemotherapy with paclitaxel. J Natl Cancer Inst 93(23): 1806–1811.

[292] Tajima T (2010) Laser acceleration and its future. Proc Jpn Acad Ser B Phys Biol Sci 86(3):147–157.

[293] Takeda K, Takai Y, Narazaki K, Mitsuya M, Umezawa R, Kadoya N, Fujita Y, Sugawara T, Kubozono M, Shimizu E, Abe K, Shirata Y, Ishikawa Y, Yamamoto T, Kozumi M, Dobashi S, Matsushita H, Chida K, Ishidoya S, Arai Y, Jingu K, Yamada S (2012) Treatment outcome of high-dose image-guided intensity-modulated radiotherapy using intra-prostate fiducial markers for localized prostate cancer at a single institute in Japan. Radiat Oncol 7:105. doi:10.1186/1748-717X-7-105.

[294] Tao Y, Zhang P, Girdler F, Frascogna V, Castedo M, Bourhis J, Kroemer G, Deutsch

E (2008) Enhancement of radiation response in p53-deficient cancer cells by the Aurora-B kinase inhibitor AZD1152. Oncogene 27(23):3244–3255.

[295] Tao Y, Leteur C, Calderaro J, Girdler F, Zhang P, Frascogna V, Varna M, Opolon P, Castedo M, Bourhis J, Kroemer G, Deutsch E (2009) The aurora B kinase inhibitor AZD1152 sensitizes cancer cells to fractionated irradiation and induces mitotic catastrophe. Cell Cycle 8(19):3172–3181.

[296] Tao Y, Bardet E, Rosine D, Rolland F, Bompas E, Daly-Schveitzer N, Lusinchi A, Bourhis J (2013) Phase I trial of oral etoposide in combination with radiotherapy in head and neck squamous cell carcinoma-GORTEC 2004-02. Radiat Oncol 8:40. doi:10.1186/ 1748-717X-8-40.

[297] Taylor RC, Cullen SP, Martin SJ (2008) Apoptosis: controlled demolition at the cellular level. Nat Rev Mol Cell Biol 9(3):231–241.

[298] Terasima T, Tolmach LJ (1963) X-ray sensitivity and DNA synthesis in synchronous populations of HeLa cells. Science 140(3566):490–492.

[299] Thiery JP, Acloque H, Huang RY, Nieto MA (2009) Epithelial- mesenchymal transitions in development and disease. Cell 139(5):871–890. doi:10.1016/j.cell.2009.11.007.

[300] Thorwarth D, Geets X, Paiusco M (2010) Physical radiotherapy treatment planning based on functional PET/CT data. Radiother Oncol 96(3):317–324.

[301] Timmerman R, Paulus R, Galvin J, Michalski J, Straube W, Bradley J, Fakiris A, Bezjak A, Videtic G, Johnstone D, Fowler J, Gore E, Choy H (2010) Stereotactic body radiation therapy for inoperable early stage lung cancer. JAMA 303(11): 1070–1076. doi:10.1001/ jama.2010.261.

[302] Tishler RB, Geard CR, Hall EJ, Schiff PB (1992) Taxol sensitizes human astrocytoma cells to radiation. Cancer Res 52(12): 3495–3497.

[303] Toulany M, Dittmann K, Kruger M, Baumann M, Rodemann HP (2005) Radioresistance of K-Ras mutated human tumor cells is mediated through EGFR-dependent activation of PI3 K-AKT pathway. Radiother Oncol 76(2):143–150.

[304] Turesson I, Nyman J, Holmberg E, Oden A (1996) Prognostic factors for acute and late skin reactions in radiotherapy patients. Int J Radiat Oncol Biol Phys 36(5):1065–1075.

[305] Tutt A, Robson M, Garber JE, Domchek SM, Audeh MW, Weitzel JN, Friedlander M, Arun B, Loman N, Schmutzler RK, Wardley A, Mitchell G, Earl H, Wickens M, Carmichael J (2010) Oral poly(ADP-ribose) polymerase inhibitor olaparib in patients with BRCA1 or BRCA2 mutations and advanced breast cancer: a proof-of-concept trial. Lancet 376(9737):235–244. doi:10.1016/S0140-6736(10)60892-6.

[306] Unger C, Damenz W, Fleer EA, Kim DJ, Breiser A, Hilgard P, Engel J, Nagel G, Eibl H (1989) Hexadecylphosphocholine, a new ether lipid analogue. Studies on the antineoplastic activity in vitro and in vivo. Acta Oncol 28(2):213–217.

[307] Valastyan S, Weinberg RA (2011) Tumor metastasis: molecular insights and evolving

paradigms. Cell 147(2):275–292. doi:10. 1016/j.cell.2011.09.024.

[308] van den Bent MJ, Carpentier AF, Brandes AA, Sanson M, Taphoorn MJ, Bernsen HJ, Frenay M, Tijssen CC, Grisold W, Sipos L, Haaxma-Reiche H, Kros JM, van Kouwenhoven MC, Vecht CJ, Allgeier A, Lacombe D, Gorlia T (2006) Adjuvant procarbazine, lomustine, and vincristine improves progression-free survival but not overall survival in newly diagnosed anaplastic oligodendrogliomas and oligoastrocytomas: a randomized European Organisation for Research and Treatment of Cancer phase III trial. J Clin Oncol 24(18):2715–2722. doi:24/18/2715.

[309] van Herk M (2004) Errors and margins in radiotherapy. Semin Radiat Oncol 14(1):52–64.

[310] Vandenabeele P, Galluzzi L, Vanden Berghe T, Kroemer G (2010) Molecular mechanisms of necroptosis: an ordered cellular explosion. Nat Rev Mol Cell Biol 11(10):700–714.

[311] Vees H, Steiner C, Dipasquale G, Chouiter A, Zilli T, Velazquez M, Namy S, Ratib O, Buchegger F, Miralbell R (2012) Target volume definition in high-risk prostate cancer patients using sentinel node SPECT/CT and 18 F-choline PET/CT. Radiat Oncol 7:134. doi:10.1186/1748-717X-7-134.

[312] Velenik V, Ocvirk J, Music M, Bracko M, Anderluh F, Oblak I, Edhemovic I, Brecelj E, Kropivnik M, Omejc M (2011) Neoadjuvant capecitabine, radiotherapy, and bevacizumab (CRAB) in locally advanced rectal cancer: results of an open-label phase II study. Radiat Oncol 6(1):105.

[313] Vink SR, Lagerwerf S, Mesman E, Schellens JH, Begg AC, van Blitterswijk WJ, Verheij M (2006) Radiosensitization of squamous cell carcinoma by the alkylphospholipid perifosine in cell culture and xenografts. Clin Cancer Res 12(5):1615–1622.

[314] Vink SR, van Blitterswijk WJ, Schellens JH, Verheij M (2007) Rationale and clinical application of alkylphospholipid analogues in combination with radiotherapy. Cancer Treat Rev 33(2):191–202.

[315] Vogelius IR, Westerly DC, Aznar MC, Cannon GM, Korreman SS, Mackie TR, Mehta MP, Bentzen SM (2011) Estimated radiation pneumonitis risk after photon versus proton therapy alone or combined with chemotherapy for lung cancer. Acta Oncol 50(6):772–776. doi:10.3109/0284186X.2011.582519.

[316] Vogler M, Dinsdale D, Dyer MJ, Cohen GM (2009) Bcl-2 inhibitors: small molecules with a big impact on cancer therapy. Cell Death Differ 16(3):360–367.

[317] Vorwerk H, Hess CF (2011) Guidelines for delineation of lymphatic clinical target volumes for high conformal radiotherapy: head and neck region. Radiat Oncol 6:97. doi:10.1186/ 1748-717X-6-97.

[318] Vredenburgh JJ, Desjardins A, Kirkpatrick JP, Reardon DA, Peters KB, Herndon JE 2nd, Marcello J, Bailey L, Threatt S, Sampson J, Friedman A, Friedman HS (2012) Addition of bevacizumab to standard radiation therapy and daily temozolomide is associated with minimal toxicity in newly diagnosed glioblastoma multiforme. Int J Radiat Oncol Biol Phys 82(1):58–66. doi:10.1016/j. ijrobp.2010.08.058.

[319] Wachsberger P, Burd R, Dicker AP (2003) Tumor response to ionizing radiation combined with antiangiogenesis or vascular targeting agents: exploring mechanisms of interaction. Clin Cancer Res 9(6):1957–1971.

[320] Wakatsuki M, Ohno T, Iwakawa M, Ishikawa H, Noda S, Ohta T, Kato S, Tsujii H, Imai T, Nakano T (2008) p73 protein expression correlates with radiation-induced apoptosis in the lack of p53 response to radiation therapy for cervical cancer. Int J Radiat Oncol Biol Phys 70(4):1189–1194. doi:10.1016/j.ijrobp. 2007.08.033.

[321] Walsh L, Gillham C, Dunne M, Fraser I, Hollywood D, Armstrong J, Thirion P (2011) Toxicity of cetuximab versus cisplatin concurrent with radiotherapy in locally advanced head and neck squamous cell cancer (LAHNSCC). Radiother Oncol 98(1):38–41. doi:10.1016/j.radonc.2010.11.009.

[322] Walter F, la Fougere C, Belka C, Niyazi M (2012) Technical Issues of [(18)F]FET-PET Imaging for Radiation Therapy Planning in Malignant Glioma Patients—A Review. Front Oncol 2:130. doi:10.3389/fonc.2012.00130.

[323] Weber U, Kraft G (2009) Comparison of carbon ions versus protons. Cancer J 15(4):325– 332.doi:10.1097/PPO.0b013e3181b01935.

[324] Weidner AM, van Lin EN, Dinter DJ, Rozema T, Schoenberg SO, Wenz F, Barentsz JO, Lohr F (2011) Ferumoxtran-10 MR lymphography for target definition and follow-up in a patient undergoing image-guided, dose-escalated radiotherapy of lymph nodes upon PSA relapse. Strahlenther Onkol 187(3):206–212. doi:10.1007/s00066-010-2195-1.

[325] Wernicke AG, Dicker AP, Whiton M, Ivanidze J, Hyslop T, Hammond EH, Perry A, Andrews DW, Kenyon L (2010) Assessment of Epidermal Growth Factor Receptor (EGFR) expression in human meningioma. Radiat Oncol 5:46. doi:10. 1186/1748-717X-5-46.

[326] Wesbuer S, Lanvers-Kaminsky C, Duran-Seuberth I, Bolling T, Schafer K-L, Braun Y, Willich N, Greve B (2010) Association of telomerase activity with radio-and chemosensitivity of neurobl- astomas. Radiat Oncol 5(1):66.

[327] Wiezorek T, Brachwitz T, Georg D, Blank E, Fotina I, Habl G, Kretschmer M, Lutters G, Salz H, Schubert K, Wagner D, Wendt TG (2011) Rotational IMRT techniques compared to fixed gantry IMRT and tomotherapy: multi-institutional planning study for head-and-neck cases. Radiat Oncol 6:20. doi:10. 1186/1748-717X-6-20.

[328] Wild-Bode C, Weller M, Rimner A, Dichgans J, Wick W (2001) Sublethal irradiation promotes migration and invasiveness of glioma cells: implications for radiotherapy of human glioblas- toma. Cancer Res 61(6):2744–2750.

[329] Willett CG, Boucher Y, di Tomaso E, Duda DG, Munn LL, Tong RT, Chung DC, Sahani DV, Kalva SP, Kozin SV, Mino M, Cohen KS, Scadden DT, Hartford AC, Fischman AJ, Clark JW, Ryan DP, Zhu AX, Blaszkowsky LS, Chen HX, Shellito PC, Lauwers GY, Jain RK (2004) Direct evidence that the VEGF-specific antibody bevacizumab has antivascular effects in human rectal cancer. Nat Med 10(2):145–147. doi:10.1038/nm988.

[330] Williams KJ, Telfer BA, Brave S, Kendrew J, Whittaker L, Stratford IJ, Wedge SR (2004) ZD6474, a potent inhibitor of vascular endothelial growth factor signaling, combined with radiotherapy: schedule-dependent enhancement of antitumor activity. Clin Cancer Res 10(24):8587–8593.

[331] Woodward WA, Chen MS, Behbod F, Alfaro MP, Buchholz TA, Rosen JM (2007) WNT/b-catenin mediates radiation resistance of mouse mammary progenitor cells. Proc Natl Acad Sci 104(2):618–623. doi:10.1073/pnas.0606599104.

[332] Wurschmidt F, Petersen C, Wahl A, Dahle J, Kretschmer M (2011) [18F]fluoroethyl choline-PET/CT imaging for radiation treatment planning of recurrent and primary prostate cancer with dose escalation to PET/CT-positive lymph nodes. Radiat Oncol 6:44. doi:10.1186/1748-717X-6-44.

[333] Wynn TA (2008) Cellular and molecular mechanisms of fibrosis. J Pathol 214(2): 199–210. doi:10.1002/path.2277.

[334] Xavier S, Piek E, Fujii M, Javelaud D, Mauviel A, Flanders KC, Samuni AM, Felici A, Reiss M, Yarkoni S, Sowers A, Mitchell JB, Roberts AB, Russo A (2004) Amelioration of radiation-induced fibrosis. J Biol Chem 279(15):15167–15176. doi:10.1074/ jbc. M309798200.

[335] Xing L, Thorndyke B, Schreibmann E, Yang Y, Li TF, Kim GY, Luxton G, Koong A (2006) Overview of image-guided radiation therapy. Med Dosim 31(2):91–112.

[336] Xiong H, Liao Z, Liu Z, Xu T, Wang Q, Liu H, Komaki R, Gomez D, Wang LE, Wei Q (2012) ATM Polymorphisms predict severe radiation pneumonitis in patients with non-small cell lung cancer treated with definitive radiation therapy. Int J Radiat Oncol Biol Phys 85(4):1066–1073. doi:10.1016/j.ijrobp.2012.09.024.

[337] Yan H, Parsons DW, Jin G, McLendon R, Rasheed BA, Yuan W, Kos I, Batinic-Haberle I, Jones S, Riggins GJ, Friedman H, Friedman A, Reardon D, Herndon J, Kinzler KW, Velculescu VE, Vogelstein B, Bigner DD (2009) IDH1 and IDH2 mutations in gliomas. N Engl J Med 360(8):765–773. doi:10.1056/NEJMoa0808710.

[338] Yang S, Wu J, Zuo Y, Tan L, Jia H, Yan H, Zhu X, Zeng M, Ma J, Huang W (2010) ZD6474, a small molecule tyrosine kinase inhibitor, potentiates the anti-tumor and anti-metastasis effects of radiation for human nasopharyngeal carcinoma. Curr Cancer Drug Targets 10(6):611–622.

[339] Yaromina A, Zips D (2010) Bio-IGRT-biological image-guided radiotherapy. Nuklearmedizin 49(Suppl 1):S50–S52.

[340] Yin H, Glass J (2011) The phenotypic radiation resistance of CD44?/CD24(-or low) breast cancer cells is mediated through the enhanced activation of ATM signaling. PLoS ONE 6(9):e24080. doi:10.1371/journal.pone.0024080.

[341] Yogo A, Sato K, Nishikino M, Mori M, Teshima T, Numasaki H, Murakami M, Demizu Y, Akagi S, Nagayama S, Ogura K, Sagisaka A, Orimo S, Nishiuchi M, Pirozhkov AS, Ikegami M, Tampo M, Sakaki H, Suzuki M, Daito I, Oishi Y, Sugiyama H, Kiriyama H, Okada H, Kanazawa S, Kondo S, Shimomura T, Nakai Y, Tanoue M, Sasao H, Wakai D, Bolton PR, Daido H (2009) Application of laser-accelerated pro-

tons to the demonstration of DNA double-strand breaks in human cancer cells. Appl Phys Lett 94(18):181502–181503.

[342] Youle RJ, Strasser A (2008) The BCL-2 protein family: opposing activities that mediate cell death. Nat Rev Mol Cell Biol 9(1):47–59.

[343] Young JC, Agashe VR, Siegers K, Hartl FU (2004) Pathways of chaperone-mediated protein folding in the cytosol. Nat Rev Mol Cell Biol 5(10):781–791. doi:10.1038/nrm1492.

[344] Zabludoff SD, Deng C, Grondine MR, Sheehy AM, Ashwell S, Caleb BL, Green S, Haye HR, Horn CL, Janetka JW, Liu D, Mouchet E, Ready S, Rosenthal JL, Queva C, Schwartz GK, Taylor KJ, Tse AN, Walker GE, White AM (2008) AZD7762, a novel checkpoint kinase inhibitor, drives checkpoint abrogation and potentiates DNA-targeted therapies. Mol Cancer Ther 7(9):2955–2966. doi:10.1158/1535-7163.MCT-08-0492.

[345] Zerp SF, Stoter R, Kuipers G, Yang D, Lippman ME, van Blitterswijk WJ, Bartelink H, Rooswinkel R, Lafleur V, Verheij M (2009) AT-101, a small molecule inhibitor of anti-apoptotic Bcl-2 family members, activates the SAPK/JNK pathway and enhances radiation-induced apoptosis. Radiat Oncol 4:47. doi:10.1186/1748-717X-4-47.

[346] Zhang K, Phan SH (1996) Cytokines and pulmonary fibrosis. Biol Signals 5(4):232–239.

[347] Zlobinskaya O, Dollinger G, Michalski D, Hable V, Greubel C, Du G, Multhoff G, Roper B, Molls M, Schmid TE (2012) Induction and repair of DNA double-strand breaks assessed by gamma-H2AX foci after irradiation with pulsed or continuous proton beams. Radiat Environ Biophys 51(1):23–32. doi:10.1007/s00411-011-0398-1.

[348] Zschenker O, Raabe A, Boeckelmann IK, Borstelmann S, Szymczak S, Wellek S, Rades D, Hoeller U, Ziegler A, Dikomey E, Borgmann K (2010) Association of single nucleotide polymor- phisms in ATM, GSTP1, SOD2, TGFB1, XPD and XRCC1 with clinical and cellular radiosensitivity. Radiother Oncol 97(1): 26–32.

Chapter 23

Scenario Drafting for Early Technology Assessment of Next Generation Sequencing in Clinical Oncology

S. E. P. Joosten[1], V. P. Retèl[2], V. M. H. Coupé[1], M. M. van den Heuvel[3], W. H. van Harten[2,4]

[1]Department of Clinical Epidemiology and Biostatistics, VU University Medical Centre Amsterdam, 1081 HZ Amsterdam, The Netherlands
[2]Department of Psychosocial Research and Epidemiology, Netherlands Cancer Institute-Antoni van Leeuwenhoek Hospital, 1066 CX Amsterdam, The Netherlands
[3]Department of Thoracic Oncology, Netherlands Cancer Institute-Antoni van Leeuwenhoek Hospital, 1066 CX Amsterdam, The Netherlands
[4]School of Governance and Management, University of Twente, MB-HTSR, PO Box 2177500 AE Enschede, The Netherlands

Abstract: Background: Next Generation Sequencing (NGS) is expected to lift molecular diagnostics in clinical oncology to the next level. It enables simultaneous identification of mutations in a patient tumor, after which targeted therapy may be assigned. This approach could improve patient survival and/or assist in controlling healthcare costs by offering expensive treatment to only those likely to benefit. However, NGS has yet to make its way into the clinic. Health Technology Assessment can support the adoption and implementation of a novel technology, but at this early stage many of the required variables are still unknown. Methods: Scenario drafting and expert elicitation via a questionnaire were used to identify factors that may act as a barrier or facilitate adoption of NGS-based molecular diagnostics. Attention was paid to predominantly elicit quantitative answers, allowing their use in future modeling of cost-effectiveness. Results: Adequately informing patients and physicians, the latters' opinion on clinical utility and underlying evidence as well as presenting sequencing results within a relevant timeframe may act as pivotal facilitators. Reimbursement for NGS-based testing and accompanying therapies (both general and in case of off-label prescription) was found to be a potential barrier. Competition on the market and demonstrating clinical utility may also be challenging. Importantly, numerous quantitative values for variables related to each of these potential barriers/facilitators, such as such as desired panel characteristics, willingness to pay or the expected number of targets identified per person, were also elicited. Conclusions: We have identified several factors that may either pose a barrier or facilitate the adoption of NGS in the clinic. We believe acting upon these findings, for instance by organizing educational events, advocating new ways of evidence generation and steering towards the most cost-effective solution, will accelerate the route from bench-to-bedside. Moreover, due to the methodology of expert elicitation, this study provides parameters that can be incorporated in future cost-effectiveness modeling to steer the development of NGS gene panels towards the most optimal direction.

Keywords: Health Technology Assessment, Next Generation Sequencing, Clinical Oncology, Personalized, Challenges

1. Background

In recent years, the cost and time required for large scale sequencing have rapidly decreased, catalyzing an increased understanding of genetic variation in both health and disease. Relatively cheap next generation sequencing (NGS) may confer great benefit in a clinical setting as well, especially in oncology[1]. Many institutes are currently developing NGS-based gene panels, which investigate the presence of multiple mutations in a single tumor at once. Subsequently, a specific targeted therapy may be assigned thereby potentially improving clinical outcome[2].

While many experts advocate that simultaneous testing of genes also has the potential to be more cost-effective than performing sequential single-gene assays, this has yet to be shown[3]. We define a NGS gene panel as "a multiplex predictive test which explores limited regions of tumor DNA/RNA for aberrations that can be used as a molecular target for therapy".

Meanwhile, NGS has reached the molecular diagnostic market and is expected to slowly replace single-gene molecular diagnostic tests[4]. Currently, within the Netherlands, hospitals have started with the implementation of NGS for diagnostics, using techniques ranging from single gene testing to small, medium or large NGS panels. Beyond biology, the adoption of NGS for large scale molecular diagnostics will also depend on a variety of organizational, societal and economic factors[5][6]. For instance, will hospitals be able to supply tissue meeting NGS requirements? Are physicians up to date on pharmacogenomics to use such a test in the clinic? And importantly, can society afford personalized medicine at all, given the costs associated with sequencing as well as extremely expensive targeted[5][6]? Due to the increased pressure to control ever-rising healthcare costs, reliable input regarding novel technologies on these factors is becoming increasingly more important. To our knowledge there are as yet no widely accepted national policies on NGS-based panels apart from the French initiative to centralize services for a specified number of molecular tests in regional centers under the Institut National du Cancer (INCa) umbrella.

A commonly used methodology to estimate and evaluate the impact of a novel technology is Health Technology Assessment (HTA), which is increasingly being used to support policy and reimbursement decisions regarding medical interventions[7]. Early stage TA can help to expedite further development and guide the adoption of a promising technology in the clinic[8]. We have previously performed such an early TA assessment for the introduction and adoption of a 70- gene prognosis-signature for breast cancer[9][10]. As part of this assessment, to fill in evidence gaps in cost-effectiveness analysis, we used scenario drafting as originally developed by Royal Dutch Shell. By describing potential directions of development, Shell is able to anticipate events possibly affecting their market position and timely adapt corporate strategy[11]–[13]. In case of the 70-gene array, we drafted several scenarios that represented likely patterns of its diffusion across the health care system focusing on features that were still likely to change during development, such as clinical, economic, patient-related, and organizational parameters[10]. Some of these were subsequently incorporated into a cost-effectiveness analysis[14].

In this paper, we report on scenario drafting concerning the adoption and implementation of NGS gene panels in clinical oncology among professionals. Our objective was first; to identify critical barriers and facilitators that may affect the speed of adoption of such panels in clinical practice and second; to estimate values of quantitative parameters for future cost-effectiveness modeling.

2. Methods

2.1. Background Research

We first interviewed in-house experts (Netherlands Cancer Institute) specialized in (molecular) diagnostics, patient management and/or next-generation sequencing to identify variables that are likely to affect the speed of adoption of NGS-panels (**Figure 1**). More info was gathered using Pubmed and Google Scholar, by searching for recent papers using (combinations of) the terms "cancer"/"oncology"/"tumor"/"clinical" + "personalized medicine", "precision medicine", "genomic medicine", "stratified medicine", "targeted therapy", "tailored therapy", "pharmacogenomics", "next-generation sequencing", "capture-based sequencing", "multiplex sequencing", "molecular diagnostics", "companion diagnostics", "genetic testing", "predictive biomarkers", "economics", "cost-effectiveness", "perspectives", "costs", "implementation", "challenges", "reimbursement", "storage", "data", "patients", "physicians". This resulted in thousands of papers often discussing the same topics. We selected papers for our background research that discussed multiple issues surrounding adoption and implementation of NGS simultaneously, highlighted the perspective of several stakeholders, were written in English and published no longer than 10 years ago, resulting in a set of 106 papers.

2.2. Scenario Drafting

Using all the gathered background information, we drafted one baseline

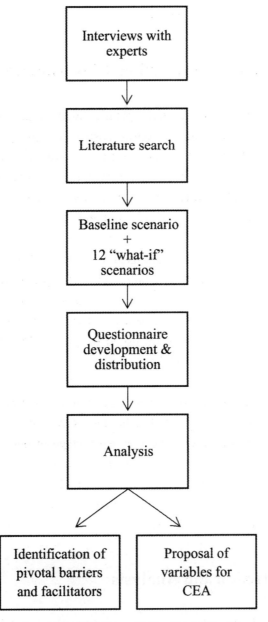

Figure 1. Overview of methodology. CEA = Cost-effectiveness analysis.

scenario describing the diffusion of NGS gene panels for personalized cancer treatment in general and twelve "what if" scenario deviations, which represent developments that may positively or negatively affect the speed of diffusion. Next, we drafted a questionnaire to elicit expert opinion on the specifics and likelihood of our "what-if" scenarios.

2.3. Questionnaire Construction & Distribution

First, forty-one questions were specifically designed to elicit quantitative answers in order to use our data in future cost-effectiveness modeling. Since we are planning to perform such modeling for at least colorectal cancer (CRC), non-small cell lung cancer (NSCLC) and melanoma, we often posed questions for each patient population separately. Input from Netherlands Cancer Institute (NKI) employees was used to prevent ambiguity in language.

Next, subsets of questions were used to construct three questionnaires (Additional file 1), each one specifically tailored to the expertise of physicians, biologists or policy workers. All versions were accompanied by the same cover letter providing background on NGS gene panels and explaining the purpose of our research. At the end, respondents were asked to rate the likelihood of the twelve scenarios on a scale from 0%–100%.

The questionnaires were distributed via email to a sample of NKI employees and external (partly international) stakeholders. Given the complexity of NGS-based diagnostics and in view of the very early stage of development and uncertainty surrounding clinical utility, we decided to focus on technical experts and clinicians first. External recipients had been in previous contact with the hospital or were selected because of published work on related matters. After a week, a reminder was sent to non-responders.

2.4. Data Collection and Analysis

A database of respondents answers was created using Adobe Acrobat X Pro and variation among expert opinions was assessed visually using colored 2D-dotplots as well as by descriptive statistics using IBM SPSS statistics. If answers were illegible these were excluded from our analysis and we also assessed whether (missing) values could be attributed to a certain respondent subgroup (e.g. profession, specialization, internal/external).

2.5. Consent Statement

This study was made possible by elicitation of expert' opinion via a questionnaire. The procedure was verified with the protocol review committee. Participation was on voluntary basis and filled-in questionnaires were anonymized prior to analysis. Upon invitation, experts were informed that their answers would be used anonymously to improve scenarios. No patients nor children, parents or guardians were involved.

2.6. Ethics Statement

According to institutional guidelines, it was verified with the protocol review committee that no ethical review nor consent was needed for this study.

3. Results

Questions posed in our survey often relate to several scenarios simultaneously, therefore we have clustered results into the following domains: social factors; technical factors; market access; clinical utility & evidence generation and reimbursement. For every domain we first report the estimated likelihood of scenario occurrence in percentages (**Table 2**) and next we discuss our findings on associated parameters (**Table 3**) and their relevance for cost effectiveness modeling. Summarizing these findings, we have labeled a scenario as a potential facilitator or barrier. All scores are represented as mean results ± standard deviation. In some cases absolute numbers are mentioned to depict clear disagreement among respondents.

3.1. Respondent Characteristics

In total, 29 questionnaires were completed by 14 physicians (specialized in general oncology, pulmonology, dermatology or pathology), 11 biologists (research and diagnostics), three policy workers and one epidemiologist; 12 from within and 17 from outside the NKI (**Table 1**).

Table 1. Respondent characteristics.

Profession		Respondents (n)	
		NKI	External
Physicians	Oncologist	5	4
	Other[a]	4	1
Biologist	Research	2	5
	Diagnostics	0	4
Policy		0	3
Epidemiologist		1	0
Total		12	17

Respondent specifics are described here, distinguishing between Netherlands Cancer Institute employees (NKI) and external respondents. 4 respondents were situated outside the Netherlands.[a] Other: specializations beyond medical oncology included pathology (2), pulmonology (1), dermatology (1) or surgery (1).

3.2. Social Factors

The likelihood of scenario 1 occurrence within 5 years, in which patients will be interested in NGS panels and will demand lots of information on this molecular approach was estimated at 66.5% (±28.1) (**Table 2**).

When presented questions related to this "what-if" scenario, clinicians among respondents estimated that this will entail 65.3% (±32.1) of patients suffering from metastatic cancer, compared to 28.3% (±29.2) of patients with non-metastasized disease (**Table 3**). Respondents whom themselves are skeptical about using NGS for adjuvant treatment, estimated larger differences between the former two patient groups (Additional file 2). Additionally, they felt that 78.2% (±16.1) and 41.5% (±26.6) of those patients respectively would be willing to enroll in a clinical trial on a new targeted therapy. The number of extra minutes during a patient's first consult to adequately inform them about NGS-based genetic testing was thought to lie around 13.2 (±12.4) minutes. Physicians themselves likely require extra education on NGS as well, estimated at 25.1 (±26.1) hours.

Scenario 2, also related to social acceptability, described a situation in which physicians will remain unconvinced of the clinical benefit of large scale sequencing.

Table 2. Baseline-and what-if scenarios.

Baseline scenario: "Within 5–10 years, NGS gene panels will become common practice for personalized treatment in oncology"

Domain	What-if scenarios (likelihood ± SD)	Effect	Barrier/ facilitator
Social	1. Patient perspective (66.5 ± 28.1; n = 13) Patients will demand lots of information on NGS-based panels, but will nevertheless be very interested in using them. 2. Medical professional perspective (16.5 ± 8.8; n = 10 and 64.0 ± 8.9; n = 5) Medical professionals remain unconvinced of the clinical benefit that can be gained using NGS-panels and targeted therapy.	Higher uptake and more compliance	Pivotal facilitators
Technical	3. Organization (84.4 ± 18.5; n = 25) The time required for preparation, NGS and analysis of a biopsy will decrease so that patients will receive results within ten days after biopsy. 4. FF versus FFPE (86.8 ± 13.1; n = 11 and 16.2 ± 9.4; n = 13) If reliable sequencing results can only be obtained by using FF tissue, the use of NGS-based panels will remain limited.	Higher uptake and less failures	
Reimbursement	5. Reimbursement (40.3 ± 24.1; n = 18) A 'minimal requirements' agreement between institutes developing NGS-based gene panels has resulted in national reimbursement policy of such panels.	Less uptake	Pivotal barriers
Clinical utility and evidence generation	6. Clinical Utility (50.4 ± 31.4; n = 25) Demonstrating clinical utility of NGS-panels will take at least a couple more years, adoption of this technology will only succeed once that point is reached. 7. Actionable targets (55.2 ± 23.7; n = 26) The number of mutations identified by NGS panels that can actually be targeted by therapy, remains limited. 8. Off-label prescription (49.2 ± 31.1; n = 18) The medical community becomes more lenient towards off-label treatment. 9. Revised evidence generation (65.5 ± 27.9; n = 29) Evidence from less time-consuming clinical studies than RCT III, will be considered valid to include new targets in NGS-based gene panels	No improved survival and slow release of new target/therapy combinations	

Market access	10. Competition from a different field (45.0 ± 21.7; n = 25) Another type of technology enters the Dutch healthcare, decreasing the popularity of NGS-based gene panels.	Less uptake
	11. Competition within the field (64.2 ± 21.9; n = 12) Another NGS-based panel outcompetes the NKI-panel, regardless of its additional features.	
	12. Intellectual property (45.6 ± 28.7; n = 25) Competitors offering NGS-based panels will be reluctant to share new biological insights generated by NGS-panels with each other, thereby decelerating the improvement of clinical utility for patients.	

Twelve potential deviations from a baseline scenario in which NGS-based gene panels are implemented in clinical oncology. Respondents were asked to rate the likelihood of their occurrence on a scale from 0%–100%. Since several scenarios were presented to relevant professions only, combined with some missing values, the number of respondents per scenario varied

The majority of respondents (10 out of 15) believed this scenario has a 16.5% (±8.8) chance of occurring, while some (5/15) believed 64.0% (±8.9) to be a more realistic number (**Table 2**).

Detailed questions on scenario 2 revealed that respondents estimate 84.9% (±23.6) of physicians to adopt NGS gene panels if such panels have at least been validated by a phase 3 randomized controlled trial (**Table 3**). However, estimates of adoption decline in case of lower level studies (e.g. 62.3% ±20.3 for a prospective observational study; 39.6% ±22.6 for a retrospective observational study; 16.7% ±8.6 for lower levels of evidence). 39% of respondents themselves believe that NGS gene panels should only be offered to patients with advanced disease, but an equal percentage believe NGS should already be offered as an adjuvant solution. Others (22%) found level of evidence, toxicity and benefit the most important indicators for use, irrespective of stage.

3.3. Technical Factors

Respondents rated the likelihood of scenario 3, describing a maximum of ten days turn-over time from biopsy to results, at 84.4% (±18.5). When asked for their own preferences, a maximum of 17.8 (±21.3) days was indicated (**Table 2**).

Table 3. Parameters and corresponding questions.

Domain	Parameter	Q	Average ±SD
Social factors	Patients interested in NGS (prim/meta)	Q1	28.3 ± 29.2/65.3 ± 32.1
	Patients interested in trial (prim/meta)	Q2	41.5 ± 26.6/78.2 ± 16.1
	Consult extra (min)	Q3	13.2 ± 12.4
	Education extra (hrs.)	Q10	25.1 ± 26.1
	NGS Adoption given: RCT3	Q6	84.9 ± 23.6
	Pros. observational		62.3 ± 20.3
	Retro. observational		39.6 ± 22.6
	Lower levels		16.7 ± 8.6
Technical Factors	Max. turnover rate (days)	Q9	17.8 ± 21.3
	Dutch institutes able to supply FF	Q16	50.5 ± 36.5
	Min. sensitivity/specificity	Q15	90.5 ± 5.7/89.0 ± 9.7
	Max. failure rate	Q17	18.4 ± 20.1
	Re-biopsydecline: CRC	Q18	33.3 ± 23.6
	NSCLC		30.0 ± 22.9
	Melanoma		8.5 ± 5.9
	Re-biopsyunfeasible: CRC	Q19	19.2 ± 11.1
	NSCLC		22.9 ± 16.0
	Melanoma		9.3 ± 10.0
	Min. storage tissue (yrs.)	Q14	24.2 ± 22.1
	Min. storage NGS results (yrs.)	Q13	22.6 ± 21.4
Reimbursement	Pay extra for NGS panel (euro)	Q12	380.8 ± 316.6
	Probability opt for NGS panel if €1000	Q40	44.0 ± 44.0
Clinical utility and evidence generation	Nb. Targets per patient	Q37	6.6 ± 7.5
	Nb. new therapies in five years	Q29	22.5 ± 20.4
	Off-label therapy required	Q22	30.2 ± 26.5
	Physicians willing to prescribe off-label	Q23	44.6 ± 31.6
	Probability reimbursement off-label	Q27	28.0 ± 32.0
	Lenient towards off-label (yrs.)	Q26	9.8 ± 12.4
Market access	Min. years NGS common practice	Q33	6.5 ± 6.3
	Min. years competition other technology	Q35	9.6 ± 5.5

Depicted are the mean results (percentages unless stated otherwise) and standard deviations on quantitative parameters, in order of appearance. Column Q refers to the number of the corresponding questions in the questionnaire (Additional file 1). NGS next generation sequencing, Prim primary cancer, Meta metastatic cancer, FF fresh frozen [tissue preservation].

NGS gene panels can vary in all kind of characteristics, including what type of tissue preservation (formalin-fixed paraffin embedded-FFPE-or fresh frozen-FF-biopsies) they can handle. When presented with scenario 4, in which only FF tissue would be able to generate reliable sequencing results, some respondents (11 out of 24) estimated a 86.8% (±13.1) chance that this requirement will limit NGS adoption by medical professionals. Others (13 out of 24) found scenario 4 less likely to occur and estimated its likeliness to occur at 16.2% (±9.4). This distinction was also found among physicians alone: 8 out of 11 estimated a 83,8% (±19.2) chance of scenario occurrence, while the remaining opted for a 14,0% (±8.9) chance.

An important parameter for scenario 4, the percentage of Dutch institutes capable of supplying FF biopsies, was estimated at 50.5% (±36.5) (**Table 3**). Other questions into technical parameters that may affect both scenarios 3 and 4 revealed preferences for a minimal sensitivity/specificity of 90.5% (±5.7) and 89.0% (±9.7) respectively and a maximally acceptable failure rate (e.g. in case of too little DNA available) of 18.4% (±20.1). If re-biopsy would be required to obtain reliable results, respondents expect a percentage of patients to decline (eg. 33.3% ±23.6 in CRC; 30.0% ±22.9 in NSCLC; 8.5% ±5.9 in melanoma). Re-biopsy may even be unfeasible in a certain number of cases (19.2% ±11.1 in CRC; 22.9% ±16.0 in NSCLC; 9.3% ±10.0 in melanoma). Respondents believed that residual tissue should be stored for minimally 24.2 (±22.1) years. For future reference, sequencing results carrying information beyond the scope of current treatment should be kept for at least 22.6 years (±21.4).

3.4. Reimbursement

Scenario 5 depicts a situation where opposing institutes draw up a "minimal requirements" agreement on NGS gene panels and consequently a national reimbursement policy is implemented. Likelihood of scenario occurrence was estimated at 40.3% (±24.1) (**Table 2**).

Addressing a related parameter, respondents felt that NGS-panel-compared to single gene diagnostics would justify €380.8 (±316.6) additionally (**Table 3**). The probability to opt for an FFPE-based NGS panel if priced at €1000 averaged at 44% (±44.0).

3.5. Clinical Utility & Evidence Generation

Scenario 6, in which the route to demonstrating clinical utility still requires several years, was assessed 50.4% (±31.4) likely. Scenario 7 described a theoretical limiting factor to that route, in which the number of therapeutic targets identified by NGS panels would remain limited. The chance of this scenario occurring was estimated at 55.2% ±23.7 (**Table 2**).

Related to these scenarios, several parameters estimates were elicited (**Table 3**). Presented with the characteristics of the NKI-panel, respondents would expect to find 6.6 (±7.5) potential targets per patient. Also, they believe that in the following 5 years, 22.5 (±20.4) novel and approved targeted therapies (for new targets) will hit the market. Furthermore, they estimated that in 30.2% (±26.5) of cases using NGS, a target for which off-label treatment is available will be identified.

Scenario 8, in which the medical community would become more lenient towards prescribing off-label medication, was found 49.2% (±31.1) likely to occur (**Table 2**).

Under circumstances as described above, respondents expect 44.6% (±31.6) of physicians to be willing to prescribe off-label therapy (regardless of reimbursement) (**Table 3**). The propensity of respondents themselves to do so varied given the level of evidence supporting a target/therapy combination and stage of disease (**Table 4**). They felt that the chance of reimbursement for off-label treatment is low (28.0% ± 0.32%) and that the medical community will minimally need 9.8 (±12.4) years to become more lenient towards it.

Some respondents pointed out that targeted therapies require novel/alternative study designs for evidence generation. Respondents estimated that there is a 65.5% (±27) chance that revised evidence generation will be generally accepted, as described in scenario 9 (**Table 2**).

Roughly half of respondents themselves consider evidence from prospective-(46%) or retrospective observational studies (50%) valid to base medical decisions on. 14% chose the option "Lower levels of evidence" and 18% ticked

Table 4. Respondent propensity to prescribe off-label therapy.

Level of evidence	Adjuvant (n = 16)	Metastatic (n = 26)
At least validated by an RCT3 in another type of cancer and an observational study for the type cancer you intent to treat	6/16; 37.5%	7/26; 27.0%
At least validated by a RCT3 for another type of cancer	2/16; 12,5%	3/26; 11.5%
At least validated by an observational study in another type of cancer	4/16; 25%	6/26; 23.1%
Other, namely never	2/16; 12.5%	1/26; 0.04%
Other, namely descriptive:	"tissue-based labeling should be changed" (1/16; 6.25%), "Bayesian approach should be used" (1/16; 6.25%)	"only as part of a trial" (2/26; 0.08%) and 7 individual comments (0,04%each) including "Based on RCTII data", "Based on RCTII with molecularly selected patients", "Casuistic evidence from other disease entities", "Any time", "tissue-based labeling should be changed", "Bayesian approach should be used", "Depending on costs"

Respondents were presented with the following hypothetical situation: "A NGS gene panel was only able to identify one molecular target in a patient's tumour. However, the corresponding targeted therapy has not been registered for that type of cancer yet, thus off-label treatment may be the only option" They were then asked based on what level of evidence and stage of disease they would prescribe the therapy. The question regarding the metastatic setting was asked in all versions of the questionnaire, while the question for the adjuvant setting was only posed in the physicians and policy version. Therefore, the number of respondents per column differs.

"Other" which some supplemented with suggestions such as basket-and adaptive protocols as acceptable designs. 72% of respondents rated the alternative endpoint progression-free-survival valid to base medical decisions upon, compared to 52% in case of time-to-progression, −41% in case of disease-free-survival (41%) and −41% in case of response rate.

3.6. Market Access

Respondents estimated a 45.0% (±21.7) chance that an alternative technology to NGS will enter the market and decrease NGS popularity, as described in scenario 10. Scenario 11, in which NGS competitors' propensity to share generated biological insight was described as reluctant, was deemed 45.6% (±28.7) to occur (**Table 2**).

Addressing parameters specific to these scenarios, respondents estimated that it will minimally take 6.5 (±6.3) years before NGS gene panels become widely implemented in the clinic and that another technology is likely to take over the market within 9.6 (±5.5) years (**Table 3**). According to some (60%), acquired resistance to therapy may be a limiting factor of adoption of NGS. A competing technology will probably still be based on sequencing, but complemented by proteomics/immunotherapy or diagnostics on circulating tumor cells. Novel drug sensitivity assays were also mentioned.

4. Discussion

Using scenario drafting on the basis of expert elicitation, we have been able to identify a number of critical factors that may affect the speed of adoption of NGS gene panels in clinical oncology as well as variables that may be incorporated in future cost-effectiveness modeling.

The outlook of patients and physicians towards this novel technology appears to be one of the pivotal facilitators of adoption of NGS panels in the clinic. Although not asked to patients themselves, our results indicated that physicians estimation was that patients' perspective on NGS panels is likely to be highly positive (~66.5%), coinciding with studies on pharmacogenomics/genetics that did include patients in their study population[15][16]. Popularity amongst patients will probably be positively related to stage of disease, although this distinction seemed related to respondents' personal opinions. Thus, further investigations into patients' perspective may be advisable, both in general as well as to confirm the validity of respondents' estimations. Nonetheless, our results do imply that social factors among patients are likely favorable towards the implementation of NGS panels in the clinic.

We also found that most physicians (~85%) are probably willing to use NGS panels in clinical practice, given validated evidence from RCTs. Lower levels of evidence are likely to have a large negative impact on adoption rates. Naturally, such stringent levels of evidence come at a cost. However, opting for a prospective observational study compared to a RCT might save time, money and effort, while still convincing the majority (~60%) of physicians. Importantly, the average physician will require ~25h of extra training on pharmacogenomics before being able to use NGS panels clinically. Thus, organizing educational activities will definitely be required prior to NGS implementation. Fortuitously, advancing physicians' knowledge on pharmacogenomics is likely to increase adoption rates even further, as previously stated by Stanek et al. (2012)[17]. Thus, while most physicians stand positive towards NGS, investing in the level of supporting evidence as well as education on NGS panels may even increase the speed of its diffusion.

Next to estimating that the adoption of NGS will benefit from current social perspectives, experts also found it highly feasible that analysis of biopsies can be performed within a clinically relevant timeframe of 10 days. Thus, achievability of timely logistics may also be labeled as a so-called facilitator of diffusion.

However, obtaining a biopsy in itself and whether acquired tissue will meet the criteria for NGS-based analysis may be troublesome on some occasions. While previous investigations have concluded that most European institutes are able to supply FF biopsies meeting standards for RNA/DNA analysis[9][18], our respondents' opinions regarding this matter varied extensively. Thus, obtaining and preserving such biopsies may still require a learning curve for a large number of hospitals and could potentially pose a barrier for widespread adoption of NGS panels. The 90.5% sensitivity, 89.0% specificity or 18.4% maximum failure rate described in this article may serve as a useful guideline during development regarding decisions on the trade-off between user-friendliness and publically desired technical specifications and as such, may help in increasing adoption rates.

One of the general barriers for NGS implementation and adoption includes low probability of reimbursement. This could pose a major barrier for implementation, since costs associated with NGS testing-while dropping-and targeted therapies themselves are still not affordable for patients themselves. According to our findings, even combined efforts to promote reimbursement policy are unlikely to succeed (~40.3%). Thus, the necessity to steer the development of such panels towards the most cost-effective solution, thereby increasing likelihood of reimbursement, is obvious and highlights the potential of early Technology Assessment. Furthermore, the probability to opt for an FFPE-based NGS panel if priced at €1000 was averaged at 44%. Recently, Kilambi and colleagues (2014) found that the willingness-to-pay (WTP) for accurate test information regarding colorectal cancer screening was approximately $1800[19]. Thus, it appears that WTP has a wide variance and could be interesting for further research.

Furthermore, demonstrating the effectiveness of guiding therapy via NGS panels also may pose a problem. While respondents expect to identify 6.6 molecular targets per patient, the number of actionable drug targets may actually remain limited. In 30.2% of cases, off-label prescription will be required, which most physicians would be willing to supply albeit depending on stage of disease and level of evidence. While perhaps helpful in some cases, these situations actually underline the need for accelerated evidence generation on drug efficacy as to increase the number of registered therapies on the market. Almost all of our respondents deemed lower levels of evidence than traditional RCTs valid to base medical decisions upon and without encouragement towards that direction, some even advocated the need for more flexible (eg. basket/adaptive protocols) and molecularly orientated designs. A recent review by Sargent and Korn (2014) affirmed that there has already been a major shift in the paradigm surrounding cancer clinical trial designs in the past decade, in which molecular classification is gaining in popularity[20]. Indeed, this topic is seldom discussed at scientific-meetings and in literature. Any such efforts are likely to benefit the clinical utility of NGS gene panels as well and may perhaps even be pivotal in their road to success.

Nonetheless, it will take approximately 6.5 years before NGS gene panels become common in clinical oncology and competition on the market can be expected to be fierce. Since our respondents believe that there is a considerable chance (45,0%) that another novel technology will rapidly become more popular, even within 9,6 years, the window of opportunity for NGS gene panels is small. Thus, timely reaching the market may be crucial for developers. We believe that our findings and suggestions can contribute to that process.

However, our results also face several limitations. Since NGS for diagnostics is rather complex to begin with, some topics such as data warehouse and

-integration, were not incorporated in our research yet as they require the in-depth expertise of completely different stakeholders. Some groups, such as patients, clinical geneticists, pharmaceutical companies or health insurers were not included in our study and should be approached in future research. Furthermore, our results are at risk for response bias, since respondents are likely to have an increased interest in NGS a priori. Since we decided not to focus on a particular NGS panel for the generalizability of our results, some questions elicited vastly different opinions or outcomes. Next to the response bias, there might also be a framing bias; a person's choice between alternatives depends on how these alternatives are framed. Although there has been a pilot series of 6 responders from different disciplines where we tested the wording in case of suggestiveness, it was not completely possible to prevent. In particular, scenarios were framed positively or negatively to evoke the responder to his or her opinion, yet this may have also led to suggestiveness of the response. Large standard deviations due to (un) intentional ambiguity in language or small sample size, disagreement or outliers can make it difficult to draw clear-cut conclusions.

5. Conclusions

To our notion, we are the first to methodologically assess NGS, mapping out both quantitative and qualitative aspects that may influence adoption of this novel technology in the clinic.

We believe our findings enable readers involved in NGS implementation to anticipate pivotal events of social, technical, clinical and financial nature (**Table 2**) and if applicable, alter their strategy to improve success. For instance, by meeting the technical specifications desired by physicians or opting for development of user-friendly FFPE-capable panels. Increasing adoption may also be achieved via hosting education events (**Table 5**). Perhaps even more important, will be to tackle anticipated barriers for adoption. For instance, further efforts will be required to accelerate, demonstrate and perhaps improve clinical utility of NGS panels (**Table 5**).

In addition, our drafted scenarios and estimates on accompanying parameters may be used for (the setup of) cost-effectiveness modeling (**Table 3**). Such

Table 5. Recommendations to promote adoption of NGS in clinical oncology.

Domain	Recommendation
Social	• Further investigate patients' perspective • Organize additional training on pharmacogenomics for physicians.
Technical	• Use desired technical specifications as a guideline for development of a NGS panel. • Develop user-friendly FFPE-capable NGS panels.
Reimbursement	• Further investigate willingness-to-pay • Set cost-effectiveness as a high priority to facilitate reimbursement.
Clinical utility and evidence generation	• Advocate novel evidence generation designs.
Market access	• Enter the market rapidly to maximize window of opportunity

FFPE fresh frozen paraffin embedded [tissue preservation].

data is a valuable starting-point at this early stage of development, since traditional resources of information are not yet available. Importantly, modeling outcomes alongside development could steer NGS towards the most optimal outcome. As reimbursement probability was also found to be low in our study, we believe such efforts should receive high priority.

To conclude, we have taken the first steps towards scientific input for reimbursement decisions, thereby potentially accelerating the route from bench-to-bedside.

6. Additional Files

Additional file 1: Questionnaire. Description: This is the full version of the questionnaire, as presented to physicians. Questions also posed in the biologists' version are marked by "Bio" and questions also posed in the policy version are marked by "Pol". (PDF 724 kb)

Additional file 2: Relationship between physicians' opinion on when to offer NGS to patients and their estimations on popularity of NGS among patients. Description: Depicted results correspond to questions 1 and 7 in the questionnaire (Additional file 1). Respondents' estimations on popularity of NGS among patients may have been biased by their own views (DOCX 12 kb)

7. Abbreviations

CRC: colorectal cancer; FF: fresh frozen; FFPE: formalin-fixed paraffin embedded; HTA: health technology assessment; NGS: next generation sequencing; NKI: Netherlands cancer institute; NSCLC: non-small cell lung cancer; RCT: randomized controlled trial; WTP: willingness-to-pay.

Competing Interests

Authors declare no conflict of interest regarding the work described in this manuscript.

Authors' Contributions

SJ held in-house interviews, designed the questionnaire, analyzed results and drafted the manuscript. VR held in-house interviews, supported development of the questionnaire, analyzed results and co-drafted the manuscript. VC helped to develop the questionnaire to elicit variables suitable for cost-effectiveness analysis, critically revised the manuscript and supervised the project. MvdH helped to develop the questionnaire, provided insights on results from a clinical viewpoint and critically revised the manuscript. WvH conceived the work, coordinated the project and helped drafting the manuscript. All authors read, revised and approved the manuscript.

Authors' Information

SJ is a master student with a background in molecular oncology as well as healthcare policy. VR has a PhD in health technology assessment. VC is an assistant professor in health economic modeling in cancer. MvdH is a chest physician specializing in oncology. WvH is a physician, professor in health technology assessment and member of the board of the NKI.

Acknowledgements

We would like to thank all respondents that took the time to fulfill and/or forward our questionnaire as well as Manuela Joore from the University of Maastricht and all NKI in-house experts for their constructive criticism on our work.

Source: Joosten S E P, Retèl V P, Coupé V M H, *et al*. Scenario drafting for early technology assessment of next generation sequencing in clinical oncology[J]. Bmc Cancer, 2016, 16(1):1–10.

References

[1]   Stratton MR, Campbell PJ, Futreal PA. The cancer genome. Nature. 2009; 458(7239):719–724. doi:10.1038/nature07943.

[2]   Diamandis M, White N, Yousef G. Personalized medicine: marking a new epoch in cancer patient management. Mol Cancer Res. 2010;8(9):1175–1187. doi:10.1158/ 1541-7786.mcr-10-0264.

[3]   Phillips KA, Ann Sakowski J, Trosman J, Douglas MP, Liang S-YY, Neumann P. The economic value of personalized medicine tests: what we know and what we need to know. Genet Med. 2014;16(3):251–257. doi:10.1038/gim.2013. 122.

[4]   Vrijenhoek T, Kraaijeveld K, Elferink M, De Ligt J, Kranendonk E, Santen G, *et al*. Next-generation sequencing-based genome diagnostics across clinical genetics centers: implementation choices and their effects. Eur J Hum Genet. 2015; 23(9):1270.

[5]   Green ED, Guyer MS. National Human Genome Research I. Charting a course for genomic medicine from base pairs to bedside. Nature. 2011; 470(7333):204–213. doi:10.1038/nature09764.

[6]   Institute of Medicine. Genome-Based Diagnostics. Demonstrating Clinical Utility in Oncology: Workshop Summary. National Academies Press (US). 2013.

[7]   Goodman C. Introduction to health technology assessment. Retrieved from United States National Library of Medicine, National Institutes of Health website: http:// www.nlm.nih.gov/nichsr/hta101/HTA_101_FINAL_7-23-14.pdf 2004. Accessed 28th May 2015.

[8]   Douma K, Karsenberg K, Hummel M, Bueno-de-Mesquita J, Van Harten W. Methodology of constructive technology assessment in health care. Int J Technol Assess Health Care. 2007; 23(2):162–168. doi:10.1017/ S0266462307070262.

[9]   Bueno-de-Mesquita J, Van Harten W, Retel V, van't Veer L, Van Dam F, Karsenberg K, *et al*. Use of 70-gene signature to predict prognosis of patients with node-negative breast cancer: a prospective community-based feasibility study (RASTER). Lancet Oncol. 2007; 8(12):1079–1087. doi:10.1016/ S1470-2045(07)70346-7.

[10] Retèl VP, Bueno-de-Mesquita JM, Hummel MJ, van de Vijver MJ, Douma KF, Kar-

senberg K, *et al.* Constructive Technology Assessment (CTA) as a tool in coverage with evidence development: the case of the 70-gene prognosis signature for breast cancer diagnostics. Int J Technol Assess Health Care. 2009; 25(1):73–83. doi:10. 1017/s0266462309090102.

[11] Royal Dutch Shell Company. 40 years of shell scenarios (anniversary brochure) 2013.

[12] Wack P. Scenarios: unchartered waters ahead. Harv Bus Rev. 1985; 63(5):73–89.

[13] Wack P. Scenarios: shooting the rapids. Harv Bus Rev. 1985; 63(6):139–150.

[14] Retèl VP, Joore MA, Linn SC, Rutgers EJ, Van Harten WH. Scenario drafting to anticipate future developments in technology assessment. BMC Res Notes. 2012; 5:442. doi:10.1186/1756-0500-5-442.

[15] Gray SW, Hicks-Courant K, Lathan CS, Garraway L, Park ER, Weeks JC. Attitudes of patients with cancer about personalized medicine and somatic genetic testing. J Clin Oncol. 2012; 8(6):329. doi:10.1200/jop.2012.000626.

[16] Henneman L, Vermeulen E, Van El C, Claassen L, Timmermans D, Cornel M. Public attitudes towards genetic testing revisited: comparing opinions between 2002 and 2010. Eur J Hum Genet. 2013; 21(8):793–799. doi:10.1038/ ejhg.2012.271.

[17] Stanek E, Sanders C, Taber K, Khalid M, Patel A, Verbrugge R, *et al.* Adoption of pharmacogenomic testing by US physicians: results of a nationwide survey. Clin Pharmacol Ther. 2012;91(3):450–458. doi:10.1038/clpt.2011.306.

[18] Mook S, Bonnefoi H, Pruneri G, Larsimont D, Jaskiewicz J, Sabadell MD, *et al.* Daily clinical practice of fresh tumour tissue freezing and gene expression profiling; logistics pilot study preceding the MINDACT trial. Eur J Cancer. 2009; 45(7):1201-1208. doi:10.1016/j.ejca.2009.01.004.

[19] Kilambi V, Johnson F, González J, Mohamed A. Valuations of genetic test information for treatable conditions: the case of colorectal cancer screening. Value Health. 2014; 17(8):838–845. doi:10.1016/j.jval.2014.09.001.

[20] Sargent DJ, Korn EL. Decade in review-clinical trials: Shifting paradigms in cancer clinical trial design. Nat Rew Clin Oncol. 2014; 11(11):625–626.doi:10. 1038/ nrclinonc.2014.167.

Chapter 24

Mathematical Models for Translational and Clinical Oncology

**Ralf Gallasch, Mirjana Efremova, Pornpimol Charoentong,
Hubert Hackl, Zlatko Trajanoski**

Biocenter, Division of Bioinformatics, Innsbruck Medical University, Innrain 80,
6020 Innsbruck, Austria

Abstract: In the context of translational and clinical oncology, mathematical models can provide novel insights intotumor-related processes and can support clinical oncologists in the design of the treatment regime, dosage, schedule, toxicity and drug-sensitivity. In this review we present an overview of mathematical models in this field beginning with carcinogenesis and proceeding to the different cancer treatments. By doing so we intended to highlight recent developments and emphasize the power of such theoretical work. We first highlight mathematical models for translational oncology comprising epidemiologic and statistical models, mechanistic models for carcinogenesis and tumor growth, as well as evolutionary dynamics models which can help to describe and overcome a major problem in the clinic: therapy resistance. Next we review models for clinical oncology with a special emphasis on therapy including chemotherapy, targeted therapy, radiotherapy, immunotherapy and interaction of cancer cells with the immune system. As evident from the published studies, mathematical modeling and computational simulation provided valuable insights into the molecular mechanisms of cancer, and can help to improve diagnosis and prognosis of the disease, and pinpoint novel therapeutic targets.

1. Introduction

Cancer is still one of the leading causes of death in the world and major efforts have been undertaken to improve diagnosis and therapy of common cancer types. Recently developed technologies (*i.e.* next generation sequencing) give us unprecedented opportunities to study individual cancer samples at the molecular level and to identify genomic variants and rearrangements[1]. This information will build the basis for the stratification of patients, and for personalized or precision medicine. The increasing complexity of the generated data utilizing various high-throughput technologies for characterizing the genome, epigenome, transcriptome, proteome, metabolome, and interactome pose considerable challenges and therefore plethora of bioinformatics methods and tools for the analysis have been developed[2]. However, the real value of the disparate datasets can be truly exploited only if the data is integrated and will then enable one to comprehensively study molecular mechanisms of cancer cells.

One possibility for data integration is the use of mathematical models. Modeling has been successfully applied in physiology for many decades but only recently the quality and the quantity of biomolecular data became available for the development of causative and predictive models. Due to their importance in cancer mathematical models have also been in the focus of theoretical investigators. For example application of theoretical techniques and the postulation of the "two hit" hypothesis in the early 70s led to the identification of tumor-suppressor genes[3]. Later, in a landmark paper it was shown that cancer results from evolutionary processes occurring within the body[4].

In the context of translational (*i.e.* from bench to bedside, or in other words: transforming scientific discoveries arising from laboratory to clinical applications) and clinical oncology, mathematical models can provide novel insights into tumor growth and progression, into tumor-related processes such as angiogenesis, the immune response, and the interaction with the tumor microenvironment, and into the development of drug resistance. Furthermore, modeling can support the clinical oncologists in the design of the treatment regime, dosage, schedule, toxicity and drug-sensitivity. Common treatments against the different types of cancers include surgery, radiation therapy, chemotherapy, targeted therapy or combinations of those to limit the progression of malignant disease, eradicate tumor cells and prolong survival. The information gained from mathematical models can also help in the development and efficacy of clinical trials and treatment protocols, and can accelerate the progress of clinical research in fighting cancer.

To the best of our knowledge there is currently no review study on mathematical models focusing on translational and clinical oncology applications except for a similar attempt made by Swierniak *et al.*[5] few years ago. We therefore initiated this work to provide an overview of the field and stimulate the discussion and the development of novel models. While mechanistic models have proven extremely valuable and provided novel insights, there are not considered here and we refer the readers to recent reviews[6]–[8]. Given the wealth of published studies using mathematical models in cancer, we by no means intended to provide a comprehensive picture. Rather, we selected several topics we believe are of relevance for the readers. Wherever possible, we refer to additional reviews in order to guide interested researchers.

We first highlight mathematical models for translational oncology comprising epidemiologic and statistical models, mechanistic models for carcinogenesis and tumor growth, as well as evolutionary dynamics models[9], which can help to describe and overcome a major problem in the clinic: therapy resistance. Next we review models for clinical oncology. It should be noted that a survey of application of modeling results in clinics was beyond the scope of this review. Rather, we provide an overview of the models with a special emphasis on therapy including chemotherapy, targeted therapy, radiotherapy, immunotherapy and interaction of cancer cells with the immune system. **Table 1** shows the specific categories and the publications used in this work.

1.1. Mathematical Models for Translational Oncology

1.1.1. Carcinogenesis and Tumor-Growth Models

Early models that aimed to explain the dynamics of cancer progression were

Table 1. Categories and mathematical models in translational and clinical oncology reviewed in this paper.

Translational oncology	Clinical oncology
Biological processes	Treatment options
Carcinogenesis	Chemotherapy
[3][10]–[17]	[61]–[70]
Tumor-growth	Targeted therapy
[18]–[27]	[58][72][73][75]–[78]
Clonal evolution	Radiotherapy
[37][38][41]–[46]	[79]–[81]
Therapy resistance	Tumor immune-cell interaction/immunotherapy
[47]–[59]	[82]–[88]

based on experimental and epidemiological data, which indicated that the cancer incidence is often rapidly increased with age and simple patterns could be observed at the population level. Fisher and Hollomon[10] presented a multicellular model in which mutations occur in different cells within the same cell population and only the combination of all mutations leads to cancer development. As an alternative to this theory, Nordling[11] suggested that mutations must occur sequentially in the same cell for transformation into cancer cell.

Most mathematical models of cancer progression descend from Armitage and Doll's[12] multistage theory, which include major concepts for how to think about incidence, carcinogenesis, and progression. The theory states that carcinogenesis progresses through series of genomic alterations in a single cell and the age-specific incidence of cancers is predicted to increase with a power of age that is one less than the number of alterations. Two other studies, using data comparing inherited and non-inherited cases in colon cancer[13] and retinoblastoma[3], provided additional empirical evidence for the multistage theory. Knudson used a statistical analysis of the incidence of retinoblastoma in children to explain the role of tumor suppressor genes in sporadic and inherited cancers. This work was later extended to a two-stage stochastic model for the process of cancer initiation and progression[14], which lead to important subsequent work[15][16] that helped with characterization of other suppressor genes such as APC in colon cancer and TP53, which is mutated in several human tumors.

Even though these models provided accurate descriptions of cancer incidence data, they were unable to relate the data with the functional changes associated with tumor progression. Since then the understanding of the molecular mechanisms underlying tumor initiation and progression has improved[17] and mechanistic models that use biological knowledge and biophysical laws to quantify and predict cancer progression were developed.

The growth and development of solid tumors occurs in two stages-avascular and vascular. The early spatio-temporal models[18][19] of avascular tumor growth describe the interactions between tumor cell population and nutrients and calculate the nutrient concentrations as a function of tumor spheroid radius that is changing due to the rate of cell proliferation. Significant progress was made with the development of new models[20][21] that introduced the interrelated concepts of cell movement and pressure.

Since tumor induced angiogenesis *i.e.* the growth of a network of blood vessels, is a crucial component of solid tumor growth, the basic models have been expanded to account for tumor growth during angiogenesis and the increase of tumor availability associated with the expanding vasculature. In order to make a transition from avascular to vascular growth, tumors may secrete diffusible substances called tumor angiogenic factors (TAF). The earliest continuum models of tumor angiogenesis[22] describe the growth of a capillary network in terms of capillary tip densities and capillary sprout densities in response to TAF. The mathematical models in angiogenesis have mostly focused on describing endothelial cell migration and proliferation through the extracellular matrix[23]–[27]. A comprehensive overview of models in this area can be found in[28]. Mathematical modeling of blood flow in tumor-induced capillary networks has been described in more recent studies[29]–[31].

The concept that the successful formation of a tumor depends on vascularization has resulted in developing cancer therapies designed to inhibit the tumor vasculature in order to deprive the tumor from oxygen and nutrients. Several models have focused on exploring the efficiency of such anti-angiogenic treatments[32]–[34]. Using methods of optimal control theory to analyze drug dosing and treatment strategies these studies showed that the combination with other forms of therapy would be beneficial.

1.1.2. Clonal Evolution Models and Therapy Resistance

An important conceptual breakthrough in understanding cancer lies in Darwinian and ecological theories: cancer progression is an evolutionary process that results from accumulation of genetic and epigenetic variations in somatic cells[35][36]. Experimental evidences and recent advances in genetic sequencing technologies that allowed identification of the genetic alterations in a cancer cell-have revealed the complexity and heterogeneity of cancer progression and have stimulated the use of evolutionary-based approaches in the study of cancer.

Several methods of population dynamics and evolutionary game theory were applied to account for the elementary principles of evolution that lead to tumor initiation and progression. In the earliest models, mutations accumulate in a population of constant or variable size, and they consider only one or two mutations[37][38]. Newer models are now being used to investigate how the sequence and timing of mutations and the environmental conditions influence tumor progression[39][40]. An in-depth review of models that describe the evolutionary dynamics of cancer can be found in[41].

Several studies have focused on the waiting time to cancer development, which may be defined as the time from the first presence of neoplasm, until a critical number of hits (driver mutations) are accumulated and initiate the growth of carcinoma. Beerenwinkel et al.[42] developed one of the first models that was based on genomic studies of colorectal cancer patients. They related the waiting time to the population size, mutation rate, and the advantage of the driver mutations and showed that selective advantage of mutations has the largest effect on the evolutionary dynamics of tumorigenesis. In a similar manner, Bozic et al.[43], by fitting their model to glioblastoma and pancreatic cancer data, estimated that driver mutations give an average fitness advantage of 0.4%.

Another characteristic of evolutionary processes is the influence of the local cellular environment on the tumor progression. The progress of tumor is characterized not only by the genetic and epigenetic changes accumulating in the cells, but also by the dynamic interactions between cells within the tumor and between the cells and the constantly changing microenvironment. The microenvironment provides a selective fitness landscape that includes competing for limited resources and active intracellular (initiation of cell proliferation and cell death) and extra-cellular control mechanisms (the immune system) that aim to restore homeostasis.

There are several studies that utilize mathematical modeling to predict and quantify the interactions of the tumor cells with the surrounding environment during tumor progression[44][45]. Gatenby et al.[46] developed a model of carcinogenesis according to which the tumor cells have to overcome six microenvironment barriers that appear as tumor cells proliferate. They proposed that the nature and sequence of the alterations during carcinogenesis are determined by the specific microenvironmental properties that prevent proliferation within changing adaptive landscapes.

An important clinical problem in cancer research that can be analyzed using modeling techniques is the development of resistance to targeted therapies. Resistance to drugs may develop as a consequence of genetic events such as point mutations or gene amplifications. The emergence of resistance to therapy as a result from a single mutational effect has been first introduced in a model of Coldman and Goldie[47]. More recent studies have also used point mutations to explain the evolutionary dynamics of drug resistant cancer cells[48]–[51]. Other models studied gene amplification as one of the mechanisms that has a strong influence on the evolution of drug resistance[52]–[56].

Foo et al.[57] designed a methodology that can be used to investigate optimal drug dosing schedules to avoid resistance conferred by one (epi) genetic mutation. In a recent study, Diaz et al.[58] showed that tumors became resistant to anti-EGFR antibodies as a result of emergence of resistance mutations in KRAS and other genes that were present in clonal subpopulation within the tumors before the initiation of the treatment. Analyzing data from 20 melanoma patients who received targeted therapy, Bozic et al.[59] found that simultaneous administration of two drugs is much more effective than sequential therapy. The improved understanding of the evolutionary dynamics of cancer provided by these models can have practical implications in the design and administration of new cancer therapeutics.

In summary, using the overwhelming amount of generated knowledge in tumor biology, mathematical modelers have succeeded in formalizing this knowledge and make it usable for simulations. Moreover, the published models represent a unique basis for testing novel hypotheses which are otherwise difficult or even impossible to test. For example, it is very difficult to obtain samples from early cancer stages or longitudinal samples in order to study the development of tumor heterogeneity. The models presented above enable researchers to address questions which were previously not possible and by using iterative cycles of simulations and experimentation ultimately lead to novel knowledge (**Figure 1**). Moreover, the maturity of the tools and the availability of data in public databases are additionally supporting the translation of this knowledge into clinical practice.

1.2. Mathematical Models for Clinical Oncology

1.2.1. Chemotherapy and Targeted Therapy

Chemotherapy is widely used therapy against cancer. Proliferating cells undergo different phases during the cell cycle including DNA replication and cell division and different chemotherapeutic compounds are affecting cells in different

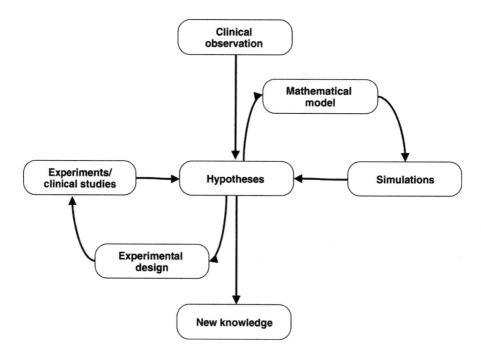

Figure 1. Cycles of experiments and modeling for gaining new knowledge. Experiments and clinical studies are closely coupled with mathematical modeling and simulations and require multiple cycles of iterations.

phases. The greatest challenge associated with chemotherapy is that not only cancer cells but also normal dividing cells are affected. In contrast, targeted cancer therapy[60] is aimed at specific molecular targets and is therefore more effective and has fewer side effects.

Fister *et al.*[61] developed a model that try to solve the problem of maximizing the effect on cancer cells but also maximizing the survival of the host cells. The mathematical model shows that if shorter periods of treatment are used it is possible to use higher doses of the drug and destroy more cancer cells without causing excess damage to the host cells. A more complex model is the cellular automaton model of Byrne *et al.*[62]. It is a multi-scale model that has a vascular layer, a cellular layer and an intracellular layer. With this model it is possible to get detailed spatio-temporal information about the tumor and the healthy tissue. In general three results are possible with the model; the tumor is eliminated, the tumor continues grow, or an oscillation. It is possible to combine different treatments in one model. The model of de Pillis *et al.*[63] based on a previous model[64] combines different treatments and shows that if the chemotherapy is stopped a system with a undetectable tumor can return to a high tumor state.

The combination of different treatments is one possibility to eliminate the patient's tumor. Jackson *et al.*[65] introduced two different types of cells and investigated the tumors response to different chemotherapeutic strategies. It was possible to estimate the largest size of a tumor that can be eradicated by a bolus injection. With only one cell population the results of bolus and continues drug were similar. With two populations, one of them drug resistant, the continuous infusion increased the time to cure. This indicates that it is important to tailor treatment strategies.

Another interesting aspect is the use of growth factors in the model from Panetta and Adam[66]. They showed that the use of growth factors in their model increases the cell killing up to 20%. Based on the model of Anderson and Chaplain[27] McDougall[29] developed a model where the blood viscosity, pressure drop and mean capillary radii can be varied of the surrounding vessels of a solid tumor can be analyzed. The model shows that if there are highly interconnected vessels around the tumor there is a low drug delivery to the tumor itself. It shows that it is important to consider the vasculature around the tumor to find the optimal chemotherapy strategy.

The strategy of chemotherapy in combination with other treatments is being increasingly used. Powathil addressed this in recent publications[67]–[69] and showed ways to simulate and improve protocols of chemotherapy. It was demonstrated that the cytotoxic effect is dependent on many factors like timing of the drug delivery, time delay between the doses, heterogeneities of the cell cycle, the spatial distribution of the tumor and the surrounding microenvironment. It is noteworthy that these issues have been also investigated in older studies, e.g. using models of phase-specificity of chemotherapeutic drugs published in the 1990s[70]. In this section different methods were shown to model chemotherapy and effects that can lead to a better treatment strategy.

Most targeted cancer therapies use monoclonal antibodies directed against tumor-specific surface proteins or small-molecule drugs against intracellular targets (e.g. tyrosin kinases)[71]. Billy et al.[72] developed a model that simulates a treatment on the angiogenesis of tumors by gene therapy. The gene therapy is delivered by adenoviruses and influences, the antagonist of vascular endothelial growth factor, endostatin. The simulation showed that there is a critical treatment dose which is important to improve the efficacy.

TGF-β is a cytokine that has an immunosuppressive effect. In the model of Kirschner et al.[73] it was shown that a treatment with initial delivery of double stranded RNA into tumor cells that is cut by the enzyme Dicer into 21–23 segments known as siRNA inhibits TGF-β production and leads to a controlled oscillatory tumor behavior. Using a combination of experimental data and a mathematical model about the resistance against the monoclonal antibody panitumumab based on the Luria-Delbrück model[74], Diaz et al.[58] tested the development of mutations conferring resistance to the antibody. The simulation results suggested a combination of therapies where at least two pathways will be required. The use of ex-vivo activated alloreactive cytotoxic-T-lymphocytes (CTL) is another possibility to direct target the tumor. Kronik et al.[75] developed a mathematical model to investigate the effect of directly administered CTL to glioblastomas. They showed that most sensitive parameters were the death rate of CTLs, the initial size of the tumor and the maximal growth rate.

Nanda et al.[76] developed a mathematical model simulating the drug imatinib mesylate that was approved in 2002 by the FDA for use in newly diagnosed cases of chronic myelogenous leukemia. The results show that a high dosing level from the beginning is optimal. Another interesting aspect of targeted therapy is the use of oncolytic viruses. Wein *et al.*[77] showed in their model that a single intratumoral injection in a solid tumor is not enough to effectively spread the virus. Also important is the suppression of the immunemediated clearance of the virus. In the work of Mok *et al.*[78] two additional modifications are shown through mathematical modeling of herpes simplex viruses first the decreasing of the binding affinity of the virus and second the effective diffusion coefficient of the virus through degradation of the tumor extracellular matrix.

1.2.2. Radiotherapy

The aim of radiotherapy is to destroy the tumor cells but not the host cells. This is possible if the tumor cells are more sensitive to irradiation than the host cells. Mathematical modeling can show strategies and improve treatment protocols to obtain an optimal patient treatment. In this sense Rockne *et al.*[79] present a model to investigate the response to various schedules and dose distribution on a virtual tumor. The advantage in the mathematical simulation is that the effect of radiation can be observed continuously. The model suggests that a radiation dose on daily basis is more effective than several treatments per day.

Another important aspect is the general response of cells to radiation. Richard *et al.*[80] used a cellular automaton model to investigate these mechanisms after low doses of radiation. Enderling *et al.*[81] developed a model that simulates the recurrence after radiotherapy. In the 2D simulations it was shown that if premalignant cells reside in the breast post-surgery and survive radio-therapy this cells could be the reason for a recurrence.

1.2.3. Tumor Immune-Cell Interaction and Immunotherapy

The immune system plays an important role in tumor progression. Immune processes with different components like chemokines, cytokines or different cell types that work together are highly complex and intertwined. Mathematical modeling has already provided deeper insights and helped to get fundamental knowledge and improve patient's treatment. For example De Boer et al.[82] developed a detailed model where they were able to show tumor regression and tumor growth dependent on the antigenicity of tumor-immune interaction. Tumour-infiltrating cytotoxic lymphocytes (TICLs) play an important role in tumor-immune interaction. Matzavinos et al.[83] developed a spatio-temporal model to investigate the interaction of TICLs and tumors. It is possible to simulate the spatio-temporal dynamics of TICLs in a solid tumor. Kirschner et al.[84] developed a model that includes immunotherapy with cultured immune cells that have anti-tumor reactivity and additionally IL-2. In simulations a total eradiation of the tumor was only possible with the immune therapy. In the model of de Pillis et al.[85] the cytolytic effectiveness of tumor specific T-cells was the most sensitive parameter. Following the simulation results the efficacy of the CD8+ T cells and the response to immunotherapy was correlating.

One therapy against superficial bladder cancer is the treatment with Bacillus Calmette-Guerin (BCG). Rentsch et al.[86] showed with their mathematical model that the dose of BCG and the treatment interval have a positive correlation of tumor extension. Wei[87] investigated this immunotherapy with a mathematical model and showed that the infection rate and the growth rate of the tumor are the most important parameters for a successful treatment. Rihan et al.[88] investigated the effect of adoptive cellular immunotherapy and found out that only a combination of the treatment with IL-2 can be used to clear the tumor.

In summary, major contributions for clinical oncology have been made by the modeling community. However, although many models were designed and tested for clinical applications, the use in routine setting is sparse. One way to overcome this is to develop models for very specific applications and rigorously test the performance and the predictive power. Furthermore, the use of the available knowledge should be also part of the decision process. We envision a computational decision support system which is using clinical data, molecular data, publicly available data, as well as simulation results of mathematical models to reach a decision for therapeutic strategy.

2. Conclusion

In this review we presented an overview of mathematical models for translational oncology and clinical oncology beginning with carcinogenesis and proceeding to the different cancer treatments. By doing so we intended to highlight recent developments in the field and emphasize the power of this theoretical work. As demonstrated in a number of studies, mathematical modeling and computational simulation can provide valuable insights into the molecular mechanisms of cancer, can improve diagnosis and prognosis of the disease, and pinpoint novel therapeutic targets. As can be seen in **Figure 1**, it is often difficult to attribute the generation of new knowledge either to the modeling or to the experimental work. Regardless the origin, the insights obtained from such cycles of experiments and modeling can improve our understanding of the complexity of cancer progression and eventually be used to stop or at least slow down the processes of tumor initiation, evolution and resistance to therapies.

Competing Interests

The authors declare that they have no competing interests.

Authors' Contribution

RG, ME, PC, HH, and ZT carried out literature search and wrote the manuscript. ZT conceived the study. All authors read and approved the final manuscript.

Acknowledgements

This work was supported by the Austria Science Fund (Projects Doktoratskolleg W11 Molecular Cell Biology and Oncology and SFB F21 Cell Proliferation and Cell Death in Tumors), the Tiroler Standortagentur (Bioinformatics Tyrol), and by the Austrian Research Promotion Agency (FFG), project Oncotyrol. We apologize to the authors of papers not cited in this review due to space constraints.

Source: Gallasch R, Efremova M, Charoentong P, *et al*. Mathematical models for translational and clinical oncology[J]. Journal of Clinical Bioinformatics, 2013, 3(1):1–8.

References

[1]   Vogelstein B, Papadopoulos N, Velculescu VE, Zhou S, Diaz LA Jr, Kinzler KW: Cancer genome landscapes. Science 2013, 339:1546–1558.

[2]   Pabinger S, Dander A, Fischer M, Snajder R, Sperk M, Efremova M, Krabichler B, Speicher MR, Zschocke J, Trajanoski Z: A survey of tools for variant analysis of next-generation genome sequencing data. Brief Bioinform 2013.

[3]   Knudson AG Jr: Mutation and cancer: statistical study of retinoblastoma. Proc Natl Acad Sci USA 1971, 68:820–823.

[4]   Nowell PC: The clonal evolution of tumor cell populations. Science 1976, 194: 23–28.

[5]   Swierniak A, Kimmel M, Smieja J: Mathematical modeling as a tool for planning anticancer therapy. Eur J Pharmacol 2009, 625:108–121.

[6]   Lowengrub JS, Frieboes HB, Jin F, Chuang Y-L, Li X, Macklin P, Wise SM, Cristini V: Nonlinear modelling of cancer: bridging the gap between cells and tumours. Nonlinearity 2010, 23:R1–R9.

[7]   Byrne HM, Alarcon T, Owen MR, Webb SD, Maini PK: Modelling aspects of cancer dynamics: a review. Philos Transact A Math Phys Eng Sci 2006, 364:1563–1578.

[8]   Deisboeck TS, Wang Z, Macklin P, Cristini V: Multiscale cancer modeling. Annu Rev Biomed Eng 2011, 13:127–155.

[9]   Stransky B, de Souza SJ: Modeling tumor evolutionary dynamics. Front Physiol 2012, 3:480.

[10]   Fisher JC, Hollomon JH: A hypothesis for the origin of cancer foci. Cancer 1951, 4:916–918.

[11]   Nordling CO: A new theory on cancer-inducing mechanism. Br J Cancer 1953, 7:68–72.

[12]   Armitage P, Doll R: The age distribution of cancer and a multi-stage theory of carcinogenesis. Br J Cancer 1954, 8:1–12.

[13]   Ashley DJ: The two "hit" and multiple "hit" theories of carcinogenesis. Br J Cancer 1969, 23:313–328.

[14]   Moolgavkar SH, Knudson AG Jr: Mutation and cancer: a model for human carcinogenesis. J Natl Cancer Inst 1981, 66:1037–1052.

[15]   Luebeck EG, Moolgavkar SH: Multistage carcinogenesis and the incidence of colorectal cancer. Proc Natl Acad Sci U S A 2002, 99:15095–15100.

[16]   Gatenby RA, Vincent TL: An evolutionary model of carcinogenesis. Cancer Res 2003, 63: 6212–6220.

[17]   Hanahan D, Weinberg RA: The hallmarks of cancer. Cell 2000, 100:57–70.

[18] Greenspan H: Models for the growth of a solid tumor by diffusion. Stud Appl Math 1972, 52:317–340.

[19] McElwain DLS, Ponzo PJ: A model for the growth of a solid tumor with non-uniform oxygen consumption. Math Biosci 1977, 35:267–279.

[20] Greenspan HP: On the growth and stability of cell cultures and solid tumors. J Theor Biol 1976, 56:229–242.

[21] Byrne HM, Chaplain MAJ: Modelling the role of cell-cell adhesion in the growth and development of carcinomas. Math Comput Model 1996, 24:1–17.

[22] Balding D, McElwain DL: A mathematical model of tumour-induced capillary growth. J Theor Biol 1985, 114:53–73.

[23] Byrne HM, Chaplain MA: Mathematical models for tumour angiogenesis: numerical simulations and nonlinear wave solutions. Bull Math Biol 1995, 57:461–486.

[24] Chaplain MA: Mathematical modelling of angiogenesis. J Neurooncol 2000, 50:37–51.

[25] Chaplain MA, Stuart AM: A model mechanism for the chemotactic response of endothelial cells to tumour angiogenesis factor. IMA J Math Appl Med Biol 1993, 10:149–168.

[26] Levine HA, Pamuk S, Sleeman BD, Nilsen-Hamilton M: Mathematical modeling of capillary formation and development in tumor angiogenesis: penetration into the stroma. Bull Math Biol 2001, 63:801–863.

[27] Anderson AR, Chaplain MA: Continuous and discrete mathematical models of tumor-induced angiogenesis. Bull Math Biol 1998, 60:857–899.

[28] Mantzaris NV, Webb S, Othmer HG: Mathematical modeling of tumor-induced angiogenesis. J Math Biol 2004, 49:111–187.

[29] McDougall SR, Anderson ARA, Chaplain MAJ, Sherratt JA: Mathematical modelling of flow through vascular networks: implications for tumour-induced angiogenesis and chemotherapy strategies. Bull Math Biol 2002, 64:673–702.

[30] Stéphanou A, McDougall SR, Anderson ARA, Chaplain MAJ: Mathematical modelling of the influence of blood rheological properties upon adaptative tumour-induced angiogenesis. Math Comput Model 2006, 44:96–123.

[31] Stéphanou A, McDougall SR, Anderson ARA, Chaplain MAJ: Mathematical modelling of flow in 2D and 3D vascular networks: applications to anti-angiogenic and chemotherapeutic drug strategies. Math Comput Model 2005, 41:1137–1156.

[32] D' Onofrio A, Gandolfi A: Tumour eradication by antiangiogenic therapy: analysis and extensions of the model by Hahnfeldt *et al.* (1999). Math Biosci 2004, 191:159–184.

[33] Ledzewicz U, Schaettler H: Anti-angiogenic therapy in cancer treatment as an optimal control problem. SIAM J Control Optim 2007, 46(3):1052–1079.

[34] Hahnfeldt P, Panigrahy D, Folkman J, Hlatky L: Tumor development under angiogenic signaling: a dynamical theory of tumor growth, treatment response, and postvascular dormancy. Cancer Res 1999, 59:4770–4775.

[35] Merlo LMF, Pepper JW, Reid BJ, Maley CC: Cancer as an evolutionary and ecological process. Nat Rev Cancer 2006, 6:924–935.

[36] Greaves M, Maley CC: Clonal evolution in cancer. Nature 2012, 481:306–313.

[37] Haeno H, Iwasa Y, Michor F: The evolution of two mutations during clonal expansion. Genetics 2007, 177:2209–2221.

[38] Nowak MA, Michor F, Komarova NL, Iwasa Y: Evolutionary dynamics of tumor suppressor gene inactivation. Proc Natl Acad Sci USA 2004, 101:10635–10638.

[39] Gerstung M, Eriksson N, Lin J, Vogelstein B, Beerenwinkel N: The temporal order of genetic and pathway alterations in tumorigenesis. PLoS One 2011, 6:e27136.

[40] Durrett R, Schmidt D, Schweinsberg J: A waiting time problem arising from the study of multi-stage carcinogenesis. Ann Appl Probab 2009, 19:676–718.

[41] Attolini CS-O, Michor F: Evolutionary theory of cancer. Ann N Y Acad Sci 2009, 1168:23–51.

[42] Beerenwinkel N, Antal T, Dingli D, Traulsen A, Kinzler KW, Velculescu VE, Vogelstein B, Nowak MA: Genetic progression and the waiting time to cancer. PLoS Comput Biol 2007, 3:e225.

[43] Bozic I, Antal T, Ohtsuki H, Carter H, Kim D, Chen S, Karchin R, Kinzler KW, Vogelstein B, Nowak MA: Accumulation of driver and passenger mutations during tumor progression. Proc Natl Acad Sci U S A 2010, 107:18545–18550.

[44] Quaranta V, Rejniak KA, Gerlee P, Anderson ARA: Invasion emerges from cancer cell adaptation to competitive microenvironments: quantitative predictions from multiscale mathematical models. Semin Cancer Biol 2008, 18:338–348.

[45] Lee H-O, Silva AS, Concilio S, Li Y-S, Slifker M, Gatenby RA, Cheng JD: Evolution of tumor invasiveness: the adaptive tumor microenvironment landscape model. Cancer Res 2011, 71:6327–6337.

[46] Gatenby RA, Gillies RJ: A microenvironmental model of carcinogenesis. Nat Rev Cancer 2008, 8:56–61.

[47] Goldie JH, Coldman AJ: A mathematic model for relating the drug sensitivity of tumors to their spontaneous mutation rate. Cancer Treat Rep 1979, 63:1727–1733.

[48] Michor F, Nowak MA, Iwasa Y: Evolution of resistance to cancer therapy. Curr Pharm Des 2006, 12:261–271.

[49] Komarova N: Stochastic modeling of drug resistance in cancer. J Theor Biol 2006, 239:351–366.

[50] Komarova NL, Wodarz D: Drug resistance in cancer: principles of emergence and

prevention. Proc Natl Acad Sci U S A 2005, 102:9714–9719.

[51] Basanta D, Gatenby RA, Anderson ARA: Exploiting evolution to treat drug resistance: combination therapy and the double bind. Mol Pharm 2012, 9:914–921.

[52] Swierniak A, Smieja J: Analysis and optimization of drug resistant and phase-specific cancer chemotherapy models. Math Biosci Eng MBE 2005, 2:657–670.

[53] Kimmel M, Axelrod DE: Mathematical models of gene amplification with applications to cellular drug resistance and tumorigenicity. Genetics 1990, 125:633–644.

[54] Kimmel M, Swierniak A, Polanski A: Infinite-dimensional model of evolution of drug resistance of cancer cells. J Math Syst Estim Contr 1998, 8(1):1–16.

[55] Smieja J, Swierniak A: Different models of chemotherapy taking into account drug resistance stemming from gene amplification. Int. J. Appl Math Comp Sci 2003, 13.3:297–306.

[56] Harnevo LE, Agur Z: Drug resistance as a dynamic process in a model for multistep gene amplification under various levels of selection stringency. Cancer Chemother Pharmacol 1992, 30:469–476.

[57] Foo J, Michor F: Evolution of resistance to targeted anti-cancer therapies during continuous and pulsed administration strategies. PLoS Comput Biol 2009, 5:e1000557.

[58] Diaz LA Jr, Williams RT, Wu J, Kinde I, Hecht JR, Berlin J, Allen B, Bozic I, Reiter JG, Nowak MA, Kinzler KW, Oliner KS, Vogelstein B: The molecular evolution of acquired resistance to targeted EGFR blockade in colorectal cancers. Nature 2012, 486:537–540.

[59] Bozic I, Reiter JG, Allen B, Antal T, Chatterjee K, Shah P, Moon YS, Yaqubie A, Kelly N, Le DT, Lipson EJ, Chapman PB, Diaz LA Jr, Vogelstein B, Nowak MA: Evolutionary dynamics of cancer in response to targeted combination therapy. Elife 2013, 2:e00747.

[60] Sawyers C: Targeted cancer therapy. Nature 2004, 432:294–297.

[61] Fister KR, Panetta JC: Optimal control applied to cell-cycle-specific cancer chemotherapy. SIAM J Appl Math 2000, 60:1059–1072.

[62] Byrne HM, Owen MR, Alarcon T, Murphy J, Maini PK: Modelling the response of vascular tumours to chemotherapy: a multiscale approach. Math Models Methods Appl Sci 2006, 16:1219–1241.

[63] De Pillis LG, Gu W, Radunskaya AE: Mixed immunotherapy and chemotherapy of tumors: modeling, applications and biological interpretations. J Theor Biol 2006, 238:841–862.

[64] De Pillis L, Radunskaya A: A mathematical model of immune response to tumor invasion. In Proc Second MIT Conf Comput Fluid Solid Mech KJ Bathe Ed Fluid Solid Mech Comput: Solid; 2003.

[65] Jackson TL, Byrne HM: A mathematical model to study the effects of drug resistance and vasculature on the response of solid tumors to chemotherapy. Math Biosci 2000, 164:17–38.

[66] Panetta JC, Adam J: A mathematical model of cycle-specific chemotherapy. Math Comput Model 1995, 22:67–82.

[67] Powathil GG, Adamson DJA, Chaplain MAJ: Towards predicting the response of a solid tumour to chemotherapy and radiotherapy treatments: clinical insights from a computational model. PLoS Comput Biol 2013, 9:e1003120.

[68] Powathil G, Kohandel M, Sivaloganathan S, Oza A, Milosevic M: Mathematical modeling of brain tumors: effects of radiotherapy and chemotherapy. Phys Med Biol 2007, 52:3291–3306.

[69] Powathil GG, Gordon KE, Hill LA, Chaplain MAJ: Modelling the effects of cell-cycle heterogeneity on the response of a solid tumour to chemotherapy: biological insights from a hybrid multiscale cellular automaton model. J Theor Biol 2012, 308:1–19.

[70] Cojocaru L, Agur Z: A theoretical analysis of interval drug dosing for cell-cycle-phase-specific drugs. Math Biosci 1992, 109:85–97.

[71] Bozic I, Allen B, Nowak MA: Dynamics of targeted cancer therapy. Trends Mol Med 2012, 18:311–316.

[72] Billy F, Ribba B, Saut O, Morre-Trouilhet H, Colin T, Bresch D, Boissel J-P, Grenier E, Flandrois J-P: A pharmacologically based multiscale mathematical model of angiogenesis and its use in investigating the efficacy of a new cancer treatment strategy. J Theor Biol 2009, 260:545–562.

[73] Kirschner DE, Jackson TL, Arciero JC: A mathematical model of tumor-immune evasion and siRNA treatment. Discrete Contin Dyn Syst-Ser B 2003, 4:39–58.

[74] Dewanji A, Luebeck EG, Moolgavkar SH: A generalized Luria-Delbrück model. Math Biosci 2005, 197:140–152.

[75] Kronik N, Kogan Y, Vainstein V, Agur Z: Improving alloreactive CTL immunotherapy for malignant gliomas using a simulation model of their interactive dynamics. Cancer Immunol Immunother CII 2008, 57:425–439.

[76] Nanda S, Moore H, Lenhart S: Optimal control of treatment in a mathematical model of chronic myelogenous leukemia. Math Biosci 2007, 210:143–156.

[77] Wein LM, Wu JT, Kirn DH: Validation and analysis of a mathematical model of a replication-competent oncolytic virus for cancer treatment: implications for virus design and delivery. Cancer Res 2003, 63:1317–1324.

[78] Mok W, Stylianopoulos T, Boucher Y, Jain RK: Mathematical modeling of herpes simplex virus distribution in solid tumors: implications for cancer gene therapy. Clin Cancer Res Off J Am Assoc Cancer Res 2009, 15:2352–2360.

[79] Rockne R, Alvord EC, Rockhill JK, Swanson KR: A mathematical model for brain tumor response to radiation therapy. J Math Biol 2008, 58:561–578.

[80] Richard M, Kirkby KJ, Webb RP, Kirkby NF: A mathematical model of response of cells to radiation. Nucl Instruments Methods Phys Res Sect B Beam Interactions Mater Atoms 2007, 255:18–22.

[81] Enderling H, Anderson ARA, Chaplain MAJ: A model of breast carcinogenesis and recurrence after radiotherapy. PAMM 2007, 7:1121701–1121702.

[82] De Boer RJ, Hogeweg P, Dullens HF, De Weger RA, Den Otter W: Macrophage T lymphocyte interactions in the anti-tumor immune response: a mathematical mode. J Immunol Baltim Md 1950 1985, 134:2748–2758.

[83] Matzavinos A, Chaplain MAJ, Kuznetsov VA: Mathematical modelling of the spatio-temporal response of cytotoxic T-lymphocytes to a solid tumour. Math Med Biol J IMA 2004, 21:1–34.

[84] Kirschner D, Panetta JC: Modeling immunotherapy of the tumor-immune interaction. J Math Biol 1998, 37:235–252.

[85] De Pillis LG, Radunskaya AE, Wiseman CL: A validated mathematical model of cell-mediated immune response to tumor growth. Cancer Res 2005, 65:7950–7958.

[86] Rentsch CA, Biot C, Gsponer JR, Bachmann A, Albert ML, Breban R: BCG-mediated bladder cancer immunotherapy: identifying determinants of treatment response using a calibrated mathematical model. PLoS One 2013, 8:e56327.

[87] Wei H-C: A numerical study of a mathematical model of pulsed immunotherapy for superficial bladder cancer. Jpn J Ind Appl Math 2013, 30:441–452.

[88] Rihan FA, Safan M, Abdeen MA, Abdel Rahman D: Qualitative and computational analysis of a mathematical model for tumor-immune interactions. J Appl Math 2012, Article ID 475720:19.

Chapter 25

Associations between Clinical and Sociodemographic Data and Patterns of Communication in Pediatric Oncology

Marina Kohlsdorf[1], Áderson Luiz Costa Junior[2]

[1]University Uni Ceub, Brasília, Brazil
[2]University of Brasília, Brasília, Brazil

Abstract: Pediatric communication directly contributes to treatment adherence, fewer symptoms, better clinical responses, healthier treatment adaptation and management of psychosocial issues. This study aimed to evaluate associations between the clinical and sociodemographic data of caregivers and children and the communicative patterns of pediatricians. Three oncohematology physicians and 44 child-caregiver dyads took part, with audio recording of 146 medical consultations. The physicians interacted more often with older children, offering more guidance, clarifying doubts, and asking for information. The number of questions from children and caregivers was positively correlated with the physician's communicative behaviors. However, there was no association between the age of the children and the number of doubts of the patients. The diagnosis, treatment time, family income, marital status and caregiver's level of education were associated with the amount of interaction provided by physicians to the children and caregivers. This study offers subsides relevant to psychosocial interventions that may improve communication in pediatric oncohematology settings.

Keywords: Cancer in Children, Physician-Patient Relationship

1. Background

Health communication may be defined as a relational process, crucial to the success of the treatment, based on cultural and sociohistorical aspects, in which information and its comprehension are exchanged between people (Gabarra and Crepaldi 2011; Wassmer et al. 2004; Zwaanswijk et al. 2011). This complex interaction has been studied with validated tools: Roter Interaction Analysis System (Wissow, Larson, Anderson & Hadjiisky, 2005), Verona Coding Definitions of Emotional Sequences (Vatne et al. 2010a, b), Rating Scales for Emphatic Communication in Medical Interviews-REM (Nicolai et al. 2007), Communication Assessment Tool-CAT (Makoul et al. 2008), and the Paediatric Consultation Assessment Tool (Howells et al. 2010). However, none of these tools have been translated and validated to Brazilian Portuguese, which prevents researchers from using them in data collection and highlights the need for studying health communication in Brazil from an objective and observable way.

The literature has focused on communication in pediatric settings in the last three decades due to the fact that this process is strongly related to quality of life, treatment adherence, symptom management, satisfaction with health service, fewer outpatient returns and better coping with treatment related difficulties (Ammentorp et al. 2011; Coyne and Gallagher 2011; Croom et al. 2011; Drotar 2009; Sleath et al. 2012).

A desirable interaction during pediatric medical consultations may include: (a) provision of tailored information by physicians, using adapted language; (b) approaching psychosocial issues related to health care (such as daily care and consequently changes in the family routine, expenses related to the treatment, caregiver's anxiety related to clinical responses); (c) emphasizing the active role of physicians, parents, and patients during the interaction; and (d) provision of social support and empathy by pediatricians (Gabarra and Crepaldi 2011; Wassmer et al. 2004; Zwaanswijk et al. 2011).

There is, however, a lack of professional training during medical undergraduate courses that could provide the necessary skills regarding communication in pediatric settings, since it demands specific abilities related to the triad interaction (Rider et al. 2008). The literature shows that the insufficient amount of communicative training during medical undergraduate courses, along with parents' worries about protecting the child from suffering, leads to a disregard for the pediatric patients' contributions during consultations, with them participating mainly in small talk or providing only basic health information (Taylor et al. 2010; Vaknin and Zisk-Rony 2010; Washington et al. 2012). Therefore, more studies concerning the process of pediatric communication are needed, in order to understand its characteristics, which could lead to psychosocial and educational interventions focused on a more efficient interaction.

The literature presents studies concerning associations between the child's clinical condition, social/demographic data and pediatric communication patterns, which are relevant to deepen the understanding of factors that may influence interaction during medical consultations. Studies conducted in the United States of America and in the United Kingdom have highlighted that, considering the characteristics of the caregivers, pediatricians tend to share more decisions and provide more information, of better quality, to white parents (Fiks et al. 2010; Moseley et al. 2006) with higher levels of education (Brinkman et al. 2011; Washington et al. 2012; Zwaanswijk et al. 2011), and higher monthly incomes (Taylor et al. 2010).

Considering communication between physicians and children during medical consultations, the literature shows age as a major differential in pediatric settings, although children at the age of four already understand information about self care, identify symptoms and organs, have doubts and concerns about treatment, and feel emotional responses related to their condition (Gordon et al. 2010; Knighting et al. 2010; Märtenson and Fägers-kiöld 2007; Märtenson et al. 2007; Vatne et al. 2010a, b). Older children receive more information from pediatricians and answer more questions directed toward them by physicians (Gabarra and Crepaldi 2011; Stivers 2011, 2012; Stivers and Majid 2007; Taylor et al. 2010; Zwaanswijk et al. 2011).

In addition to age, the level of education of the caregiver and child as well as the prognosis, the race and gender of the child appear to be relevant characteristics: pediatricians communicate more and better with white and female children, with parents and children with higher educational levels and also with children with better prognosis regarding treatment (Drotar 2009; Gabarra and Crepaldi 2011; Stivers 2011, 2012; Stivers and Majid 2007; Taylor et al. 2010; Zwaanswijk et al. 2011). Conversely, studies from Fiks et al. (2010) and Wissow et al., (2005) showed no associations between communicative patterns and sociodemographic data of parents and children.

Although the studies presented in this paper show relevant results concerning communication and sociodemographic data, there are some features that were not included in their analyses, such as type of diagnosis, marital status of the caregivers, and time since diagnosis of chronic conditions, characteristics that may be relevant when considering communication during medical consultations. Furthermore, the pediatric oncohematologic milieu presents a very specific and complex condition which includes various psychosocial demands, long-term treatment and family challenges that demands a better understanding related to the communication between physicians, children and caregivers. It is also relevant to note that there are few studies in the Brazilian literature related to pediatric communication, and none of them analyzes the relationship between the personal characteristics of children and caregivers and the way in which physicians communicate with them.

Therefore, this study aimed to analyze associations between communicative patterns from physicians in pediatric settings and sociodemographic data of caregivers and children. Specifically, the authors hypothesized that the physicians might establish a better communication toward parents with higher income and higher levels of education, as well as toward older children with advanced schooling.

2. Method

2.1. Participants

Participants in this study were three physicians of a pediatric cancer hospital, aged 49, 34 and 32 years, with seven, 11 and 26 years of medical practice. They were respectively two women and one man, however there were no noticeable differences in communicative patterns among these three participants. The public hospital in which data were collected has a pediatric oncohematology team consisting of ten physicians: two of them were not working at the time of data collection, one of them was in the process of retirement, and two were moving to other services in following weeks. Of the five physicians left, only three had stable clinical practice schedules that allowed the collection of data.

In addition to these pediatricians, 47 caregiver-child dyads were invited to participate in the research, with three refusals. Therefore, 44 dyads participated, including 41 mothers, one aunt, one grandmother and one father. Inclusion criteria were related to the age of the child (between 4 and 12 years), the age of the caregiver (over 18 years) and dyads in the first semester of treatment for childhood cancer, considering that the first 6 months is the most difficult period, including psychosocial changes for the family, lengthy hospitalizations, a large amount of information related to care and treatment and weekly or biweekly medical visits (Kohlsdorf, 2012). The exclusion criteria were children with other chronic health conditions, cancer relapse or sequelae, speaking difficulties or that were not clinically improving from the disease. **Table 1** shows the characteristics of the parents and children.

2.2. Instruments

In the study, 146 consultations were audio recorded and observed in person by the main researcher. The medical visits lasted between 6 m 30 s and 37 m 36 s (mean 19 m 23 s; SD = 13.01). During the consultations, the researcher used an observational protocol, developed ad hoc for the study and presented in Appendix A, in which relevant aspects of the communication were written down e.g., the position of the caregiver, child and physician in the room, and other behaviors that could be relevant for the data analysis, such as whether a participant left the room.

2.3. Procedure

Data Collection

Over 18 months, 146 medical visits for childhood cancer were directly audio

Table 1. Characteristics of the caregiver and child.

Characteristics of the caregiver and child	Frequency
Child's age	
4 to 6 years	21
7 to 10 years	15
11 to 12 years	08
Mean (SD)	7.3 years (2.6)
Child's schooling	
Primary or none	20
First year to sixth year	24
Child's gender	
Male	22
Female	22
Diagnosis	
Leukemia or lymphoma	25
Solid tumors	19
Time since diagnosis	
1 month	14
2 to 4 months	25
4 to 6 months	06
Mean (SD)	2.03 months (1.52)
Caregiver's age	
22 to 35 years	22
36 to 56 years	22
Mean (SD)	35 years (7,9)
Caregiver's education level	
Elementary school	09
Middle school	11
High school	13
College	11
Caregiver's marital status	
Married/cohabiting	24
Single/divorced/widowed	20
Household income	
Low income	26
Medium income	14
High income	04

recorded. The data were classified by the main researcher into 11 categories regarding the communication of the pediatrician with the children and the caregivers, focusing especially on the exchange of information and doubts.

Inter-rater reliability rate regarding the frequencies of communicative behaviors was calculated between two observers: the main researcher and the auxiliary researcher. Thirty percent of all the recorded consultations were randomly chosen and analyzed to provide this reliability, achieving between 55% and 76% concordance (mean 64.20%; SD = 5.03). Disagreements between the two observers related to the data were solved by a third researcher, unaware of the answers given by each observer. This observer works as a psychology professor, has experience in research related to the field of expertise and was mentoring this research. Intra-rater reliability was also calculated for all data recorded and performed solely by the main researcher, which achieved between 75.7% and 95% (mean 84.55%; SD = 4.13). The reliability index was conducted according to Danna and Matos (2006).

2.4. Data Analysis

This cross-sectional and descriptive research focused on statistical associations between nine characteristics from the dyad child-caregiver and eleven communicative categories observed during pediatric consultations. Based on studies available in the literature, nine variables from the dyad child-parent were chosen corresponding to the sociodemographic data presented in **Table 1**, regarding the age, schooling and gender of the child, time since diagnosis, cancer diagnosis, household income, and age, education level, and marital status of the caregiver.

A total of eleven communicative categories were developed by the researchers ad hoc for this study, corresponding to the other variables in this research. Following the proposal of Bardin (1977), the main researcher and the auxiliary researcher listened twice to all the recorded consultations and made an individual list of categories. Each researcher worked independently to develop this first list of communicative behaviors, excluding repetitive issues and/or broadening these categories to include similar themes. Then, these initial lists were compared in order to achieve a second list with the same categories, including their operational definition. Finally, both researchers listened one last time to all the consultations to check for new categories or any necessary adjustments.

Each communicative category was analyzed based on its frequency during the consultations in order to provide statistical data analysis. The six categories focused on physician-child communication and the five categories focused on physician-caregiver communication are described in Appendix B.

The Statistical Package for Social Sciences (SPSS) was used (version 13). Considering the frequencies obtained for each quantitative variable, Shapiro-Wilk normality tests were performed and all data showed $p \leq 0.002$, therefore non-parametric tests were applied in the data analysis, including Spearman's correlations, the Mann Whitney U test, and the Kruskal-Wallis test. Results in which $p \leq 0.05$ were considered statistically significant.

2.5. Ethical Considerations

This study was approved by the Ethics Committee of the Foundation for Research and Education in Health Sciences under registration number 289/2009. All audio recordings and other information were sealed in a confidential, password-protected archive. The research took place in a hospital that provides cancer treatment for children and adolescents. All participants physicians, caregivers and children, through their parents were first approached and invited to participate in the study, by signing an Informed Consent form.

3. Results

Table 2 and **Table 3** show the results of the Spearman's correlations, regarding communication with the children and caregivers.

The age of the child was positively and moderately associated with the amount of physicians' behaviors directed toward the patient, regarding guidance to children ($r = 0.46$; $p < 0.01$), asking about doubts ($r = 0.45$; $p < 0.01$) and obtaining information from the child ($r = 0.54$; $p < 0.01$); it was also negatively and moderately associated with protesting. Time since diagnosis was weakly and negatively associated with protesting ($r = -0.32$; $p = 0.01$).

Table 2. Correlations between Sociodemographic and Clinical Dimensions and Pediatrician's Communicative Behaviors towards the Child.

	Child's age	Time since diagnosis	Guidance for child	Asks child about doubts	Child's doubts	Protesting	Child's schooling	Bonding with child
Time since diagnosis	r = −0.29							
	p < 0.01							
Guidance for child	r = 0.46	r = −0.01						
	p < 0.01	p = 0.37						
Asks child about doubts	r = 0.45	r = −0.05	r = 0.64					
	p < 0.01	p = 0.11	p < 0.01					
Child's doubts	r = −0.01	r = 0.13	r = 0.49	r = 0.23				
	p = 0.76	p = 0.73	p < 0.01	p < 0.01				
Protesting	r = −0.32	r = 0.18	r = 0.17	r = −0.14	r = 0.15			
	p = 0.01	p = 0.03	p < 0.01	p = 0.26	p = 0.27			
Child's schooling	r = 0.81	r = −0.26	r = 0.52	r = 0.50	r = 0.24	r = −0.17		
	p < 0.01	p < 0.01	p < 0.01	p < 0.01	p = 0.02	p = 0.05		
Bonding with child	r = −0.12	r = 0.23	r = 0.44	r = 0.28	r = 0.38	r = 0.13	r = 0.13	
	p = 0.41	p = 0.02	p < 0.01	p < 0.01	p < 0.01	p = 0.62	p = 0.25	
Obtaining information from the child	r = 0.54	r = −0.11	r = 0.64	r = 0.57	r = 0.24	r = −0.10	r = 0.62	r = 0.30
	p < 0.01	p = 0.04	p < 0.01	p < 0.01	p = 0.03	p = 0.27	p < 0.00	p = 0.01

Table 3. Correlations between Sociodemographic and Clinical Dimensions and Pediatrician's Communicative Behaviors towards the Caregiver.

	Child's age	Time since diagnosis	Guidance to caregiver	Asks caregiver about doubts	Caregiver's doubts	Caregiver's age	Bonding with caregiver
Time since diagnosis	$r = -0.29$						
	$p < 0.01$						
Guidance to caregiver	$r = 0.12$	$r = -0.21$					
	$p = 0.02$	$p = 0.02$					
Asks caregiver about doubts	$r = 0.09$	$r = -0.11$	$r = 0.50$				
	$p = 0.07$	$p = 0.06$	$p < 0.01$				
Caregiver's doubts	$r = -0.07$	$r = 0.01$	$r = 0.68$	$r = 0.32$			
	$p = 0.38$	$p = 0.79$	$p < 0.01$	$p < 0.01$			
Caregiver's age	$r = 0.29$	$r = 0.03$	$r = 0.08$	$r = -0.03$	$r = 0.17$		
	$p < 0.01$	$p = 0.96$	$p = 0.33$	$p = 0.54$	$p = 0.03$		
Bonding with caregiver	$r = -0.08$	$r = 0.08$	$r = 0.31$	$r = 0.43$	$r = 0.12$	$r = -0.01$	
	$p = 0.43$	$p = 0.51$	$p < 0.01$	$p = 0.01$	$p = 0.09$	$p = 0.21$	
Obtaining information from caregiver	$r = 0.05$	$r = -0.25$	$r = 0.55$	$r = 0.18$	$r = 0.20$	$r = 0.03$	$r = 0.13$
	$p = 0.57$	$p < 0.01$	$p < 0.01$	$p = 0.03$	$p = 0.01$	$p = 0.69$	$p = 0.30$

Physician's guidance directed toward the child was moderately associated with the following behaviors: asking about doubts ($r = 0.64$; $p < 0.01$) and bonding with the child ($r = 0.44$; $p < 0.01$), expression of doubts ($r = 0.49$; $p < 0.01$), protesting ($r = 0.17$; $p < 0.01$), obtaining information from the child ($r = 0.64$; $p < 0.01$) and the child's schooling ($r = 0.52$; $p < 0.01$). Pediatrician's behavior related to asking about the child's doubts was positively and weakly associated with the child's questions ($r = 0.23$; $p < 0.01$). Doubts verbalized by children were positively associated with the child's schooling ($r = 0.24$; $p = 0.02$), bonding ($r = 0.38$; $p < 0.01$), and obtaining information from the child ($r = 0.24$; $p = 0.03$), however it is relevant to pointing out that this behavior had no association with the child's age ($r = 0.01$; $p = 0.76$).

Table 3 shows that the time since diagnosis was weakly and negatively associated with guidance directed toward the caregivers ($r = -0.21$; $p = 0.02$) and obtaining information from them ($r = -0.25$; $p < 0.01$). Guidance for the caregivers also showed relevant associations with clarifying the caregivers' doubts ($r = 0.50$; $p < 0.01$), questions raised by the caregivers ($r = 0.68$; $p < 0.01$), bonding ($r = 0.31$; $p < 0.01$) and asking information from the caregivers ($r = 0.55$; $p < 0.01$). Despite the obtained results, it is relevant to point out that pediatrician's behavior related to asking about caregiver's doubts was positively and moderately associated with questions expressed by the caregiver ($r = 0.32$; $p < 0.01$), and also positively and weakly associated with obtaining information from the caregiver ($r = 0.18$; $p = 0.03$). **Table 4** shows an analysis of communicative behaviors and marital status, diagnosis, and the child's gender.

According to **Table 4**, marital status was related to physician's guidance to caregivers ($t[143] = 1.78$; $p = 0.05$), asking the child about doubts ($t[143] = 2.38$; $p < 0.01$), and questions from caregivers ($t[143] = 2.38$; $p < 0.01$), with married parents presenting higher means. The diagnosis also seemed to be associated with physician's guidance directed towards the caregiver ($t[144] = 3.41$; $p < 0.001$), questions from children ($t[144] = 2.61$; $p < 0.001$) and caregivers ($t[144] = 3.59$; $p = 0.001$). The child's gender was not associated with any communicative behavior. **Table 5** shows an analysis of associations between communicative behaviors, caregiver's level of education and monthly income.

Table 5 highlights relevant associations between the caregiver's level of

Table 4. Associations Between Physician's Communicative Behaviors, Caregiver's Marital Status, Diagnosis, and Child's Gender.

	Marital Status		Diagnosis		Child's gender	
	Single or divorced	Married	Leukemia or Lymphoma	Solid tumors	Female	Male
Physician's guidance to child - M(SD)	6.78 (9.51)	8.51 (8.20)	9.49 (9.54)	5.68 (7.51)	7.36 (9.1)	8.24 (8.71)
	t[143] = 1.17; p = 0.24		t[144] = 2.63; p = 0.15		t[144] = 0.59; p = 0.38	
Physician's guidance to caregiver - M(SD)	32.1 (23.25)	39.49 (26.48)	41.93 (30.9)	29 (12.37)	35.5 (23.4)	36.75 (27.21)
	t[143] = 1.78; p = 0.05		t[144] = 3.41; p < 0.001		t[144] = 0.29; p = 0.52	
Asks child about doubts - M(SD)	0.54 (1.27)	1.12 (1.58)	0.96 (1.57)	0.79 (1.47)	0.96 (1.57)	0.79 (1.47)
	t[143] = 2.38; p < 0.01		t[144] = 0.69; p = 0.81		t[144] = 0.66; p = 0.52	
Asks caregiver about doubts - M(SD)	1.21 (1.75)	1.53 (1.89)	1.73 (1.89)	0.98 (1.67)	1.50 (1.91)	1.26 (1.73)
	t[143] = 1.07; p = 0.45		t[144] = 2.47; p = 0.16		t[144] = 0.77; p = 0.35	
Child's doubts - M(SD)	1.12 (2.00)	1.12 (2.15)	1.53 (2.54)	0.68 (1.23)	1.19 (2.15)	1.09 (2.03)
	t[143] = 0.002; p = 0.75		t[144] = 2.61; p < 0.001		t[144] = 0.29; p = 0.71	
Caregiver's doubts - M(SD)	6.32 (4.96)	10.16 (8.66)	10.16 (8.61)	6.12 (4.73)	7.76 (5.97)	9.00 (8.71)
	t[143] = 3.31; p < 0.01		t[144] = 3.59; p = 0.001		t[144] = 1.02; p = 0.50	
Protesting - M(SD)	2.18 (4.91)	2.60 (4.78)	2.73 (5.57)	1.97 (5.15)	2.01 (5.09)	2.81 (5.11)
	t[143] = 0.46; p = 0.80		t[144] = 1.78; p = 0.28		t[144] = 0.99; p = 0.08	
Physician's bonding with the child - M(SD)	9.75 (5.44)	9.38 (5.49)	11.41 (5.30)	7.32 (4.74)	10.18 (6.16)	8.81 (4.38)
	t[142] = 0.70; p = 0.40		t[143] = 4.84; p = 0.46		t[143] = 1.56; p = 0.10	
Physician's bonding with the caregiver - M(SD)	2.70 (3.62)	2.47 (2.78)	2.91 (2.63)	2.21 (3.73)	2.32 (2.37)	2.91 (3.92)
	t[142] = 0.43; p = 0.83		t[143] = 1.31; p = 0.67		t[143] = 1.07; p = 0.20	
Obtaining information from child - M(SD)	3.63 (4.48)	3.99 (3.57)	4.20 (4.31)	3.42 (3.60)	3.92 (4.4)	3.76 (3.54)
	t[142] = 0.53; p = 0.91		t[143] = 1.16; p = 0.53		t[143] = 0.24; p = 0.28	
Obtaining information from caregiver - M(SD)	9.78 (5.82)	9.91 (5.20)	9.28 (5.23)	10.61 (5.71)	10.22 (6.21)	9.49 (4.49)
	t[142] = 0.14; p = 0.56		t[143] = 1.45; p = 0.78		t[143] = 0.81; p = 0.02	

Table 5. Associations between Communicative Behaviors and the Caregiver's level of education and Monthly Income.

	Caregiver's level of education				Monthly income		
	None, primary grade	Junior high school	High school	College	Low income	Medium income	High income
Physician's guidance to child - M(SD)	3.92 (5.11)	5.46 (7.27)	10.7 (11.1)	10.04 (7.8)	7.4 (9.7)	8.52 (7.8)	6.75 (7.1)
	$F[3,144] = 5.39; p = 0.002$				$F[2,144] = 0.33; p = 0.72$		
Physician's guidance to caregiver - M(SD)	25.69 (14.1)	24.57 (10.8)	46.82 (25.9)	47.04 (25.5)	32.3 (19.7)	34.1 (23.5)	60.94 (39.4)
	$F[3,144] = 11.07; p < 0.001$				$F[2,144] = 9.96; p < 0.001$		
Asks child about doubts - M(SD)	0.46 (1.42)	0.54 (1.17)	1.16 (1.77)	1.21 (1.28)	0.88 (1.57)	0.96 (1.5)	0.38 (0.62)
	$F[3,144] = 2.57; p = 0.05$				$F[2,144] = 0.97; p = 0.38$		
Asks caregiver about doubts - M(SD)	1.15 (1.89)	0.63 (1.22)	1.87 (2.05)	2.04 (1.84)	1.36 (1.93)	1.48 (1.7)	1.19 (1.6)
	$F[3,144] = 5.42; p = 0.001$				$F[2,144] = 0.16; p = 0.85$		
Child's doubts - M(SD)	1.12 (2.01)	0.52 (0.91)	1.27 (2.27)	1.86 (2.87)	1.01 (1.86)	1.39 (2.5)	0.88 (1.71)
	$F[3,144] = 2.60; p = 0.05$				$F[2,144] = 0.61; p = 0.54$		
Caregiver's doubts - M(SD)	6.31 (4.73)	5.74 (4.04)	9.38 (7.27)	12.93 (10.9)	6.76 (4.96)	8.37 (7.3)	16.6 (12.1)
	$F[3,144] = 7.27; p < 0.001$				$F[2,144] = 14.09; p < 0.001$		
Protesting - M(SD)	2.73 (6.87)	1.63 (3.08)	3.31 (5.67)	1.89 (3.15)	2.05 (4.74)	2.8 (5.26)	11.25 (6.5)
	$F[3,144] = 1.06; p = 0.36$				$F[2,144] = 0.53; p = 0.59$		
Physician's bonding with child -M(SD)	8.88 (5.88)	7.30 (5.55)	9.91 (3.85)	13.29 (5.18)	8.07 (5.1)	11.6 (5.1)	11.25 (6.5)
	$F[3,143] = 8.25; p < 0.001$				$F[2,143] = 7.63; p = 0.001$		
Physician's bonding with caregiver - M(SD)	1.81 (1.79)	1.20 (1.99)	3.30 (4.16)	4.43 (2.95)	2.28 (3.5)	2.65 (2.5)	3.88 (3.13)
	$F[3,143] = 8.36; p < 0.001$				$F[2,143] = 1.70; p = 0.19$		
Obtaining information from child - M(SD)	3.15 (2.55)	3.52 (3.96)	4.59 (5.24)	3.71 (2.79)	3.85 (4.18)	3.8 (4.21)	3.69 (2.39)
	$F[3,143] = 0.87; p = 0.46$				$F[2,143] = 0.01; p = 0.98$		
Obtaining information from caregiver - M(SD)	9.69 (5.03)	8.89 (6.24)	11.50 (4.94)	8.96 (5.01)	10.17 (5.8)	8.63 (4.8)	11.69 (5.1)
	$F[3,143] = 2.09; p = 0.01$				$F[2,143] = 2.22; p = 0.01$		

education, monthly income and communicative behaviors. The caregiver's level of education was associated with physician's guidance towards the child ($F[3,144] = 5.39$; $p = 0.002$) and caregiver ($F[3,144] = 11.07$; $p < 0.001$), asking about the child's ($F[3,144] = 2.57$; $p = 0.05$) and caregiver's doubts ($F[3,144] = 5.42$; $p = 0.001$), the child's questions ($F[3,144] = 2.60$; $p = 0.05$), the caregiver's doubts ($F[3,144] = 7.27$; $p < 0.001$), pediatrician's bonding with the child ($F[3,143] = 8.25$; $p < 0.001$) and caregiver ($F[3,143] = 8.36$; $p < 0.001$) and also obtaining information from the caregiver by the physician ($F[3,143] = 2.09$; $p = 0.01$). All behaviors with higher means were among the caregivers with a high school or college degree level of education.

Monthly income was associated with physician's guidance to caregiver ($F[2,144] = 9.96$; $p < 0.001$), questions from parents ($F[2,144] = 14.09$; $p < 0.001$), pediatrician's bonding with the child ($F[2,143] = 7.63$; $p = 0.001$), and also obtaining information from the caregiver by the physician ($F[2,143] = 2.22$; $p = 0.01$). The means in all of these behaviors were elevated for caregivers with higher income.

4. Discussion

The results showed that older children with advanced schooling received more interaction, since these variables were associated with more guidance from the physician directed toward the child and more frequently asking about doubts and obtaining information, data also found in the literature (Gabarra and Crepaldi 2011; Gordon et al. 2010; Knighting et al. 2010; Märtenson and Fägerskiöld 2007; Märtenson et al. 2007; Stivers 2011, 2012; Stivers and Majid 2007; Taylor et al. 2010; Vatne et al. 2010a, b; Zwaanswijk et al. 2011).

Pediatrician's behavior related to asking about doubts of the child (e.g., "Do you wanna ask anything, honey?" or "Any questions? Think carefully, ok?") was positively and weakly associated with questions from the child, which may suggest that this specific and simple behavior from the physician could be crucial to promote verbalization of the patients. It is also relevant to state that this physician's behavior was moderately and positively related to child's schooling and age, indicating sociodemographic characteristics that influence communicative behaviors by the physician towards the child. It should be highlighted that there was more interaction between the older children and the pediatricians, which may also have contributed to a better communicative process. The literature, however, highlights that 4-year-old patients can already understand elementary health care behaviors, identify symptoms and, therefore, should contribute within an active role in health related processes, endorsing the need for including these patients during medical consultations (Gordon et al. 2010; Knighting et al. 2010; Märtenson and Fägerskiöld 2007; Märtenson et al. 2007; Vatne et al. 2010a, b).

Considering communication between pediatricians and children, this study also presented relevant associations between several of the physician's behaviors directed towards the patients, including guidance, asking about doubts, bonding, and obtaining information. The results seem to indicate a group of communicative behaviors that usually occur together during the interaction, or, in other words, that pediatricians could have a personal communicative pattern and/or that this interaction is strongly influenced by the child's behavior, stimulating other subsequent interactions.

When considering the interaction between physicians and children, the present study showed no associations between the amount of doubts verbalized by the patients and their age, however, this behavior was associated with the child's schooling, bonding, and the physician obtaining information and asking about doubts. This data highlights the relevance of pediatrician's behavior that may promote child's inclusion in the communication, however, it is important to point out that pediatric cancer treatment may generate clinical conditions such as pain, nausea, and sleepiness which directly influence the interaction with the child (Kohlsdorf, 2012).

Considering communication between the physicians and caregivers, monthly income and caregiver's level of education were associated with better communication by the pediatrician, with parents with higher income and higher levels of education receiving more guidance, bonding, and being more frequently asked for information. These results are similar to those found in the literature (Brinkman et al. 2011; Fiks et al. 2010; Moseley et al. 2006; Taylor et al. 2010; Washington et al. 2012; Zwaanswijk et al. 2011). In addition to these results, the present study showed associations between marital status and better communication with physicians, considering guidance from pediatricians, and the amount of questions raised by the parents.

Clinical conditions also seem to play a relevant role in communicative patterns. In the present study, the type of diagnosis was related to physician's guidance to the children, asking about the caregiver's doubts, bonding and the amount of questions asked by the children and parents. It should be noted that children with solid tumors may have a specific clinical condition with more intense symptoms such as pain, physical impairment or injuries and surgery which may influence the condition of the child during consultations and, as a consequence, the interaction between the patients and pediatricians (Kohlsdorf, 2012). In addition, time since diagnosis was negatively associated with guidance and asking for information, suggesting that caregivers receive more information during the early stages of the treatment. The positive and weak associations between caregiver's doubts and asking caregivers for information might suggest a relevant pattern from physicians when including parents in communication. All these results are consistent with the literature, however, the gender of the child was not associated with pediatrician's communicative patterns in the present study, which is not consistent with the existing literature (Drotar 2009; Gabarra and Crepaldi 2011; Stivers 2011, 2012; Stivers and Majid 2007; Taylor et al. 2010; Zwaanswijk et al. 2011).

5. Conclusions

This study has some limitations that should be mentioned. First, the number of participating physicians was very small and, therefore, the results cannot be generalized to larger samples and different health conditions. It would be relevant to investigate patterns of pediatric communication with broader and multicentric samples in order to better characterize this phenomena, as well as studying samples from multiple health care settings. However, as already stated in the Method section, few professionals were available in the public health service in which this study was conducted, and all potential and recruitable participants were approached.

In addition, other variables related to the organization of the health care service were not included in this research, with these variables possibly moderating communication in pediatric settings. For example, it is possible to highlight that the amount of patients in the waiting room, the delay regarding examinations and bureaucratic procedures lead to less time for communication (Kohls-dorf, 2012). These factors may be confounding variables, which also moderate communication, beyond the sociodemographic data itself.

Furthermore, as a cross-sectional and descriptive study, it was not possible to assume causality effects among the variables, which restricts the possibilities to apply these data directly to the health communication milieu. Inter-rater reliability scores were low, which could have undermined the internal validity concerning this study. However, it should be highlighted that intra-rater reliability obtained high scores and that the field experience in health psychology and behavior observation was very different between the two observers. These two aspects may explain the low scores obtained, as already proposed by Danna and Matos (2006).

Finally, it should be stated that none validated tools to measure emphatic communication in clinical contexts have been employed in this study. Although the works of Wissow et al. (2005), Nicolai et al., (2007), Makoul et al., (2008), Vatne et al. (2010a, b) and also Howells et al. (2010) provided these tools, none of them have been adapted, translated and validated for the language and country in which this study took place, which explains the impossibility of using these scales.

Even with these limitations, this study presents contributions regarding associations between the clinical and sociodemographic data of children and caregivers, and communication patterns established by physicians. This should be taken into account when considering professional training during graduate courses, in order to provide tailored skills that may suit individual communicative patterns, since the literature highlights the lack of appropriate professional training (Rider et al. 2008). It is also relevant to point out the need of psychosocial interventions that may contribute to include children of very early ages, considering that the patients should not be excluded from pediatric interaction (Taylor et al. 2010; Vaknin and Zisk-Rony 2010; Washington et al. 2012). The data showed in the present study may be useful in planning educational interventions in health settings, focused on the staff as well as parents and children, and it may be relevant to highlight the need of more academic discussions regarding the pediatric communication process.

Future research should study other sociodemographic variables that may influence interaction during medical consultations, including the characteristics of the pediatricians and the variables related to the organization of the healthcare services, with a larger sample size and other clinical and sociodemographic variables of children and caregivers, in order to contribute towards a better quality of care in pediatric settings.

Competing Interests

The authors declare that they have no competing interests.

Authors' Contributions

MK carried out data collection, data analysis and drafted the manuscript. ALCJ was the professor advisor in the research, contributed to data analysis and also drafted the manuscript. All authors read and approved the final manuscript.

Source: Kohlsdorf M, Áderson Luiz Costa Junior. Associations between clinical and sociodemographic data and patterns of communication in pediatric oncology [J]. Psicologia Reflexao E Critica, 2016, 29(1):1–10.

References

[1] Ammentorp J, Kofoed PE, Laulund LW. Impact of communication skills training on parents perceptions of care: Intervention study. J Adv Nurs. 2011; 67(2): 394–400. http://dx.doi.org/10.1111/j.1365-2648.2010.05475.x.

[2] Bardin L. Análise de conteúdo. Lisboa: Edições; 1977. p.70.

[3] Brinkman WB, Hartl J, Rawe LM, Sucharew H, Britto MT, Epstein JN. Physicians' shared decision-making behaviors in attention-deficit/hyperactivity disorder care. Arch Pediatr Adolesc Med. 2011; 165(11):1013–19.

[4] Coyne I, Gallagher P. Participation in communication and decision-making: Children and young people's experiences in a hospital setting. J Clin Nurs. 2011; 20:2334–43. http://dx.doi.org/10.1111/j.1365-2702.2010.03582.x.

[5] Croom A, Wiebe DJ, Berg CA, Lindsay R, Donaldson D, Foster C, et al. Adolescent

and parent perceptions of patient-centered communication while managing type 1 diabetes. J Pediatr Psychol. 2011; 36(2):206–215. http://dx.doi.org/10.1093/jpepsy/jsq 072.

[6] Danna MF, Matos MA. Fidedignidade nas observações. Em Danna, M.F. & Matos, M.A., Aprendendo a observar (141–156). São Paulo: Edicon; 2006.

[7] Drotar D. Physician behavior in the care of pediatric chronic illness: Association with health outcomes and treatment adherence. J Dev Behav Pediatr. 2009; 30(3):246–254. http://dx.doi.org/10.1097/DBP.0b013e3181a7ed42.

[8] Fiks AG, Localio AR, Alessandrini EA, Asch DA, Guevara JP. Shared decision-making in pediatrics: A national perspective. Pediatrics. 2010; 126(2):306–314.

[9] Gabarra LM, Crepaldi MA. A comunicação médico-paciente pediátrico-família na perspectiva da criança. Psicologia Argumento. 2011; 29(65):209–218.

[10] Gordon BK, Jaaniste T, Bartlett K, Perrin M, Jackson A, Sandstrom A, et al. Child and parental surveys about pre-hospitalization information provision. Child Care Health-Dev.2010;37(5):727–733.http://dx.doi.org/10.1111/j.1365-2214.2010.01190.x.

[11] Howells RJ, Davies HA, Silverman JD, Archer JC, Mellon AF. Assessment of doctors' consultation skills in the paediatric setting: The Paediatric Consultation Assessment Tool. Arch Dis Child. 2010; 95:323–329.

[12] Knighting, K., Rowa-Dewar, N., Malcolm, C., Kearney, N. & Gibson, F. (2010). Children's understanding of cancer and health behaviors. Child: Care, health and development. 289–299. http://dx.doi.org/10.1111/j.1365-2214.2010.01138.x.

[13] Kohlsdorf M. Proposta de pré-consulta comportamental: análise da comunicação médico-cuidador-paciente em onco-hematologia pediátrica, Doctoral Thesis. Brasília: Universidade de Brasília; 2012.

[14] Makoul M, Krupat E, Chang C. Measuring patients views of physician communication skills: Development and testing of the Communication Assessment Tool. Patient Educ Couns. 2008; 67:333–342.

[15] Märtenson EK, Fägerskiöld AM. A review of children's decision-making competence in health care. J Clin Nurs. 2007; 17(23):3131-41.http://dx.doi.org/10.1111/j.1365-2702.2006.01920.x.

[16] Märtenson EK, Fägerskiöld AM, Berteró CM. Information exchange in paediatric settings: An observational study. Paediatr Nurs. 2007; 19(7):40–43.

[17] Moseley KL, Clark SJ, Gebremariam A, Sternthal MJ, Kemper AR. Parent's trust in their child's physician: Using an Adapted Trust in Physician Scale. Ambul Pediatr. 2006; 6(1):58–61.

[18] Nicolai J, Demmel R, Hagen J. Rating scales for the assessment of empathic communication in medical interviews (REM): Scale development, reliability and validity. J Clin Psychol Med Settings. 2007; 14:367–375.

[19] Rider EA, Volkan K, Hafler JP. Pediatric resident's perceptions of communication

competencies: Implications for teaching. Med Teach. 2008; 30(7):208–217.

[20] Sleath B, Carpenter DM, Slota C, Williams D, Tudor G, Yeatts K, et al. Communication during pediatric asthma visits and self-reported asthma medication adherence. Pediatrics. 2012; 130(4):1–7. http://dx.doi.org/10.1542/ peds.2012-0913.

[21] Stivers T. Negotiating who presents the problem: Next speaker selection in pediatric encounters. J Commun. 2011; 51(2):252–282.

[22] Stivers T. Physician-child interaction: When children answer physicians' questions in routine medical encounters. Patient Educ Couns. 2012; 87:3–9.

[23] Stivers T, Majid A. Questioning children: Interactional evidence of implicit bias in medical interviews. Soc Psychol Q. 2007; 70(4):424–441.

[24] Taylor S, Haase-Casanovas S, Weaver T, Kidd J, Garralda EM. Child involvement in the paediatric consultation: A qualitative study of children and carers' views. Child Care Health Dev. 2010; 36(5):678–685.

[25] Vaknin O, Zisk-Rony RY. Including children in medical decisions and treatments: Perceptions and practices of healthcare providers. Child Care Health Dev. 2010;37(4):533–539. http://dx.doi.org/10.1111/j.1365-2214.2010.01153.x.

[26] Vatne TM, Finset A, Ornes K, Ruland CM. Application of the Verona Coding Definitions of Emotional Sequences (VR-CoDES) on a pediatric data set. Patient Educ Couns. 2010a; 80:399–404.

[27] Vatne TM, Slaughter L, Ruland CM. How children with cancer communicate and think about symptoms. J Pediatr Oncol Nurs. 2010b; 27(1):24–32. http://dx.doi.org/ 10.1177/1043454209349358.

[28] Washington D, Yeatts K, Sleath B, Ayala GX, Gillette C, Williams D, et al. Communication and education about triggers and environmental control strategies during pediatric asthma visits. Patient Educ Couns. 2012; 86:63–69.http://dx.doi.org/10.1016/j.pec. 2011.04.015.

[29] Wassmer E, Minnaar G, Aal NA, Atkinson M, Gupta E, Yuen S, et al. How do paediatricians communicate with children and parents? Acta Paediatr. 2004; 93(11): 1501–1506. http://dx.doi.org/10.1111/j.1651-2227.2004.tb02637.x.

[30] Wissow LS, Larson S, Anderson J, Hadjiisky E. Pediatric residents' responses that discourage discussion of psychosocial problems in primary care. Pediatrics. 2005; 115(6): 1569–1578. http://dx.doi.org/10.1542/peds.2004-1535.

[31] Zwaanswijk M, Tates K, van Dulmen S, Hoogerbrugge PM, Kamps WA, Beishuizen A, et al. Communicating with child patients in pediatric oncology consultations: A vignette study on child patients', parents', and survivors' communication preferences. Psycho-Oncology. 2011; 20:269–277. http://dx.doi.org/10.1002/pon.1721.

Chapter 26

Contrast-Enhanced [18F] Fluorodeoxyglucose-Positron Emission Tomography/Computed Tomography in Clinical Oncology: Tumor-, Site-, and Question-Based Comparison with Standard Positron Emission Tomography/Computed Tomography

Silvia Morbelli[1], Raffaella Conzi[2], Claudio Campus[3], Giuseppe Cittadini[2], Irene Bossert[1], Michela Massollo[1], Giuseppe Fornarini[4], Iolanda Calamia[1], Cecilia Marini[5], Francesco Fiz[1], Chiara Ghersi[1], Lorenzo E Derchi[2], Gianmario Sambuceti[1]

[1]Nuclear Medicine Unit, IRCCS AOU San Martino-IST, Department of Health Sciences, University of Genoa, Largo R Benzi, 10, Genoa 16132, Italy
[2]Department of Radiology, IRCCS AOU San Martino-IST, Genoa, Italy
[3]Italian Institute of Technology (IIT), Genoa, Italy
[4]Department of Medical Oncology, IRCCS AOU San Martino-IST, Genoa, Italy
[5]Institute of Molecular Bioimaging and Physiology, CNR, Genoa-Milan, Italy

Abstract: Background: The present study aimed to evaluate the added value of contrast-enhanced computed tomography (ceCT) in comparison to standard, non-enhanced CT in the context of a combined positron emission tomography (PET)/CT examination by means of a tumor-, site-, and clinical question-based approach. Methods: Analysis was performed in 202 patients undergoing PET/CT consisting of a multiphase CT protocol followed by a whole-body PET. The Cochran Q test was performed, followed by a multiple comparisons correction (McNemar test and Bonferroni adjustment), to compare standard and contrast-enhanced PET (cePET/CT). Histopathology or clinical-radiologic follow-up greater than 1 year was used as a reference. Results: cePET/CT showed significantly different results with respect to standard PET/CT in head and neck and gastrointestinal cancer (P = 0.02 and 0.0002, respectively), in the evaluation of lesions located in the abdomen (P = 0.009), and in the context of disease restaging (P = 0.003). In all these clinical scenarios, adding ceCT resulted in a distinct benefit, by yielding a higher percentage of change in patient management. Conclusion: These data strongly underline the importance of strictly selecting patients for the combined exam. In particular, patient selection should not be driven solely by mere tumor classification, but should also account for the clinical question and the anatomical location of the neoplastic disease, which can significantly impact patient management.

Keywords: PET/CT, Contrast-Enhanced PET/CT, [18F] Fluorodeoxyglucose, Head and Neck Cancer, Gastrointestinal Cancer

1. Background

Since the early 1990s, functional imaging with positron emission tomography (PET) has been the fastest growing diagnostic modality in oncology[1][2]. In particular, PET with [18F] fluorodeoxyglucose (FDG), which exploits the increased glucose uptake and metabolism by the rapidly proliferating cancer cells, has opened a new field in clinical imaging and is widely used for staging, restaging, therapeutic response monitoring, and prognostic evaluation in patients affected by several types of cancers. However, PET imaging alone is unable to provide precise anatomical localization. Moreover, its utility is often limited by the contextual presence of augmented, non-disease-related glucose uptake in several anatomical districts. These findings can range from the physiologically increased uptake in organs, such as the heart, liver, voluntary muscles, and brain, to paraphysiological scenarios, such as FDG hyperaccumulation in skeletal repair sites, in the active ovarian follicle, and within the active bone marrow[3]. Inflammation is per se a common cause of increased glucose use[3][4].

Over the last decades, hybrid imaging, encompassing combined PET and computed tomography (CT) in a single scanner has become commercially available. Its emergence has had a major impact on diagnostic performance of oncology patients[4], enabling the physician to acquire both metabolic and anatomical imaging data in a single diagnostic session[2].

Modern PET/CT scanners incorporate the latest CT technology, thus technically allowing the execution of multiphase, high-quality CT imaging. Recently, there have been several reports of the possible superiority of contrast-enhanced PET (cePET)/contrast-enhanced CT (ceCT) over standard PET/CT in different clinical settings, including disease staging, restaging, presurgical evaluation, and treatment planning of different tumor types[5]–[10]. However, in the vast majority of PET/CT scans, the CT component is performed with low current setting and without intravenous contrast, its purpose being to allow an attenuation-weighted reconstruction of the PET sinograms and obtain an anatomical correlation of radiotracer distribution. Indeed, the adoption of a low-dose, contrast-free CT protocol has been guided mostly by practical considerations, so as to reduce radiation burden, reduce patient discomfort, and minimize scanning time, thus increasing the number of exams that a center can perform on daily basis. Also, the lack of large prospective trials and the absence of clinical guidelines have prevented a systematic application of this dual-mode imaging using an evidence-based approach.

It has, however, to be considered that the analyses performed in the vast majority of published studies are mainly focused on a tumor-based approach[5]–[10] in the absence of a more 'translational' evaluation of the feasibility of such a powerful, but practically complex, imaging modality. In fact, the potential advantages of executing the CT part of a PET/CT scan with protocol encompassing contrast administration are related to the greater anatomical details given by ceCT, and its improved characterization of millimetric lesions and the delineation of known lesions with respect to surrounding tissues (*i.e.* the identification of infiltrative behavior). These latter aspects may be more strictly related to each patient's specific clinical history (site of disease and clinical question) rather than to the mere classification of tumor type. For these reasons, we hypothesized that a more comprehensive approach would help to identify patients that are more likely to benefit from cePET/CT imaging. This approach should account not only for tumor histopathology, but also for the site of known/suspected lesions and for the clinical question. Thus, the aim of the present study was to evaluate the additional diagnostic value of ceCT in comparison to standard, non-enhanced CT in the context of a combined PET/CT examination by means of a tumor-, site-, and clinical question-based approach.

2. Methods

2.1. Patients

Between September 2007 and June 2011, 202 patients were referred to our institution for the execution of multimodal PET/CT, including both non-enhanced and contrast-enhanced diagnostic CT. Clinical indication comprised diagnosis of suspected oncologic disease, diagnosis of a suspected recurrence, and staging, restaging, or post-therapy evaluation of a known oncologic disease. All patients accepted the use of imaging data for research purposes by providing written informed consent that was approved by the local regulatory bodies. Patient characteristics are summarized in **Table 1**. In these patients, the indications for adding a multiphase ceCT to the standard PET/CT exam protocol were: (1) new patients with no state-of-the-art, whole-body staging examination available; (2) equivocal or insufficient results of previous examinations; (3) precise assessment of tumor extent before local radiation therapy; (4) post-therapy assessment of an inpatient who required restaging with both ceCT and PET/CT.

2.2. Positron Emission Tomography/Computed Tomography Scanning

Patients were prepared and standard PET/CT exams were performed according to the European guidelines[11]. Briefly, patients fasted overnight prior to

Table 1. Patient characteristics.

	Whole patient group (n = 202)	Histopathological confirmation (n = 73)
Age (years)	61.9 ± 14.9	54.2 ± 17.3
Gender (M/F)	120/82	43/30
Tumor type[a,b]		
Lung cancer	38	30
Head and neck cancer	22	14
Gastrointestinal cancer[c]	31	7
Breast cancer	21	4
Lymphoma	36	9
Melanoma	19	2
Multiple melanoma	15	5
Other[d]	18	2
Clinical question[b]		
Diagnosis	22	10
Staging	20	11
Restaging[e]	33	18
Response to chemotherapy	58	6
Response to radiotherapy	18	6
Post-surgery evaluation	11	0
Surveillance	40	22

Values are mean ± standard deviation. [a]Two patients were not affected by any oncologic disease after histologic confirmation. [b]Tumor type and clinical questions correspond to the groups submitted to the tumor-based and question-based analyses. [c]Including esophageal, gastric, and colorectal cancer. [d]Gynecologic malignancy (n = 8), testicular cancer (n = 2), sarcoma (n = 3), low-differentiated neuroendocrine carcinoma (n = 4), thymoma (n = 1). [e]Suspected relapse or patients with potentially resectable metastatic disease.

the intravenous administration of FDG; this was performed in a quiet room, with the patient lying in a recumbent position and asked not to move. Blood glucose was measured before tracer injection was administered, to ensure blood glucose levels < 160mg/dl. The dose of FDG varied between 350MBq and 450MBq, depending on the patient's weight, and was injected through a peripheral vein catheter. To minimize artifacts caused by the presence of radioactive urine in the excretory system, patients were asked to drink 500ml–1000ml of water 1 h prior to image acquisition and to void just before the scan. No urinary bladder catheterization was used. Whole-body imaging was performed using a combined PET/CT scanner (BioGraph 16 Hi-Rez PET/CT scanner; Siemens AG, Erlangen, Germany). The technical parameters of the 16-detector row, helical CT scanner included a gantry rotation speed of 0.5s and a table speed of 24mm per gantry rotation. The PET component of the combined imaging system had an axial view of 16.2cm (per bed position), with an interslice spacing of 3.75mm in one bed position. The transaxial field of view and pixel size of the reconstructed PET images were 58.5cm and 4.57mm, respectively, with a matrix size of 128×128. Data acquisition started 60 ± 10 minutes after intravenous tracer administration. First, unenhanced, low-dose CT was performed at 140kV and 40mA for emission-based attenuation correction, immediately followed by a PET scan, which was executed in three-dimensional (3D) mode, with a 3-min acquisition per bed position. The scan was performed starting from the orbital plane on to the mid-thigh, except for those cases where the clinical history demanded a whole-body, head-to-toes scan (e.g. multiple myeloma or melanoma). Attenuation-corrected PET images were reconstructed by means of an ordered-subset expectation maximization, iterative reconstruction algorithm (three iterations, eight subsets). Finally, diagnostic ceCT was performed for the same axial coverage. The entire ceCT data set was automatically fused with the 3D PET images using the integrated software interface provided by the manufacturer (syngo Image Fusion; Siemens AG, Erlangen, Germany) to create contrast-enhanced anatomical images superimposed with FDG uptake. We did not experience significant fusion mismatch as the ceCT was performed immediately after the PET emission scan, while the patient was maintaining the same position.

2.3. Contrast-Enhanced Computed Tomography Technique

The CT scan was performed immediately after completion of PET acquisition, planned with the same scout view. In most cases, a pre-contrast diagnostic scan was not acquired and the standard acquisition protocol consisted of an arterial phase scan of the upper abdomen, starting 35s after the start of contrast injection, followed by a portal phase scan, extended from the skull base to the symphysis pubis, starting 70s after the administration of the intravenous contrast. The scan parameters were as follows. Arterial phase: slice thickness of 5mm, pitch 0.8, tube rotation speed 0.5s, 120kV, reference 175mA. A dose modulation system was applied to optimize total exposure according to the patient's body size; an additional set of 1-mm thick slices was reconstructed to obtain high-resolution, multiplanar reformations. Portal phase: slice thickness 5mm, pitch 0.8, tube rotation speed 0.5s, 120kV, reference 175mA with the same modulation system; 2-mm thick slices at 1.5mm intervals were reconstructed for multiplanar reformations.

In selected cases, a delayed scan was performed at equilibrium or in the urographic phase, according to the clinical question. In the follow-up of known lesions or in patients with lymphoproliferative disorders and with previous negative imaging examination, only the portal phase scan was obtained, so as to reduce the dose administered to the patient.

Iodinated contrast medium, with a concentration of 350mg/ml, was injected using a power injector at a flow rate of 3ml/s and a dose of 80ml–130ml, depending on body weight, followed by 40ml of saline at the same flow rate. Contrast medium administration protocols and measures aiming to prevent contrast-related adverse effects were performed according to the guidelines of the European Society of Urogenital Radiology[12].

Standard, 5-mm thick images were used for rapid evaluation by the radiologist and for reviewing by the referring physician, while thinner slices were used for multiplanar imaging of vessels, bone (ribs and spine), and for high-resolution scanning of lung and liver lesions.

2.4. Image Interpretation

Positron emission tomography, ceCT, and fused images were reconstructed for review on a dedicated computer workstation (syngo Image Fusion; Siemens AG, Erlangen, Germany).

Initially, PET/low-dose CT and multiphase diagnostic CT images were evaluated independently by two experienced nuclear medicine specialists and by two experienced CT radiologists, respectively. All readers had access to the patient's clinical history, but were blinded to the other modality results. Subsequently, fused, cePET/CT images were evaluated in consensus, by the combined team of radiologists and nuclear physicians. This latter consensus report was compared with the previous evaluations to determine the additional value of diagnostic CT on PET/CT image interpretation.

In the evaluation of FDG-PET/CT, a lesion was considered positive whenever it showed a non-physiological increase of FDG uptake. In particular, the diagnosis of a PET-positive lesion was also supported by a maximum standardized uptake (SUV_{max}) value of at least 2.5 or by an FDG uptake exceeding the surrounding background tissue, the blood pool radioactivity, or the average liver uptake. However, the differentiation between malignant and benign lesion was not based solely on SUV_{max}, as the qualitative assessment of increased FDG uptake areas played a major role in the clinical reporting. For instance, if a lesion showed clearly abnormal focal FDG avidity but displayed a SUV_{max} lower than the 2.5 threshold (e.g. due to partial volume effect in small-sized lesions), that lesion was deemed malignant.

On diagnostic ceCT-only images, detection of a pathologic lesion was performed according to published criteria[13]–[16]. For example, lymph node (LN) assessment in the neck, thorax, and abdomen was based on size criteria (1-cm short-axis diameter threshold). However, the presence of peripheral low attenuation, suggesting a fatty hilum within a LN, was considered a benign sign, regardless of node size. Finally, criteria such as abnormal enhancement, central necrosis, irregular borders, and the presence of infiltrative behavior were used to characterize soft tissue lesions. Consensus interpretation of the PET/ceCT exam was performed according to the following criteria: (1) positive lesions were diagnosed when an abnormal area of focal FDG uptake, as observed in PET images, corresponded to an abnormal finding on CT; (2) LNs with increased glucose uptake were deemed positive for metastatic spread even if they were smaller than 1cm in short-axis diameter; (3) conversely, LNs with no detectable tracer uptake were deemed negative for metastatic spread, even if they were larger than 1cm in short-axis diameter; (4) in all the remaining cases, the two readers decided to emphasize either functional information from the PET or morphological information from the ceCT on a case-by-case basis, according to type and site of disease and in relation to the patient's clinical history. For example, in cePET/CT images, small pathological lesions, such as millimetric lung metastases, which often lack FDG accumulation, were evaluated on the basis of the ceCT results.

2.5. Standard of Reference

The final diagnosis was obtained from the results of the histopathologic examination, obtained following surgery or biopsy (73 patients, 147 lesions), or clinical/radiological 12-month follow-up or, again, on the basis of tumor marker levels or on the evolutionary pattern of known findings at subsequent imaging (129 patients, 450 lesions). Follow-up information included physical examination, laboratory tests, tumor markers, other independent imaging studies, such as multislice CT, magnetic resonance imaging, FDG-PET/CT, 18 F-NaF PET/CT, X-ray studies, and bone scans.

The criteria used as the standard of reference were: (1) laboratory findings, such as increasing tumor markers; (2) combination of either negative follow-up imaging findings and negative clinical findings or positive clinical findings with decreasing lesion size after therapy, as determined by subsequent imaging studies; (3) increasing lesion size or metabolic activity in the course of follow-up; (4) subsiding of pathological findings on follow-up PET/CT studies combined with negative clinical follow-up.

2.6. Statistical Analysis

Statistical analysis was carried out using the 'R' software program[17] and the DiagnosisMed software package[18].

We performed patient-based and lesion-, site-, tumor-, and question-based analyses of the cePET/CT results compared with PET/CT. **Table 1** and **Table 2** list the tumor type, clinical question, and site of disease that were used in the tumor-, question-, and site-based analyses.

A lesion was included in the analysis if at least one of the three modalities (cePET/CT, ceCT, PET/CT) deemed it positive or if it was considered as non-pathologic at these three modalities but resulted positive at a subsequent histopathologic analysis.

Sensitivity, specificity, positive predictive value, negative predictive value

Table 2. Distribution of lesions.

	Lesions included in the analysis (n = 597)	Histopathological confirmation (n = 147)
Tumor type[a,b]		
Lung cancer	104	40
Head and neck cancer	61	32
Gastrointestinal cancer[c]	129	24
Breast cancer	60	6
Lymphoma	125	20
Melanoma	26	10
Multiple melanoma	32	3
Other[d]	60	12
Clinical question[b]		
Diagnosis	22	10
Staging	20	11
Restaging[e]	33	18
Response to chemotherapy	58	6
Response to radiotherapy	18	6
Post-surgery evaluation	11	0
Surveillance	40	22
Site of disease[b]		
Neck	93	33
Thorax	110	49
Abdomen	220	45
Skeleton-bone marrow	174	20
Lymph nodes[f]	198	32

Values are mean ± standard deviation. [a]Two patients were not affected by any oncologic disease after histologic confirmation. [b]Tumor type, clinical questions, and disease sites correspond to the groups submitted to the tumor-based and question-based analyses. [c]Including esophageal, gastric, and colorectal cancer. [d]Gynecologic malignancy (n = 8), testicular cancer (n = 2), sarcoma (n = 3), low-differentiated neuroendocrine carcinoma (n = 4), thymoma (n = 1). [e]Suspected relapse or patients with potentially resectable metastatic disease. [f]Lymph nodes were computed twice: according to their position in the body and independently from their position.

(NPV), accuracy, likelihood ratios, diagnostic odds ratio, error rate, and Youden's index were calculated using standard statistical formulae, and the 95% confidence interval was determined for each parameter. Differences among imaging modalities were assessed with the Cochran Q test, followed by multiple comparisons using the McNemar test with continuity correction and Bonferroni adjustment. Probability values inferior to 0.05 were considered as statistically significant. The value of adding a diagnostic CT to the standard PET/CT protocol was also evaluated in terms of the impact on patient management, following the information derived from the cePET/CT exam only. This evaluation was performed on a patient basis for each tumor type and clinical question.

In order to better characterize the additional value of ceCT with respect to the low-dose PET/CT study, the management-changing findings were classified into the following categories: (1) metabolism-related; (2) site-related; (3) dimension-related; (4) related to local infiltration or additional findings on ceCT.

Category 1 referred to the improved characterization of a lesion that presented no increment in FDG uptake or whose uptake did not reach the significance threshold. Category 2 encompassed the scenario of a more accurate interpretation of lesions due to improved localization of abnormal FDG uptake, which also allowed a better distinction between abnormal and physiological FDG uptake. Category 3 was applied to the cases of identification of pathologic lesions with size falling below PET image resolution. Finally, category 4 referred to the evaluation of infiltrative behavior or to meaningful findings that had gone undetected at the standard PET/CT scan.

3. Results

Overall diagnostic accuracy and patient-based analysis Positron emission tomography/CT, ceCT, and combined cePET/CT correctly classified (true positive plus true negative) 173, 153, and 179 patients, respectively. The Cochran Q test evidenced a significant difference in the comparison of the three techniques (Cochran Q = 26.08, degrees of freedom (df) = 2, P = 2 × 10^{-6}). However, a pairwise comparison using continuity-corrected McNe-mar tests with Bonferroni adjustment revealed that cePET/CT was not significantly different with respect to

PET/CT alone (McNemar chi-squared test = 1.5625, df = 1, P = 0.21). Although not reaching significance, cePET/CT presented better sensitivity, NPV, negative likelihood ratio (NLR) and Youden's index, when compared to PET/CT. Patient-based performance comparisons between PET/CT and combined cePET/CT are shown in **Table 3**.

3.2. Overall Lesion-Based Analysis

A total of 597 lesions were detected. Among these, 431, 385, and 467 lesions were correctly evaluated (true positive plus true negative) by PET/CT, ceCT and combined cePET/CT, respectively. The Cochran Q test evidenced a significant difference between the three techniques (Cochran Q = 58.3969, df = 2, P < 10^{-12}). A pairwise comparison using continuity-corrected McNemar tests with Bonferroni adjustment revealed that the evaluation with cePET/CT yielded significantly different results with respect to PET/CT (McNemar chi-squared test = 30.96, df = 1, adjusted P < 0.05). Performance comparisons between PET/CT and cePET/CT are shown in **Table 4**; cePET/CT showed better sensitivity, NPV, NLR, and You den's index compared to PET/CT. However, PET/CT showed a slightly better specificity than cePET/CT.

Table 3. Patient-based performance comparisons between PET/CT and cePET/CT.

	PET/CT	cePET/CT
Sensitivity (%)	92.79 (86.42–96.30)	98.20 (93.67–99.50)
Specificity (%)	76.92 (67.28–84.38)	76.55 (67.02–84.76)
Positive predictive value (%)	83.06 (75.49–88.65)	83.85 (76.56–89.18)
Negative predictive value (%)	89.74 (81.05–94.71)	97.22 (90.43–99.23)
Positive likelihood ratio	4.02 (2.75–5.88)	4.26 (2.92–6.20)
Negative likelihood ratio	0.09 (0.05–0.18)	0.02 (0.01–0.09)
Diagnostic odds ratio	41.67 (16.96–115.67)	174.43 (41.26–1593.39)
Error rate (%)	14.36 (10.19–19.86)	11.39 (7.71–16.51)
Accuracy (%)	85.64 (80.14–89.81)	88.61 (83.49–92.29)
Youden's index	0.6972 (0.700–0.6940)	0.7512 (0.7541–0.7483)

PET, positron emission tomography; CT, computed tomography; cePET/CT, contrast-enhanced PET/CT.

Table 4. Lesion-based analysis: performance comparisons between PET/CT and cePET/CT.

	PET/CT	cePET/CT
Sensitivity (%)	80.54 (76.41–84.10)	91.38 (88.25–93.74)
Specificity (%)	54.45 (47.37–61.36)	50.26 (43.24–57.28)
Positive predictive value (%)	78.99 (74.80–82.63)	79.61 (75.72–83.02)
Negative predictive value (%)	56.83 (49.59–63.79)	73.28 (65.12–80.12)
Positive likelihood ratio	1.77 (1.50–2.09)	1.84 (1.58–2.13)
Negative likelihood ratio	0.36 (0.28–0.45)	0.17 (0.12–0.24)
Diagnostic odds ratio	4.93 (3.39–7.21)	10.63 (6.85–16.84)
Error rate (%)	27.81 (24.36–31.53)	21.78 (18.65–25.26)
Accuracy (%)	72.19 (68.47–75.64)	78.22 (74.74–81.35)
Youden's index	0.349 (0.352–0.347)	0.416 (0.418–0.414)

Estimated parameters corresponding to each technique are presented with a 95% confidence interval shown within parentheses. PET, positron emission tomography; CT, computed tomography; cePET/CT, contrast-enhanced PET/CT.

3.3. Tumor-Based Lesion Analysis

Table 5 lists the different types of tumor in which lesion-based performance comparison was executed between PET/CT and cePET/CT. The latter imaging modality showed significantly different results with respect to standard PET/CT in head and neck cancer (McNemar chi-squared test = 5.9, df = 1, P = 0.02) and gastrointestinal cancer (McNemar chi-squared test = 13.1, df = 1, P = 0.0002) patients. **Table 6** lists the corresponding sensitivity and specificity values.

3.4. Site-Based Analysis of Lesions

Five anatomical districts, including neck, thorax, abdomen, skeletal-bone marrow, and LNs (regardless of body region), were evaluated in each patient. Contrast-enhanced PET/CT results were significantly different with respect to standard PET/CT in the abdominal region (McNemar chisquared test = 6.8, df = 1, P = 0.009). As expected, in the subset of patients with abdominal lesions, the largest subgroup was represented by patients with colorectal cancer (n = 21) followed

Table 5. Statistical difference (P values) between the performance of PET/CT and ce-PET/CT for each analyzed tumor type, site of disease, and clinical question.

	P value
Tumor type	
Lung cancer	0.12
Head and neck cancer	0.02
Gastrointestinal cancer[a]	0.0002
Breast cancer	0.09
Lymphoma	0.24
Melanoma	0.16
Multiple melanoma	0.08
Other[b]	0.33
Site of disease	
Neck	0.096
Thorax	0.36
Abdomen	0.009
Skeleton-bone marrow	0.33
Lymph nodes	0.44
Clinical question	
Diagnosis	0.39
Staging	0.09
Restaging[c]	0.003
Response to chemotherapy	0.13
Response to radiotherapy	0.1
Post-surgery evaluation	0.54
Surveillance	0.51

[a]Including esophageal, gastric, and colorectal cancer. [b]Gynecologic malignancy n = 8, testicular cancer n = 2, sarcoma n = 3, low-differentiated neuroendocrine carcinoma n = 4, thymoma n = 1. [c]Suspected relapse or patients with potentially resectable metastatic disease. PET, positron emission tomography; CT, computed tomography; cePET/CT, contrast-enhanced PET/CT.

Table 6. Performance of PET/CT and cePET/CT in tumors, sites of disease, and clinical questions whose diagnostic results were significantly different between the two imaging modalities.

	PET/CT	cePET/CT
Tumor type		
Head and neck cancer		
Sensitivity (%)	71.33 (63.64–77.97)	82.67 (75.81–87.89)
Specificity (%)	46.30 (33.69–59.39)	48.15 (35.39–61.15)
Gastrointestinal cancer[a]		
Sensitivity (%)	71.25 (60.54–80.01)	95.00 (87.84–98.04)
Specificity (%)	84.21 (62.43–94.48)	89.47 (68.61–97.06)
Site of disease		
Abdomen		
Sensitivity (%)	97.53 (91.44–99.32)	92.59 (84.77–96.56)
Specificity (%)	46.15 (23.21–70.86)	92.31 (66.69–98.63)
Questions		
Restaging[b]		
Sensitivity (%)	83.96 (75.81–89.74)	96.23 (90.70–98.52)
Specificity (%)	78.37 (52.33–92.50)	78.57 (52.41–92.43)

Estimated parameters corresponding to each technique are presented with 95% confidence interval within parentheses. [a]Including esophageal, gastric, and colorectal cancer. [b]Suspected relapse or patients with potentially resectable metastatic disease. PET, positron emission tomography; CT, computed tomography; cePET/CT, contrast-enhanced PET/CT.

by non-Hodgkin lymphoma patients (n = 12), while subgroups comprising patients affected by other tumor types were smaller (five esophageal, five breast, two ovarian, and four lung cancers, two melanomas, one neuroendocrine tumor). Table 6 lists the corresponding sensitivity and specificity values.

3.5. Question-Based Analysis of Lesions

Table 1 lists the different clinical questions, submitted independently from the lesion-based performance comparisons between PET/CT and cePET/CT. The results of cePET/CT were significantly different with respect to standard PET/CT when the scenario of disease restaging was considered (McNemar chi-squared test = 8.5, df = 1, P = 0.003). Again, among patients submitted for restaging, the largest subgroup of patients was represented by the patients with colorectal cancer (n = 14) while all other patient subgroups were smaller (three head and neck, three breast, four lung and one ovarian cancers, five melanomas, three non-Hodgkin lymphomas). **Table 6** lists the corresponding sensitivity and specificity values.

3.6. Impact on Patient Management

Findings that were detected only at the cePET/CT imaging modality resulted in a change of management for 15 of the 202 patients (7.4%). In particular, three patients initiated a previously unplanned therapy, six patients avoided inappropriate surgery, while a previously decided medical treatment was spared in four patients. In two patients, the use of cePET/CT significantly modified the radiotherapy protocol. Adding ceCT produced more distinct benefits, *i.e.* yielded a greater percentage of clinical management modifications in selected tumor types and clinical questions. In fact, the incremental value of this diagnostic technique rose to 22% in patients with head and neck cancer (5/23) and in 16% of patients with gastrointestinal cancer (5/31). Finally, when patients were grouped using the clinical question criterion, the additional value of diagnostic ceCT was more evident in the disease restaging setting (8/33 patients, 24.2%). These patients, submitted to cePET/CT for restaging purposes, were respectively affected by head and neck cancer (n = 2), gastrointestinal cancer (n = 2), lung cancer (n = 1), non-Hodgkin lymphoma (n = 1), breast cancer (n = 1), and poorly differentiated neuroendocrine carcinoma (n = 1).

The 15 patients whose management was changed by cePET/CT, were classified according to the previously explained management-changing findings categorization, as follows: category 1 = six patients; category 2 = three patients; category 3 = five patients; category 4 = one patient. Representative cases are shown in **Figures 1–3**.

4. Discussion

The present analysis does not support the routine use of cePET/CT. In fact, our study confirms that, when clinically indicated, PET/CT executed with low-dose

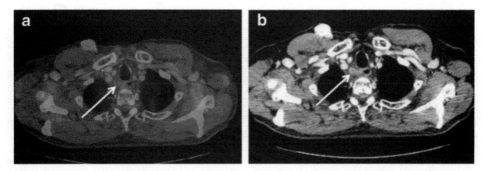

Figure 1. A 65-year-old male patient affected by pharyngeal cancer with lymph nodal relapse (secondary disease relapse: the first relapse in the neck lymph nodes had been treated with surgery and radiotherapy one year before). (a) Axial, contrast-enhanced, full-dose CT shows a small lymph node, which seems to infiltrate the upper esophagus. (b) As evident from contrast-enhanced PET/CT fused images, this lymph node does not display increased FDG uptake. Subsequent endoesophageal ultrasound biopsy confirmed the presence of lymph node metastasis. The patient was then submitted to chemotherapy. CT, computed tomography; PET, positron emission tomography; FDG, [^{18}F] fluorodeoxyglucose.

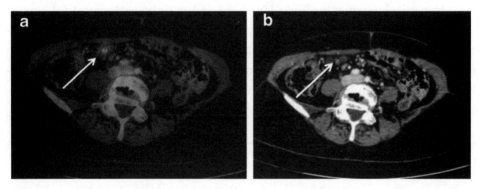

Figure 2. A 54-year-old female patient previously submitted for surgical treatment for primary colon cancer and with a known, single liver metastasis. This patient underwent contrast-enhanced PET/CT for the exclusion of other metastatic lesions, as she was a candidate for surgical resection of the hepatic localization. (a) Axial, contrast-enhanced, full-dose CT shows a suspicious 8-mm solid lesion close to the small bowel. (b) The lesion is highly FDG-avid on contrast-enhanced PET/CT. However, the pathologic nature of this finding is clearly evident only on contrast-enhanced CT, whereas using standard CT, it could have been deemed as unspecific bowel FDG-activity. This patient thus avoided inappropriate surgical treatment and was referred for chemotherapy. PET, positron emission tomography; CT, computed tomography; FDG, [^{18}F] fluorodeoxyglucose.

CT is adequate for the workup of FDG-avid tumor types[2]. However, our analysis demonstrated that ceCT could improve the diagnostic potential of hybrid imaging in specific clinical scenarios, where it can significantly impact patient management.

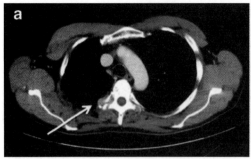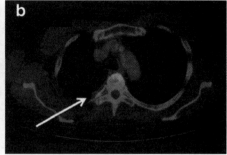

Figure 3. A 51-year-old male patient, presenting tumor marker increase after surgery for lung cancer. (a) Axial, contrast-enhanced, full-dose CT showed a paravertebral lesion, which was slightly enlarged and significantly more hyperemic with respect to a previous CT scan. (b) The lesion showed very mild FDG uptake; it was, however, classified as highly suspicious on the basis of the contrast-enhanced CT component of the exam. Biopsy confirmed the presence of lung adenocarcinoma metastasis. Accordingly, the patient was referred for radiotherapy. CT, computed tomography; FDG, [18F] fluorodeoxyglucose.

In particular, patients affected by head and neck or gastrointestinal cancer, and patients undergoing PET/CT for evaluation of abdominal lesions and for restaging purposes, seem to receive a greater benefit from imaging protocols including both PET and ceCT. A greater diagnostic accuracy of cePET/CT has been indeed reported in both head and neck and gastrointestinal cancer patients, with sensitivity and specificity comparable with our results.

4.1. Head and Neck Cancer

Haerle *et al.* demonstrated that cePET/CT is superior to PET/CT with regard to pathologically confirmed N0 versus N + status in head and neck cancer patients[19]. In this study, sensitivity and specificity for correct N classification were respectively 70.7% and 50% for PET/CT and 85.5% and 45.5% for cePET/CT. Similarly, Yoshida *et al.* reported the superiority of cePET/CT over PET/CT in the detection of head and neck malignancies[20]. Overall, these results are consistent with the fact that the interpretation of FDG-PET/CT findings in the neck can be challenging because of the numerous areas of physiologic FDG uptake and also due to the frequently observed pitfalls in post-treatment PET/CT imaging (e.g. slight homogeneous FDG uptake at the tracheostomy site or due to post-treatment edema of the mucosal surfaces). Besides the complexity of neck anatomy, other aspects related to each specific patient can also be advocated. In fact, Haerle *et al.*

highlighted a statistically significant correlation between SUVmax and the degree of necrosis in the involved neck LNs[19]. Actually, while the presence of central necrosis in neck LNs is considered as a reliable sign of LN metastasis at ceCT, these nodes are often disregarded by non-enhanced PET/CT because of the lack of FDG uptake in the necrotic, hypocellular tissue. The presence of necrotic LNs can be predicted in some cases, being more frequent in human papillomavirus-associated head and neck squamous cell carcinoma[19]. Accordingly, in the present study, more than one-third of patients whose management was changed by cePET/CT had PET-negative or only faintly positive lesions, whose presence could have been predicted before the exam. This finding confirms that patients can be selected for cePET/CT on the basis of their specific clinical history.

4.2. Gastrointestinal Cancer and Abdominal Imaging

Dirisamer *et al.* showed that the sensitivity and specificity of PET/CT in colorectal cancer rose from 85% to 100% and from 70% to 81%, respectively, when contrast medium was added to the CT component of the exam[21]. More importantly, these authors showed that the significant increase in sensitivity (which is similar to the one highlighted in the present study) was due to a misdetection of 67% of the metastases at the standard PET/CT exam. Interestingly enough, these metastases were smaller than 8mm in the majority of cases (94%). Indeed, small metastatic lesions from colon cancer, located within the liver or in the lung parenchyma, can show absent or only modest tracer uptake at PET/CT. Contrast enhancement is particularly effective when evaluating lesions within the liver, as it allows the spotting and classification of lesions as positive, small, and faintly FDG-avid, otherwise missed by standard PET/CT. In this type of patient, other reasons for false-negative PET/CT results are millimetric peritoneal metastatic spread or small peritoneal lesions located in proximity to areas of non-specific FDG uptake, which are common in the intestinal tract[22]. In the present study, the potential usefulness of cePET/CT in the evaluation of patients with gastrointestinal cancer is further testified by the fact that patients with colorectal cancer represented the largest subgroup both in patients with abdominal lesions and in patients submitted for restaging. In these two groups, we independently demonstrated a significantly greater diagnostic accuracy of cePET/CT with respect to standard PET/CT.

4.3. Restaging in Suspected Cases or Known Disease Relapse

Both these findings (tiny lesions or lesions close to sites of physiologic FDG uptake), whenever undetected by PET/CT, may significantly undermine the correct management of patients. Accordingly, these reasons account for more than one-half of cePET/CT findings that demanded a change of therapeutic strategy in patients included in the present study and are indeed especially relevant as they can avoid inappropriate surgery. On the other hand, ceCT alone showed limited capability in differentiating disease recurrence from post-radio-therapy tissue reaction, while PET/CT displayed a good performance in telling apart these two settings, owing to its intrinsic capacity to identify viable tumor tissue[23]. Overall, both very small lesions, which are likely to produce false-negatives at PET/CT, and local, post-therapy changes, which are likely to prove a diagnostic challenge at ceCT alone, are particularly relevant in patients submitted to medical imaging for restaging or for the preoperative workup of metastatic lesions, candidates for surgical resection. Altogether, these findings strongly suggest that restaging of patients with gastrointestinal cancer could be one of the main indications for cePET/CT use.

4.4. Patient Selection Based on Criteria Other Than Tumor Type

Despite the advantages of cePET/CT highlighted here and in previous studies, the use of cePET/CT is still not justified for clinical routine examinations due to higher costs, increased radiation burden, and potential adverse drug reaction to the intravenous contrast medium. Moreover, to obtain an accurate fusion of the two image sets, ceCT should be performed without repositioning the patient. This demands the presence of a physician for immediate image assessment after the standard PET/CT examination, thus resulting in a lowered patient throughput, because of additional time requirements for image review[24]. Therefore, given the demands for FDG-PET/CT and the number of available PET/CT scanners, the diffusion of cePET/CT as a 'one-stop-shop' examination for all patients submitted to PET/CT does not presently appear to be the most appropriate choice.

In this scenario, our approach pinpoints the situations where cePET/CT could be of benefit, not only on the basis of tumor type, but also according to the criteria related to the site of lesions and to the clinical question. This multiple parameter statistical analysis further defines the subsets of patients that can be candidates for cePET/CT, on the basis of their specific clinical history. The present study suggests that these patients have to be specifically identified, for example, in the context of oncologic, multidisciplinary, disease-management team discussions.

4.5. Limitations

The present study has several limitations. It was a single-center, retrospective study whose results may have been influenced by its study population, including cancer patients with both initial and recurrent disease. Moreover, due to ethical reasons, the histologic verification of metastasis was not performed for all distant lesions. However, as in other studies, the presence of metastasis was verified with a 1-year imaging follow-up, to ensure the highest possible confidence. We should also underline that we did not directly compare the diagnostic performance of PET/CT with separate CT as we focused on the specific added value of ceCT with respect to standard PET/CT. Finally, as many workstations and several freeware software programs allow to fuse PET and ceCT images, and as ceCT is becoming more and more a 'frontline' investigation, a further question concerns the different diagnostic accuracy of combined cePET/CT obtained in a single session with respect to the off-line image fusion of PET images with a recently obtained CT scan. This issue, which is crucial and the object of active work and discussion within radiological and nuclear medicine societies, is presently beyond the aims of our study and deserves further specific investigation.

5. Conclusion

We have highlighted a significant benefit of adding ceCT to PET/CT hybrid imaging in patients with head and neck or gastrointestinal cancer. This imaging modality was particularly helpful in the setting of disease restaging, in the presence of increased tumor markers, or in the case of metastatic lesions candidate for surgical treatment. Similarly, regardless of tumor type, lesions located within the abdomen were also more correctly classified thanks to the help of diagnostic ceCT. The present study could not highlight such a significant benefit in the general population of oncology patients submitted to standard FDG-PET/CT, which should be preferred when clinically indicated. Accordingly, these data strongly underline the importance of strictly selecting patients for the combined exam. In the age of personalized medicine and multidisciplinary approaches in oncology patients, the present results allow us to propose a clinical, history-related criterion when selecting candidates for cePET/CT, thus allowing the right imaging workup for the right patient without lowering patient throughput and without causing an unjustified increase in radiation burden.

Competing Interests

The authors declare that they have no competing interest.

Authors' Contributions

SM, RF, GS, GC, LE: data acquisition, study concept and design, analysis and interpretation of the data and text writing. CC: statistics, and interpretation of the data and text writing. CG: FDG production, interpretation of the data and critical revision of the text. GF: study concept and design, interpretation of the data and critical revision of the text. IB,mm, FF,cm and IC: analysis and interpretation of the data and critical revision of the text. All authors read and approved the final manuscript.

Acknowledgements

The authors are grateful to Mr Michele Sita' for his administrative assistance.

Source: Morbelli S, Conzi R, Campus C, *et al*. Contrast-enhanced [¹⁸ F] fluorodeoxyglucose-positron emission tomography/computed tomography in clinical oncology: tumor-, site-, and question-based comparison with standard positron emission tomography/computed tomography[J]. Cancer Imaging the Official Publication of the International Cancer Imaging Society, 2014, 14(1):1–10.

References

[1] Kostakoglu L, Agress H Jr, Goldsmith SJ: Clinical role of FDG PET in evaluation of cancer patients. Radiographics 2003, 23:315–340.

[2] Beyer T, Townsend DW, Brun T, Kinahan PE, Charron M, Roddy R, Jerin J, Young J, Byars L, Nutt R: A combined PET/CT scanner for clinical oncology. J Nucl Med 2000, 41:1369–1379.

[3] Cook GJ, Maisey MN, Fogelman I: Normal variants, artefacts and interpretative pitfalls in PET imaging with 18-fluoro-2-deoxyglucose and carbon-11 methionine. Eur J Nucl Med 1999, 26:1363–1378.

[4] Bar-Shalom R, Yefremov N, Guralnik L, Gaitini D, Frenkel A, Kuten A, Altman H, Keidar Z, Israel O: Clinical performance of PET/CT in evaluation of cancer: additional value for diagnostic imaging and patient management. J Nucl Med 2003, 44:1200–1209.

[5] Pfannenberg AC, Aschoff P, Brechtel K, Müller M, Bares R, Paulsen F, Scheiderbauer J, Friedel G, Claussen CD, Eschmann SM: Low dose non-enhanced CT versus standard dose contrast-enhanced CT in combined PET/CT protocols for staging and therapy planning in non-small cell lung cancer. Eur J Nucl Med Mol Imaging 2007, 34:36–44.

[6] Tateishi U, Maeda T, Morimoto T, Miyake M, Arai Y, Kim EE: Non-enhanced CT versus contrast-enhanced CT in integrated PET/CT studies for nodal staging of rectal cancer. Eur J Nucl Med Mol Imaging 2007, 34:1627–1634.

[7] Rodríguez-Vigil B, Gómez-León N, Pinilla I, Hernández-Maraver D, Coya J, Martín-Curto L, Madero R: PET/CT in lymphoma: prospective study of enhanced full-dose PET/CT versus unenhanced low-dose PET/CT. J Nucl Med 2006, 47:1643–1648.

[8] Strobel K, Heinrich S, Bhure U, Soyka J, Veit-Haibach P, Pestalozzi BC, Clavien PA, Hany TF: Contrast-enhanced 18 F-FDG PET/CT: 1-stop-shop imaging for assessing the respectability of pancreatic cancer. J Nucl Med 2008, 49:1408–1413.

[9] Kitajima K, Murakami K, Yamasaki E, Domeki Y, Kaji Y, Fukasawa I, Inaba N, Suganuma N, Sugimura K: Performance of integrated FDG-PET/contrast enhanced CT in the diagnosis of recurrent ovarian cancer: comparison with integrated FDG-PET/non-contrast-enhanced CT and enhanced CT. Eur J Nucl Med Mol Imaging 2008, 35:1439–1448.

[10] Kitajima K, Suzuki K, Nakamoto Y, Onishi Y, Sakamoto S, Senda M, Kita M, Sugimura K: Low-dose non-enhanced CT versus full-dose contrast-enhanced CT in integrated PET/CT studies for the diagnosis of uterine cancer recurrence. Eur J Nucl Med Mol Imaging 2010, 37:1490–1498.

[11] Boellaard R, O'Doherty MJ, Weber WA, Mottaghy FM, Lonsdale MN, Stroobants SG, Oyen WJ, Kotzerke J, Hoekstra OS, Pruim J, Marsden PK, Tatsch K, Hoekstra

CJ, Visser EP, Arends B, Verzijlbergen FJ, Zijlstra JM, Comans EF, Lammertsma AA, Paans AM, Willemsen AT, Beyer T, Bockisch A, Schaefer-Prokop C, Delbeke D, Baum RP, Chiti A, Krause BJ: FDG PET and PET/CT: EANM procedure guidelines for tumour PET imaging: version 1.0. Eur J Nucl Med Mol Imaging 2010, 37:181–200.

[12] Morcos SK, Thomsen HS, Webb JA: Contrast-media-induced nephrotoxicity: a consensus report: contrast media safety committee, European society of urogenital radiology (ESUR). Eur Radiol 1999, 9:1602–1613.

[13] Castelijns JA: Diagnostic radiology in head and neck oncology. Curr Opin Oncol 1990, 2:557–561.

[14] Aronberg DJ, Glazer HS, Sagel SS: MRI and CT of the mediastinum: comparisons, controversies, and pitfalls. Radiol Clin North Am 1985, 23:439–448.

[15] Austin JH, Müller NL, Friedman PJ, Hansell DM, Naidich DP, Remy-Jardin M, Webb WR, Zerhouni EA: Glossary of terms for CT of the lungs: recommendations of the nomenclature committee of the fleischner society. Radiology 1996, 200:327–331.

[16] Meyers MA: Dynamic radiology of the abdomen: normal and pathologic anatomy. 5th edition. New York: Springer-Verlag; 1999.

[17] R Development Core Team: The R project for statistical computing. Available from: http://www.R-project.org/(accessed 21 January 2013).

[18] Brasil P, Diagnosis Med: Diagnostic test accuracy evaluation for medical professionals: R package version 0.2.3. 2011. Available from: http://cran.r-project. org/src/ contrib/Archive/DiagnosisMed/(accessed 21 January 2013).

[19] Haerle SK, Strobel K, Ahmad N, Soltermann A, Schmid DT, Stoeckli SJ: Contrast-enhanced 18 F-FDG-PET/CT for the assessment of necrotic lymph node metastases. Head Neck 2011, 33:324–329.

[20] Yoshida K, Suzuki A, Nagashima T, Lee J, Horiuchi C, Tsukuda M, Inoue T: Staging primary head and neck cancers with (18)F-FDG PET/CT: is intravenous contrast administration really necessary? Eur J Nucl Med Mol Imaging 2009, 36:1417–1424.

[21] Dirisamer A, Halpern BS, Flöry D, Wolf F, Beheshti M, Mayerhoefer ME, Langsteger W: Performance of integrated FDG-PET/contrast-enhanced CT in the staging and restaging of colorectal cancer: comparison with PET and enhanced CT. Eur J Radiol 2010, 73:324–328.

[22] Dirisamer A, Halpern BS, Flöry D, Wolf F, Beheshti M, Mayerhoefer ME, Langsteger W: Staging pathways in recurrent colorectal carcinoma: is contrast-enhanced 18 F-FDG PET/CT the diagnostic tool of choice. J Nucl Med 2008, 49:354–361.

[23] Kitajima K, Murakami K, Yamasaki E, Domeki Y, Tsubaki M, Sunagawa M, Kaji Y, Suganuma N, Sugimura K: Performance of integrated FDG PET/contrast-enhanced CT in the diagnosis of recurrent colorectal cancer: comparison with integrated FDG PET/non-contrast-enhanced CT and enhanced CT. Eur J Nucl Med Mol Imaging

2009, 36:1388–1396.

[24] Antoch G, Freudenberg LS, Beyer T, Bockisch A, Debatin JF: To enhance or not to enhance? 18 F-FDG and CT contrast agents in dual-modality 18 F-FDG PET/CT. J Nucl Med 2004, 45(Suppl 1):56S–65S.

Chapter 27

Lack of Timely Accrual Information in Oncology Clinical Trials: A Cross-Sectional Analysis

Aaron P. Mitchell[1,2], Bradford R. Hirsch[1], Amy P. Abernethy[1,3]

[1]Duke Cancer Institute & Center for Learning Health Care, Duke Clinical Research Institute 2400 Pratt St, Durham, NC 27705, USA
[2]Department of Internal Medicine, Duke University Hospital, 2301 Erwin Road, Rm 8254DN, Durham, NC 27710, USA
[3]Duke University Medical Center, Box 3436, Durham, NC 27710, USA

Abstract: Background: Poor accrual is a significant barrier to the successful completion of oncology clinical trials; half of all phase 3 oncology trials close due to insufficient accrual. Timely access to accrual data fosters an understanding of successful trial design and can be used to inform the design of new clinical trials prospectively. Accrual statistics are available within research networks, such as the cancer cooperative groups, but comprehensive data reflecting the overall portfolio of cancer clinical trials are lacking. As a demonstration case, the purpose of this study was to quantify the public availability of accrual data across all recent renal cell carcinoma (RCC) trials. Methods: The database for the Aggregate Analysis of ClinicalTrials.gov (AACT) summarizes all trials registered between October 2007 and September 2010. In total, 108 trials of pharmacologic therapy for RCC were included. Accrual data on these trials were gathered via ClinicalTrials.gov (CTG), a manual review of resulting publications, and online surveys sent to principle investigators or trial coordinators. Results: In total, 26% (20 of 76) of trials listing a government, academic, or cooperative group (GAC) sponsor responded to the survey vs 0% (0 of 32) of those listing only industry sponsors. Across all methods, accrual data were available for only 40% (43 of 108) of trials, including 37% (28 of 76) of GAC trials and 47% (15 of 32) of industry trials. Moreover, 87% (66 of 76) of GAC trials were ongoing (open, actively recruiting, or of unknown status) vs 75% (24 of 32) of industry trials, while 9% (10 of 108) of trials were terminated or suspended. Conclusions: Despite extensive efforts (surveys, phone calls, CTG abstraction, publication searches), accurate accrual data remained inaccessible for 60% of the RCC trial cohort. While CTG reports trial results, ongoing accrual data are also critically needed. Poor access to accrual data will continue to limit attempts to develop a national summary of clinical trials metrics and to optimize the cancer clinical research portfolio.

Keywords: Accrual, Cancer, Clinical Trials, ClinicalTrials.gov, Renal Cell Carcinoma

1. Background

We must improve accrual of study participants to clinical trials. Successful accrual ensures the appropriate use of limited research resources by enabling study completion. It also indicates the perceived value of a trial's clinical questions and methodologies; efficient accrual signals that the results of a study are likely to be important and impactful.

Within oncology, poor accrual is a leading barrier to progress in clinical research[1]. Half of all phase 3 oncology trials close because of insufficient accrual[2], with only 2% of cancer patients participating[3][4]. Surveys and observational studies have identified trial characteristics that may predict accrual success, including cancer type, number of inclusion criteria, use of a placebo arm, randomization strategy, proximity to an academic center, and a managed care environment[2][5]–[8]. However, a detailed model of accrual success is lacking.

It is difficult to identify ways to align research priorities, trial methodologies, and recruitment networks to optimize accrual until, through a study of past experiences, we identify practices that positively affect accrual rates. Necessarily, the effective study of past clinical research requires that clinical trial results, most importantly data regarding recruitment rates and targets, be made publicly available in a timely fashion.

Monitoring of, and reaction to, past and ongoing accrual patterns enables the prospective improvement of accrual rates. At the institutional level, others have found that close monitoring of accrual, "aid[s] in continuously tracking and troubleshooting clinical trial accrual' and have called for 'a continuous feedback loop of information for sustaining the pipeline of clinical trials[9]". The ability to track accrual on a larger scale across all clinical trials may yield similar improvements.

The systems in place for clinical trial reporting might be inadequate to facilitate the needed level of data transparency and availability. Currently, data are available only in pockets; for example, accrual to federally funded cancer cooperative group trials can be characterized, but these data are not publicly available and are difficult to interpret without access to trials run by different sponsors. In response to this problem, the development of registries, such as ClinicalTrials.gov (CTG), has been mandated by the US Food and Drug Administration (FDA) to capture data on the clinical research portfolio; the mandate acknowledges the importance of developing comprehensive data repositories that can be leveraged in order to maximize our societal investment in clinical research.

ClinicalTrials.gov requires registration of all phase 2 to 4 interventional drug or device trials that are conducted (in whole or in part) in the United States or are conducted under an investigational new drug application or investigational device exemption. Since its expansion under the FDA Amendments Act of 2007, Section 801, results reporting has also been mandatory. Required results include, at minimum, (1) adverse events, (2) outcome measures, (3) participant baseline characteristics, and (4) participant flow, which describes the number of subjects enrolling in and completing the trial. To comply with the law, results must be finalized within 1 year of the end of data collection[10].

These data, if updated and aggregated in a timely fashion, could be used to identify trial factors and strategies that produce successful achievement of recruitment goals. For example, prior studies have shown that streamlining the trial design process would increase successful accrual[1], and that development of a model for predicting accrual success would enable the early identification of trials unlikely to achieve sufficient accrual, allowing for trial redesign and saving scarce research resources[2]. For CTG to succeed as a public repository, facilitating research transparency, and for it to be useful in the secondary analysis of clinical trials, it is necessary that data reported on CTG be accurate, complete, and up-to-date.

The purpose of our research effort was to determine whether publicly available clinical trial data are sufficient to develop a comprehensive understanding of accrual. We tested the hypothesis that incomplete and delayed reporting of clinical trials would result in low availability of accrual data through public channels. As a proof of concept, we selected a manageable cohort of trials for thorough analysis. Renal cell carcinoma (RCC) was chosen, owing to the rapid evolution of treatments in the field and the number of trials supporting novel agents (seven new drugs from 2005 through 2012)[11].

2. Methods

The Clinical Trials Transformation Initiative, a public-private partnership between Duke University and the FDA, recently created the AACT (Aggregate Analysis of ClinicalTrials.gov) database, a searchable database of trials registered in ClinicalTrials.gov (CTG) and intended to facilitate analysis of the clinical trials portfolio[12]–[14]. Detailed methods describing the creation of the AACT, including the oncology specific dataset, have been reported previously[12]. The final oncology dataset included 8,942 trials registered on CTG between 2007 and 2010. Analysis of the AACT database identified 108 trials focused on pharmacologic therapy for RCC.

We used CTG as the initial data source, since accrual data are supposed to be available there by public mandate. All clinical trials registered on CTG initially include an anticipated accrual goal, denoted as 'estimated enrollment'. For either ongoing or completed trials, this figure may be updated to reflect the actual number of trial subjects accrued, denoted "enrollment". Those trials that presented "enrollment" rather than "estimated enrollment" figures on CTG were counted as having reported accrual data. Additionally, the dates of the end of data collection, denoted "primary completion date", and trial status (pre-enrollment, completed, terminated, and so on) are investigator-reported figures listed for each trial on

CTG. These data were abstracted in June 2012.

Owing to low rates of reporting on CTG, additional efforts were made to extract accrual data from other publicly available sources. This led to the implementation of a supplemental structured survey of clinical trial teams and a review of resulting publications for accrual data (see Additional file 1). Approval from the institutional review board was obtained before beginning the survey. For the majority of trials registered on CTG, one or more persons are listed as the principal investigators or trial coordinators; email addresses for each of these persons were obtained either directly from CTG or from institutional websites or other publications authored by the same persons. Other trials did not list investigators but instead listed a "contact person"; in such cases, our survey was sent to these persons. At least one functional email address (no "bounce-back" message when the survey was sent) was ultimately available for all but five trials; for four of these trials, the relevant parties were contacted using phone numbers listed on CTG, and for one trial, no contact information was available.

In March of 2012, a survey was sent via email to the contacts, as described, requesting information about accrual rates, trial sponsor, and completion status. For each trial, the survey was sent to each available email address, whether this was only one or more than one. For no trial did we receive more than one survey response. If the survey was not completed within two weeks, a reminder email was sent and then an attempt at telephone contact was made.

PubMed and Google Scholar were used to search for resulting publications. For each trial, separate searches, including (1) the ClincalTrials.gov identifier number, (2) the study title as listed on CTG, and (3) the names of persons listed as principle investigators or trial coordinators, were conducted. Resulting abstracts or papers were searched for reported accrual figures. The date of the last abstraction was 23 June 23 2012.

3. Results and Discussion

Abstraction from CTG yielded accrual data for 8% (6 of 76) of trials listing a government, academic, or cooperative group sponsor (GAC trials) and 47% (15 of 32) of trials listing an industry sponsor. The survey response rate was 26% (20 of 76) for GAC and 0% (0 of 32) for industry trials. The PubMed review provided additional data from 3% (2 of 76) of GAC and 0% (0 of 32) of industry trials. Overall, accrual data were obtained for only 40% (43 of 108) of trials, including 37% (28 of 76) of GAC and 47% (15 of 32) of industry trials (**Table 1**).

According to CTG records, 87% (66 of 76) of GAC trials registered between 2007 and 2010 were still ongoing (open, actively recruiting, or of unknown status) at the time of abstraction in June 2012 vs 75% (24 of 32) of industry trials (**Table 1**). Across all sponsors, more trials were terminated or suspended (9%, 10 of 108) than were completed (7%, 8 of 108).

In total, 62% (67 of 108) of the trials had reached their primary completion date by the time we conducted data abstraction. Accrual data were available for 46% (29 of 67) of the trials past their primary completions dates, and for 34% (14 of 41) of the trials that had not yet reached primary completion, 25% (27 of 108) were more than one year past their primary completion date (**Table 2**). Of trials more than one year past primary completion, 32% (6 of 19) of GAC trials and 75% (6 of 8) of industry trials had reported accrual data on CTG.

4. Conclusions

Data presently available via CTG are inadequate, as they are often incomplete

Table 1. Availability of updated accrual data by source (left) and clinical trial status as listed on ClinicalTrials.gov.

| Primary sponsor | Total trials | Source of accrual information | | | | Trial status per CTG | | | | |
		Survey	ClinicalTrials.gov	Publication	Not available	Completed	Recruiting	Open; ongoing or not recruiting	Unknown	Terminated or suspended
GAC	76	20 (26)	6 (8)	2 (3)	48 (63)	3 (4)	46 (61)	11 (14)	9 (12)	7 (9)
Industry	32	0 (0)	15 (47)	0 (0)	17 (53)	5 (16)	9 (28)	15 (47)	0 (0)	3 (9)
Total	108	20 (19)	21 (19)	2 (2)	65 (60)	8 (7)	55 (51)	26 (24)	9 (8)	10 (9)

Percentages shown in parentheses. Government, Academic, or Cooperative group.

Table 2. Accrual reporting on ClinicalTrials.gov by clinical trials more than 1 year past date of primary completion.

Primary sponsor	Total trials	Trials >1 year past primary completion	Final accrual data reported on ClinicalTrials.gov	Final accrual data not reported on ClinicalTrials.gov
Government, academic, or cooperative group	76	19	6 (32)	13 (68)
Industry	32	8	6 (75)	2 (25)
Total	108	27	12 (44)	15 (56)

Percentages shown in parenthesis.

and difficult to obtain. In our cohort of RCC trials, only 19% (21 of 108) reported accrual information on CTG, while 56% (15 of 27) did not report accrual on CTG despite being more than 1 year past the date of primary completion, in violation of federal reporting requirements. After expanding our data acquisition to include surveys, phone calls, and publication searches, accrual data for RCC trials remained largely unavailable. The results of this study demonstrate that access to trial results remains a barrier to research on accrual patterns; even with the time and capability to search the web manually for published results and contact trial investigators by telephone individually, we were able to obtain accrual figures for only 40% of the cohort of RCC trials. Factors contributing to the low response rate included a reluctance to release this information to unknown parties and possible time constraints among research teams.

Participant accrual remains a challenge to clinical research. Without adequate data, we will struggle to improve the completion of trials, devise, and implement new strategies to enhance accrual, and monitor impact. Detailed clinical trial data need to be available, in order to support our societal investment in research. Furthermore, data should be available quickly, as a "real-time approach" of adapting to accrual patterns may be optimal[9].

To facilitate trial completion, we must better understand drivers of accrual by developing systems to monitor ongoing accrual success. Accrual statistics are available within research networks, such as the cancer cooperative groups, but they are not comprehensive or publicly available. Some regionalized efforts have made impressive progress in systematically monitoring accrual[8], and have begun to identify systemic drivers of accrual rates and clinical trial success[7][15]. However, this work has been limited to trials under US National Cancer Institute sponsorship, and therefore does not describe the full breadth of the clinical trial infrastructure. For a comprehensive understanding, such research must have access to and include accurate data on all clinical trials.

ClinicalTrials.gov is well positioned to meet these needs, as one of its objectives is to facilitate standardized reporting of trial characteristics and results. It requires reporting of accrual figures; however, such results are not required until 1 year after data collection, precluding the study of ongoing trials[13]. Additionally, compliance with CTG reporting is poor, with only 10% to 22% of registered trials meeting mandatory requirements[16][17]. Compliance with results reporting is particularly low for phase II trials (10% compared with 32% of phase III trials) and publicly funded trials (8% compared with 40% of industry funded trials)[17]. Though we used a different metric for results reporting that focused only on accrual data, our comparable result of 40% reporting reaffirms an ongoing need to for improvement.

Although greater transparency in recruitment may allow for improvement in accrual over the long term, there may also be drawbacks. Early public availability of accrual figures for ongoing trials might lead to withdrawal of funding for those trials with slower than expected recruitment. While this might help to funnel resources towards trials more likely to produce meaningful results, it could also result in financial stress at the institutional level. It is also possible that patients might decide to enroll in trials based upon publicly reported accrual rates, potentially further depressing accrual in trials that are already accruing poorly; we lanticipate that this is an unlikely scenario.

Efforts to increase the timeliness and completeness of reporting will help CTG meet its full potential as a central clearing house of clinical trial data, capable of supporting vital analysis of our research priorities and conduct. A requirement that clinical trial data be updated at predefined intervals would significantly increase the quality of data available in CTG. As clinical researchers, study sponsors, and a community at large, it is important that we share this information, recognizing its importance in advancing the conduct of clinical trials.

5. Additional File

Additional file 1: Survey outline.

6. Abbreviations

AACT: Aggregate Analysis of ClinicalTrials.gov; CTG: ClinicalTrials.gov; FDA: US Food and Drugs Administration; GAC: government, academic, or cooperative group; RCC: Renal cell carcinoma.

Competing Interests

The authors disclose the following conflicts of interest: Aaron Mitchell-none; Bradford Hirsch research funding (Pfizer, Dendreon, Bristol-Meyers Squibb); Amy Abernethy compensated leadership role (Advoset, American Academy of Hospice and Palliative Medicine, Orange Leaf Associates), compensated advisory role (Novartis, Bristol-Myers Squibb, Pfizer), research funding (Alexion, Kanglaite, Biovex, DARA BioSciences, Mi-Co, Genentech, Helsinn Therapeutics, Lilly, Bristol-Myers Squibb, Amgen, Pfizer); This work was unfunded. No other party was involved in the design and conduct of the study, data analysis, or preparation or review of the manuscript.

Authors' Contributions

APM conducted survey, data collection, and results analysis, and drafted the manuscript. BRH performed results analysis and drafted the manuscript. APA formulated the study and helped to draft the manuscript. All authors read and approved the final manuscript.

Authors' Information

Dr. Abernethy had full access to all of the data in the study and takes responsibility for the integrity of the data and the accuracy of the data analysis.

Source: Mitchell A P, Hirsch B R, Abernethy A P. Lack of timely accrual information in oncology clinical trials: a cross-sectional analysis[J]. Trials, 2014, 15(1):1768–1773.

References

[1] Cheng SK, Dietrich MS, Dilts DM: A sense of urgency: evaluating the link between clinical trial development time and the accrual performance of cancer therapy evaluation program (NCI-CTEP) sponsored studies. Clin Cancer Res 2010, 16(22):5557–5563.

[2] Schroen AT, Petroni GR, Wang H, Gray R, Wang XF, Cronin W, Sargent DJ, Benedetti J, Wickerham DL, Djulbegovic B, Slingluff CL Jr: Preliminary evaluation of factors associated with premature trial closure and feasibility of accrual benchmarks in phase III oncology trials. Clin Trials 2010, 7(4):312–321.

[3] Murthy VH, Krumholz HM, Gross CP: Participation in cancer clinical trials: race-, sex-, and age-based disparities. JAMA 2004, 291(22):2720–2726.

[4] Sateren WB, Trimble EL, Abrams J, Brawley O, Breen N, Ford L, McCabe M, Kaplan R, Smith M, Ungerleider R, Christian MC: How sociodemographics, presence of oncology specialists, and hospital cancer programs affect accrual to cancer treatment trials. J Clin Oncol 2002, 20(8):2109–2117.

[5] Schroen AT, Petroni GR, Wang H, Thielen MJ, Gray R, Benedetti J, Wang XF, Sargent DJ, Wickerham DL, Cronin W, Djulbegovic B, Jr Slingluff CL: Achieving sufficient accrual to address the primary endpoint in phase III clinical trials from U.S. Cooperative Oncology Groups. Clin Cancer Res 2012, 18(1):256–262.

[6] McDonald AM, Knight RC, Campbell MK, Entwistle VA, Grant AM, Cook JA, Elbourne DR, Francis D, Garcia J, Roberts I, Snowdon C: What influences recruitment to randomised controlled trials? A review of trials funded by two UK funding agencies. Trials 2006, 7:9.

[7] Carpenter WR, Weiner BJ, Kaluzny AD, Domino ME, Lee S-YD: The effects of managed care and competition on community-based clinical research. Med Care 2006, 44(7):671–679.

[8] Carpenter WR, Tyree S, Wu Y, Meyer AM, DiMartino L, Zullig L, Godley PA: A surveillance system for monitoring, public reporting, and improving minority access to cancer clinical trials. Clin Trials 2012, 9(4):426–435.

[9] Kanarek NF, Kanarek MS, Olatoye D, Carducci MA: Removing barriers to participation in clinical trials, a conceptual framework and retrospective chart review study. Trials 2012, 13:237.

[10] Tse T, Williams RJ, Zarin DA: Reporting "basic results" in ClinicalTrials.gov. Chest 2009, 136(1):295–303.

[11] Hutson TE: Targeted therapies for the treatment of metastatic renal cell carcinoma: clinical evidence. Oncologist 2011, 16(Suppl 2):14–22.

[12] Tasneem A, Aberle L, Ananth H, Chakraborty S, Chiswell K, McCourt BJ, Pietrobon R: The database for aggregate analysis of ClinicalTrials.gov (AACT) and subsequent regrouping by clinical specialty. PLoS ONE 2012, 7(3):e33677.

[13] Califf RM, Zarin DA, Kramer JM, Sherman RE, Aberle LH, Tasneem A: Characteristics of clinical trials registered in ClinicalTrials.gov, 2007–2010. JAMA 2012, 307(17):1838–1847.

[14] Hirsch B, Califf R, Cheng S: The state of the oncology clinical trials portfolio: insights from a systematic analysis of ClinicalTrials.gov. JAMA Intern Med, 173(11):972–979.

[15] Carpenter WR, Fortune-Greeley AK, Zullig LL, Lee S-Y, Weiner BJ: Sustainability and performance of the National Cancer Institute's Community Clinical Oncology Program. Contemp Clin Trials 2012, 33(1):46–54.

[16] Gopal RK, Yamashita TE, Prochazka AV: Research without results: inadequate public reporting of clinical trial results. Contemp Clin Trials 2012, 33(3):486–491.

[17] Prayle AP, Hurley MN, Smyth AR: Compliance with mandatory reporting of clinical trial results on ClinicalTrials.gov: cross sectional study. BMJ 2012, 344: d7373.

Chapter 28

Testing the Treatment Effect on Competing Causes of Death in Oncology Clinical Trials

Federico Rotolo[1], Stefan Michiels[1,2]

[1]Gustave Roussy, Service de Biostatistique et d'Épidémiologie, F-94805 Villejuif, France
[2]Univérsité Paris-Sud, F-94805 Villejuif, France

Abstract: Background: Chemotherapy is expected to reduce cancer deaths (CD), while possibly being harmful in terms of non-cancer deaths (NCD) because of toxicity. Peto's log-rank test is popular in the medical literature, but its operating characteristics are barely known. We compared this test to the most common ones in the statistical literature: the cause-specific hazard test and Gray's test on the hazard of the subdistribution. We investigated for the first time the impact of reclassifications of causes of death (CoD) after recurrences, and of misclassification of CoD. **Methods:** We present a simulation study in which we varied the censoring rate and the correlation between CD and NCD times, we generated recurrence times to study the role of the reclassification of CoD, and we added 20% misclassified CoD. We considered four scenarios for the treatment effect: none; none for CD and negative for NCD; positive for CD and none for NCD; positive for CD and negative for NCD. We applied the three tests to a randomized clinical trial evaluating adjuvant chemotherapy in 1,867 patients with non-small-cell lung cancer. **Results:** Most often the three tests well preserved their nominal size, Gray's test did not when the treatment had an effect on the competing CoD. With a high rate of misclassified CoD, Gray's and the cause-specific tests lost much of their power, whereas the Peto's test had the highest power. The cause-specific test had inflated size for NCD when the treatment was beneficial for CD with many misclassified CoD, but had the highest power for NCD when the treatment had no effect on CD, and had similar power to Peto's test for CD when the treatment had no effect on NCD. Gray's test performed best when the effect on the two CoD was opposite. The higher the censoring, the lower the rejection probabilities of all the tests and the smaller their differences. **Conclusions:** In this first head-to-head comparison of the three tests, the cause-specific test often proved to be the most reliable. Comparing results with and without misclassification of the CoD, Peto's test was the least influenced by the presence of such misclassification.

Keywords: Competing Risks, Peto's Test, Cause of Death, Cancer Death, Cumulative Incidence Function, Cause-Specific Hazard, Gray's Test

1. Background

The analysis of survival data in the presence of competing risks has been a widely debated topic for many decades in both the statistical[1]-[5] and the medical literature[6]-[11]. Interest in the subject gained momentum in the 1990s, when two main approaches emerged: an approach based on the cause-specific hazard function and another based on the cumulative incidence function and its associated hazard of the subdistribution. For a detailed discussion see[12] for example. An issue of particular importance in clinical research is testing the effect of covariates typically the treatment on competing causes of death. Different solutions have been proposed. The most common ones in the statistical literature are the log-rank test for the cause-specific hazard[1][13] and nonparametric and semiparametric tests for the cumulative incidence function (CIF)[14][15]. However, Peto and the Early Breast Cancer Trialists' Collaborative Group proposed the log-rank sub- traction method in the context of oncology[16]-[19], which is quite popular in the clinical literature and especially in meta-analyses: see for instance references[20]-[24]. This test imputes deaths to the cancer whenever the cause is unknown or when they occur after a recurrence, whatever the recorded cause. It calculates cause-specific mortality as the difference between overall mortality and that attributable to other causes. The authors assert that this approach makes the test unbiased for the assessment of the effect on cancer mortality.

The comparison of different methods from a theoretical point of view and via simulation studies is being considered with increasing interest in the literature. Putter *et al.*[3] offered a detailed and insightful review of competing risks methodology. Dignam *et al.*[10] and Dignam and Kocherginsky[25] focused on point estimation of the treatment effect according to different modeling approaches. Pintilie[26] provided a simulation study, with independent variables of the times to death by cause, showing that the tests based on the cause-specific hazard Wald, score and likelihood-ratio have the correct size and power, in the absence of any effect on the competing event. Using simulations, Freidlin and Korn[27] compared the cause-specific log-rank test to Gray's non-parametric test[14] for the CIF. They concluded that the former preserves its nominal size better and has greater power than the latter, even with positively correlated event times. Williamson *et al.*[28] extended these results showing that Gray's test has greater power in the case of very different degrees of negative correlation between competing event times in the two treatment arms. Ruan and Gray[29] studied Peto's test both analytically and in simulations with independent survival times. They proved that it has good properties when the rates of competing events are similar, whereas it has an inflated size and poor power otherwise.

For the first time we present in this article a simulation study to compare head-to-head Peto's log-rank subtraction test to the log-rank test on the cause-specific hazard, and to Gray's test based on the CIF in a broad set of clinical scenarios. In order to investigate the effect of different classifications of the cause of death established by Peto's test, we used a simulation method that allows relapse times to be generated in addition to cancer-death (CD) and non-cancer-death (NCD) times. We simulated data with negative, null, and positive correlations, thereby covering an exhaustive range of dependence assumptions. This study is the first which investigates the impact of censoring and, most importantly, of misclassification of causes of death on the behaviour of these tests.

The clinical problem motivating this study was the evaluation of the efficacy of adjuvant chemotherapy for patients with non-small-cell lung cancer in the International Adjuvant Lung Cancer Trial (IALT)[30][31]. Its interest is to test whether chemotherapy has a beneficial effect on the occurrence of CD, taking into account the fact that patients can meanwhile die of other causes, and that an increased risk of NCD is possible in the treatment arm, due to chemotherapy toxicity.

In the next section, we present the test statistics of interest. Then, we provide details on the simulation study and its results. Finally, we present the IALT study and the results of the tests for CD and NCD.

2. Methods

2.1. Tests for Competing Causes of Death

There are different approaches to dealing with duration data in the presence of competing events, such as cause-specific death and death from other causes. In a latent failure time perspective, there is a random variable T_i for the time to each possible event, but only the time to the first event can be recorded. The hazard function of the marginal distribution of each T_i is usually called the cause-specific hazard. Testing the treatment effect on the cause-specific hazard allows one to evaluate the net effect of covariates on each event; even though quite intuitive, this strategy has been criticized because it compares the treatment arms in terms of the risk of each event type while ignoring all the others. Gray[14] proposed an alternative approach, based on the CIF, which takes into account all types of events. As the hazard of the CIF incorporates information on all the competing risks, testing the effect of the treatment on the incidence of each type of event also reflects its effect on all the others. As variations of the risk of each event reverberate on the hazards of competitors, it is advised to consider their results in combination with the analysis of all cause-specific hazards[4]. Moreover, due to its mathematical definition, the hazard of the CIF requires that patients who experience an event remain in the risk sets of the other types of event. For a detailed discussion of this topic, we refer to Section 3 of[3] and Chapters 4 to 6 of[12].

Consequently, there are also several approaches for testing the effect of a treatment on competing events. We restricted ourselves to considering three of the most popular ones: the cause-specific and the Gray tests, which receive most of the attention through methodological research, and the Peto test, which is quite common in the medical literature. We aim to compare them in several clinically relevant situations.

2.1.1. Peto (Pe)

The log-rank subtraction test proposed and further described by Peto[16][17] consists in a piecewise (with respect to time) version of the log-rank test, performed separately by cause of death. It is said to be a subtraction method because the quantities used to compute the test statistic are first calculated for overall mortality and for NCD. Those concerning CD are then obtained by taking the difference between the former two. Another relevant peculiarity of this approach is that all deaths due to an unknown cause and all those occurring after a relapse are ascribed to the cancer, even if explicitly declared as due to another cause.

2.1.2. Cause-Specific (CS)

Historically, the simplest and most naive approach adopted reflects the idea of considering only the relevant events for each cause of death, while treating all the competing events as independent censoring. This leads to the use of the log-rank test on the cause-specific hazard[1][13], which is approximately equivalent to the score test of the cause-specific Cox model which itself is asymptotically equivalent to the Wald and likelihood-ratio tests in the same model.

2.1.3. Gray (Gr)

Another popular approach in the context of competing risks is the one based on the CIF, for which the assumption of independence of the competing events is not required. The hazard associated with the CIF, called the hazard of the subdistribution, also takes into account the occurrence of competing events. In particular, when a subject experiences a competing event, his/her time to the relevant event is not censored and he/she remains in the risk set. Gray's nonparametric test[14], used in our study, is asymptotically equivalent to the Wald test on the regression parameter in the Cox model of the hazard of the subdistribution[15] when there is no censoring.

2.2. Plots

In the example presented later on, we will show the cumulative risk and incidence curves for all, non-cancer and cancer deaths by treatment arm. They will be plotted by means of three methods corresponding to the three tests for the treatment effect. The first, corresponding to the cause-specific test, is the Nelson-Aalen method for the (cause-specific) cumulative risk[32][33]. In the case of cause-specific risks, only deaths declared due to the cause of interest are considered as events by the Nelson-Aalen estimator, while all other deaths are censored (assuming non informative censoring). The plots in the second group are the Peto estimator of the (cause-specific) cumulative yearly rates; in these plots all deaths following a recurrence are classified as CD, as well as those of an unknown cause. NCDs preceded by a recurrence are censored when a recurrence occurs. According to the Peto method, first the survival probability is computed per year for the 2 arms combined. Then the survival probability for each arm is obtained by adding to it or subtracting from it a quantity which depends on the logarithm of the yearly risk ratio[16][17]. Finally, the Aalen-Johansen estimates of the CIFs[34], corresponding to the Gray test, are plotted. It is noteworthy that, in the case of overall survival, one minus the CIF corresponds to the Kaplan-Meier estimate.

2.3. Simulation Study

Testing the efficacy of the therapy on the time to CD and NCD is the focus of the researcher's interest. Sometimes, the classification of causes of deaths implicitly requires the occurrence of a recurrence (Rec). Although the treatment evaluation is done directly on times to CD and NCD, the tests differ in the manner of classifying causes of death. In particular, the Peto test requires information on the times to recurrence.

We first considered the times to CD and NCD (**Figure 1**). We generated them by using two exponential distributions, possibly with positive or negative dependence. We obtained them in two steps. First, a bivariate normal random variable $Z = \left(Z_1, Z_2\right)^{\mathsf{T}}$ was generated with unit means, unit variances and correlation

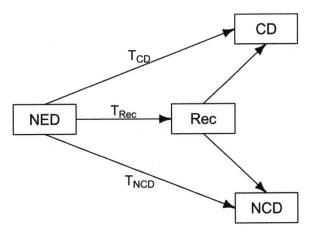

Figure 1. Event history structure used for data simulation. T: time to different events. NED: no evidence of disease after initial treatment. Rec: recurrence; CD: cancer death; NCD: non-cancer death.

ρ. Then, the times to death were computed as $T_{CD} = -\log\big(\Phi(Z_1)\big)/\lambda_{CD}$ and $T_{NCD} = -\log\big(\Phi(Z_2)\big)/\lambda_{NCD}$, where $\Phi(\cdot)$ is the standard normal distribution function[27]. Thus, $T_{CD} \sim \text{Exp}(\lambda_{CD})$ and $T_{NCD} \sim \text{Exp}(\lambda_{NCD})$. In the control group of the IALT trial, which we describe below, we estimated that the CD rate is about five-fold higher than the NCD rate. Therefore, we set $\lambda_{CD} = \sqrt{5} \approx 2.24$ and $\lambda_{NCD} = 1/\sqrt{5} \approx 0.45$ The time to death for each subject is then $T_D = \min(T_{CD}, T_{NCD})$. Finally, we assumed that, conditional on the time to CD, the time to recurrence T_{Rec} follows a uniform distribution between 0 and T_{CD}. Hence, a recurrence is observed whenever $T_{Rec} < T_D$ and is censored only when $T_{Rec} > T_{NCD}$. This method allowed us to study the effect of the reclassification done by Peto: in our simulations about half of the NCD were preceded by a recurrence. We did not consider the case of unknown causes of death, which were very marginal in our real dataset.

Here we present different scenarios concerning the treatment effect. Figure A.1 in the Additional file 1 shows, for the first scenario, the correlations obtained between the event times, depending on ρ, the correlation of the underlying normal random variables: the relation is roughly linear and setting the parameter ρ can be considered almost equivalent to setting the correlation between CD and NCD times. On the other hand, this does not affect the correlation between CD and recurrence times, which can be shown to be constantly $\sqrt{3/5} = 0.77$. In this respect, no difference exists between the scenarios. In order to investigate the properties of the tests in a wide range of situations, we chose five values for ρ, covering very negative and very positive dependence, passing through weak and no dependence: −0.75, −0.375, 0, 0.375, 0.75.

We examined four clinical situations for the effect of the treatment on the occurrence of death from cancer and from other causes:

1) a null effect on both CD and NCD ($HR_{CD} = HR_{NCD} = 1$),

2) a null effect on CD ($HR_{CD} = 1$) and an increased NCD risk ($HR_{NCD} = 1.25$),

3) a reduction of the risk of CD ($HR_{CD} = 0.8$) and a null effect on NCD ($HR_{NCD} = 1$),

4) a reduction of the risk of CD ($HR_{CD} = 0.8$) and an increased NCD risk ($HR_{NCD} = 1.25$).

The first scenario is the complete null scenario, *i.e.* the one in which both the null hypotheses of no treatment effect are true. The second is the most pessimistic, where the treatment is toxic and ineffective. The third scenario is the ideal target for a treatment in oncology, which just reduces the risk of CD. Finally, the fourth one is a scenario that could occur for chemotherapy and radiotherapy regimens in oncology, as their efficacy against CD implies a cost in terms of an increased NCD hazard. The hazard ratios for the treatment effect in the four scenarios are illustrated in **Figure 2**. In addition to the situation with complete data, we replicated simulations with 25% and 50% of censored observations. Censoring times were generated from uniform random variables between zero and a given bound. For each scenario, the choice of this upper bound was made numerically in order to attain the desired proportion of censored times to death. As in clinical practice the causes of death can be misrecorded, we also reperformed all the tests after inverting the cause (CD *vs.* NCD) of 20% of deaths.

2.4. The International Adjuvant Lung Cancer Trial

The IALT recruited 1,867 patients who underwent complete surgical resection

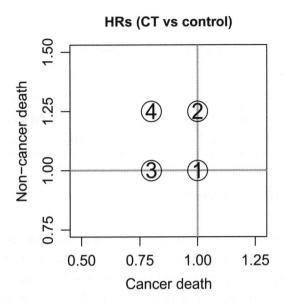

Figure 2. Hazard ratios in the simulation study. Hazard ratios for cancer death and non-cancer death in the four scenarios used for the simulation study.

of non-small-cell lung cancers. They were randomly assigned to cisplatin-based adjuvant chemotherapy (932) or the control (935) group and were followed up for 10 years (median: 7.5 years). The International Adjuvant Lung Cancer Trial Collaborative Group[30] and Arriagada et al.[31] showed that adjuvant chemotherapy provides a benefit in terms of both overall and disease-free survival at 5 years. As shown in **Table 1**, 1,168 (62.6%) out of 1,867 patients died during follow up, 578 in the experimental and 590 in the control arm. Among all the recorded deaths, 918 (78.6%) were ascribed to lung cancer, 179 (15.3%) to other causes, and 71 (6.1%) to unknown causes. Among the 197 patients who died of non-cancer causes, 71 had a recurrence recorded; among the 71 patients who died of unknown causes, 26 had a recurrence recorded. In total, 97 deaths that occurred after a recurrence and declared due to non-cancer or unknown causes were reclassified as due to the cancer by the Peto method.

The Ethics Committee of Kremlin-Bicêtre hospital in France France (Comité de Protection des Personnes Îlede-France VII) approved the protocol on January 9, 1995. When the study began in 1995, informed consent was obtained from each patient according to the regulations of the participating country; in 1999, all participants were required to give written informed consent.

Table 1. Causes of deaths by treatment arm in the IALT study.

	Chemotherapy	Control	Total	
Cancer Deaths	438	480	918	
Non-Dancer Deaths	107	72	179	(Of which 71 after a relapse)
Deaths from unknown cause	33	38	71	(Of which 26 after a relapse)
All Deaths	578	590	1168	

3. Results and Discussion

As described above, we considered four scenarios for the treatment effect, five possible degrees of dependence between the times to CD and NCD, three possible proportions of censoring, and presence or absence of misclassification of the cause of death. For each of these $4 \times 5 \times 3 \times 2 = 120$ situations, 10 000 data sets of size 1000 were generated. The three tests were performed for each of them and the empirical rejection probabilities at a 5% nominal size were computed across the 10 000 replications. The null hypothesis of no treatment effect holds in scenarios 1 and 2 for CD and in scenarios 1 and 3 for NCD. In these cases the empirical rejection probabilities stand for the empirical size of the tests. On the contrary, in all the other situations, the hypothesis does not hold and the rejection probabilities represent the empirical power of the tests. Of note, the rate of miclassified causes of death (20%) is quite high with respect to clinical real life, but it is useful in this context to study its role in a somehow extreme situation.

In the null scenario, *i.e.* in the absence of any treatment effect on both causes of death, all the tests have empirical rejection probabilities that are very close to the nominal size of 5% (range: 0.04–0.06; Additional file 1: Table A.1 and Figure A.2) and their use is equivalent. Furthermore, none of censoring, correlation between causes of death, and misclassification of causes of death (Additional file 1: Table A.2 and Figure A.3) affect the results.

In the second scenario, we considered the case where the therapy is not effective for reducing CD, but it is harmful in terms of NCD, because of toxicity. **Figure 3** shows the main results with complete data, whereas full details with 25% and 50% censored observations are provided in Additional file 1: Table A.3 and Figure A.4. Let's first consider the results when there is no misclassification of the

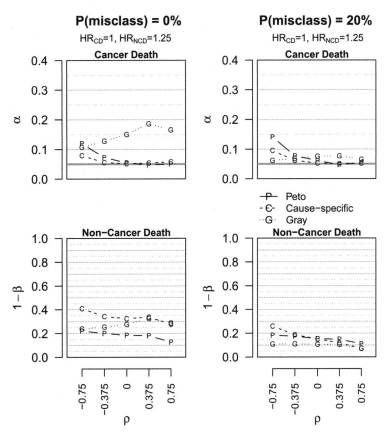

Figure 3. Empirical size and power of the tests in scenario 2. Empirical size (α) and power $(1 - \beta)$ of the tests for CD and NCD in scenario 2 ($HR_{CD} = 1$, $HR_{NCD} = 1.25$). The data are simulated without censored observations. The plots on the first line concern CD, those on the second line NCD. The plots on the left are for data with correct causes of death (P(misclass) = 0%), those on the right for data with 20% of misclassified causes of death (P(misclass) = 20%). The bold grey horizontal line corresponds to the 0.05 level and ρ to the correlation.

cause of death. Under these conditions results show that for complete data Gr (Gray test) has an overinflated size for CD ($0.10 < \alpha < 0.19$, complete data), whereas the other two tests have better empirical sizes in general ($0.04 < \alpha \leq 0.12$ for Pe [Peto test] and $0.05 < \alpha < 0.08$ for CS [Cause-Specific test], complete data). Due to the set-up of our simulation study with a CD rate about 5-fold higher than a NCD rate, the three tests have moderate power for detecting an effect for NCD ($0.12 < 1 - \beta < 0.41$, complete data), with CS out-performing its two competitors and Pe being the least powerful ($1 - \beta < 0.23$). As censoring increases, all the rejection probabilities decrease in general and get closer and closer to each other, so that the differences between them become less and less pronounced. CS seems to be the most reliable choice in this context. In the case that 20% of the causes of death are misrecorded (see also Additional file 1: Figure A.5 and Table A.4), the size of Gr is more correct ($\alpha \in [0.06, 0.08]$, complete data) and the three tests loose power for detecting the effect on NCD, notably CS ($1 - \beta < 0.26$) and Gr ($1 - \beta < 0.13$).

Scenario 3 represents the target situation for a cancer treatment that is just effective on CD, without any effect on NCD. Under these conditions and without misclassified causes of death, the results in **Figure 4** (see also Additional file 1: Figure A.6 and Table A.5) suggest that Gr has the lowest power for CD ($0.54 < 1$

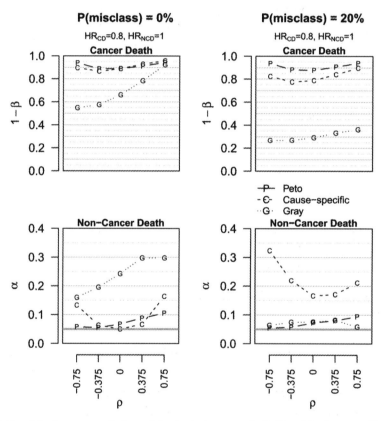

Figure 4. Empirical power and size of the tests in scenario 3. Empirical power ($1 - \beta$) and size (α) of the tests for CD and NCD in scenario 3 ($HR_{CD} = 0.8$, $HR_{NCD} = 1$). The data are simulated without censored observations. The plots on the first line concern CD, those on the second line NCD. The plots on the left are for data with correct causes of death (P(misclass) = 0%), those on the right for data with 20% of misclassified causes of death (P(misclass) = 20%). The bold grey horizontal line corresponds to the 0.05 level and ρ to the correlation.

$- \beta < 0.93$ for Gr, while $0.86 < 1 - \beta$ for Pe and CS; complete data) and often by far the highest size for NCD ($0.16 < \alpha$; complete data). CS and Pe are largely equivalent for CD. Either CS or Pe is preferable for NCD ($0.05 < \alpha < 0.17$ for CS, $0.05 < \alpha < 0.11$ for Pe; complete data), depending on the correlation. Again, censoring causes a contraction of the empirical rejection probabilities, irrespective of whether the null hypothesis holds or not. In this scenario Pe and CS are broadly equivalent, whereas Gr should not be preferred. When introducing miclassification of the cause of 20% of deaths (see also Additional file 1: Figure A.7 and Table A.6), CS is less powerful for CD ($0.77 < 1 - \beta$; complete data) and has very inflated size for NCD ($0.10 < \alpha < 0.33$); Gr has very poor power for CD ($1 - \beta < 0.37$, complete data) but is more correct for NCD ($0.04 < \alpha < 0.09$); again, Pe is less sensitive to misclassification as it reclassifies at least some of the deaths as due to the cancer when a recurrence occurs, irrespective of the declared cause.

Finally, **Figure 5** (see also Additional file 1: Figure A.8 and Table A.7) provides empirical powers if the treatment has a beneficial effect on the risk of CD, but at a cost of a harm in terms of NCD hazard. Gr is uniformly the most powerful in this scenario. In particular, for NCD it is in general 35%–40% more powerful than its competitors ($0.62 < 1 - \beta < 0.89$ for Gr, $0.16 < 1 - \beta < 0.74$ for CS and $0.22 < 1 - \beta < 0.40$ for Pe; complete data). The rejection probabilities are far more similar for CD, with high power ranging from 0.73 to 1.00 for all tests (complete data). In all the scenarios, the tests are generally more powerful for CD than for NCD because the baseline hazard for CD is considerably higher than for NCD ($\lambda_{CD} = 5 \times \lambda_{NCD}$). Even though censoring attenuates differences between the three tests, Gr is undoubtedly preferable under these conditions. On the other hand, Gr has the highest loss of power due to misclassification of the cause of death (see also Additional file 1: Figure A.9 and Table A.8) notably for CD ($1 - \beta < 0.57$, complete data); for NCD the widest power loss is for CS ($1 - \beta < 0.09$).

In the International Adjuvant Lung Cancer Trial, the separate evaluation of the chemotherapy effect on the risks of CD and NCD is of primary interest. Plots on the first line of **Figure 6** show the Nelson-Aalen estimate of the cumulative risk (a), the cumulative yearly rates estimated by the Peto method (b), and the cumulative incidence function (c), respectively, for overall mortality by treatment arm. Note that, as no competing event exists for overall survival, plot 6(c) corresponds to one minus the Kaplan-Meier estimate. Chemotherapy seems to provide a benefit

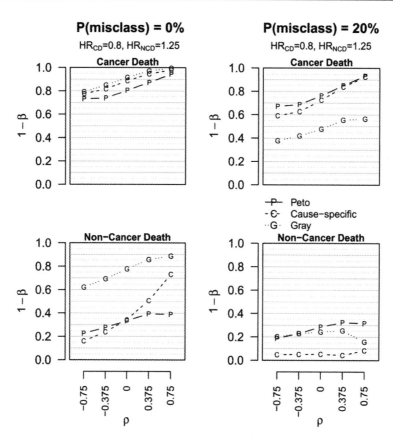

Figure 5. Empirical power of the tests in scenario 4. Empirical power $(1 - \beta)$ of the tests for CD and NCD in scenario 4 ($HR_{\text{CD}} = 0.8$, $HR_{\text{NCD}} = 1.25$). The data are simulated without censored observations. The plots on the first line concern CD, those on the second line NCD. The plots on the left are for data with correct causes of death (P(misclass) = 0%), those on the right for data with 20% of misclassified causes of death (P(misclass) = 20%).

up to five years after randomization, and then the two curves overlap. Under a proportional hazards assumption, the estimated hazard ratio between the chemotherapy and the control groups is 0.95 (95% CI: 0.84–1.06) and the log-rank test has a p-value equal to 0.34. Note that, for the sake of simplicity, we did not adjust for any of the prognostic factors used in previous publications about the IALT study. The desired and expected action of cisplatin-based chemotherapy is to reduce the risk of CD, while having no effect or moderately increasing the risk of NCD. **Figures 6(g)-6(i)** show the same quantities as (a)-(c) but only for CD; you can see that risk and incidence are constantly less in the chemotherapy group than in the control group. On the other hand, **Figures 6(d)-6(f)** show that the two treatment arms are overall equivalent with respect to non-cancer mortality; an

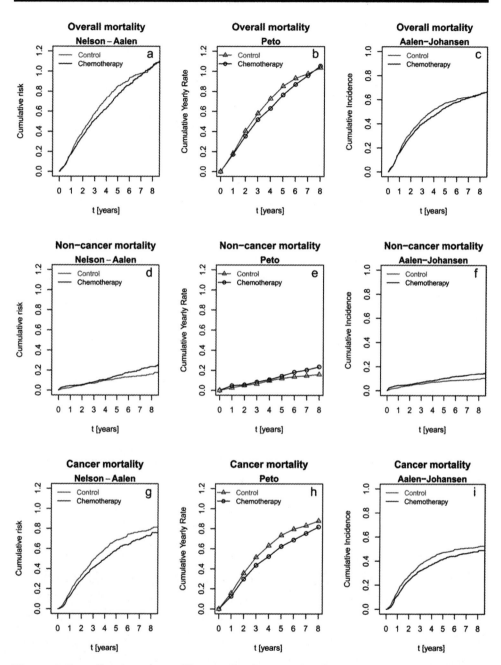

Figure 6. Overall and cause-specific mortality for control and treatment arms in the IALT trial. First column [(a), (d), (g)]: Nelson-Aalen estimates of the cumulative hazards. Second column [(b), (e), (h)]: Peto estimates of the cumulative yearly rates. Third column [(c), (f), (i)]: Aalen-Johansen estimates of the cumulative incidence functions. First line [(a)-(c)]: overall mortality. Second line [(d)-(f)]: non-cancer mortality. Third line [(g)-(i)]: cancer mortality.

Table 2. Results of the three tests for the treatment effect on CD and NCD, in the IALT study.

	CD		NCD	
	X^2	(p-val)	X^2	(p-val)
Pe	3.72	(0.054)	4.77	(0.029)
CS	3.44	(0.064)	4.19	(0.041)
Gr	4.52	(0.033)	5.89	(0.015)

The values of the test statistics (X^2) are provided together with the associated p-values (p-val).

increased NCD rate and incidence are observed for the experimental group after five years. Then, we compared the results of testing the effect of chemotherapy on the competing causes of death by means of the three test statistics considered thus far: Pe, CS and Gr (**Table 2**). The increase observed in NCD in the treatment arm [see **Figure 6(d)**] is significant according to the three tests: $p = 0.029$ for Pe, $p = 0.041$ for CS and $p = 0.015$ for Gr. One should keep in mind that the Pe reclassifies as CD a total of 97 deaths: 26 NCDs which could attenuate the differences between treatment arms and 71 deaths from an unknown cause. These deaths from an unknown cause are censored for both causes of death by CS, whilst they make up a third group according to Gr.

The difference in survival in favor of the treatment arm, which is non-significant for overall survival, is significant or borderline for CD, with p-values ranging from 0.033 to 0.064. This suggests that the effects on the risks of CD and NCD are in opposite directions, and that they compensate each other, at least partially, when all deaths due to any cause are considered together. Gr, based on the CIF, detects a statistically significant difference at a 5% level ($p = 0.033$), whereas the other two are borderline but not significant ($p = 0.054$ for Pe, $p = 0.064$ for CS). Most likely, the net increase (*i.e.* in the cause-specific hazard) in the risk of NCD in the chemotherapy arm contributes to reducing the incidence of CD in that group, amplifying the reduction in the risk of CD when measured in terms of the CIF, although the differences between the test statistics are small.

Both the CS and the Pe tests treat death from other causes as independent censoring, which is not realistic in most practical situations. Gr does not require such an assumption but on the other hand its estimated effect on each competing event reflects also the effect on the others. Thus, both the approaches have a possible drawback, but none of the two prevailed clearly in the simulation study: assuming independent censoring can be a serious issue in the case of strong correlation, whereas using the hazard of the subdistribution can be misleading whenever the treatment changes the hazard of only one of the competing events.

The main innovation and the motivation of the present work was to study the operating characteristics of the test by Peto, which is largely used in the medical literature, though almost absent in statistical publications. We aimed at comparing the test by Peto to the most common ones in the statistical literature, *i.e.* the test on the cause-specific hazard and the test on the hazard of the subdistribution by Gray. These two tests have already been compared head to head previously (see notably[27] and [28]). The main reason for this is that, despite the fact that these two tests address different questions, these are closely linked to each other and in our experience the interest of physicians in a clinical trial is somewhere in-between. Furthermore, to the best of our knowledge, the behavior of these tests in presence of misclassification of the cause of death had never been studied before; we think that the knowledge of such an aspect for the three tests is of primary importance for their practical use.

As our aim was to compare the tests across objectively characterized scenarios, we also investigated how the power and level of the tests could depend on the correlation between times to death from different causes, which has a precise clinical meaning. For example, positive correlation corresponds to comorbidity, which is quite common in advanced diseases. Negative correlation, too, is interesting as this could correspond to the effect of a standard of care therapy with different modalities that impact both disease control and toxicity. In the adjuvant context for lung cancer, for instance, all patients undergo surgery, either segmentectomy, or lobectomy or pneumonectomy: the greater the portion of lung resected, the lower the risk of relapses (and then of CD) but the higher the risk of pulmonary complications (and then of NCD).

4. Conclusions

Testing the treatment effect on the cause-specific death rate requires paying attention to the effect on the competing events. We considered three popular tests among several existing ones: a test based on recurrence data proposed by Peto, the cause-specific test and the cumulative incidence test proposed by Gray.

We performed a simulation study in four clinically relevant scenarios, with negatively correlated, uncorrelated and positively correlated event times, and with two censoring proportions in addition to complete data. We also generated recurrence times in order to bring to the fore the effects of classifying the cause of death in different ways. The recurrence times, conditional on the time to cancer deaths, followed a uniform distribution, which we considered a reasonable hypothesis. Further, we compared results to those obtained in the case of a high rate of misclassified causes of death.

All the three tests adequately preserved their nominal size when the treatment was completely ineffective. Gr seemed to be the most reliable in the situation of a therapy that reduced the risk of CD and increased that of NCD, provided that causes of death are correctly recorded; otherwise, it performed substantially worse and Pe should be recommended. In all the other situations Gr had the poorest performances, both in terms of the preservation of the nominal size and in terms of power. CS should be preferred whenever the treatment is expected to be ineffective against the risk of CD and possibly harmful in terms of NCD. A cancer treatment is required to be effective against the risk of CD but not against that of NCD. In that case, Pe was comparable to CS, except that CS had very high size for NCD in the presence of a high rate of misrecorded causes of death. In our study, Pe did not outperform its competitors in any situation in which the causes of death were correctly classified, whereas it was often the most reliable when the misclassification rate was high.

No clear pattern linked to the dependence between time variables emerged from our study. Censoring always reduces the rejection probabilities of all the tests, notably under the alternative hypothesis. Consequently, the tests are less and less powerful as censoring increases and their differences are less and less pronounced as well.

In the IALT study, the three tests suggested possible harm due to toxicity; Gr was firmly in favor of a benefit versus the risk of CD, whereas CS and Pe were borderline. We showed how the natural graphical representations for the three tests are the Nelson-Aalen estimate of the cumulative cause-specific hazard, the cumulative yearly rates as estimated by Peto, and the Aalen-Johansen estimate of the cumulative incidence function.

This study is the first to compare the operating characteristics of the log-rank test by Peto to those of the two best established tests in the statistical literature. The method used to simulate the data is innovative in that it takes into account the occurrence of recurrences and, at the same time, it is capable of generating both negatively and positively dependent times. This allowed us to study the effect of the reclassification of the causes of death proposed by Peto, without the requirement of assuming independence between CD and NCD. To keep things simple, we chose not to generate times to death from unknown causes. In such cases, multiple imputations or inverse probability weighting techniques exist (see for instance[35]).

5. Additional File

Additional file 1: Figures A.1 to A.9 and Tables A.1 to A.8. Detailed results of the simulation study: Correlation between the simulated event times (Figure A1) and empirical rejection probabilities of the tests in the four scenarios, with and without misclassified causes of death (Figures A2–A9 and Tables A1–A8).

6. Abbreviations

CD: Cancer death; CIF: Cumulative incidence function; CS: Cause-specific test; Gr: Gray's test; IALT: International Adjuvant Lung cancer Trial; NCD: Non-cancer death; Pe: Peto test; Rec: Recurrence.

Competing Interests

The authors declare that they have no competing interests.

Authors' Contributions

FR and SM conceived the study and developed the simulation model. FR was responsible for the simulation study and drafted the manuscript. FR and SM contributed to the interpretation of results and critically revised the report. Both authors read and approved the final manuscript.

Acknowledgements

The authors are grateful to Thierry Le Chevalier, Institut Gustave-Roussy, Villejuif, France, and the IALT Collaborative Group for providing the IALT data set. They further thank Boris Freidlin, Paula Williamson and Ruwanthi Kolamunnage Dona for their valuable elucidations and for sharing their R code for generating correlated survival times. They are grateful to Ariane Dunant for her precious work of critical and attentive revision. The authors thank Vanessa Rousseau for her R code on the Peto method and Lorna Saint Ange for editing the article.

Source: Rotolo F, Michiels S. Testing the treatment effect on competing causes of death in oncology clinical trials[J]. Bmc Medical Research Methodology, 2014, 14(1):1–11.

References

[1]   Prentice RL, Kalbfleisch JD, Peterson AV, Flournoy N, Farewell VT, Breslow NE: The analysis of failure times in the presence of competing risks. *Biometrics* 1978, 34(4):541–554.

[2]   Gooley T, Leisenring W, Crowley J, Storer B: Estimation of failure probabilities in the presence of competing risks: new representations of old estimators. *Stat Med* 1999,30(6):695–705.doi:10.1002/(SICI)1097025819990330 18:6<695::AID-SIM60> 3.0.CO;2-O.

[3]   Putter H, Fiocco M, Geskus RB: Tutorial in biostatistics: competing risks and multi-state models. *Stat Med* 2007, 26(11):2389–2430. doi:10.1002/sim.2712.

[4]   Allignol A, Schumacher M, Wanner C, Drechsler C, Beyersmann J: Understanding competing risks: a simulation point of view. *BMC Med Res Methodol* 2011, 11(1):86. doi:10.1186/1471-2288-11-86.

[5]   Koller M, Raatz H, Steyerberg E, Wolbers M: Competing risks and the clinical community: irrelevance or ignorance? *Stat Med* 2012, 31(11–12):1089–1097.

doi:10.1002/sim.4384.

[6] Klein JP, Shu YY: Multi-state models for bone marrow transplantation studies. *Stat Methods Med Res* 2002, 11:117–139. doi:10.1191/0962280202sm277ra.

[7] Lim H, Zhang X, Dyck R, Osgood N: Methods of competing risks analysis of end-stage renal disease and mortality among people with diabetes. *BMC Med Res Methodol* 2010, 10(1):97. doi:10.1186/1471-2288-10-97.

[8] Deslandes E, Chevret S: Joint modeling of multivariate longitudinal data and the dropout process in a competing risk setting: application to icu data. *BMC Med Res Methodol* 2010, 10(1):69. doi:10.1186/1471-2288-10-69.

[9] Chappell R: Competing risk analyses: how are they different and why should you care? *Clin Cancer Res* 2012, 18(8):2127–2129.doi:10.1158/1078-0432. CCR-12-0455.

[10] Dignam JJ, Zhang Q, Kocherginsky M: The use and interpretation of competing risks regression models. *Clin Cancer Res* 2012, 18(8):2301–2308. doi:10.1158/1078-0432.CCR-11-2097.

[11] Rauch G, Kieser M, Ulrich S, Doherty P, Rauch B, Schneider S, Riemer T, Senges J: Competing time-to-event endpoints in cardiology trials: a simulation study to illustrate the importance of an adequate statistical analysis. *Eur J Prev Cardiol* 2014, 21(1):74–80. doi:10.1177/2047487312460518.

[12] Pintilie M: *Competing Risks: A Practical Perspective*. New York: Wiley; 2006. doi: 10.1002/9780470870709.

[13] Gaynor JJ, Feuer EJ, Tan CC, Wu DH, Little CR, Straus DJ, Clarkson BD, Brennan MF: On the use of cause-specific failure and conditional failure probabilities: examples from clinical oncology data. *J Am Stat Assoc* 1993, 88(422):400–409. doi:10.1080/01621459.1993.10476289.

[14] Gray RJ: A class of k-sample tests for comparing the cumulative incidence of a competing risk. *Ann Stat* 1988, 16(3):1141–1154.

[15] Fine JP, Gray RJ: A proportional hazards model for the subdistribution of a competing risk. *J Am Stat Assoc* 1999, 94(446):496–509.

[16] Early Breast Cancer Trialists' Collaborative Group: *Treatment of Early Breast Cancer: Worldwide Evidence 1985-1990, vol. 1*. Oxford: Oxford University Press; 1990.

[17] Early Breast Cancer Trialists' Collaborative Group: Effects of radiotherapy and surgery in early breast cancer an overview of the randomized trials. *New Engl J Med* 1995, 333(22):1444–1456. doi:10.1056/NEJM199511303332202.

[18] Early Breast Cancer Trialists' Collaborative Group: Tamoxifen for early breast cancer: an overview of the randomised trials. *Lancet* 1998, 351(9114):1451–1467. doi:10.1016/S0140-67369711423-4.

[19] Early Breast Cancer Trialists' Collaborative Group: Effects of chemotherapy and hormonal therapy for early breast cancer on recurrence and 15-year survival: an

overview of the randomised trials. *Lancet* 2005, 365:1687–1717. doi:10.1016/S0140-67360566544-0.

[20] Bourhis J, Overgaard J, Audry H, Ang KK, Saunders M, Bernier J, Horiot J-C, Maître AL, Pajak TF, Poulsen MG, O'Sullivan B, Dobrowsky W, Hliniak A, Skladowski K, Hay JH, Pinto LH, Fallai C, Fu KK, Sylvester R, Pignon J-P: Hyperfractionated or accelerated radiotherapy in head and neck cancer: a meta-analysis. *Lancet* 2006, 368(9538):843–854. doi:10.1016/S0140-67360669121-6.

[21] Pignon J, Bourhis J, Domenge C, Designé L: Chemotherapy added to locoregional treatment for head and neck squamous-cell carcinoma: three meta-analyses of updated individual data. *Lancet* 2000, 355(9208):949–955. doi:10.1016/S0140-67360090011-4.

[22] Pignon J-P, le Maître A, Maillard E, Bourhis J: Meta-analysis of chemotherapy in head and neck cancer (MACH-NC): an update on 93 randomised trials and 17,346 patients. *Radiother Oncol* 2009, 92(1):4-14.doi:10.1016/j.radonc. 2009.04.014.

[23] Early Breast Cancer Trialists' Collaborative Group: Effects of radiotherapy and of differences in the extent of surgery for early breast cancer on local recurrence and 15-year survival: an overview of the randomised trials. *Lancet* 2005, 366(9503):2087l. doi:10.1016/S0140-67360567887-7.

[24] Early Breast Cancer Trialists' Collaborative Group: Relevance of breast cancer hormone receptors and other factors to the efficacy of adjuvant tamoxifen: patient-level meta-analysis of randomised trials. *Lancet* 2011, 378(9793):771–784. doi:10.1016/S0140-67361160993-8.

[25] Dignam JJ, Kocherginsky MN: Choice and interpretation of statistical tests used when competing risks are present. *J Clin Oncol* 2008, 26(24):4027–4034. doi:10.1200/JCO.2007.12.9866.

[26] Pintilie M: Dealing with competing risks: testing covariates and calculating sample size. *Stat Med* 2002, 21(22):3317–3324. doi:10.1002/sim.1271.

[27] Freidlin B, Korn EL: Testing treatment effects in the presence of competing risks. *Stat Med* 2005, 24(11):1703–1712. doi:10.1002/sim.2054.

[28] Williamson PR, Kolamunnage-Dona R, Tudur Smith C: The influence of competing-risks setting on the choice of hypothesis test for treatment effect. *Biostatistics* 2007, 8(4):689–694. doi:10.1093/biostatistics/kxl040.

[29] Ruan PK, Gray RJ: A method for analyzing disease-specific mortality with missing cause of death information. *Lifetime Data Anal* 2006, 12(1):35–51. doi:10. 1007/s10985-005-7219-2.

[30] International Adjuvant Lung Cancer Trial Collaborative Group: Cisplatin-based adjuvant chemotherapy in patients with completely resected non-small-cell lung cancer. *New Engl J Med* 2004, 350(4):351. doi:10.1056/NEJMoa031644.

[31] Arriagada R, Dunant A, Pignon J-P, Bergman B, Chabowski M, Grunenwald D,

Kozlowski M, Le Péchoux C, Pirker R, Pinel M-IS, Tarayre M, Le Chevalier T: Long-Term results of the international adjuvant lung cancer trial evaluating adjuvant Cisplatin-Based chemotherapy in resected lung cancer. *J Clin Oncol* 2010, 28(1):35–42. doi:10.1200/JCO.2009.23.2272.

[32] Nelson W: Theory and applications of hazard plotting for censored failure data. *Technometrics* 1972, 14(4):945–966. doi:10.1080/00401706.1972.10488991.

[33] Aalen O: Nonparametric inference for a family of counting processes. *Ann Stat* 1978, 6(3):701–726. doi:10.1214/aos/1176344198.

[34] Aalen OO, Johansen S: An empirical transition matrix for non-homogeneous markov chains based on censored observations. *Scand J Stat* 1978, 5(3):141–150.

[35] Moreno-Betancur M, Latouche A: Regression modeling of the cumulative incidence function with missing causes of failure using pseudo-values. *Stat Med* 2013, 32(18):3206–3223. doi:10.1002/sim.5755.

Chapter 29

Postmastectomy Radiotherapy: An American Society of Clinical Oncology, American Society for Radiation Oncology, and Society of Surgical Oncology Focused Guideline Update

Abram Recht[1], Elizabeth A. Comen[2], Richard E. Fine[3], Gini F. Fleming[4],
Patricia H. Hardenbergh[5], Alice Y. Ho[2], Clifford A. Hudis[2],
E. Shelley Hwang[6], Jeffrey J. Kirshner[7], Monica Morrow[2],
Kilian E. Salerno[8], George W. Sledge[9], Lawrence J. Solin[10],
Patricia A. Spears[11], Timothy J. Whelan[12], Mark R. Somerfield[13],
Stephen B. Edge[8]

[1]Beth Israel Deaconess Medical Center, Boston, MA
[2]Memorial Sloan Kettering Cancer Center, New York
[3]West Clinic Comprehensive Breast Center, Germantown, TN
[4]University of Chicago Medical Center, Chicago, IL
[5]Shaw Regional Cancer Center, Edwards, CO
[6]Duke University Medical Center, Durham, NC
[7]Hematology Oncology Associates of Central New York, East Syracuse
[8]Roswell Park Cancer Institute, Buffalo, NY

[9]Stanford University Medical Center, Palo Alto, CA

[10]Albert Einstein Healthcare Network, Philadelphia, PA

[11]North Carolina State University, Raleigh, NC

[12]Juravinski Cancer Centre, McMaster University, Hamilton, Ontario, Canada

[13]American Society of Clinical Oncology, Alexandria, VA

Abstract: Purpose. A joint American Society of Clinical Oncology, American Society for Radiation Oncology, and Society of Surgical Oncology panel convened to develop a focused update of the American Society of Clinical Oncology guideline concerning use of postmastectomy radiotherapy (PMRT). **Methods.** A recent systematic literature review by Cancer Care Ontario provided the primary evidentiary basis. The joint panel also reviewed targeted literature searches to identify new, potentially practice-changing data. **Recommendations.** The panel unanimously agreed that available evidence shows that PMRT reduces the risks of locoregional failure (LRF), any recurrence, and breast cancer mortality for patients with T1-2 breast cancer with one to three positive axillary nodes. However, some subsets of these patients are likely to have such a low risk of LRF that the absolute benefit of PMRT is outweighed by its potential toxicities. In addition, the acceptable ratio of benefit to toxicity varies among patients and physicians. Thus, the decision to recommend PMRT requires a great deal of clinical judgment. The panel agreed clinicians making such recommendations for individual patients should consider factors that may decrease the risk of LRF, attenuate the benefit of reduced breast cancer-specific mortality, and/or increase risk of complications resulting from PMRT. When clinicians and patients elect to omit axillary dissection after a positive sentinel node biopsy, the panel recommends that these patients receive PMRT only if there is already sufficient information to justify its use without needing to know additional axillary nodes are involved. Patients with axillary nodal involvement after neoadjuvant systemic therapy should receive PMRT. The panel recommends treatment generally be administered to both the internal mammary nodes and the supraclavicular-axillary apical nodes in addition to the chest wall or reconstructed breast.

1. Introduction

The American Society of Clinical Oncology (ASCO) guideline for the use of postmastectomy radiotherapy (PMRT) was published in 2001.[1] This update of that guideline, completed in collaboration with the American Society for Radiation Oncology (ASTRO) and the Society of Surgical Oncology (SSO), focuses on key areas of ongoing controversy, including the use of PMRT for patients with one to three positive lymph nodes, use of PMRT for patients undergoing neoadjuvant systemic therapy (NAST), and selected technical aspects of PMRT, particularly the extent of regional nodal irradiation (RNI). The question of whether PMRT is indicated in women with T1-2 tumors and a positive sentinel node biopsy (SNB) who do not undergo completion axillary lymph node dissection (ALND) is also discussed.

The use of PMRT has been widely accepted for patients with four or more positive lymph nodes,[2][3] but there is still controversy regarding the value of PMRT for those with one to three positive nodes. In 2014, the Early Breast Cancer Trialists' Collaborative Group (EBCTCG) published an updated meta-analysis of the effects of PMRT.[4] Its findings were summarized in a recent review by Cancer Care Ontario (CCO), which was reviewed by the panel (**Table 1**).[5] There were 22 trials that in aggregate accrued 8,135 women between 1964 and 1986 who were randomly assigned to receive or not receive radiotherapy to the chest wall and regional lymph nodes after mastectomy and axillary surgery. Our panel focused on the results for the 3,786 women who underwent axillary dissection, defined as: inclusion in a protocol requiring at least an anatomic level I to II dissection, a median of 10 nodes examined in the study population, or individual patient data showing 10 or more recovered nodes. The EBCTCG performed additional subset analyses of those trials in which systemic therapy was routinely administered. Among the 1,133 patients with one to three positive nodes who had undergone axillary dissection and received systemic therapy, the 10-year rate of isolated LRF (defined as local recurrence without simultaneous or preceding distant failure) was 21.0% without irradiation and 4.3% with PMRT (P < 0.001). The 10-year rate for any recurrence (locoregional or distant) was 45.5% without irradiation and 33.8% with irradiation (P < 0.001), and the respective 20-year rates of breast cancer mortality were 49.4% and 41.5% (P = 0.01; relative risk, 0.78). There were no differences in the benefits of PMRT for patients with one positive node compared with those with two or three positive nodes with regard to any first recurrence or breast cancer mortality. However, the median follow-up for all patients in the meta-analysis was only 9.4 years, which means that relatively small numbers of patients were observable at 20 years.

733

Table 1. Results of the Fifth Cycle of the EBCTCG Review of the Role of PMRT.

Nodal Status	No. of Patients	10-Year Local Recurrence Risk		20-Year Breast Cancer Mortality			20-Year Any-Cause Mortality		
		RT v no RT (%)	P	RT v no RT (%)	RR	P	RT v no RT (%)	RR	P
Mastectomy plus axillary dissection to C level II (14 trials)									
Negative	700	3.0 v 1.6	>0.1	28.8 v 26.6	1.18	>0.1	47.6 v 41.6	1.23	0.03
Positive	3,131	8.1 v 26.0	<0.001	58.3 v 66.4	0.84	0.001	65.4 v 70.4	0.89	0.01
One to three positive	1,314	3.8 v 20.3	<0.001	42.3 v 50.2	0.80	0.01	53.5 v 56.5	0.89	>0.1
One to three positive plus systemic therapy	1,133	4.3 v 21.0	<0.001	41.5 v 49.4	0.78	0.01	52.6 v 55.5	0.86	0.08
C Four positive nodes	1,772	13.0 v 32.1	<0.001	70.7 v 80.0	0.87	0.04	75.1 v 82.7	0.89	0.05
C Four positive nodes plus systemic therapy	1,677	13.6 v 31.5	<0.001	70.0 v 78.0	0.89	0.08	74.9 v 82.0	0.90	>0.1
Mastectomy plus axillary sampling (nine trials)									
Negative	870	3.7 v 17.8	<0.001	32.0 v 35.8	0.97	>0.1	46.1 v 49.9	1.00	>0.1
Positive	2,541	6.3 v 37.2	<0.001	55.6 v 68.2	0.74	<0.001	63.1 v 71.8	0.79	<0.001
Mastectomy only (four trials)									
Clinically negative	2,896	16.1 v 35.4	<0.001	50.8 v 53.1	0.97	>0.1	62.8 v 61.8	1.06	>0.1
Clinically positive	1,481	18.0 v 45.0	<0.001	56.6 v 63.3	0.86	0.03	67.1 v 71.5	0.91	>0.1

NOTE. Data adapted with permission[5]. Abbreviations: EBCTCG, Early Breast Cancer Trialists' Collaborative Group; PMRT, postmastectomy radiotherapy; RR, relative risk; RT, radiotherapy.

The most recent EBCTCG meta-analysis provides evidence that PMRT is highly effective at preventing LRF and, in an era of intermediate to high risk for recurrence, reduces the risk of patients with one to three nodes developing distant metastases and dying as a result of breast cancer. However, more recent evidence suggests that these findings may not be directly applicable to all patients with one to three positive nodes in the current era, when many of these patients are at much lower risk for recurrence. The trials included by the EBCTCG were predominantly conducted in the 1970s and 1980s. Rates of LRF and any recurrence reported in this meta-analysis were considerably higher than those reported in many contemporaneous and later series. Multiple studies from North America, Europe, and Asia of patients treated with mastectomy and systemic therapy without irradiation since 1990 have reported much lower 5 to 10 year actuarial LRF rates, with the most recent series usually reporting local LRF rates lower than 10% (**Table 2**). The divergence between the rates reported by the EBCTCG and contemporary series seems to have increased over time since the original ASCO PMRT guideline was published.

This trend of decreasing LRF rates over time likely results from multiple factors. These include decreasing average tumor sizes and a smaller average number of positive lymph nodes than that reported in some of the earlier randomized trials of PMRT[23]; a higher average number of resected lymph nodes in axillary lymph node dissections in more recent years, reflecting more complete axillary clearance; and the use of increasingly effective systemic therapy regimens. The trials included in the EBCTCG meta-analysis were primarily conducted in the 1970s and 1980s, with a median of fewer than 10 resected lymph nodes. Chemotherapy was most commonly cyclophosphamide, methotrexate, and fluorouracil; methotrexate plus fluorouracil; or single-agent cyclophosphamide or melphalan (Data Supplement Table 1).[4] Only a few trials included early doxorubicin- containing regimens. Ovarian irradiation was used in three trials. Tamoxifen was often administered for short courses (eg, for only 1 year in the Danish trial for postmenopausal women[24]), and generally, patients did not receive both tamoxifen and chemotherapy. The results of the trials included in the meta-analysis thus do not reflect the advances in systemic therapy made since 1986 and hence are not representative of current practice. These advances include the advent of adjuvant use of taxanes, dose-dense chemotherapy schedules, supportive care measures that improve chemotherapy adherence, adjuvant trastuzumab and other human epidermal

Table 2. LRF Rates Without RT After Modified Radical Mastectomy and Chemotherapy (with or without endocrine therapy) in Modern Series of Patients With pT1-2N1 Breast Cancer With Median Follow-Up of C5 Years.

Institution	Accrual Dates	No. of Patients	Median Follow-Up (months)	Measure	Rate (%)
MDACC[6]	1975-1994	466	116	10-year actuarial	14
ECOG[7]	1978-1987	1,018	145	10-year actuarial	13
NSABP[8]	1984-1994	2,957	133	10-year actuarial	13
BCCA[9]	1989-1997	821	92	10-year actuarial	17
Ankara, Turkey[10]	1990-2004	326	70	Crude	4
MGH[11]	1990-2004	165	84	10-year actuarial	11
Shikoku, Japan[12]	1990-2002	248	82	8-year actuarial	5*
Kaohsiung, China[13]	1990-2008	155	102	10-year actuarial	11†
Seoul, Korea[14]	1992-2004	401	68	10-year actuarial	20†
CALGB 9344[15]	1994-1997	254	67	Crude	8
MSKCC[16]	1995-2006	924	84	5-year actuarial	4†
Tampa, FL[17]	1996-2007	204	66	Crude	10
EIO[18]	1997-2001	262	120	10-year actuarial	10*
MDACC[19]	1997-2002	266	90	10-year actuarial	4
Cleveland Clinic[20]	2000-2007	271	62	5-year actuarial	9†
MDACC[21]	2000-2007	385	84	10-year actuarial	7
Tianjin, China[22]	2001-2005	368	86	8-year actuarial	11

NOTE. Rates include patients with both isolated LRF and simultaneous LRF and distant metastases, unless otherwise noted Abbreviations: BCCA, British Columbia Cancer Agency; CALGB, Cancer and Leukemia Group B; ECOG, Eastern Cooperative Oncology Group; EIO, European Institute of Oncology; LRF, locoregional failure; MDACC, MD Anderson Cancer Center; MGH, Massachusetts General Hospital; MSKCC, Memorial Sloan Kettering Cancer Center; NSABP, National Surgical Adjuvant Breast and Bowel Project; RT, radiotherapy. *Isolated locoregional recurrences only; †Not stated whether isolated or total locoregional recurrence rate reported

growth factor receptor 2-targeted drugs for patients with human epidermal growth factor receptor 2-positive cancers, adjuvant aromatase inhibitor therapy for postmenopausal women, combined endocrine blockade (ovarian ablation plus aromatase inhibitor therapy) in premenopausal women, and the use of prolonged adjuvant hormonal therapy (eg, 10 years of tamoxifen or 5 years of tamoxifen followed by 5 years of aromatase inhibitor therapy). As adjuvant systemic therapy improves, the risk of LRF is likely to decrease, and hence, the benefits seen of PMRT might decrease in both relative and absolute terms.

In view of the importance of the question of whether the benefits of PMRT (including its impact on overall survival) outweigh its known toxicities for this large group of patients with cancer, ASCO convened a guideline update panel in collaboration with ASTRO and SSO to provide recommendations for the use of PMRT in patients with T1 and T2 tumors (≤5cm) and one to three involved nodes. On the basis of its discussion of the current concerns of clinicians and recent publications, [25]-[27]and with the approval of the ASCO Breast Cancer Guideline Advisory Group co-chairs, the panel also addressed recommendations regarding the use of PMRT for patients undergoing SNB without ALND and for those treated with NAST and the optimal extent of RNI.

2. Focused Guideline Update Questions

Question 1: Is PMRT indicated in patients with T1-2 tumors with one to three positive axillary lymph nodes who undergo ALND?

Question 2: Is PMRT indicated in patients with T1-2 tumors and a positive SNB who do not undergo completion ALND?

Question 3: Is PMRT indicated in patients presenting with clinical stage I or II cancers who have received NAST?

Question 4: Should RNI include the internal mammary (IMNs) and/or supraclavicular-axillary apical nodes when PMRT is used in patients with T1-2 tumors with one to three positive axillary nodes?

3. Methods

3.1. Guideline Update Process

ASCO uses a signals approach to facilitate guideline updating. This approach is intended to identify new, potentially practice-changing data that might translate into revised practice recommendations. The approach relies on targeted literature searching and the expertise of ASCO guideline panel members to identify signals. The Methodology Supplement published with this article provides additional information about the signals approach.

The 2014 publication of the EBCTCG meta-analysis[4] provided the signal for this focused update. Based in large part on this signal, the ASCO Breast Cancer Advisory Group ranked updating the ASCO PMRT guideline question concerning use of PMRT for patients with one to three positive lymph nodes as a high priority. To that end, a joint ASCO-ASTRO-SSO panel was formed to review the evidence and formulate updated recommendations for practice.

The systematic review of literature by the CCO of locoregional therapy for locally advanced breast cancer guideline provided the primary evidentiary basis for the ASCO guideline focused update.[5] The CCO literature searches identified systematic reviews, meta-analyses, randomized controlled trials, cohort studies, and clinical practice guidelines that studied locoregional therapy for locally advanced breast cancer. For studies to be included in the analysis, the CCO required them to have at least 50 patients, have a prospective design, and provide a statistical comparison of the interventions of interest. At the request of ASCO, CCO guideline staff conducted an updated search of the CCO systematic review. The yield from the updated CCO search was reviewed for new, potentially practice-changing data.

Two additional targeted searches were conducted by the ASCO Guidelines Division staff to identify systematic reviews, meta-analyses, and randomized controlled trials of PMRT in women who had received neoadjuvant chemotherapy and of technical aspects of PMRT, especially RNI. A third targeted literature search and review was conducted to identify single-center and multi-institutional prospective and retrospective studies of patients treated since the PMRT trials in the EBCTCG meta-analysis were completed. Inclusion criteria for this targeted review were: retrospective or prospective study published between January 2001 and July 2015, patients accrued from 1985 or later, 150 or more patients explicitly identified with T1-2 cancers with one to three positive nodes, patients not treated with neoadjuvant chemotherapy, and median follow-up 48 months or longer.

The entire panel contributed to the development of the guideline, provided critical review, and finalized the guideline recommendation. All ASCO guidelines are reviewed and approved by the ASCO Clinical Practice Guidelines Committee. This focused update was reviewed by the ASTRO Guidelines Committee and approved by the ASTRO Board of Directors; the update was also reviewed by the SSO Breast Cancer Disease Site Work Group and approved by the SSO Quality Committee and Executive Council.

3.2. Guideline Disclaimer

The clinical practice guideline and other guidance published herein are provided by ASCO to assist providers in clinical decision making. The information herein should not be relied upon as being complete or accurate, nor should it be considered as inclusive of all proper treatments or methods of care or as a statement of the standard of care. With the rapid development of scientific knowledge, new evidence may emerge between the time information is developed and when it is published or read. The information is not continually updated and may not reflect the most recent evidence. The information addresses only the topics specifically identified herein and is not applicable to other interventions, diseases, or stages of disease. This information does not mandate any particular course of medical care. Furthermore, the information is not intended to substitute for the independent professional judgment of the treating provider, because the information does not account for individual variation among patients. Recommendations reflect high, moderate, or low confidence that the recommendation reflects the net effect of a given course of action. The use of words like "must," "must not," "should," and "should not" indicates that a course of action is recommended or not recommended for either most or many patients, but there is latitude for the treating physician to select other courses of action in individual cases. In all cases, the selected course of action should be considered by the treating provider in the context of treating the individual patient. Use of the information is voluntary. ASCO provides this information on an as-is basis and makes no warranty, express or implied, regarding the information. ASCO specifically disclaims any warranties of merchantability or fitness for a particular use or purpose. ASCO assumes no responsibility for any injury or damage to persons or property arising out of or related to any use of this information or for any errors or omissions.

This guideline reflects the most recent information as of the submission date. For the most recent information or to submit new evidence, please visit www.asco.org/pmrtguideline and the ASCO Guidelines Wiki (www.asco.org/guidelineswiki).

3.3. Guideline and Conflicts of Interest

The expert panel was assembled in accordance with the ASCO Conflict of Interest Management Procedures for Clinical Practice Guidelines summarized at www.asco.org/rwc). Members of the panel completed the ASCO disclosure form, which requires disclosure of financial and other interests that are relevant to the subject matter of the guideline, including relationships with commercial entities that are reasonably likely to experience direct regulatory or commercial impact as a result of promulgation of the guideline. Categories for disclosure include: employment; leadership; stock or other ownership; honoraria, consulting or advisory role; speaker's bureau; research funding; patents, royalties, other intellectual property; expert testimony; travel, accommodations, expenses; and other relationships. In accordance with these procedures, the majority of the members of the panel did not disclose any such relationships.

4. Recommendations

4.1. Clinical Question 1

Is PMRT indicated in patients With T1-2 tumors with one to three positive axillary lymph nodes who undergo ALND?

4.1.1. Updated Recommendations

Recommendation 1a The panel unanimously agreed that the available evidence shows that PMRT reduces the risks of LRF, any recurrence, and breast cancer mortality for patients with T1-2 breast cancer with one to three positive axillary nodes (type: evidence based; evidence quality: high; strength of recommendation: strong). However, some subsets of these patients are likely to have such a low risk of LRF that the absolute benefit of PMRT is outweighed by its potential toxicities (type: evidence based; evidence quality: intermediate; strength of recommendation: strong). In addition, the acceptable ratio of benefit to toxicity varies among patients and physicians. Thus, the decision to recommend PMRT or not requires a great deal of clinical judgment. The panel agreed clinicians making such recommendations for individual patients should consider factors that may decrease the risk of LRF, attenuate the benefit of reduced breast cancer-specific mortality, and/or increase the risk of complications resulting from PMRT. These factors include: patient characteristics (eg, age > 40–45 years, limited life expectancy because of older age or comorbidities, or coexisting conditions that might increase the risk of complications), pathologic findings associated with a lower tumor burden (eg, T1 tumor size, absence of lymphovascular invasion, presence of only a single positive node and/or small size of nodal metastases, or substantial response to NAST), and biologic characteristics of the cancer associated with better outcomes and survival and/or greater effectiveness of systemic therapy (eg, low tumor grade or strong hormonal sensitivity; type: informal consensus; evidence quality: intermediate; strength of recommendation: moderate). There are several risk-adaptive models that physicians may find useful in explaining the benefits of PMRT during shared decision making with patients. However, the panel found insufficient evidence to endorse any specific model or to unambiguously define specific patient subgroups to which PMRT should not be administered (type: no recommendation; evidence quality: low; strength of recommendation: weak). Further research is needed on how to accurately estimate individuals' risk of LRF and hence their potential reductions in LRF and breast cancer mortality.

Recommendation 1b The decision to use PMRT should be made in a multidisciplinary fashion through discussion among providers from all treating disciplines early in a patient's treatment course (soon after surgery or before or soon after the initiation of systemic therapy), either in the context of a formal tumor board or by referral (type: informal consensus; evidence quality: insufficient; strength of recommendation: strong).

Recommendation 1c Decision making must fully involve the patient, whose values as to what constitutes sufficient benefit and how to weigh the risk of complications against this in light of the best information the treating physicians can provide regarding PMRT in her situation must be respected and incorporated into the final treatment choice (type: informal consensus; evidence quality: insufficient;

strength of recommendation: strong).

4.1.2. Literature Review and Analysis

The grouping of patients with breast cancer in relation to the number of involved axillary nodes (eg, zero, one to three, four to nine, or [10) is of long standing in clinical trials and has been codified in the American Joint Committee on Cancer and Union for International Cancer Control TNM staging systems. However, these divisions have arguably been made much less important by improved understanding of the biology of breast cancer. Certainly, there is likely little difference in prognosis or benefit of therapy for women with three versus four positive nodes, but there may well be substantial difference between those with a single node with minimal metastatic burden and those with three nodes with bulky metastases. In addition, the prognostic and therapeutic impacts of a particular number of positive nodes may be different in patients who undergo SNB without ALND than in those who undergo ALND, because the total number of positive nodes may only be inferred if only SNB is performed (Clinical Question 2 provides a discussion of the use of PMRT for patients treated with SNB without completion ALND). Nonetheless, although such division of patients into groups on the basis of the number of involved nodes may be less operationally useful than in the past, it remains deeply embedded within the structure of clinical trial design, data analysis, and staging, making it difficult to avoid addressing the issue of the value of PMRT without using this categorization. Therefore, the panel focused its attention on patients with one to three positive nodes while recognizing that distinctions between the historic nodal prognostic groups are increasingly difficult to justify.

The recent EBCTCG meta-analysis provides considerable evidence that for patients with T1-2 tumors with one to three nodes PMRT reduces the risk of developing any recurrence and dying as a result of breast cancer and markedly reduces the risk LRF. However, as previously noted, the LRF rate in patients not undergoing irradiation in the trials reported in the EBCTGC (21%) was higher than that seen in most studies using more modern surgery and more contemporary adjuvant systemic therapies (most studies report LRF rates ranging from 4% to 10%; **Table 2**), leading the panel to question the generalizability of the EBCTCG results to all patients. Hence, not all patients treated with current standard axillary dissection and modern systemic therapy regimens will likely benefit sufficiently from PMRT to justify its use. Although morbidities resulting from PMRT have diminished over time because of improved radiation treatment planning and delivery techniques, compared with those used at the time of the trials reported in the EBTCG meta-analysis, [28] they are not negligible. Some, such as radiation-induced cardiac disease[29]–[32] and cancers, [33] may take decades to appear; hence, their ultimate rates with modern PMRT techniques cannot yet be ascertained. RNI may increase the risk of lymphedema, especially in patients who also undergo ALND. [26][34]Furthermore, many more patients now undergo breast reconstructive surgery. Administration of PMRT can worsen cosmetic results and increase the risk of both short and long-term complications.[35] [36] Therefore, if it can be determined that the risk of LRF is low for certain subgroups of patients, then by inference any reduction in breast cancer mortality would be low or negligible, making PMRT unadvisable in such patients.

Previous estimates of the value of irradiation in patients treated with breast- conserving surgery have suggested that radiation treatment has reduced impact on survival when it changes the risk of local recurrence risk by less than 10%. [37]Comparable data are not available for patients with one to three positive nodes in the EBCTCG meta-analysis, although some studies support that smaller reductions in regional recurrence can reduce breast cancer mortality (as discussed in Clinical Question 4). Furthermore, individual clinicians and patients will differ on the precise level of benefit (either a reduction in LRF, any recurrence, or breast cancer mortality) they feel is sufficient to justify PMRT, even if its impact could be accurately calculated. In addition, some have argued that the total risk of relapse would be a better surrogate or proxy than LRF to guide this decision making, because PMRT may eradicate areas of disease not destroyed by systemic therapy that could result in eventual tumor dissemination but may not manifest themselves clinically at those sites before (or after) systemic relapse. Hence, the panel cannot set a specific threshold for a risk of LRF that would justify the use or omission of PMRT.

Because the absolute benefit of PMRT seems likely to be greater for those patients with a higher risk of recurrence, the panel supports the use of a risk-adaptive strategy to guide patient selection for PMRT that attempts to balance the potential benefits of PMRT against its potential harms. Such a calculation should be based on: patient characteristics predicting for a lower risk of LRF or shorter life expectancy or an increased risk of complications, pathologic findings predicting a smaller tumor burden after definitive surgery, biologic factors predicting better outcome and survival, and the expected effectiveness of planned systemic therapy in order to balance benefits against harms. Evidence regarding the importance of individual factors is often based on older studies and limited data and is often contradictory. The effect of these factors in different studies often varies substantially. Until more definitive evidence is available, using its best clinical opinion, the panel recommends that such a strategy or risk estimation include assessment of patient age as it affects the risk of LRF, [7][10][21][22][38][39] estimated life expectancy in relation to age and comorbid conditions that might reduce life expectancy[40]–[44] or increase the risk of complications, [45]–[49]tumor size, [6][7]axillary lymph node burden (number of positive nodes,[9],[16],[19],[22] nodal ratio,[10],[20],[22],[38] and size of nodal tumor deposits [16][17][19]), tumor grade, [11][16][20][22][38][50]lymphovascular invasion, [10][16][21][22][38][51]biomarker or receptor status, [7][8][16][22][38][52]–[56]and planned systemic therapy (Data Supplement provides discussions of these and additional factors, such as margin status[57][58] and extranodal extension[16][19][20]). Several groups have proposed prognostic models to estimate the risk of LRF after mastectomy by combining several of these factors.[10][16][20][22][38] Although the panel cannot endorse any specific model, because the models have yet to be validated, physicians may find them useful in explaining the benefits of PMRT. Further research is needed on these models and how to accurately estimate an individual's risk of LRF and hence the potential reduction in LRF and breast cancer mortality.

Finally, the panel noted that the United Kingdom Medical Research Council SUPREMO (Selective Use of Postoperative Radiotherapy After Mastectomy) trial[59] randomly allocated approximately 1,600 patients with high-risk node-negative disease and one to three positive nodes (including when found after neoadjuvant chemotherapy) from June 2006 to April 2013 to receive PMRT or not. The results of this trial may eventually help determine which patients are most likely to benefit from PMRT when modern systemic therapy and surgery are used.

4.2. Clinical Question 2

Is PMRT indicated in patients with T1-2 tumors and a positive SNB who do not undergo completion ALND?

4.2.1. Recommendation

For patients with clinical T1-2 tumors with clinically negative nodes, SNB is now generally performed at the time of mastectomy, with omission of ALND if the nodes are negative. ALND has generally been performed if the nodes are positive, but there is increasing controversy about whether this is always necessary, especially if there is limited disease in the affected nodes. The panel recognizes that some clinicians omit axillary dissection with one or two positive sentinel nodes in patients treated with mastectomy. This practice is primarily based on extrapolation of data from randomized trials of patients treated exclusively or predominantly with breast-conserving surgery and whole-breast irradiation or breast plus axillary irradiation. In such cases where clinicians and patients elect to omit axillary dissection, the panel recommends that these patients receive PMRT only if there is already sufficient information to justify its use without needing to know that additional axillary nodes are involved (type: informal consensus; evidence quality: weak; strength of recommendation: moderate).

4.2.2. Literature Review and Analysis

The discussion of Clinical Question 1 was based on the assumption that patients had undergone level I to II ALND. However, it is not clear whether the clinical implications of positive nodes found on SNB are the same as those for patients undergoing ALND, because the extent of surgery is smaller, and there is a substantial chance of additional positive nonsentinel nodes remaining in the patient treated with SNB alone. The 2014 ASCO Panel on Sentinel Lymph Node Biopsy discussed the role of ALND for patients undergoing mastectomy (in Clinical Question 2.2 of its guideline). [60]It concluded the following: "Clinicians may offer ALND for women with early-stage breast cancer with nodal metastases found on SNB who will undergo mastectomy. Type: evidence based; benefits outweigh harms. Evidence quality: low. Strength of recommendation: weak." However, that panel did not discuss whether this applied equally to patients who are or are not likely to receive PMRT.

Some clinicians question the need for ALND after mastectomy in women based on extrapolation of the findings from three trials that randomly assigned patients with positive sentinel nodes to undergo ALND or no further axillary surgery.

The ACOSOG (American College of Surgeons Oncology Group) Z0011 trial in-cluded 856 patients with one or two sentinel node micro or macro metastases un-dergoing breast-conserving therapy, including whole-breast irradiation. [61][62] At a median follow-up of 6.3 years, there was no difference between patients allocated to ALND or no ALND with regard to locore-gional recurrence or survival. A small percentage of patients underwent axillary irradiation in violation of the protocol, but the effect of this on outcome is not known. [63]The IBCSG (International Breast Cancer Study Group) 23–01 trial included 931 women with one or two sentinel node micrometastases; those with macrometastases were excluded. [64]Similar to the ACOSOG Z0011 trial, patients were randomly assigned to undergo SNB alone or completion ALND. Patients who had undergone mastectomy were eligible and constituted 9% of the study population (84 patients). Breast irradiation without nodal irradiation was administered to 81% of those treated with breast conserving surgery, but PMRT was not administered to those who had undergone mastectomy. This trial also showed no difference in rate of regional or distant failure between the arms at a median follow-up of 5 years. Of note, there were no regional nodal recurrences in 42 patients treated with mastectomy who did not receive PMRT or ALND. Finally, the EORTC (European Organisation for Research and Treatment of Cancer) 0981–22023 trial AMAROS [After Mapping of the Axilla, Radiothe-rapy or Surgery]) compared ALND with breast plus axillary irradiation in 1,525 women with one or two sentinel node micro or macrometastases. [65]Most had un-dergone breast-conserving surgery and whole-breast irradiation, but 18% of the participants had undergone mastectomy, of whom approximately one third had also received chest wall irradiation. There were no significant differences in any measure of recurrence or mortality at a median follow-up of 6.1 years. Rates of nodal failure in the patients who had undergone mastectomy were not separately reported for this trial. However, in both studies, the total number of women treated with mastectomy was small.

Hence, at present, some physicians feel that ALND can be omitted for pa-tients undergoing mastectomy who have similar findings on SNB to those of pa-tients eligible for the randomized trials, particularly if PMRT is administered, whereas others feel ALND should still be performed. Although there are insuffi-cient data to support or refute these opinions, the panel agreed that it is inappro-priate to subject patients to the potential acute and long-term toxicities of PMRT (including rare but potentially fatal second cancers and cardiac events) without careful consideration of whether these are justified compared with the potential toxicities of ALND. The decision as to how to integrate ALND and PMRT for an individual patient should be a multidisciplinary effort that considers the treatment program as a whole. Thus, PMRT should be administered if there is otherwise sufficient evidence to warrant its use when ALND is omitted and the potential toxicities of PMRT are felt to be justified, and ALND should be used when the totality of the evidence is not yet sufficient for administering PMRT. That is, clinicians should ask themselves: "Would I recommend PMRT for this patient if she had undergone simultaneous ALND, and there were no additional nodal metastases in the nonsentinel nodes?" If the answer is no, ALND should be performed. This discussion should ideally occur before surgery, especially because this could guide patient decision making about reconstruction choices if reconstruction is desired.

4.3. Clinical Question 3

Is PMRT indicated in patients with clinical stage I or II cancers who have received NAST?

4.3.1. Updated Recommendation

Patients with axillary nodal involvement that persists after NAST (eg, less than a complete pathologic response) should receive PMRT. Observational data suggest a low risk of locoregional recurrence for patients who have clinically negative nodes and receive NAST or who have a complete pathologic response in the lymph nodes with NAST. However, there is currently insufficient evidence to recommend whether PMRT should be administered or can be routinely omitted in these groups. The panel recommends entering eligible patients in clinical trials that examine this question (type: informal consensus; evidence quality: low; strength of recommendation: weak).

4.3.2. Literature Review and Analysis

Neoadjuvant chemotherapy was initially limited to patients with unresectable locally advanced disease to allow mastectomy to be performed. Such patients then generally received PMRT. Whether PMRT is indicated in women with resectable early-stage breast cancer who have received neoadjuvant chemotherapy or endocrine therapy is an issue of increasing importance. There are few studies of the risks of LRF in such patients in relation to either pre-or post-treatment clinical and pathologic features. [66]-[69]The interpretation of these data are further complicated by the varying use of axillary ultrasound and biopsy before initiation of systemic therapy to enhance detection of clinically positive nodes before NAST and by the downstaging of nodal status by NAST (ie, a complete pathologic response in an individual with pre-NAST positive nodes that were detected on imaging only). The influence of potential risk factors for LRF may be different in patients undergoing NAST and those undergoing surgery before systemic therapy.

The panel agrees that, on the basis of currently available data, patients with persistently involved nodes on ALND after NAST have a sufficiently high risk of LRF to recommend that they receive PMRT, although there are as yet no data from randomized trials showing the effect of such treatment on long-term breast cancer mortality rates. Rates of LRF in patients with residual invasive cancer in the breast but negative axillary nodes after NAST are inconsistent across studies. Although patients with no residual disease in either the breast or axillary nodes seem to have low rates of LRF, there are insufficient data to exclude the possibility that certain subgroups of these patients may still benefit from PMRT (eg, those who had biopsy-proven axillary nodal involvement before chemotherapy or those with tumors with aggressive biologic features). Hence, the panel did not believe that recommendations for or against the use of PMRT could be made with confidence for these latter two groups at this time. The panel recommends entering these patients in clinical trials if available. There are currently two ongoing major multicenter trials in North America for patients with biopsy-proven axillary node involvement before NAST. The NRG Oncology Group 9353 trial, which opened in August 2013, randomly allocates patients with positive axillary fine-needle aspiration cytology or core biopsy before chemotherapy who undergo mastectomy or breast-conserving surgery and have negative nodes on ALND or SNB to either no irradiation or PMRT including the chest wall or reconstructed breast and RNI (if they undergo mastectomy) or breast irradiation or breast plus RNI (if they undergo breast-conserving surgery; ClinicalTrials.gov identifier NCT01872975). The Alliance for Clinical Trials in Oncology A011202 trial addresses another question relevant to patients undergoing NAST, namely, whether patients with a positive

SNB after chemotherapy have a different outcome when treated with ALND or axillary radiation therapy without additional surgery (ClinicalTrials.gov identifier NCT01901 094). Unfortunately, there are no such trials for patients without biopsy-proven nodal involvement before NAST who are found to have pathologically negative axillary nodes after NAST.

4.4. Clinical Question 4

Should RNI include both the IMNs and supraclavicul araxillary apical nodes when PMRT is used in patients with T1-2 tumors with one to three positive axillary nodes?

4.4.1. Updated Recommendation

The panel recommends treatment generally be administered to both the IMNs and the supraclavicular-axillary apical nodes in addition to the chest wall or reconstructed breast when PMRT is used for patients with positive axillary lymph nodes. There may be subgroups that will experience limited, if any, benefits from treating both these nodal areas compared with treating only one or perhaps treating only the chest wall or reconstructed breast. There is insufficient evidence at this time to define such subgroups in detail. Additional research is needed to identify them (type: informal consensus; evidence quality: intermediate; strength of recommendation: moderate).

4.4.2. Literature Review and Analysis

The panel agreed the critical question to address in this update should be whether to administer PMRT or not and not to focus on issues of what areas should be treated or how to deliver treatment. However, the panel also deemed it necessary to discuss the issue of RNI in patients with one to three positive nodes in view of the recent publications of the French, Canadian, and European prospective randomized trials and a large Danish retrospective study on this topic.[25]–[27][70]

The minimum mandatory target volumes for PMRT that were agreed upon by the panel are the chest wall and supraclavicular-axillary apical nodes in current practice. There remains controversy over when the IMNs and level I and II axillary nodes should be deliberately included. The radiation fields in 20 of the 22 trials in the EBCTCG meta-analysis showing benefit with PMRT included the IMNs, usually with additional regional nodes.[5]

Two randomized trials, conducted by the Canadian Cancer Trials Group (previously the National Cancer Institute of Canada) and the EORTC evaluated the addition of irradiation of the supraclavicular nodes, axillary apical nodes, and IMNs to whole-breast irradiation after breast-conserving surgery (both trials) or after chest wall or no chest wall irradiation after mastectomy (in the EORTC trial only).[26][27] A randomized trial conducted in France addressed the question of the addition of IMN irradiation to chest wall, supraclavicular, and axillary apical nodal irradiation.[25] All three trials included patients with node positive and node-negative breast cancers. Finally, a non-randomized study from Denmark compared results in node-positive patients with right-sided cancers who, according to Danish national guidelines, were to receive IMN irradiation in addition to the breast or chest wall and supraclavicular infraclavicular nodes with results in patients with left-sided cancers, who were not to undergo IMN irradiation. Overall findings of these four studies are summarized in **Table 3**. All found 1%–5% reductions in rates of relapse and breast cancer-specific and overall mortalities in patients receiving more extensive irradiation. Some of these differences were statistically significant (eg, overall survival in the EORTC and Danish studies).

Together, these studies support the effectiveness of RNI. However, their interpretation is complicated by differences in their exact design and in their detailed findings. For example, the French trial included only patients treated with mastectomy; the Canadian trial included only those undergoing breast-conserving surgery; and the EORTC trial mainly included patients treated with breast-conserving surgery, but 24% of patients were treated with mastectomy. All three randomized trials included patients with negative axillary nodes, but the proportions in each trial were different (25%, 10%, and 44% in the French, Canadian, and EORTC trials, respectively). Any patient with negative nodes with a central- or inner-quadrant primary was eligible for the French and EORTC trials, whereas only node-negative patients with high-risk features were eligible for the Canadian trial

Table 3. Outcome in Studies of Nodal Irradiation.

Study	SFRO[25]	EORTC[27]	NCIC[26]	Danish[70]
Dates of accrual	1991-1997	1996-2004	2000-2007	2003-2007
No. of patients	1,332	4,004	1,832	3,089
Median follow-up (years)	8.6	10.9	9.5	8.9
Irradiated sites	Chest wall + SC-IC ± IMN	Breast and chest wall ± SC-IC-IMNs	Breast ± SC-IC-IMNs	Breast and chest wall + SC-IC ± IMNs
Disease-free survival,%	50% and 53%	69% and 72%	77% and 82%	NR
Distant disease-free survival	NR	75% and 78%	83% and 87%	70% and 73%
Breast cancer-specific mortality	NR	14% and 12%	12% and 10%	23% and 21%
Overall survival	59% and 63%	81% and 82%	91% and 92%	72% and 76%

NOTE. Results given first for more limited irradiation and then for more extensive irradiation. All results for the Danish study given at 8 years; all others given at 10 years. Abbreviations: EORTC, European Organisation for Research and Treatment of Cancer; IC, infraclavicular or axillary apex; IMN, internal mammary node; NCIC, National Cancer Institute of Canada; NR, not reported; SC, supraclavicular; SFRO, Société Francaise de Radiation Oncologique.

(tumor ≥ 5cm, tumor ≥ 2cm with ≤ 10 axillary nodes removed, estrogen receptor (ER) negative, histologic grade 3, or lymphovascular invasion present). In the EORTC trial, patients who had undergone mastectomy underwent RNI versus no RNI according to random allocation; chest wall irradiation was administered at the discretion of the treating physicians. The use of systemic therapy and radiation field guidelines and techniques also varied. For example, the IMNs in the first five intercostal spaces were included in the French trial, the first three intercostal spaces in the Canadian trial, and the first three intercostal spaces in the EORTC trial, except for patients with lower inner-quadrant tumors, in whom the first five intercostal spaces could be included. Finally, all patients in the French trial underwent supraclavicular-infraclavicular nodal irradiation, with IMN irradiation being randomly assigned. However, the MA.20 and EORTC trials assigned patients to irradiation of both the supraclavicular-infraclavicular area and IMN nodes or to no nodal irradiation, so the effects of treating these two sites could not be separately evaluated.

Mindful of the limitations of subgroup analyses, reporting of results also differed substantially among these trials, particularly with regard to plausible prognostic or predictive factors. The French trial did not report results for patients with one to three positive nodes separately from those with more involved nodes. Crude rates of any breast cancer event were reduced from 20% to 16% in the MA.20 trial and from 33% to 30% in the EORTC trial with the addition of RNI, with respective reductions in overall death rates of 1% and 2%. However, there was no difference in overall survival at 8 years (83%) between the two groups in the Danish study (subgroup treatment interactions were not reported). Results in relation to receptor status were reported only for the MA.20 trial. Ten-year disease-free survival rates in the control and RNI arms for patients with ER-positive tumors were 79% and 81%, respectively, which were not significantly different; 10-year overall survival rates were 84% in both arms. However, for patients with ER-negative tumors, 10-year disease-free survival rates were significantly different in the control and RNI arms (71% and 82%, respectively); 10-year overall survival rates were 74% and 81%, respectively. The EORTC trial found no difference in death rates between the control and RNI arms when chemotherapy alone was used (28% and 30%, respectively) or in patients not receiving systemic therapy (14% and 13%, respectively). However, although there was no significant difference in mortality with the addition of RNI for patients receiving endocrine therapy alone (a reduction from 21% to 18%), there was a statistically significant reduction in patients receiving both endocrine therapy and chemotherapy (from 20% to 15%). It is not yet clear whether these different results in different subgroups resulted from chance alone or reflect important clinical distinctions.

The consensus of the panel, on the basis of the EBCTCG meta-analysis and the Canadian and EORTC RNI trials, is that both the IMN and supraclavicular-axillary apical areas should generally be treated when PMRT is used. However, certain subgroups may experience limited benefit from such treatment, and as noted, treating the supraclavicular and IMN areas can result in additional toxicities, with pulmonary and cardiac morbidities being particular concerns even with improved radiotherapy techniques. Additional analyses of these trials and other studies are needed to determine which patients should undergo irradiation of only one or neither of these areas.

In general, the full axilla is not irradiated in those who have had ALND, because recurrence in the dissected axilla is rare, and its inclusion may further increase toxicities, particularly lymphedema.[71] However, there are circumstances where full axillary irradiation may be considered, such as when ALND is not performed or after ALND in cases with extensive bulky involvement. There are insufficient data to propose recommendations in this area at present.

5. Discussion

The panel recommends strongly that input from all clinicians as well as the patient is needed to yield the best results from PMRT. This is best achieved through discussion among providers early in the patient's treatment course (before or soon after surgery and before or soon after the initiation of systemic therapy), either in the context of a formal tumor board or by referral to the surgical, medical, and radiation oncologists caring for the patient. Patients vary in how much they wish to participate in decision making, but ultimately, their values determine whether the potential long-term benefits of PMRT are sufficient to outweigh potential short and long-term risks of adverse effects.

Additional information, including a Data Supplement, a Methodology Supplement, evidence tables, and clinical tools and resources are, in part, published with this article and can all be found at www.asco.org/pmrt-guideline and www.asco.org/guidelineswiki. Patient information is available there and at www.cancer.net. Visit www.asco.org/guidelineswiki to provide comments on the guideline or to submit new evidence.

Acknowledegment

We thank Gary Freedman, Stephen Grobmyer, I. Craig Henderson, Nancy Klauber-DeMore, Gary Lyman, and Eleftherios Mamounas for kindly reviewing draft versions of the joint guideline manuscript. We also thank the American Society of Clinical Oncology Clinical Practice Guidelines Committee, the American Society for Radiation Oncology Clinical Affairs and Quality Committee and Board of Directors, and the Society of Surgical Oncology Quality Committee and Executive Committee for their thoughtful reviews of and insightful comments on this guideline document. The panel also thanks Glenn Fletcher of the Cancer Care Ontario Program in Evidence-Based Care, and Eva Culakova, Gary Lyman, and Marek S. Poniewierski of the Fred Hutchinson Cancer Research Center for their assistance with the literature searches and Brittany Harvey for administrative assistance.

Author Contributions

Administrative support: Clifford A. Hudis, Mark R. Somerfield

Manuscript writing: All authors

Final approval of manuscript: All authors

Authors' Disclosures of Potential Conflict of Interest

Postmastectomy Radiotherapy: An American Society of Clinical Oncology, American Society for Radiation Oncology, and Society of Surgical Oncology Focused Guideline Update

The following represents disclosure information provided by authors of this manuscript. All relationships are considered compensated. Relationships are self-held unless noted. I = Immediate Family Member, Inst = My Institution. Relationships may not relate to the subject matter of this manuscript. For more information about ASCO's conflict of interest policy, please refer to www.asco.org/rwc or jco.ascopubs.org/site/ifc.

Abram Recht

Consulting or Advisory Role: CareCore, US Oncology

Research Funding: Genomic Health (Inst)

Elizabeth A. Comen

Honoraria: Navigant Consulting, Kantar Health, Grey Global Group, ClearView Healthcare Partners, Decision Resources, Gerson Lehrman Group

Richard E. Fine

No relationship to disclose

Gini F. Fleming

Research Funding: Corcept Therapeutics (Inst)

Other Relationship: Aeterna Zentaris

Patricia H. Hardenbergh

Stock or Other Ownership: Chartrounds

Alice Y. Ho

No relationship to disclose

Clifford A. Hudis

Consulting or Advisory Role: Pfizer, Genentech, Novartis, Merck, Eli Lily

Other Relationship: Breast Cancer Research Foundation, American Society of Clinical Oncology

E. Shelley Hwang

No relationship to disclose

Jeffrey J. Kirshner

No relationship to disclose

Monica Morrow

Honoraria: Genomic Health

Kilian E. Salerno

No relationship to disclose

George W. Sledge Jr

Leadership: Syndax

Stock or Other Ownership: Syndax

Honoraria: Symphogen

Consulting or Advisory Role: Symphogen, Nektar, Synaffix, Radius

Research Funding: Genentech (Inst)

Travel, Accommodations, Expenses: GlaxoSmithKline, Nektar, Radius

Lawrence J. Solin

No relationship to disclose

Patricia A. Spears

Consulting or Advisory Role: Pfizer

Travel, Accommodations, Expenses: Genentech

Timothy J. Whelan

Consulting or Advisory Role: Genomic Health

Mark R. Somerfield

No relationship to disclose

Stephen B. Edge

No relationship to disclose

Source: Recht A, Comen E A, Fine R E, *et al*. Postmastectomy Radiotherapy: An American Society of Clinical Oncology, American Society for Radiation Oncology, and Society of Surgical Oncology Focused Guideline Update[J]. Journal of Clinical Oncology Official Journal of the American Society of Clinical Oncology, 2016:1–14.

References

[1] Recht A, Edge SB, Solin LJ, *et al*. Postmastectomy radiotherapy: clinical practice guidelines of the American Society of Clinical Oncology. J Clin Oncol. 2001; 19:1539–69.

[2] Tseng YD, Uno H, Hughes ME, *et al*. Biological subtype predicts risk of locoregional recurrence after mastectomy and impact of postmastectomy radiation in a large national database. Int J Radiat Oncol Biol Phys. 2015;93:622–630. doi:10.1016/j.ijrobp. 2015.07.006.

[3] Frasier LL, Holden S, Holden T, *et al*. Temporal trends in post-mastectomy radiation therapy and breast reconstruction associated with changes in National Comprehensive Cancer Network guidelines. JAMA Oncol. 2016; 2:95–101. doi:10.1001/ jamaoncol.2015.3717.

[4] McGale P, Taylor C, Correa C, *et al*. Effect of radiotherapy after mastectomy and axillary surgery on 10-year recurrence and 20-year breast cancer mortality: meta-analysis of individual patient data for 8135 women in 22 randomised trials. Lancet. 2014;383:2127–2135. doi:10.1016/S0140-6736(14)60488-8.

[5] Brackstone M, Dayes I, Fletcher GG, *et al*. Locoregional therapy of locally advanced breast cancer (LABC): program in evidence-based care evidence-based series no. 1–19. Toronto, Cancer Care Ontario, 2014.

[6] Katz A, Strom EA, Buchholz TA, *et al*. Locoregional recurrence patterns after mastectomy and doxorubicin-based chemotherapy: implications for postoperative irradiation. J Clin Oncol. 2000;18: 817–27.

[7] Recht A, Gray R, Davidson NE, *et al*. Locoregional failure 10 years after mastectomy and adjuvant chemotherapy with or without tamoxifen without irradiation: experience of the Eastern Cooperative Oncology Group. J Clin Oncol. 1999; 17: 1689–1700.

[8] Taghian A, Jeong JH, Mamounas E, *et al*. Patterns of locoregional failure in patients

with operable breast cancer treated by mastectomy and adjuvant chemotherapy with or without tamoxifen and without radiotherapy: results from five National Surgical Adjuvant Breast and Bowel Project randomized clinical trials. J Clin Oncol. 2004; 22:4247–54. doi:10.1200/JCO.2004.01.042.

[9] Truong PT, Berthelet E, Lee J, *et al.* The prognostic significance of the percentage of positive/dissected axillary lymph nodes in breast cancer recurrence and survival in patients with one to three positive axillary lymph nodes. Cancer. 2005; 103:2006–2014. doi:10.1002/cncr.20969.

[10] Yildirim E, Berberoglu U. Local recurrence in breast carcinoma patients with T(1–2) and 1–3 positive nodes: indications for radiotherapy. Eur J Surg Oncol. 2007; 33:28–32. doi:10.1016/j. ejso.2006.10.022.

[11] Macdonald SM, Abi-Raad RF, Alm El-Din MA, *et al.* Chest wall radiotherapy: middle ground for treatment of patients with one to three positive lymph nodes after mastectomy. Int J Radiat Oncol Biol Phys. 2009; 75:1297–1303. doi:10.1016/j.ijrobp.2009.01.007.

[12] Hamamoto Y, Ohsumi S, Aogi K, *et al.* Are there high-risk sub-groups for isolated locoregional failure in patients who had T1/2 breast cancer with one to three positive lymph nodes and received mastectomy without radiotherapy? Breast Cancer. 2014; 21:177–182. doi:10.1007/s12282-012-0369-7.

[13] Huang CJ, Hou MF, Chuang HY, *et al.* Comparison of clinical outcome of breast cancer patients with T1-2 tumor and one to three positive nodes with or without postmastectomy radiation therapy. Jpn J Clin Oncol. 2012;42:711–720. doi:10.1093/jjco/hys080.

[14] Kim SI, Park S, Park HS, *et al.* Comparison of treatment outcome between breast-conservation surgery with radiation and total mastectomy without radiation in patients with one to three positive axillary lymph nodes. Int J Radiat Oncol Biol Phys. 2011;80:1446–1452. doi:10.1016/j.ijrobp.2010.04.051.

[15] Sartor CI, Peterson BL, Woolf S, *et al.* Effect of addition of adjuvant paclitaxel on radiotherapy delivery and locoregional control of node-positive breast cancer: cancer and Leukemia Group B 9344. J Clin Oncol. 2005; 23:30–40.doi:10.1200/JCO.2005.12.044.

[16] Moo TA, McMillan R, Lee M, *et al.* Selection criteria for postmastectomy radiotherapy in t1-t2 tumors with 1 to 3 positive lymph nodes. Ann Surg Oncol. 2013; 20:3169–3174. doi:10.1245/ s10434-013-3117-0.

[17] Harris EE, Freilich J, Lin HY, *et al.* The impact of the size of nodal metastases on recurrence risk in breast cancer patients with 1–3 positive axillary nodes after mastectomy. Int J Radiat Oncol Biol Phys. 2013;85:609–614. doi:10.1016/j.ijrobp. 2012.05.050.

[18] Botteri E, Gentilini O, Rotmensz N, *et al.* Mastectomy without radiotherapy: outcome analysis after 10 years of follow-up in a single institution. Breast Cancer Res Treat. 2012;134:1221–1228. doi:10.1007/s10549-012-2044-2.

[19] Sharma R, Bedrosian I, Lucci A, *et al*. Present-day locoregional control in patients with t1 or t2 breast cancer with 0 and 1 to 3 positive lymph nodes after mastectomy without radiotherapy. Ann Surg Oncol. 2010;17:2899–2908.doi:10.1245/s10434-010 -1089-x.

[20] Tendulkar RD, Rehman S, Shukla ME, *et al*. Impact of postmastectomy radiation on locoregional recurrence in breast cancer patients with 1–3 positive lymph nodes treated with modern systemic therapy. Int J Radiat Oncol Biol Phys. 2012; 83:e577–e581. doi:10.1016/j.ijrobp.2012.01.076.

[21] McBride A, Allen P, Woodward W, *et al*. Locoregional recurrence risk for patients with T1,2 breast cancer with 1–3 positive lymph nodes treated with mastectomy and systemic treatment. Int J Radiat Oncol Biol Phys. 2014; 89:392–398. doi:10.1016/ j.ijrobp. 2014.02.013.

[22] Lu C, Xu H, Chen X, *et al*. Irradiation after surgery for breast cancer patients with primary tumours and one to three positive axillary lymph nodes: yes or no? Curr Oncol. 2013;20:e585-e592. doi:10.3747/co.20.1540.

[23] Cady B, Stone MD, Schuler JG, *et al*. The new era in breast cancer: invasion, size, and nodal involvement dramatically decreasing as a result of mammographic screening. Arch Surg. 1996; 131:301–308. doi:10.1001/archsurg.1996.014301 50079015.

[24] Overgaard M, Jensen MB, Overgaard J, *et al*. Postoperative radiotherapy in high-risk postmenopausal breast-cancer patients given adjuvant tamoxifen: Danish Breast Cancer Cooperative Group DBCG 82c randomised trial. Lancet. 1999; 353:1641– 1648. doi:10.1016/S0140-6736(98)09201-0.

[25] Hennequin C, Bossard N, Servagi-Vernat S, *et al*. Ten-year survival results of a ran-domized trial of irradiation of internal mammary nodes after mastectomy. Int J Radiat Oncol Biol Phys. 2013;86:860–866. [Erratum: Int J Radiat Oncol Biol Phys. 2014; 89:1145]; doi:10.1016/j.ijrobp.2013.03.021.

[26] Whelan TJ, Olivotto IA, Parulekar WR, *et al*. Regional nodal irradiation in early-stage breast cancer. N Engl J Med. 2015; 373:307–316. doi:10.1056/NEJMoa 1415340.

[27] Poortmans PM, Collette S, Kirkove C, *et al*. Internal mammary and medial supracla-vicular irradiation in breast cancer. N Engl J Med. 2015; 373:317–327. doi:10.1056/ NEJMoa1415369.

[28] Giordano SH, Kuo YF, Freeman JL, *et al*. Risk of cardiac death after adjuvant radio-therapy for breast cancer. J Natl Cancer Inst. 2005; 97:419–424. doi:10.1093/ jnci/dji067.

[29] Clarke M, Collins R, Darby S, *et al*. Effects of radiotherapy and of differences in the extent of surgery for early breast cancer on local recurrence and 15-year survival: an overview of the randomised trials. Lancet. 2005;366:2087–2106. doi:10.1016/S0140-6736(05)67887-7.

[30] McGale P, Darby SC, Hall P, *et al*. Incidence of heart disease in 35,000 women treated with radiotherapy for breast cancer in Denmark and Sweden. Radiother Oncol.

2011;100:167–175. doi:10.1016/j.radonc.2011.06.016.

[31] Darby SC, Ewertz M, McGale P, *et al*. Risk of ischemic heart disease in women after radiotherapy for breast cancer. N Engl J Med. 2013; 368:987–998. doi:10.1056/ NEJMoa1209825.

[32] Yeboa DN, Evans SB. Contemporary breast radiotherapy and cardiac toxicity. Semin Radiat Oncol. 2016; 26:71–78. doi:10.1016/ j.semradonc.2015.09.003.

[33] Grantzau T, Overgaard J. Risk of second non-breast cancer after radiotherapy for breast cancer: a systematic review and meta-analysis of 762,468 patients. Radiother Oncol. 2015; 114:56–65. doi:10.1016/j.radonc.2014.10.004.

[34] Warren LE, Miller CL, Horick N, *et al*. The impact of radiation therapy on the risk of lymphedema after treatment for breast cancer: a prospective cohort study. Int J Radiat Oncol Biol Phys. 2014;88:565–571. doi:10.1016/j.ijrobp.2013.11.232.

[35] Kelley BP, Ahmed R, Kidwell KM, *et al*. A systematic review of morbidity associated with autologous breast reconstruction before and after exposure to radiotherapy: are current practices ideal? Ann Surg Oncol. 2014; 21:1732–1738. doi:10.1245/ s10434-014-3494-z.

[36] Momoh AO, Ahmed R, Kelley BP, *et al*. A systematic review of complications of implant-based breast reconstruction with pre-reconstruction and postreconstruction radiotherapy. Ann Surg Oncol. 2014; 21:118–24. doi:10.1245/s10434-013-3284-z.

[37] Darby S, McGale P, Correa C, *et al*. Effect of radiotherapy after breast-conserving surgery on 10-year recurrence and 15-year breast cancer death: meta-analysis of individual patient data for 10 801 women in 17 randomised trials. Lancet. 2011; 378:1707–1716.

[38] Truong PT, Olivotto IA, Kader HA, *et al*. Selecting breast cancer patients with T1-T2 tumors and one to three positive axillary nodes at high postmastectomy locoregional recurrence risk for adjuvant radiotherapy. Int J Radiat Oncol Biol Phys. 2005; 61:1337–1347. doi:10.1016/j.ijrobp.2004.08.009.

[39] Yang PS, Chen CM, Liu MC, *et al*. Radiotherapy can decrease locoregional recurrence and increase survival in mastectomy patients with T1 to T2 breast cancer and one to three positive nodes with negative estrogen receptor and positive lymphovascular invasion status. Int J Radiat Oncol Biol Phys. 2010; 77:516–522. doi:10.1016/ j.ijrobp.2009.05.016.

[40] Schairer C, Mink PJ, Carroll L, *et al*. Probabilities of death from breast cancer and other causes among female breast cancer patients. J Natl Cancer Inst. 2004; 96:1311–1321. doi:10.1093/jnci/ djh253.

[41] Kendal WS. Dying with cancer: the influence of age, comorbidity, and cancer site. Cancer. 2008;112:1354–1362. doi:10.1002/ cncr.23315.

[42] Schonberg MA, Marcantonio ER, Li D, *et al*. Breast cancer among the oldest old: tumor characteristics, treatment choices, and survival. J Clin Oncol. 2010;

28:2038–2045. doi:10.1200/JCO. 2009.25.9796.

[43] Ring A, Sestak I, Baum M, *et al*. Influence of comorbidities and age on risk of death without recurrence: a retrospective analysis of the Arimidex, Tamoxifen Alone or in Combination trial. J Clin Oncol. 2011;29:4266–4272.doi:10.1200/JCO. 2011.35.5545.

[44] Schonberg MA, Davis RB, McCarthy EP, *et al*. External validation of an index to predict up to 9-year mortality of community-dwelling adults aged 65 and older. J Am Geriatr Soc. 2011;59:1444–1451. doi:10.1111/j.1532-5415.2011.03523.x.

[45] Ross JG, Hussey DH, Mayr NA, *et al*. Acute and late reactions to radiation therapy in patients with collagen vascular diseases. Cancer. 1993; 71:3744–3752. doi:10. 1002/1097-0142(19930601)71:11<3744::AID-CNCR2820711144>3.0.CO;2-C.

[46] Chen AM, Obedian E, Haffty BG. Breast-conserving therapy in the setting of collagen vascular disease. Cancer J. 2001; 7: 480–491.

[47] Phan C, Mindrum M, Silverman C, *et al*. Matched-control retrospective study of the acute and late complications in patients with collagen vascular diseases treated with radiation therapy. Cancer J.2003; 9:461–466. doi:10.1097/00130404200311000-00005.

[48] Lin A, Abu-Isa E, Griffith KA, *et al*. Toxicity of radiotherapy in patients with collagen vascular disease. Cancer. 2008;113: 648–653. doi:10.1002/cncr.23591.

[49] Lee CE, Prabhu V, Slevin NJ. Collagen vascular diseases and enhanced radiotherapy-induced normal tissue effects: a case report and a review of published studies. Clin Oncol (R Coll Radiol). 2011;23:73–78. doi:10.1016/j.clon.2010.08.030.

[50] Wallgren A, Bonetti M, Gelber RD, *et al*. Risk factors for locoregional recurrence among breast cancer patients: results from International Breast Cancer Study Group trials I through VII. J Clin Oncol.2003; 21:1205–1213.doi:10.1200/JCO.2003.03. 130.

[51] Matsunuma R, Oguchi M, Fujikane T, *et al*. Influence of lymphatic invasion on locoregional recurrence following mastectomy: indication for postmastectomy radiotherapy for breast cancer patients with one to three positive nodes. Int J Radiat Oncol Biol Phys. 2012; 83:845–852. doi:10.1016/j.ijrobp. 2011.08.029.

[52] Kyndi M, Sørensen FB, Knudsen H, *et al*. Estrogen receptor, progesterone receptor, HER-2, and response to postmastectomy radiotherapy in high-risk breast cancer: the Danish Breast Cancer Cooperative Group. J Clin Oncol. 2008; 26:1419–1426.doi:10. 1200/JCO.2007.14.5565.

[53] Kwan W, Al-Tourah AJ, Speers C, *et al*. Does HER2 status influence locoregional failure rates in breast cancer patients treated with mastectomy for pT1-2pN0 disease? Ann Oncol. 2010;21:988–993. doi:10.1093/annonc/mdp396.

[54] Mamounas EP, Tang G, Fisher B, *et al*. Association between the 21-gene recurrence score assay and risk of locoregional recurrence in node-negative, estrogen receptor-positive breast cancer: results from NSABP B-14 and NSABP B-20. J Clin Oncol. 2010; 28:1677–1683. doi:10.1200/JCO.2009.23.7610.

[55] Wang SL, Li YX, Song YW, et al. Triple-negative or HER2-positive status predicts higher rates of locoregional recurrence in node-positive breast cancer patients after mastectomy. Int J Radiat Oncol Biol Phys. 2011;80:1095–1101. doi:10.1016/j.ijrobp.2010.03.038.

[56] Kneubil MC, Brollo J, Botteri E, et al. Breast cancer subtype approximations and loco-regional recurrence after immediate breast reconstruction. Eur J Surg Oncol. 2013;39:260–265. doi:10. 1016/j.ejso.2012.12.004.

[57] Truong PT, Olivotto IA, Speers CH, et al. A positive margin is not always an indication for radiotherapy after mastectomy in early breast cancer. Int J Radiat Oncol Biol Phys. 2004; 58:797–804. doi:10.1016/S0360-3016(03)01626-2.

[58] Childs SK, Chen YH, Duggan MM, et al. Surgical margins and the risk of local-regional recurrence after mastectomy without radiation therapy. Int J Radiat Oncol Biol Phys. 2012; 84: 1133–1138. doi:10.1016/j.ijrobp.2012.02.048.

[59] Kunkler IH, Canney P, van Tienhoven G, et al. Elucidating the role of chest wall irradiation in 'intermediate-risk' breast cancer: the MRC/EORTC SUPREMO trial. Clin Oncol (R Coll Radiol). 2008; 20:31–34. doi:10.1016/j.clon.2007.10.004.

[60] Lyman GH, Temin S, Edge SB, et al. Sentinel lymph node biopsy for patients with early-stage breast cancer: American Society of Clinical Oncology clinical practice guideline update. J Clin Oncol. 2014; 32:1365–1383.doi:10.1200/JCO.2013.54.1177.

[61] Giuliano AE, McCall L, Beitsch P, et al. Locoregional recurrence after sentinel lymph node dissection with or without axillary dissection in patients with sentinel lymph node metastases: the American College of Surgeons Oncology Group Z0011 randomized trial. Ann Surg. 2010; 252:426–432. Discussion 432–433.

[62] Giuliano AE, Hunt KK, Ballman KV, et al. Axillary dissection vs no axillary dissection in women with invasive breast cancer and sentinel node metastasis: a randomized clinical trial. JAMA. 2011; 305:569–575. doi:10.1001/jama.2011.90.

[63] Jagsi R, Chadha M, Moni J, et al. Radiation field design in the ACOSOG Z0011 (Alliance) trial. J Clin Oncol. 2014; 32: 3600–3606. doi:10.1200/JCO.2014.56.5838.

[64] Galimberti V, Cole BF, Zurrida S, et al. Axillary dissection versus no axillary dissection in patients with sentinel-node micrometastases (IBCSG 23–01): a phase 3 randomised controlled trial. Lancet Oncol. 2013; 14:297–305. doi:10.1016/S1470-2045(13)70035-4.

[65] Donker M, van Tienhoven G, Straver ME, et al. Radiotherapy or surgery of the axilla after a positive sentinel node in breast cancer (EORTC 10981-22023 AMAROS): a randomised, multicentre, open-label, phase 3 non-inferiority trial. Lancet Oncol. 2014; 15:1303–1310. doi:10.1016/S1470-2045(14)70460-7.

[66] Buchholz TA, Tucker SL, Masullo L, et al. Predictors of local-regional recurrence after neoadjuvant chemotherapy and mastectomy without radiation. J Clin Oncol. 2002; 20:17–23. doi:10. 1200/JCO.20.1.17.

[67] Nagar H, Mittendorf EA, Strom EA, *et al*. Local-regional recurrence with and without radiation therapy after neoadjuvant chemotherapy and mastectomy for clinically staged T3N0 breast cancer. Int J Radiat Oncol Biol Phys. 2011;81:782–787. doi:10.1016/j.ijrobp.2010.06.027.

[68] Mamounas EP, Anderson SJ, Dignam JJ, *et al*. Predictors of locoregional recurrence after neoadjuvant chemotherapy: results from combined analysis of National Surgical Adjuvant Breast and Bowel Project B-18 and B-27. J Clin Oncol. 2012; 30:3960–3966. doi:10.1200/JCO.2011.40.8369.

[69] Krug D, Lederer B, Debus J, *et al*. Relationship of omission of adjuvant radiotherapy to outcomes of locoregional control and disease-free survival in patients with or without pCR after neoadjuvant chemotherapy for breast cancer: a meta-analysis on 3481 patients from the Gepar-trials. J Clin Oncol. 33, 2015 (suppl; abstr 1008).

[70] Thorsen LB, Offersen BV, Danø H, *et al*. DBCG-IMN: a population-based cohort study on the effect of internal mammary node irradiation in early node-positive breast cancer. J Clin Oncol. 2016; 34:314–320. doi:10.1200/JCO.2015.63.6456.

[71] Recht A, Houlihan MJ. Axillary lymph nodes and breast cancer: a review. Cancer. 1995;76:1491–1512.doi:10.1002/1097-0142(19951101)76:9<1491:AID-CNCR2820 76090 2>3.0.CO;2–8.

Chapter 30

Clinical Oncology in Resource-Limited Settings

Franco M. Buonaguro[1], Serigne N. Gueye[2], Henry R. Wabinga[3], Twalib A. Ngoma[4], Jan B. Vermorken[5], Sam M. Mbulaiteye[6]

[1]Division of Molecular Biology & Viral Oncology, Department of Experimental Oncology, Istituto Nazionale Tumori -IRCCS "Fond Pascale", Naples, Italy
[2]Division of Urology and Andrology, Grand Yoff General Hospital-Department of Surgery/Urology, University Cheikh Anta DIOP, Dakar, Senegal
[3]Department of Pathology, College of Health Sciences, Makerere University, Kampala, Uganda
[4]Ocean Road Cancer Institute, Dar es Salaam, Tanzania
[5]Department of Medical Oncology, Antwerp University Hospital, Antwerp, Belgium
[6]Infections and Immunoepidemiology Branch, Div of Cancer Epidemiology and Genetics, National Cancer Institute, National Institutes of Health, Department of Health and Human Services, 9609 Medical Center Dr, Rm. 6E118 MSC 9704, Bethesda, MD 20892–9704, USA

Abstract: Infectious Agents and Cancer is introducing a new section of Clinical Oncology with the main objective of stimulating debate through articles published in the section. Infectious diseases have been the major causes of morbidity and mortality in human populations, and have dominated the medical approach to clinical and public health. Successful efforts to control mortality from acute infections have paved the way for chronic, mostly indolent, infections to become major causes of morbidity. Cancer, hitherto thought to be rare in resource-limited settings, is becoming a major contributor. The changes in mortality patterns are due, in part, to diseases linked to rapid changes in lifestyle, urbanization, and pollution. These diseases include many of the non-infection associated cancers. However, there is a dearth of information about the burden, pathogenesis, and therapeutic approaches about cancer in resource-limited countries. There are also substantial other challenges, including economic, infrastructure, technology, and personnel. The Journal advocates for interactive local-global (lo-bal) efforts to generate relevant knowledge about cancer burden, pathogenesis, and therapeutic approaches using a bottom-up approach to sharpen the focus on local and global relevance of research and clinical and public practice, particularly in resource-limited countries. The section on Clinical Oncology in Infectious Agents and Cancer will harness these "lo-bal" strategies to reduce substantially the time from concept, discovery, and development and implementation of locally and globally applicable diagnostic and therapeutic technologies.

1. Editorial

Do we really need a clinical oncology journal focusing on resource-limited countries? Many, perhaps, would be inclined to answer "no". Resource-limited countries are faced with extraordinary burdens of acute and chronic infectious agents, malnutrition, civil disturbance, violence, and economic disparity and have to make, often, painful choices how to spend their limited resources. Intuitively, those countries should focus on identifying diseases that rank top in their morbidity surveys and learning and applying strategies for early diagnosis and treatment of those conditions. Because previous morbidity surveys have indicated that acute infections, malnutrition, and maternal conditions are the leading causes of morbidity and mortality, the argument to establish and develop clinical and basic oncology services in resource-limited countries seems weak.

Yet, morbidity and mortality from cancer is substantial in many resource-limited countries. The successful efforts to control mortality from acute infections have paved the way for chronic infections to become the major causes of morbidity in resource-limited settings. Inevitably, cancer will also become important. Infection-associated cancers already contribute to more than one-third of cancers in resource-limited settings, compared to less than one-fifth in developed countries. Concomitant increases in mortality from other diseases, which are linked to rapid changes in lifestyle, urbanization, and pollution, will undermine the gains from decreased mortality from acute infections. Clinicians working in resource-limited countries regularly encounter patients with cancer, many patients present with late symptoms. Clinicians confront the challenges to diagnose, treat and rehabilitate patients with cancer. Public health managers confront the challenges to balance resource allocation between cancer services, for which the demand is growing steeply, and the need to meet priorities imposed by acute infections, malnutrition, and maternal disease for which the demand has historically been high.

We lack robust data from well-designed and well-conducted studies in resource-limited settings, which complicates forecasting. Likewise, there is a dearth of information about pathogenesis, metabolic or genetic pathways and therapeutic approaches, which hampers efforts towards rational programs to mitigate the cancer burden in resource-limited countries. The challenges for developing evidence-based oncologic programs in resource-limited settings are broad and diverse.

However, there are many reasons to develop robust oncologic programs in resource-limited countries. These include humanitarian considerations: the need to provide a basic diagnosis, treatment or pain care and rehabilitation. Others include scientific considerations to estimate the burden, distribution, and trends of cancer and conduct in-depth studies of the biology of cancer. Basic science studies are necessary to develop targeted therapies. The increasing appreciation of the substantial contribution of chronic infections to cancer provides strong motivation to identify infection-associated cancers and to deploy infection control strategies to cancer control.

Infections have historically exerted tremendous evolutionary pressure on human populations. For example, pressure from malaria infections has left the glucose-6-phosphate dehydrogenase (G6PD) signature mutation at nucleotide 563 (Exon 6). This mutation leads to a substitution of a phenylalanine amino acid with a serine amino acid at position 188 (SER188PHE) and it is associated with G6PD deficiency anemia and reduced risk of death from malaria[1], as initially proposed by Davidson et al., 1964[2]. Similarly, other severe fatal infections, such as plague, smallpox HIV infection, have induced signature mutations, including the CCR5 deletion (*i.e.* CCR5 Δ32), which is associated with resistance to these diseases[3], but it might also increase susceptibility to other infections, such as the West Nile infections[4]. Other infections show peculiar distributions, but whether these disparities may be associated with signature mutations and/or specific concurrent infections or other local environmetal co-factors is unknown. For example, human herpesvirus 8 (HHV-8), the viral cause of Kaposi's sarcoma (KS), shows a peculiar gradient that mirrors KS incidence[5], but genetic factors for this disease as well as other cofactors, able to explain the different susceptibility to the infection, are largely unknown. Another important virus that shows disparity is hepatitis C virus (HCV) whose prevalence in Europe is <2.5%, but is extremely high in some populations including in Southern Italy where the prevalence in people >65 years of age is >30%. The incidence of hepato-cellular carcinoma incidence tracks imperfectly with HCV prevalence[6][7], but whether genetic factors or local environmental co-factors contribute is unknown. Finally, the higher incidence of colon cancer could be associated with meat consumption, as recently raised by Nobel laureate Harold zur Hausen[8]. Could the habit of eating raw meat be a factor in transmitting infections from animals to humans? The Euro-Asiatic bovines (Bos taurus) and Indian Zebu (Bos indicus) or their hybrids Bos taurus Africanus (such as Sanga or the Ugandan race Ankole-Watusi) are less susceptible to bovine infections, such as rinderpest, thus favoring them over other bovine types. Is it possible that these cows also transmit other pathogens to humans that increase the risk of cancers? Studies conducted in resource-limited settings could be informative.

While serendipitous findings, such as the discovery and identification of HPV16 in cervical cancer from African patients[9] and of several HPV18 copies in HeLa cervical cancer cells[10], have driven science in the past, such opportunities arise only in the context of ongoing sustained research activity. For example, observation of extraordinarily high incidence of penile cancers in Ugandan tribes, where penile cancer represented >40% of all male cancers was observed when research was introduced in Africa[11][12], and suggested effects of local factors. However, when civil disturbance disrupted nascent research efforts in Africa, no further scientific studies were appropriately performed and the underlying local risk factors for cancer were not identified. More recently, following the HIV epidemic, a mini-epidemic of conjunctival cancers has been reported in Africa[13], but not in the West. While the descriptive data may not lead to definitive scientific interpretation, integration of molecular data could substantially increase their relevance. Taken together, study of cancer in resource-limited settings has relevance to local communities as well as to the international community through knowledge generation[14].

For these reasons, Infectious Agents and Cancer is introducing a new section on Clinical Oncology to stimulate debate in the scientific community, along with the pharmaceutical companies, to act in concert to support nascent oncologic programs in resource-limited settings. This debate will lead to identification of the cheapest available route to a complete and effective anti-cancer regimen, for it to be pursued and implemented as for acute infectious diseases[15]. This approach will help meet the needs in limited-settings, and also bring mutual benefits to communities in wealthy countries. In a global village no one component can be left out. Wholesome clinical experience must be shared; the technological advances must be exchanged. This bottom-up approach may be referred to as the "lo- bal" strategy, where local observations are analyzed with scientific methods and the results are extrapolated for global comprehension of the phenomenon. Innovative pathogenesis studies in African populations may lead to discovery of novel genetic pathways or targets for new therapeutic approaches[16]. An integration of technological advanced oncologists with the local bio-medical community will accelerate the general scientific knowledge, while optimizing local public health programs and the general health conditions.

Young doctors from newly established Medical school lost in the bush of the dark Africa, such as at St. Mary's Hospital, Lacor, in Uganda, (**Figure 1**) have applied themselves to medical science. In one example, they showed that some protocols developed outside Africa, may not be easily or usefully translated to the local conditions, highlighting the need for better interaction between the more advanced scientific community and local teams[17][18]. The FEAST trial project, which won the BMJ Research Paper of the Year 2012[19], is an excellent example of this. In the same hospital (**Figure 1**) local clinicians and nurses were able to identify and mount rapid containment, albeit at some cost of their lives, an Ebola epidemic and "produce more scientific data on Ebola". These examples indicate a thirst to learn and practice that good medicine, even extreme in terms of economic conditions and constructive interaction with the global scientific community[20][21].

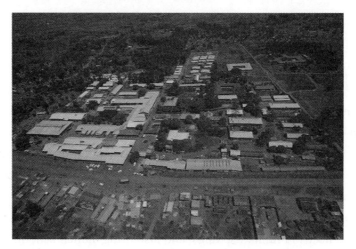

Figure 1. The St Mary's Hospital at Lacor, Gulu-Uganda.

The "lo-bal" strategy is well developed for acute infectious diseases. It will definitely foster the sharing of experiences and information between worldwide oncologist as well as the identification and development of diagnostic and therapeutic protocols globally valid in the current global village. Infectious Agents and Cancer hopes to stimulate and contribute to this debate through articles published in the section of Clinical Oncology.

Acknowledgements

The Editorial reflects the views of the Editors-in-Chief and the section Editors, on behalf of Infectious Agents and Cancer. The content is the responsibility of the authors alone and does not necessarily reflect the views of their respective employers as well as of the publisher.

Source: Buonaguro F M, Gueye S N, Wabinga H R, *et al*. Clinical oncology in resource-limited settings[J]. Infectious Agents & Cancer, 2013, 8(1):1–4.

References

[1]   Kumar V, Abbas AK, Fausto N, Aster JC: Robbins and Cotran Pathologic Basis of Disease. Expert Consult. Elsevier Health. Kindle Edition: Professional Edition; 2009.

[2] Davidson RG, Childs B, Siniscalco M: Genetic variations in the quantitative control of erythrocyte glucose-6-phosphate dehydrogenase activity. Ann Hum Genet 1964, 28:61–70.

[3] Galvani AP, Slatkin M: Evaluating plague and [[smallpox]] as historical selective pressures for the CCR5-Delta 32 HIV-resistance allele. Proc Natl Acad Sci USA 2003, 100:15276–15279.

[4] Glass WG, McDermott DH, Lim JK, Lekhong S, Yu SF, Frank WA, Pape J, Cheshier RC, Murphy PM: CCR5 deficiency increases risk of symptomatic West Nile virus infection. J Exp Med 2006, 203:35–40.

[5] Buonaguro FM, Tomesello ML, Buonaguro L, Satriano RA, Ruocco E, Castello G, Ruocco V: Kaposi's sarcoma: aetiopathogenesis, histology and clinical features. J Eur Acad Dermatol Venereol 2003, 17:138–154.

[6] Maio G, D'Argenio P, Stroffolini T, Bozza A, Sacco L, Tosti ME, Intorcia M, Fossi E, D'Alessio G, Kondili LA, Rapicetta M, Mele A: Hepatitis C virus infection and alanine transaminase levels in the general population: a survey in a southern Italian town. J Hepatol 2000, 33:116–120.

[7] Fusco M, Girardi E, Piselli P, Palombino R, Polesel J, Maione C, Scognamiglio P, Pisanti FA, Solmone M, Di Cicco P, Ippolito G, Franceschi S, Serraino D: Epidemiology of viral hepatitis infections in an area of southern Italy with high incidence rates of liver cancer. Eur J Cancer 2008, 44:847–453.

[8] Zur Hausen H: Red meat consumption and cancer: reasons to suspect involvement of bovine infectious factors in colorectal cancer. Int J Cancer 2012, 130:2475-2483.

[9] Dürst M, Gissmann L, Ikenberg H, Zur Hausen H: A papillomavirus DNA from a cervical carcinoma and its prevalence in cancer biopsy samples from different geographic regions. Proc Natl Acad Sci USA 1983, 80:3812–3815.

[10] Macville M, Schröck E, Padilla-Nash H, Keck C, Ghadimi BM, Zimonjic D, Popescu N, Ried T: Comprehensive and definitive molecular cytogenetic characterization of HeLa cells by spectral karyotyping. Cancer Res 1999, 59:141–150.

[11] Dodge OG, Owor O, Templeton AC: In Tumours in a tropical country. Edited by Templeton AC. Berlin: Springer; 1973:132–144.

[12] Tornesello ML, Buonaguro FM, Beth-Giraldo E, Kyalwazi SK, Giraldo G: Human papillomavirus (HPV) DNA in penile carcinomas and in two cell lines from high-incidence areas for genital cancers in Africa. Int J Cancer 1992, 51:587–592.

[13] Wabinga HR, Parkin DM, Wabwire-Mangen F, Nambooze S: Trends in cancer incidence in Kyadondo County, Uganda, 1960–1997. Br J Cancer 2000, 82:1585–1592.

[14] Levine AS: The epidemic of acquired immune dysfunction in homosexual men and its sequelae-opportunistic infections, Kaposi's sarcoma, and other malignancies: an update and interpretation. Cancer Treat Rep 1982, 66:1391–1395.

[15] Waning B, Diedrichsen E, Moon S: A lifeline to treatment: the role of Indian generic

manufacturers in supplying antiretroviral medicines to developing countries. J Int AIDS Soc 2010, 13:35.

[16] Mbulaiteye S: Burkitt Lymphoma: beyond discoveries. IAC 2013, 8:35.

[17] Wanyama R: Malnutrition and child morbidity and mortality. Gulu University Medical Journal 2010, 5:11–12. http://www.kampala.cooperazione.esteri.it/utlkampala/Download/GUMJ2010Final.pdf.

[18] Maitland K, Kiguli S, Opoka RO, Engoru C, Olupot-Olupot P, Akech SO, Nyeko R, Mtove G, Reyburn H, Lang T, Brent B, Evans JA, Tibenderana JK, Crawley J, Russell EC, Levin M, Babiker AG, Gibb DM: FEAST trial group mortality after fluid bolus in African children with severe infection. N Engl J Med 2011, 364:2483–2495.

[19] The FEAST trial BMJ Research Paper award. http://www.ctu.mrc.ac.uk/news_and_press_releases/news_archive/feast_bmj_award_24052012.aspx.

[20] Harden B, Dr. Matthew's Passion: The New York Magazine, February 18, 2001; 2001. http://www.nytimes.com/library/magazine/home/20010218mag-ebola.html.

[21] Dimbley J: On the Ebola frontline: the story of the doctors and nurses at St Mary's Hospital, Lacor. BBC Radio Science May 26 2002. http://www.bbc.co.uk/radio4/science/ebola.shtml.